Advanced Nutrition and Dietetics in Obesity

Advanced Nutrition and Dietetics in Obesity

Edited by

Catherine Hankey PhD RD

Series Editor

Kevin Whelan PhD RD FBDA

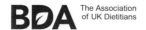 BDA The Association of UK Dietitians

WILEY Blackwell

Registered Office(s)
John Wiley & Sons, Inc., 111 River Street, Hoboken, NJ 07030, USA
John Wiley & Sons Ltd, The Atrium, Southern Gate, Chichester, West Sussex, PO19 8SQ, UK

Editorial Office
9600 Garsington Road, Oxford, OX4 2DQ, UK

For details of our global editorial offices, customer services, and more information about Wiley products, visit us at www.wiley.com.

Wiley also publishes its books in a variety of electronic formats and by print-on-demand. Some content that appears in standard print versions of this book may not be available in other formats.

Library of Congress Cataloging-in-Publication data applied for

ISBN: 9780470670767(PB)

Cover Design: Wiley

Set in 9/11.5pt Times by SPi Global, Pondicherry, India
Printed and bound in Malaysia by Vivar Printing Sdn Bhd

10 9 8 7 6 5 4 3 2 1

ADVANCED NUTRITION AND DIETETICS BOOK SERIES

Dietary recommendations need to be based on solid evidence, but where can you find this information? The British Dietetic Association and the publishers of the *Manual of Dietetic Practice* present an essential and authoritative reference series on the evidence base relating to advanced aspects of nutrition and dietetics in selected clinical specialties. Each book provides a comprehensive and critical review of key literature in the area. Each covers established areas of understanding, current controversies and areas of future development and investigation, and is oriented around six key themes:

- Disease processes, including metabolism, physiology and genetics
- Disease consequences, including morbidity, mortality and patient perspectives
- Clinical investigation and management
- Nutritional consequences of disease
- Nutritional assessment, including anthropometric, biochemical, clinical, dietary, economic and social approaches
- Nutritional and dietary management of disease

Trustworthy, international in scope, and accessible, *Advanced Nutrition and Dietetics* is a vital resource for a range of practitioners, researchers and educators in nutrition and dietetics, including dietitians, nutritionists, doctors and specialist nurses.

Contents

Preface

Obesity, which is often described using terms such as *fat*, *stout* or *corpulent*, is in fact derived from the Latin word *obesus*. Obesity is a disease, and as such has had an International Classification of Disease code since just after World War II. Despite having the status and recognition as a disease, obesity treatment has often been overlooked as a regular component of medical management. Comorbidities associated with obesity, such as type 2 diabetes, hypertension and hyperlipidaemia, have themselves been treated, while interventions that aim to reduce body weight are less rigorously and consistently employed.

The first clinical guidelines for obesity were published in 1996, advocating roles and responsibilities for a range of health professionals – including doctors (general practitioners/family physicians), nurses and dietitians – to manage obesity. In the light of these clinical guidelines, researchers sought the views of health professionals whose practice was either in the community (primary care) or in a speciality based in a hospital (secondary care). Hospital consultants across all specialities agreed that effective weight management could, without exception, improve treatment outcomes. However, none had a treatment protocol in place, suggesting that obesity management was *ad hoc*. A majority felt unable to resource weight management, suggesting that community (primary care) and general practice were more suitable as locations for treatment. General practice staff, general practitioners and practice nurses also felt that reduction in body weight would improve the health of many adults who consulted them. Once more, they themselves felt unable, for the same reasons, to address the need for weight loss as part of their care. Many considered obesity an inevitable result of aging, an intractable and persistent condition and a time-consuming issue that they were unable to treat effectively. Any treatments they considered were long term, resource intensive and only poorly effective. Sadly, these data from the 1990s have been replicated many times.

Advanced Nutrition and Dietetics in Obesity takes on the huge task of describing the aetiology of obesity across the life course. There are large sections devoted to the disease in children and in adults. Treatments including surgical, pharmacological and lifestyle interventions are considered. Prevention of weight gain and obesity, the role of the environment, new town design and transport policy too are discussed. The occurrence of obesity has reached epidemic proportions worldwide, and this text aims to provide the reader with a broad understanding of the multifactorial causes of excessive and unwanted weight gain. After reading this book, I hope the reader will feel that obesity is not a simple problem, but a global phenomenon that is multifactorial in nature, requiring a multidisciplinary approach for management and prevention. Much effort, commitment and research are still required to challenge this chronic and persistent disease.

This book is aimed at all those whose work embraces any aspect of obesity. This includes clinicians, researchers, public health experts, educators and health economics specialists. Those undertaking further studies in health and disease too may find this a useful reference and resource.

Catherine Hankey PhD RD
Senior Lecturer in Human Nutrition
University of Glasgow, UK
Editor
Advanced Nutrition and Dietetics in Obesity

This book is the third title in a series (*Advanced Nutrition and Dietetics Book Series*) commissioned as part of a major initiative between the British Dietetic Association and Wiley. Each book in the series provides a comprehensive and critical review of the key literature in a clinical area. Each book is edited by one or more experts who have themselves undertaken extensive research and published widely in the relevant topic area. Each book chapter is written by experts drawn from an international audience and from a variety of disciplines as required of the relevant chapter (e.g. dietetics, medicine, public health, psychology, biomedical sciences). A future title in this series will cover nutritional support.

The editor and I are proud to present the third title in the series, *Advanced Nutrition and Dietetics in Obesity*. We hope that it will impact on health professionals' understanding and application of nutrition and dietetics in the management and prevention of obesity. Effective weight management improves the health of both adults and children. Prevention of the chronic weight gain of adulthood in many parts of the world are essential, and approaches to address this issue so far are discussed.

Kevin Whelan PhD RD FBDA
Professor of Dietetics
King's College London, UK
Series Editor
***Advanced Nutrition and Dietetics* Book Series**

Foreword

This book is a very timely synthesis of the dimensions of the problems of obesity and how to manage them in what is rapidly now becoming the most intractable issue in both clinical management and public health across the globe. This book, written by contributors from the UK, Europe and throughout the world, comes at a time when it looks as though politicians are finally waking up to the fact that health services are already overwhelmed by the numbers of people with multiple obesity-related conditions. As healthcare professionals become ever more sophisticated at coping with the immediate risk factors of type 2 diabetes and cardiovascular disease, we still see most clinical teams neglecting obesity as the underlying driver, with all its proximal causes. Given the magnitude of the currently escalating health burden, it is timely that this book, essentially geared to the clinical teams involved in obesity prevention and treatment, is now published. The descriptions cover the full range of new ideas and evidence of both the underlying pressures on the majority of our population and how to begin to effectively manage such a challenging organisational and multidimensional problem.

Many of these expert contributors have decades of experience in trying to establish effective approaches to the management and prevention of obesity. The historical account emphasises the struggle that has gone on for decades, with the first semi-official reports on appropriate clinical schemes for managing the problem only emerging 20 years ago in both Scotland and the USA. Much of the drive, as is usual in medical management, has come with the search for suitable pharmacological strategies; nevertheless, as other chapters emphasise, the neglect of the transformation of both the dietary modification and physical activity required necessitates not only an understanding of the underlying features of appetite control but also the need for routine physical activity incorporated into most individuals' normal habits. There are very authoritative accounts of the genetic, endocrinological and clinical aspects of the epidemic in adults as well as in children, in whom obesity only emerged in the last 20 years as a major burden in paediatric practice. Although the childhood obesity epidemic seems to be slowing in many European countries, the overall prevalence of childhood overweight and obesity are still horrifying. Hence, we can expect to see vicious combinations of genetic and epigenetic influences as these children and the next generation enter adulthood, with their clinical care becoming ever more difficult. Thus, young overweight women now entering pregnancy seem unaware of the challenges that new research suggests lies in wait for their families and family practitioners. With rapidly rising rates of gestational diabetes, especially in Europe's ethnic minorities, we are already witnessing far earlier onsets of adult abdominal obesity and type 2 diabetes, with its sustained challenges for maintaining medical care of chronically sick patients. The chapters on the co-morbidities should therefore help to amplify a broader approach to the management of an array of risk factors, and this book benefits from adding musculoskeletal and psychological comorbidities to the traditional cardiovascular foci of concern.

There are very appropriate chapters first on the diagnostic criteria that should be used in both screening and monitoring clinical progress in children and adults, followed by a comprehensive description and analysis of dietary approaches that have been tried and progressively evaluated. Then come assessments of the value of pharmacological and surgical management, as well as interventions to improve physical activity levels.

Fitting all this together with the issues of obesity prevention and how this can link into clinical practice is a real challenge. This book therefore gives us both an overview and the detail that is so necessary if we are to engineer a revolution in clinical practice. One just wishes that the many integrated contributions could have been produced a decade ago, but then we would not have benefitted from so much of the new research and analyses that are presented here.

W. Philip T. James
Professor, London School of Hygiene and
Tropical Medicine
Past president of the World Obesity Federation

Editor biographies

Catherine Hankey PhD RD

Catherine Hankey is a Senior Lecturer in Human Nutrition in the School of Medicine at the University of Glasgow. Her research investigates clinical and public health aspects of obesity and weight management. Examples of research include the optimization of weight management during smoking cessation and in those with intellectual disabilities. Dr Hankey was a group member for the Scottish Intercollegiate Guidelines Network (SIGN) guideline for the Management of Obesity and the update of the SIGN prevention and management of cardiovascular disease. She is the author of the Weight Management chapter in the Manual of Dietetic Practice and is co-editing the forthcoming version of the ABC of Nutrition.

Kevin Whelan PhD RD FBDA

Kevin Whelan is the Professor of Dietetics and the Head of Department of Nutritional Sciences at King's College London. He is a Principal Investigator leading a research programme exploring the interaction between the gastrointestinal microbiota, diet and health and disease. In 2012 he was awarded the Nutrition Society Cuthbertson Medal for research in clinical nutrition and in 2017 was appointed a Fellow of the British Dietetic Association. Prof Whelan is on the editorial boards of *Alimentary Pharmacology and Therapeutics* and the *Journal of Human Nutrition and Dietetics* and is the Series Editor for the *British Dietetic Association Advanced Nutrition and Dietetics* book series.

Contributors

Ghalia Abdeen PhD
Lecturer in Nutrition
King Saud University
Riyadh, Saudi Arabia

Karen Allan PhD RD
AHP Practice Education Coordinator
NHS Education for Scotland
Edinburgh, Scotland, UK

Werd Al-Najim PhD
Postdoctoral Researcher
University College Dublin
Dublin, Ireland

Annie S Anderson PhD RD
Professor of Public Health Nutrition
University of Dundee
Dundee, UK

Daryll Archibald PhD
Research Fellow
University of Edinburgh
Edinburgh, UK

Alison Avenell MD FRCP
Professor of Health Services Research
University of Aberdeen
Aberdeen, UK

Amanda Avery PhD RD
Assistant Professor in Nutrition and Dietetics
University of Nottingham
Nottingham, UK

Panagiotis Balaskas MSc
University of Glasgow
Glasgow, UK

John E Blundell PhD
Professor of Psychobiology
University of Leeds
Leeds, UK

Emma J Boyland PhD
Lecturer in Psychological Sciences
University of Liverpool
Liverpool, UK

Wendy J Brown PhD
Professor of Physical Activity and Health
University of Queensland
Queensland, Australia

Duff Bruce MBChB FRCS
Visiting Professor of Surgery
Robert Gordon University
Aberdeen, UK

Johannes Brug PhD
Professor of Epidemiology
EMGO Institute for Health and Care Research
Amsterdam, Netherlands

Janet Cade PhD RNutr
Professor of Nutritional Epidemiology
and Public Health
University of Leeds
Leeds, UK

Magdalin Cheong MPH RD
Head of Department of Dietetics and Food Services
Changi General Hospital
Singapore

Pia Christensen PhD RD
Postdoctoral Research Associate
University of Copenhagen
Copenhagen, Denmark

Peter Clifton PhD FRACP
Professor of Nutrition
University of South Australia
Adelaide, Australia

Gianluca Lo Coco PhD
Associate Professor of Clinical Psychology
University of Palermo
Palermo, Italy

Angela M Craigie PhD RNutr
Lecturer in Cancer Prevention
University of Dundee
Dundee, UK

Helen Croker PhD RD
Clinical Research Dietitian
University College London
London, UK

Michelle Dalton PhD
Research Fellow in Psychology and Nutrition
University of Leeds
Leeds, UK

Sandra Drummond PhD RPHNutr
Senior Lecturer in Nutrition
Queen Margaret University
Edinburgh, UK

Ulf Ekelund PhD
Professor in Physical Activity and Health
Norwegian School of Sport Sciences
Oslo, Norway

Alison Gahagan PG Dip RD
Specialist Weight Management Dietitian
NHS South West London
London, UK

Paul Gately PhD
Professor of Exercise and Obesity
Leeds Beckett University
Leeds, UK

Ekavi N Georgousopoulou PhD
Adjunct Research Professional
University of Canberra
Canberra, Australia

Nazim Ghouri MD
Senior Lecturer in Cardiovascular Sciences
University of Glasgow
Glasgow, UK

Catherine Gibbons PhD
Research Fellow
University of Leeds
Leeds, UK

Sjaan R Gomersall PhD
Research Fellow
University of Queensland
Queensland, Australia

Eleanor Grieve BA MPH
Research Associate
University of Glasgow
Glasgow, UK

Catherine Hankey PhD RD
Senior Lecturer in Human Nutrition
University of Glasgow
Glasgow, UK

Katherine Hart PhD RD
Lecturer in Nutrition and Dietetics
University of Surrey
Guildford, UK

Marion Hetherington DPhil
Professor of Biopsychology
University of Leeds
Leeds, UK

Mark Hopkins PhD
Senior Lecturer in Exercise Physiology
Leeds Beckett University
Leeds, UK

Kathleen B Hrovat MS RD
Lead Nutritionist for Surgical Weight Loss
Cincinnati Children's Hospital Medical Center
Cincinnati, OH, USA

Adrienne Hughes PhD
Lecturer in Physical Activity for Health
University of Strathclyde
Glasgow, UK

Thomas H Inge MD PhD
Director of Surgical Weight Loss
Cincinnati Children's Hospital Medical Center
Cincinnati, OH, USA

Maria E Jackson PhD
Senior Lecturer
University of Glasgow
Glasgow, UK

Nathalie Jones MSc RD
Research Assistant
University of Glasgow
Glasgow, UK

Louise A Kelly PhD
Associate Professor of Exercise Science
California Lutheran University
Thousand Oaks, CA, USA

Joan Khoo MBBS MRCP
Chief and Consultant in Endocrinology
Changi General Hospital
Singapore

Neil A King PhD
Director of Research Training
Queensland University of Technology
Brisbane, Australia

Linda M Kollar MSN RN
Clinical Director of Surgical Weight Loss
Cincinnati Children's Hospital Medical Center
Cincinnati, OH, USA

Peter Kopelman MD FRCP FFPH
Principal and Professor of Medicine
St George's, University of London
London, UK

Jeroen Lakerveld PhD
Senior Researcher
EMGO Institute for Health and Care Research
Amsterdam, Netherlands

Mike Lean FRCP
Professor of Human Nutrition
University of Glasgow
Glasgow, UK

Anthony R Leeds MBBS CBiol FSBiol
Visiting Senior Fellow
University of Surrey
Guildford, UK

Wilma S Leslie PhD RGN
Research Associate
University of Glasgow
Glasgow, UK

Joreintje D Mackenbach PhD
Epidemiologist
EMGO Institute for Health and Care Research
Amsterdam, Netherlands

Louise McCombie BSc RD
Research Assistant
University of Glasgow
Glasgow, UK

Janet McNally MSc
Doctoral Research Fellow
University of Leeds
Leeds, UK

Bethan R Mead PhD
Research Fellow
University of Liverpool
Liverpool, UK

Duane D Mellor PhD APD RD
Senior Lecturer in Human Nutrition
University of Coventry
Coventry, UK

Craig A Melville MD
Professor of Intellectual Disabilities Psychiatry
University of Glasgow
Glasgow, UK

Rebecca Mete MND APD
PhD Student
University of Canberra
Canberra, Australia

Jillian M Morrison MSc RD
Specialist Paediatric Dietitian
Royal Hospital for Children
Glasgow, UK

Aileen Muir MSc
Lead Pharmacist for Governance
NHS Greater Glasgow and Clyde
Glasgow, UK

Chandani Nekitsing MSc
Doctoral Research Fellow
University of Leeds
Leeds, UK

Mary O'Kane MSc RD
Clinical Specialist Dietitian
Leeds Teaching Hospitals NHS Trust
Leeds, UK

Thomas Reinehr MD
Head of the Department
University of Witten
Witten, Germany

Lina A Ricciardelli PhD
Professor of Psychology
Deakin University
Melbourne, Australia

Clare Robertson MSc
Research Fellow
University of Aberdeen
Aberdeen, UK

Natasha P Ross MBChB MRCS
Speciality Trainee in Surgery
NHS Grampian
Aberdeen, UK

Carel W le Roux PhD FRCP FRCPath
Professor of Experimental Pathology
University College Dublin
Dublin, Ireland

Harry Rutter MB BChir
Senior Clinical Research Fellow
London School of Hygiene and Tropical Medicine
London, UK

M Guftar Shaikh MD
Consultant Paediatric Endocrinologist
Royal Hospital for Children
Glasgow, UK

Netalie Shloim PhD
Lecturer in Counselling and Psychotherapy
University of Leeds
Leeds, UK

Dimitrios Spanos PhD RD
Manager of Clinical Dietetics
Cleveland Clinic Abu Dhabi
Abu Dhabi, UAE

Laura Stewart PhD RD
Nutrition and Dietetics Service Lead
Perth Royal Infirmary
Perth, UK

Gareth Stratton PhD
Professor of Paediatric Exercise Science
Swansea University
Swansea, UK

Louise Waters PhD
Research Assistant
University of Glasgow
Glasgow, UK

Kevin Whelan PhD RD FBDA
Professor of Dietetics
King's College London
London, UK

Chris Williams PhD
Professor of Psychosocial Psychiatry
University of Glasgow
Glasgow, UK

Abbreviations

AT	Adaptive thermogenesis	BMI	Body mass index
AGB	Adjustable gastric band	BMI-SDS	Body mass index standard deviation score
AgRP	Agouti-related protein		
AHO	Albright's hereditary osteodystrophy	BDNF	Brain-derived neurotrophic factor
ADF	Alternate-day fasting	BOMSS	British Obesity and Metabolic Surgery Society
ADMF	Alternate-day modified fasting		
AAIDD	American Association on Intellectual and Developmental Disabilities	CPS-I	Cancer Prevention Study I
		CVD	Cardiovascular disease
ACS	American Cancer Society	CADM2	Cell adhesion molecule 2
ACP	American College of Physicians	CDC	Centers for Disease Control and Prevention
ACR	American College of Rheumatology		
ACSM	American College of Sports Medicine	CEBQ	Child Eating Behaviour Questionnaire
		CHASE	Child Health Heart Study in England
ADA	American Diabetes Association	CHEW	Children Eating Well
ASMBS	American Society for Metabolic and Bariatric Surgery	CCK	Cholecystokinin
		COPD	Chronic obstructive pulmonary disease
ANGELO	ANalysis Grid for Elements Linked to Obesity		
		CART	Cocaine- and amphetamine-related transcript
ARC	Arcuate nucleus		
ACMOMS	Asian Consensus Meeting on Metabolic Surgery	CBT	Cognitive behavioural therapy
		CWMO	Commercial weight management organisation
ALSWH	Australian Longitudinal Study on Women's Health		
		COMPX	Compensation index
BEBQ	Baby Eating Behaviour Questionnaire	CT	Computer tomography
		CI	Confidence interval
BLW	Baby-led weaning	CER	Continuous energy restriction
BBS	Bardet-Biedl syndrome	CNVs	Copy number variants
BMR	Basal metabolic rate	CAD	Coronary artery disease
BOCF	Baseline observation carried forward	CARDIA	Coronary Artery Risk Development in Young Adults
BDI	Beck depression inventory		
BT	Behavioural therapy	CUA	Cost utility analysis
ADRB3	Beta-3 adrenergic receptor	CBA	Cost-benefit analysis
BED	Binge eating disorder	CEA	Cost-effectiveness analysis
BIA	Bio-electrical impedance analysis	CRP	C-reactive protein
BBSRC	Biotechnology and Biological Sciences Research Council	CRM	Customer relationship management
		DHHS	Department of Health and Human Services
BCS	Body contour surgery		

DPS	Diabetes Prevention Study
DSM-IV	Diagnostic and Statistical Manual of Mental Disorders
DIT	Diet-induced thermogenesis
DALY	Disability-adjusted life year
DEXA	Dual-energy X-ray absorptiometry
DS	Duodenal switch
EAH	Eating in the absence of hunger
EF	Ectopic fat
ER	Endoplasmic reticulum
EE	Energy expenditure
EI	Energy intake
EnRG	Environmental Research framework for weight Gain prevention
EIN	Epode International Network
EFNA	European Federation of Neurological Associations
EFSA	European Food Safety Authority
EULAR	European League Against Rheumatism
EMAS	European Male Aging Study
EMA	European Medicines Agency
ENERGY	Exercise and Nutrition to Enhance recovery and Good Health for You
FBBT	Family-based behavioural treatment
FANCL	Fanconi anaemia, complementation group L
FAIM2	Fas apoptotic inhibitory molecule 2
FTO	Fat mass and obesity–associated
FFM	Fat-free mass
FDA	Food and Drug Administration
FFIT	Football Fans in Training
FEV1	Forced expiratory volume in the first
FFA	Free fatty acids
GP	general practitioner
GWA	Genome wide association
GWAS	Genome-wide association studies
GCWMS	Glasgow and Clyde Weight Management Service
GLP-1	Glucagon-like peptide-1
GCKR	Glucokinase regulatory protein
GNPDA2	Glucosamine-6-phosphate deaminase 2
QPCTL	Glutaminyl-peptide cyclotransferase-like
HR	Hazard Ratio
HBSC	Health Behaviour in School-Aged Children
HBM	Health belief model
HSE	Health Survey for England
HTA	Health technology assessment
HDL	High-density lipoprotein
HIF3A	Hypoxia inducible factor 3A gene
IWQOL	Impact of Weight on Quality of Life
ICER	Incremental cost-effectiveness ratio
INSIG2	Insulin-induced gene-2
IGF	Insulin-like growth factor
ID	Intellectual disabilities
ITT	Intention-to-treat
IL-6	Interleukin 6
IER	Intermittent energy restriction
IF	Intermittent fasting
ICAD	International Children's Accelerometry Database
IOTF	International Obesity Task Force
IPT	Interpersonal psychotherapy
IWHS	Iowa Women's Health Study
IRX3	Iroquois homeobox protein
kb	Kilobase
LAGB	Laparoscopic adjustable gastric band
LOCF	Last observation carried forward
LEP	Leptin
LEPR	Leptin receptor
LMCP	Leptin-melanocortin pathway
LRRN6C	Leucine-rich repeat neuronal 6C
LPS	Lipopolysaccharide
LCDs	Low-calorie diets
LCLDs	Low-calorie liquid diets
LCKD	Low-carbohydrate ketogenic diet
LDLR	Low-density lipoprotein receptor gene
LRP1B	Low-density lipoprotein receptor-related protein 1B
LUTS	Lower urinary tract symptoms
LYPLAL1	Lysophospholipase-like 1
MRI	Magnetic resonance imaging
MCT	Medium-chain triglyceride
MC3R	Melanocortin 3 receptor
MC4R	Melanocortin 4 receptor
MET	Metabolic energy turnover
METs	Metabolic equivalents
MSRA	Methionine sulfoxide reductase gene A
miRNA	microRNA
MEAL	mindful eating and living
MB-EAT	mindfulness-based eating awareness training
MTCH2	mitochondrial carrier 2

MTIF3	Mitochondrial translational initiation factor 3	PCOS	Polycystic ovarian syndrome
MAP2K5	Mitogen-activated protein kinase 5	PTBP2	Polypyrimidine tract binding protein 2
MVPA	Moderate-vigorous-intensity physical activity	PAGE	Population architecture using genomics and epidemiology
MI	Motivational interviewing	15KCTD15	Potassium channel tetramerisation domain containing
MDT	Multidisciplinary team		
NCEP	National Cholesterol Education Program	PWS	Prader–Willi syndrome
		POMC	Proopiomelanocortin
NHMRC	National Health and Medical Research Council	PMT	Protection motivation theory
		PRKD1	Protein kinase D1
NHANES	National Health and Nutrition Examination Survey	PPP1R3B	Protein phosphatase 1 regulatory subunit 3b
NHS	National Health Service	QALY	Quality-adjusted life year
NHLBI	National Heart, Lung, and Blood Institute	QEWP-R	Questionnaire on Eating and Weight Patterns – Revised
NICE	National Institute for Health and Clinical Excellence	RBJ	Rab and DnaJ domain-containing protein A
NOO	National Obesity Observatory	RCTs	Randomised controlled trials
NWCR	National Weight Control Registry	RT	Resistance training
NRXN3	Neurexin	REE	Resting energy expenditure
NCAN	Neurocan	RMR	Resting metabolic rate
NEGR1	Neuronal growth regulator 1	RPL27A	Ribosomal protein L27a
NPY	Neuropeptide Y	RC	Rosemary Conley
NGS	Next-generation DNA sequencing	RYGB	Roux-en-Y gastric bypass
NES	Night eating syndrome	RCPCH	Royal College of Paediatrics and Child Health
NAFLD	Non-alcoholic fatty liver disease		
NASH	Non-alcoholic steatohepatitis	SCOTT	Scottish Childhood Overweight Treatment Trial
NEFAs	Non-esterified fatty acids		
NEAT	Non-exercise activity thermogenesis	SIGN	Scottish Intercollegiate Guidelines Network
NUDT3	Nucleoside diphosphate-linked moiety X-type motif 3		
		SSRI	Selective serotonin reuptake inhibitor
NDR-UK	Nutrition and Diet Resources UK		
OSCA	Obesity Services for Children and Adolescents	SDCCAG8	Serologically defined colon cancer antigen 8
OR	Odds ratios	SCFAs	Short-chain fatty acids
OPRM1	Opioid receptor mu-1 gene	SNP	Single nucleotide polymorphism
OA	Osteoarthritis	SG	Sleeve gastrectomy
PP	Pancreatic polypeptide	SW	Slimming World
PTH	Parathyroid hormone	SCT	Social cognitive theory
Peds QL	Pediatric Quality of Life Inventory	SES	Socioeconomic status
PYY	Peptide tyrosine tyrosine	SLC39A8	Solute carrier family 39 (zinc transporter), member 8
PNPLA3	Phospholipase domain-containing protein 3		
		SFT	Solution-focused therapy
PA	Physical activity	SH2B1	Src homology 2 domain-containing adapter protein 1
PAEE	Physical activity energy expenditure		
PAL	Physical activity level	SBT	Standard behavioural therapy
PAI-1	Plasminogen activator inhibitor-1	SD	Standard deviation

SDS	Standard deviation score		VBG	Vertical banded gastroplasty
STOP Regain	Study To Prevent weight Regain		VSG	Vertical sleeve gastrectomy
SAT	Subcutaneous adipose tissue		VLCD	Very-low-calorie diet
SCOTS	SurgiCal Obesity Treatment Study		VLDL	Very-low-density lipoprotein
SR	Sustained-release		VLED	Very-low-energy diet
SOS	Swedish obesity study		VAT	Visceral adipose tissue
TNKS	Tankyrase		VF	Visceral fat
TPB	Theory of planned behaviour		WC	Waist circumference
TRF	Time-restricted feeding		WHR	Waist-to-hip ratio
TLR	Toll-like receptor		WTR	Waist-to-thigh ratio
TDEE	Total daily energy expenditure		WLMRCT	Weight Loss Maintenance Randomised Controlled Trial
TEE	Total daily energy expenditure		WW	Weight watchers
TCF7L2	Transcription factor 7-like 2		WAT	White adipose tissue
TFAP2B	Transcription factor AP-2 beta		WHS	Women's Health Study
TMEM160	Transmembrane protein 160		WHEL	Women's Healthy Eating and Living
TMEM 18	Transmembrane protein 18 gene		WINS	Women's Intervention Nutrition Study
TTM	Transtheoretical model			
TNF	Tumour necrosis factor			
UKPDS	United Kingdom Prevention of Diabetes Study		WCRF	World Cancer Research Fund
			WHO	World Health Organization
VTE	Venous thromboembolism		ZNF608	Zinc finger protein 608

SECTION 1

Introduction

Chapter 1.1

Definition, prevalence and historical perspectives of obesity in adults

Peter Kopelman
St George's, University of London, London, UK

1.1.1 Definitions of *overweight* and *obesity*

In clinical practice, body fat is most commonly and simply estimated by using a formula that combines weight and height. The underlying assumption is that most variations in weight for persons of the same height is due to fat mass. The formula most frequently used in epidemiological studies is the *body mass index* (BMI), which is weight in kilograms divided by the square of the height in metres. BMI is strongly correlated with densitometry measurements of fat mass adjusted for height in middle-aged adults. The main limitation of BMI is that it does not distinguish fat mass from lean mass. Table 1.1.1 identifies the cut-off points applied by the World Health Organisation for BMI classification in adults [1].

Although BMI is used to classify individuals as 'obese' or 'overweight', it is only a proxy measure of the underlying problem of excess fat. As a person's body fat increases, both their BMI and their future risk of obesity-related illness also rise, although there is still some uncertainty about the exact nature of the relationship, especially in children.

Measurement of body circumference is an additional indicator of health risk in an overweight or obese person: excess visceral (intra-abdominal) fat is a risk factor for long-term conditions independent of total adiposity. Waist circumference and the ratio of waist circumference to hip circumference are practical measures for assessing upper-body fat distribution.

Skinfold thickness, measured with calipers, provides a more precise assessment of body fat, especially if taken at multiple sites. Skinfolds are useful in the estimation of fatness in children, for whom standards have been published. However, the measurements are more difficult to make in adults (particularly in the very obese), are subject to considerable variation between observers, require accurate calipers and do not provide any information on abdominal and intramuscular fat. In general, they are not superior to simpler measures of height and weight. Table 1.1.2 lists the practical measures for the assessment of an obese person.

Why use BMI?

BMI is an attractive measure because it is an easy, cheap and non-invasive means of assessing excess body fat. Prior to the application of BMI, clinicians referred to 'ideal' weight tables, which were derived from the weight–height tables provided by the Metropolitan Life Insurance Company (1959), based on subsequent mortality of insured adults in the USA and Canada [2]. However, prospective epidemiological data confirmed the impreciseness of the term 'ideal' even within a North American population (despite attempts to sharpen this with measures of body frame size), and its inapplicability when applied in a global context. BMI has been used widely around the world, permitting comparisons between areas, across population subgroups and over a long period. Another advantage

Advanced Nutrition and Dietetics in Obesity, First Edition. Edited by Catherine Hankey.
© 2018 John Wiley & Sons Ltd. Published 2018 by John Wiley & Sons Ltd.

Table 1.1.1 Cut-off points applied by the World Health Organisation for the classification of overweight and obesity

BMI*	WHO classification	Popular description
<18.5	Underweight	'Thin'
18.5–24.9	Healthy weight	'Healthy'
25.0–29.9	Overweight	'Overweight'
30.0–34.9	Obesity I	'Obese'
35.0–39.9	Obesity II	'Obese'
40 or greater	Obesity III	'Morbidly or seriously obese'

*BMI is the weight in kilograms divided by the square of the height in metres.
Data sourced from http://apps.who.int/bmi/index.jsp?introPage=intro_3.html

Table 1.1.2 Clinical methods for the assessment of an individual with obesity

Characteristic of obesity measured	Methods
Body composition	BMI Underwater weighing Dual-energy X-ray absorptiometry (DEXA) Isotope dilution Bioelectrical impedance Skinfold thickness
Regional distribution of fat	Waist circumference; waist-to-hip ratio Computerised axial tomography Ultrasound Magnetic resonance imaging (MRI)
Energy intake	Dietary recall or record 'macronutrient composition' by prospective dietary record or dietary questionnaire
Energy expenditure	Doubly labelled water Indirect calorimetry (resting) Physical activity level (PAL) by questionnaire Motion detector Heart rate monitor

of BMI is the availability of published thresholds and growth references to which children's BMI can be compared. BMI in children varies with age and gender, which prevents the use of fixed thresholds as in adults [3,4]. Equivalent growth references do not exist for other measures such as waist circumference.

Interpretation of BMI: defining a 'healthy weight' for a particular society

There are methodological problems that derive from a definition based on total mortality rates. People frequently lose weight as a consequence of illness that is ultimately fatal, which was unrecognised at the time of the survey. This gives the appearance of higher mortality among those with lower weights: reverse causation. The effect can be minimised by either excluding persons with diagnoses that might affect weight and/or those who report recent weight loss, or excluding those who die during the first years of follow-up. A second major concern is confounding factors that may distort the association between body weight and mortality – cigarette smoking is of particular importance. Overweight and obesity cause or exacerbate a large number of health problems, both independently and in association with other diseases, and are among the most significant contributors to ill health [5]. Unfortunately, many of the health risks associated with increasing body weight begin their manifestation in children and young people – of great current concern is the increasing prevalence of type 2 diabetes and associated medical complications in young overweight adults. There is a close relationship between BMI and the incidence of many long-term conditions caused by excess fat: type 2 diabetes, hypertension, coronary heart disease and stroke, metabolic syndrome, osteoarthritis (OA)

Table 1.1.3 Risks and diseases associated with increasing body weight

Metabolic syndrome	30% of middle-aged people in developed countries have features of metabolic syndrome
Type 2 diabetes	90% of people with type 2 diabetes have BMI >23 kg/m²
Hypertension	5x risk in obesity
	66% hypertension linked to excess weight
	85% hypertension associated with BMI >25 kg/m²
Coronary artery disease (CAD) and stroke	3.6x increase in risk of CAD for each unit change in BMI
	Dyslipidaemia progressively develops as BMI increases from 21 kg/m² with rise in small-particle LDL
	70% of obese women with hypertension have left ventricular hypertrophy
	Obesity a contributing factor to cardiac failure in >10% patients
	Overweight/obesity plus hypertension associated with increased risk of ischaemic stroke
Respiratory effects	Neck circumference >43 cm in men and >40.5 cm in women associated with obstructive sleep apnoea, daytime somnolence and development of pulmonary hypertension
Cancers	10% of all cancer deaths among non-smokers related to obesity (30% of endometrial cancers)
Reproductive function	6% of primary infertility in women attributable to obesity
	Impotency and infertility frequently associated with obesity in men
OA	Frequent association in the elderly with increasing body weight – risk of disability attributable to OA equal to heart disease and greater to any other medical disorder among elderly
Liver and gall bladder disease	Overweight and obesity associated with non-alcoholic fatty liver disease and non-alcoholic steatohepatitis (NASH); 40% of NASH patients are obese; 20% have dyslipidaemia
	3x risk of gallbladder disease in women with BMI >32 kg/m²; 7x risk if BMI >45 kg/m²

and cancer. An overview of the association between BMI and the development of a range of diseases is given in Table 1.1.3.

Risk factors for some conditions start to increase at relatively low BMIs (e.g. hypertension and type 2 diabetes). It is found that 85% of patients with hypertension have a BMI of >25 kg/m², and 90% of those with type 2 diabetes have a BMI of >23. In 2011, an estimated 62% of adults (aged 16 and over) were overweight or obese in the UK. The risk of developing type 2 diabetes is about two times more for people who are obese as compared to lean people. Abdominal obesity is a particular risk for the cluster of diseases that have become known as the *metabolic syndrome* – type 2 diabetes, hypertension and dyslipidaemia – and is strongly linked to the risk of cardiovascular disease [6]. Most of the medical complications will not present to a medical practitioner until the age of 40 years – hence, it is difficult

to discern the immediate benefits to younger generations from modest weight loss. In prevention terms, the benefit that an individual may feel may be relatively quick to manifest, but the overall benefit to society will take years [7].

1.1.2 Prevalence and trends for obesity in adults

In the UK, data on overweight and obesity among adults (16 years and older) are derived from the Health Survey for England [3]. Results from the 2011 survey are summarised in Box 1.1.1. A comparison with international findings is given in Figure 1.1.1.

A recent review of international comparisons has collated published and unpublished studies on BMI to provide a comprehensive global dataset covering

Box 1.1.1 Summary of the results from the Health Survey of England 2011 [3]

- An estimated 62% of adults (aged 16 and over) were overweight or obese.
- Around 2% were underweight, and 3% had severe obesity (BMI 40 or greater).
- Men and women have a similar prevalence of obesity, but men are more likely to be overweight (41%, compared to 33% in women).
- The prevalence of obesity in adults rose from 15% in 1993 to 25% in 2011. Many of those in the obese category have a BMI much higher than 30. There are more women than men with extremely high BMI values.
- The prevalence of obesity and overweight changes with age, being lowest in the 16–24 years age group, and generally higher in the older age groups among both men and women.
- Women living in more deprived areas have the highest prevalence of obesity, and those living in less deprived areas have the lowest. There is no clear pattern for men.
- Women from the African American racial category appear to have the highest prevalence of obesity, and men from Chinese and Bangladeshi groups the lowest, based on the most recent data (2004). However, research has shown that BMI may overestimate obesity among Africans and underestimate obesity in South Asians.
- Using adjusted thresholds for these ethnic groups could improve obesity estimates.

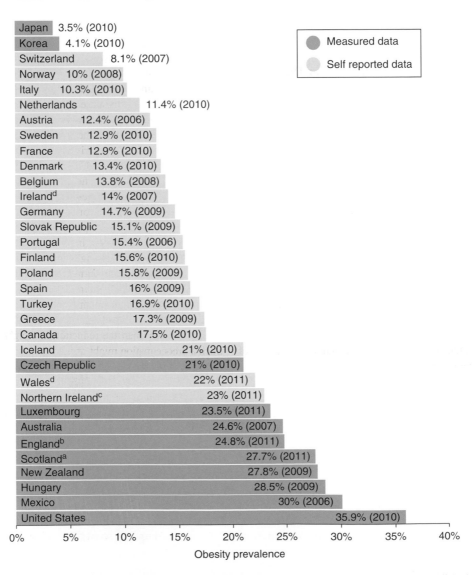

Figure 1.1.1 International comparisons of the prevalence of obesity (BMI 30 kg/m² and greater). Published with acknowledgment from Public Health England. Source: http://www.noo.org.uk/NOO_about_obesity/adult_obesity/international.

the years 1980–2008 [8]. The data was derived from both measured and self-reported estimates and included 199 countries and territories. Between 1980 and 2008, age-standardised mean global BMI increased by 0.4–0.5 kg/m^2 per decade in men and women. The reviewers noticed substantial differences across regions and gender. The region with the largest BMI rise was Oceania for both sexes, and the regions with almost flat trends or even potential decreases were Central and Eastern Europe for women and Central Africa and South Asia for men. The estimated value for the UK at 24.8% is high compared to most other countries, as is the rate of increase (almost double) during the past 25 years [3].

1.1.3 Recent history of obesity in adults

From an evolutionary point of view, excess body fat has served nature's purpose by providing a superbly efficient system for storing energy reserves. This system only became maladaptive when technological advances altered the balance between the availability of food and the body's expenditure of energy. During pre-historic times, the greatest burden for mankind was infection and famine. Natural selection rewarded the 'thrifty' genotypes of those who could store the greatest amount of fat from the least amount of food and release it as frugally as possible. Those who could store fat easily had an evolutionary advantage in the harsh environment of hunters and gatherers. This precarious food supply was gradually reduced with the advent of agriculture and domestication of animals – humankind developed the ability to grow its food, but supply still remained precarious due to the vagaries of nature and warfare.

Food shortage, famine and infection remained the biggest challenges to the world's population until the twentieth century. The current global epidemic of obesity is a problem of the late twentieth century, and now impacts across societies. Modern technological and scientific advances have resulted in an abundance of food in many countries, although many tragically still face chronic food shortages. However, it is only within the last 50 years that overweight and obesity have come to be regarded as long-term conditions associated with well-defined comorbidities; prior to this, corpulence was often regarded by many societies as desirable and a reflection of well-being.

The increasing prevalence of obesity is closely associated with the emergence of modern lifestyles in the UK and other developed countries in Europe, North America and Asia. Towards the close of the nineteenth century, medical concerns were raised about obesity. In 1900, the UK was already the world's most urbanised and one of the wealthiest countries, with a large service sector, expanding public transport network and a developing consumer culture.

Living standards continued to rise during the years between World Wars I and II (1919–1939) despite high unemployment and economic depression. With falling prices and smaller families, real incomes per capita increased by about one-third. Britain's growing prosperity was not shared equally, and substantial sections of the working class continued to suffer from undernutrition.

Sir George Newman, the Chief Medical Officer at the Ministry of Health in the UK, held 'excessive and unsuitable food combined with lack of fresh air and exercise' responsible for sowing the 'seeds of degeneration' [9]. He accepted that some persons 'no doubt' were 'under-fed' in 1931, but argued that many were 'over-fed – giving their poor bodies little rest, clogging them with yet more food'.

Doctors began to take interest in obesity, and *The Lancet* noted in 1933 that in 'these days of "slimming" there was no more popular subject of discussion among the laity than the reduction in weight' [10]. Such a preoccupation might appear incongruous at a time of economic depression, high unemployment, hunger marches and working-class poverty, but has been seen again in the present century. Between the wars, obesity was noted to be increasingly associated with the comforts of suburban middle-class life, plentiful food and a rapid rise in car ownership.

After 1939, the introduction of extensive rationing with a strict regulation on food supplies resulted in reductions of sugar, meat and fats, with consumption shifting to bread, potatoes and milk [11]. This substantial governmental intervention, which was only possible in the context of World War II, amounted to a major turning point in the history of the British diet. The policy has been described as a revolutionary transformation because it largely eliminated the disparities of energy and nutrient intake between social classes. Energy consumption declined, and physical activity levels rose among the middle classes due to longer working hours, increased walking, reduced motoring (owing to petrol rationing) and schemes such as 'Dig for Victory' [12].

Nobel laureate Robert Fogel has examined health, nutrition and technology over three centuries, concluding that a synergy between improvements in productive technology and human physiology has enabled humans to more than double their longevity and to increase their average body size by more than 50% [13]. Fogel argues that larger and healthier humans have resulted in accelerated economic growth that, in turn, has led to reduced workload and increased leisure time. Increased longevity has also resulted in increased demands for healthcare. The erosion of class differentials in food intake persisted after the end of rationing in 1954, and weight gain was no longer confined to the highest-income groups. Since the 1950s, the British diet has been characterised by ever more abundant cheap food. In recent decades, the traditional three-meals-at-home pattern has been replaced by snacking, junk foods and takeaways, contributing towards weight gain. This has been compounded by a decline in physical activity, with expanding car ownership and new forms of home-based entertainment. The increasing problem of overweight and obesity in children and adults highlight the limits of personal responsibility when considering daily food consumption. However, policies aimed at addressing this imbalance have avoided any form of regulation.

The UK's Foresight programme, in the Government Office for Science, was asked by government in 2005 to consider how society might deliver a sustainable response to obesity in the UK over the next 40 years [7]. Foresight works across government departments to analyse complex cross-cutting issues. The analysis of published evidence revealed that the causes of obesity are embedded in an extremely complex biological system, set within an equally complex societal framework. Furthermore, the scale of the challenge

to prevent obesity is substantially increased by the complex nature of the condition. The many causes of obesity argue against depending on a number of unconnected solutions to address the issue, and against focussing on single aspects because this is unlikely to bring about the scale of change required.

In 2010, a new coalition government in the UK prompted a rethink about social policies and public health. The new Secretary of State for Health launched a policy of 'nudge' when addressing the British Medical Association's conference [14]. The Right Honourable Andrew Lansley cited evidence that 'if we are constantly lecturing people and trying to tell them what to do, we will actually find that we undermine and are counterproductive in the results that we achieve'. Mr Lansley went on: 'Behaviour change is the great challenge for public health – but too often it is ignored. Public health efforts, which only try to control supply, will fail. We have to impact on demand. That means we have to change behaviour, and change people's relationships with each other and with drugs, alcohol, tobacco and food. The fact is, you can't legislate for self-esteem from Westminster. We can't pass the Elimination of Obesity Act 2010. Our Government will be a much smarter one, shunning the bureaucratic levers of the past and finding intelligent ways to encourage support and enable people to make better choices for themselves'.

Sadly, the historical evidence from public health initiatives and the complexity of the scientific basis of obesity suggests limited success from the policy of 'nudge'. As Foresight concluded, a long-term comprehensive strategy needs to incorporate a range of policies. Importantly, the implementation of such strategies may have limited impact on the current generation of adults, but lead to long-term benefit in younger generations. Benefits from integrated and sustained strategies should lead to a progressive decline in obesity prevalence across all generations and an accompanying reduction in obesity-related diseases [7].

Lessons from the history of obesity

Too often, it seems that we concentrate on the present without reflecting on lessons from the past.

The following is a summary of knowledge about the growing prevalence of overweight and obesity.

- The history of consumption and living standards in Britain during the twentieth and early twenty-first century points towards the close relationship between obesity and modern affluent lifestyles characterised by abundant food and increasingly sedentary habits.
- Extensive rationing and controls on food reversed these trends during the 1940s and early 1950s. The policy was only possible in the context of war and does not offer a practical solution for the public health problems of the early twenty-first century.
- Inter-war weight loss manuals did not pay much attention to energy counting, but rather emphasised a holistic approach to transform lifestyles by adopting healthy habits as the key to successful, permanent weight reduction.

1.1.4 Genetics of obesity

The suspicion of an inherited background to obesity has existed over many generations. Carl Van Noorden in 1907 delineated two type of obesity – exogenous and endogenous [15]. He suggested that exogenous obesity, which accounted for the majority of cases, was the consequence of external elements, namely food consumption in excess of energy expenditure. Nevertheless, the group with endogenous obesity had an intrinsic problem that led to hypometabolism. Jules Hirsch observed in the 1950s that there is a 'biochemical or biological element' to will power, basing the observation on the life-long struggle faced by many obese persons to maintain weight loss over the longer term [16]. Ethan Sims demonstrated in a prison population that the majority of inmates (over)fed 10,000 kcal/day over 200 days had difficulty in maintaining their weight gain, whereas a small number, with family history of obesity, gained weight swiftly and struggled to lose the weight once the overfeeding had ceased [17].

The seminal studies of twins by Albert Stunkard and colleagues provide additional strong evidence for an inherited basis to obesity. From the Danish Twin Registry, Stunkard identified twins who had been adopted early in life and therefore separated from their biological parents. Despite a shared environment with the adoptive parents, the adoptee twins' BMIs were more closely associated to that of their biological rather than the adoptive parents. Accordingly, most adoptees inherited their biological parents' obesity [18]. On reviewing identical twins registered by the Swedish registry, Stunkard found that identical twins had virtually the same body weight regardless of whether they had grown up together or separately [19]. A subsequent study by Bouchard and colleagues, which involved overfeeding 12 pairs of identical male twins over 100 days, demonstrated a wide variety of responses across the twin pairs; however, within each twin pair, there was little difference in the weight gained and even less difference in body fat distribution and visceral fat accumulation [20].

With the advent of molecular genetics, extensive mapping of obesity-gene mutations in rodents began in earnest. Jeffrey Friedman and colleagues cloned the gene *ob*, which encodes leptin [21]; their findings resulted in a transformation in obesity research. Thousands of articles have been published and substantial research funds invested in pursuing the relevance of leptin and related genes, including ghrelin, neuropeptide y and MCHC, in human obesity. However, the signalling pathways of molecules involved in appetite; and the genetic mutations that may interfere with these pathways. More recently, a common variant of the fat mass and obesity–associated gene *FTO* and genetic variants of DYRK18 have been associated with human obesity [22]. This is evidence that provides fuel to the argument that body weight regulation is not simply governed by 'energy in – energy out'.

Nevertheless, evidence remains that few are pre-destined to obesity, while many are predisposed to weight gain. Genetic predisposition in tandem with the development of food environments that encourage overeating and built environments that discourage energy expenditure are undoubtedly explanations for the increasing prevalence of obesity observed during the last four decades.

1.1.5 Summary box

Key points

- In clinical practice, body fat is most commonly and simply estimated by using a formula that combines weight and height – BMI. Measurement of body circumference is an additional indicator of health risk in an overweight or obese person: excess visceral (intra-abdominal) fat is a risk factor for long-term conditions independent of total adiposity.
- Overweight and obesity cause or exacerbate a large number of health problems, both independently and in association with other diseases, and are among the most significant contributors to ill health.
- Between 1980 and 2008, age-standardised mean global BMI has increased by 0.4–0.5 kg/m^2 per decade in men and women.
- The history of consumption and living standards during the twentieth and early twenty-first century points towards the close relationship between obesity and modern affluent lifestyles, characterised by abundant food intakes and increasingly sedentary habits.
- Evidence confirms that few individuals are predestined to obesity, while many are predisposed to weight gain. Genetic predisposition in tandem with the development of food environments that encourage overeating and built environments that discourage energy expenditure explain the increasing prevalence of obesity observed during the last four decades.

References

1. National Obesity Observatory, Public Health England. Available from: http://www.noo.org.uk/NOO_about_obesity/measurement, accessed August 25, 2016.
2. Metropolitan Life Insurance Company: 1983 Metropolitan height and weight tables. *Statistical Bulletin* 1983; **64**: 2–9.
3. Health and Social Care Information Centre. The Health Survey for England – 2012 trend tables. London: Health and Social Care Information Centre. 2013. Available from: http://www.hscic.gov.uk/catalogue/PUB13219.
4. De Onis M, Onyango AW, Siyam A, Nishida C, Siekmann J. Development of a WHO growth reference for school-aged children and adolescents. *Bulletin of the World Health Organization* 2007; **85**: 660–667.
5. Kopelman PG. Obesity as a medical problem. *Nature* 2000; **404**: 635–643.
6. Willet WC, Dietz WH, Colditz GA. Guidelines for healthy weights. *New England Journal of Medicine* 1999; **341**: 427–433.
7. Tackling obesity – Foresight Report. Government Office for Science 2007.
8. Finucane MM, Stevens GA, Cowan MJ, Danaei G, Lin JK, Paciorek CJ, et al. National, regional and global trends in body-mass index since 1980: systematic analysis of health examination surveys and epidemiological studies with 960 country-years and 9.1 million participants. *Lancet* 2011; **377**: 557–567.
9. Storey GO, Smith H. Sir George Newman (1870–1948). *Journal of Medical Biography* 2005; **13**: 31–38.
10. Howard C. Diet and weight. *Lancet* 1933; **222**: 1394–1395.
11. Rationing in the United Kingdom. Available from: http://en.wikipedia.org/wiki/Rationing_in_the_United_Kingdom.
12. Dig for Victory. Available from: http://www.nationalarchives.gov.uk/theartofwar/films/dig_victory.htm.
13. Fogel RW. *The Escape from Hunger and Premature Death, 1700–2100*. Cambridge: Cambridge University Press, 2004.
14. Minister rejects 'Jamie Oliver approach' on health. Available from: http://www.bbc.co.uk/news/10459744.
15. Jou C. The biology and genetics of obesity – a century of inquiries. *New England Journal of Medicine* 2014; **370**: 1874–1877.
16. Liebel RL, Rosenbaum M, Hirsch J. Changes in energy expenditure resulting from altered body weight. *New England Journal of Medicine* 1995; **322**: 621–628.
17. Salans LB, Horton ES, Sims EH. Experimental obesity in man: cellular character of the adipose tissue. *Journal of Clinical Investigation* 1971; **50**: 1005–1011.
18. Stunkard AJ, Sorensen TIA, Harris C, Teasdale TW, Chakraborty R. An adoption study of human obesity. *New England Journal of Medicine* 1986; **314**: 193–198.
19. Stunkard AJ, Harris JR, Pedersen NL, McCleam GE. The body-mass index of twins who have been reared apart. *New England Journal of Medicine* 1990; **322**: 1483–1487.
20. Bouchard C, Tremblay A, Despres JP, Nadeau A, Lupien PJ, Theriault G, et al. The response to long term overfeeding in identical twins. *New England Journal of Medicine* 1990; **322**: 1477–1482.
21. Zhang Y, Proenca R, Maffei M, Barone M, Leopold L, Friedman JM. Positional cloning of the mouse obese gene and its human homologue. *Nature* 1994; **372**: 425–431.
22. Frayling TM, Timpson NJ, Weedon MN, Zeggini M, Freathy RM, Lindgren CM, et al. A common variant in the *FTO* gene is associated with body mass index and predisposes to childhood and adult obesity. *Science* 2007; **316**: 889–894.

Chapter 1.2

Definition, prevalence and historical perspectives of obesity in children

Adrienne Hughes

University of Strathclyde, Glasgow, UK

An epidemic of childhood obesity occurred over the past few decades, affecting all age and social groups in the developed world. The prevalence of childhood obesity appears to have stabilised in some developed countries in recent years, but at an unacceptably high level. Therefore, obesity continues to be one of the most common child health problems, and a major challenge to public health. Developing countries have also experienced rising childhood obesity rates in recent years. The aim of this chapter is to summarise the evidence, using good-quality systematic reviews where available, on the worldwide prevalence of obesity among children; the development of the childhood obesity epidemic in the UK and USA; and the identification of subgroups of the population at greater risk of becoming obese. This chapter will also discuss how to define obesity in children for epidemiological purposes (i.e. to monitor and compare prevalence at the population level), whereas the criteria for diagnosing obesity in children for clinical management will be covered in Chapter 3.2.

1.2.1 Definition of obesity in children

Obesity is an excess of body fat, which is associated with increased health risks. Subjective assessment of obesity in children is inaccurate, and therefore obesity should be defined using objective methods [1]. Direct measures of adiposity, such as densitometry and dual-energy X-ray absorptiometry, are more accurate than indirect methods (e.g. waist circumference, skinfolds, body mass index, bioelectrical impedance), but are not practical for epidemiological studies or clinical use [2]. A critique of the different methods to measure adiposity and define obesity in children is available elsewhere [2,3]. There is widespread international support for the use of body mass index (BMI; ratio of body weight to height squared – kg/m^2) to define childhood obesity in epidemiological studies and in clinical practice [1–7]. Although BMI is not a direct measure of adiposity in children, it correlates well with more accurate measures of body fatness, it is practical to measure and a high BMI for age is associated with both high fat mass and increased risk to health [1–3,7–10].

As BMI varies with age and gender in children, BMI values are compared with age- and gender-specific national reference data using cut-off points in the BMI distribution (BMI percentiles or standard deviation scores, SDSs) to identify obesity in children [4]. National BMI reference data are available in many countries including the UK [4] and the USA [11]. The UK 1990 reference data represents the BMI distribution of UK children in 1990, are widely available in the form of BMI centile charts and can be used as a baseline against which subsequent obesity trends can be compared [4]. Epidemiological studies commonly use the ≥85th centile of BMI for age and gender and the ≥95th centile of BMI for age and gender based on national (country-specific) reference data as the percentiles to identify overweight and obesity in children [1].

Advanced Nutrition and Dietetics in Obesity, First Edition. Edited by Catherine Hankey.

These percentiles define overweight and obesity reasonably well, and children with BMI in the ≥95th percentile are at high risk of obesity-related conditions [1,5,7,10]. Age- and gender-specific waist circumference percentiles are available for the UK and elsewhere but have not been used in epidemiological studies to estimate obesity prevalence.

An alternative method for identifying obesity in children was developed by Cole et al. in 2000 [12]. This method provides age- and gender-specific BMI cut-offs that correspond to the adult cut-offs for obesity (i.e. BMI of 30 kg/m^2) and are based on international data collected from six countries (UK, Brazil, Hong Kong, the Netherlands, Singapore and the USA). These cut-offs, commonly referred to as the *International Obesity Task Force* (IOTF) *definition of obesity*, allow international comparisons of childhood obesity prevalence, but are not intended for clinical or national epidemiological use [12]. Detailed discussions of the ongoing debate surrounding the use of national and international methods to classify healthy weight, overweight and obesity in children are available elsewhere [1,12,13]. Briefly, both methods are widely used to define obesity in epidemiological studies; however a recent systematic review found that the IOTF method was much less sensitive (poorer accuracy) than national reference methods for detecting obesity in children [1]. The IOTF cut-offs for BMI are useful for worldwide comparisons of childhood obesity prevalence [2], but will give more conservative estimates of obesity prevalence, particularly in boys, compared to methods based on national (country-specific) reference data [1,2].

1.2.2 Trends in the prevalence of childhood obesity

Comparison of obesity rates among countries is difficult as different methods have been used to define obesity. Further differences can be due to different study designs, the range of ages of the samples included and the timing of the surveys [2]. Despite these problems, several systematic reviews have examined trends in the prevalence of childhood obesity in developed and developing countries over the past few decades [2,14–20].

The global situation

The prevalence of childhood obesity has increased markedly over the past few decades in most developed countries and in several developing countries [2,14,15,17]. Thus, obesity in children is a serious global public health problem. Prevalence is particularly high in the USA, Canada, Australia, Japan and parts of Europe, with obesity rates doubling or tripling from the 1970s to late 1990s in these countries [2,14,15]. In Europe, the highest levels are reported in the UK and many southern European countries, such as Greece, Spain, Malta, Portugal and Italy [2,14,15,18]. Parts of South East Asia and much of sub-Saharan Africa appear to have the lowest prevalence [2,14]. Some developing countries have experienced a marked increase in obesity prevalence, associated with rapid socioeconomic growth, including Brazil, Chile and urban regions of China [2,14]. Data from Brazil demonstrated a threefold increase in obesity prevalence among children and adolescents from 1974 to 1997 [14]. Obesity is more prevalent in wealthier groups and urban populations in developing countries, whereas children in the lowest SES groups are more at risk in developed countries [2,14].

Recent systematic reviews [16,18–20] have indicated that the prevalence of obesity in children has stabilised (i.e. no change in obesity prevalence) or levelled off (i.e. change in the trend from an increase towards stability or a slowing down in the increase) since the early 2000s in several developed countries including Australia, most of Europe, Japan and the USA. However, levels remain high in these countries, and childhood obesity continues to be a major public health issue. In addition, it is unclear if this stabilisation is a long-term change or a temporary phase that may be followed by a further increase [20]. Additionally, obesity prevalence has continued to rise in some countries (e.g. China and Vietnam), and recent trends for Africa, South America and much of the Middle East have not been reported [20].

Development of the obesity epidemic in the USA and UK

In the USA, the National Health and Nutrition Examination Survey (NHANES) has monitored

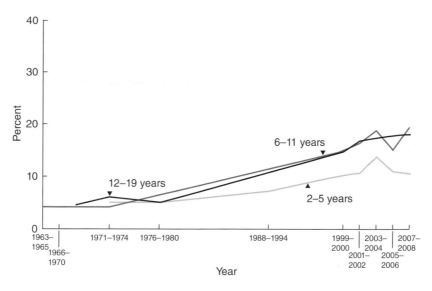

Figure 1.2.1   Trends in obesity among children and adolescents: United States, 1963–2008. Source: From reference [21].

trends in obesity prevalence among children from the 1960s (shown in Figure 1.2.1) using cross-sectional, nationally representative samples of US children [21]. The proportion of obese children and adolescents (defined as BMI ≥95th percentile on US/CDC reference charts) remained stable at 5% from mid-1960s to 1976–1980, but then trebled between 1976–1980 and 2003–2004 [21]. By 2003–2004, 14% of 2–5-year-olds, 19% of 6–11-year-olds and 17% of 12–19-year-olds in the USA were obese [21,22]. The most recent estimate of obesity prevalence based on data from the 2007–2008 NHANES indicates that 10% of children aged 2–5 years, 20% of those aged 6–11 years and 18% of adolescents aged 12–19 years were obese, suggesting that prevalence has stabilised in the USA as previously discussed, although prevalence remains high [21,23].

Childhood obesity increased markedly in the UK from the late 1980s [24–26]. Chinn reported the prevalence of obesity (defined using the IOTF method) in representative samples of English and Scottish children aged 4–11 years using three cross-sectional surveys in 1974, 1984 and 1994 [24]. Obesity prevalence did not increase from 1974 to 1984, but increased substantially from 1984 to 1994 in both English and Scottish children. Similarly, in the 1996 Health Survey for England (HSE), 11% of

6-year-olds and 17% of 15-year-olds were classed as obese (BMI ≥95th percentile). These figures were significantly higher than the 1990 UK reference standard of 5% [25], and indicated that obesity prevalence had doubled in children and trebled in adolescents (relative to the UK 1990 reference data) in a short period of time (shown in Figure 1.2.2). By the 2003 HSE, 14% of children aged 2–10 years and 21% of 11–15-year-olds were obese [27]. The most recent estimate of obesity prevalence based on the 2009 HSE indicated that 15% of 2–10-year-olds and 18% of 11–15-year-olds were obese [28], suggesting that prevalence has stabilised, albeit at a high level [26].

In addition to the rise in the proportion of children classed as 'obese', average BMI and BMI z scores have risen across paediatric populations in developed countries over the past few decades, suggesting that most children have been affected by the obesogenic environment (i.e. environments that promote obesity) [19,24,29,30]. In addition, data from measures of body composition and body fat distribution, such as skinfolds and waist circumference, indicate that total body fatness and central fatness has increased over the past few decades among children and adolescents [30–32]. A meta-analysis found significant increases in triceps and

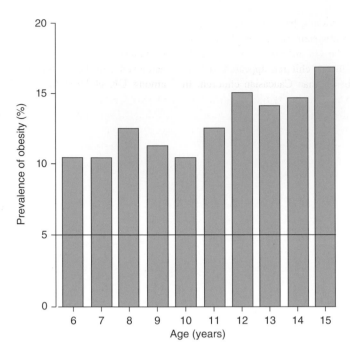

Figure 1.2.2 Prevalence of obesity (BMI>95th centile) at each age compared with expected frequency (5%, horizontal line). Source: From reference [25].

subscapular skinfold thickness and percentage body fat (estimated from skinfold measures) between 1951 and 2003 in children aged 0–18 years in developed countries, with the rate of increase becoming much steeper in the 1980s [32]. McCarthy et al. used data from cross-sectional surveys conducted in 1977, 1987 and 1997 to examine changes in waist circumference for age (a measure of central fatness) and BMI of adolescents aged 11–16 years [29]. Average waist circumference for age and BMI had increased substantially over the 10–20-year period between the surveys. In addition, waist circumference for age had increased at a faster rate than BMI. The increase in central fatness among children is particularly worrying because central fatness is strongly associated with several cardiometabolic risk factors [1,10].

Obesity prevalence by age, gender, socioeconomic status (SES) and ethnicity

The obesity epidemic has affected children of all ages, both genders, most ethnic groups and all socioeconomic backgrounds, although some groups have been affected more than others [2,30]. Several studies in the USA have observed higher obesity rates in African American and Hispanic children compared to non-Hispanic white children [22,33,34]. Hedley et al. [34] showed that the prevalence of obesity (BMI ≥ 95th percentile on US/CDC reference charts) among children aged 6–11 years was 20% in African Americans, 22% among Mexican Americans and 14% among non-Hispanic whites. Furthermore, over a 30-year period from 1971–1974 to 1999–2002, Mexican American and African American children experienced much greater increases in the prevalence of obesity than white children [33]. For example, among 6–11-year-olds, the prevalence of obesity (BMI ≥ 95th percentile) increased by 16% among Mexican Americans, by 15% among African Americans and by 10% among white children. Recent data from the 2007–2008 period indicate that ethnic differences in obesity prevalence are still evident [23].

The relationship between obesity and ethnicity in developed countries other than the USA is less clear, although there is some evidence to suggest that some ethnic minority groups may be at greater risk of obesity [30,35]. A recent systematic review [35] of studies conducted in the UK between 1980 and 2010 concluded that Chinese children appeared to have lower risk for obesity than Caucasian children. In contrast, the literature on obesity prevalence among South Asian and black children relative to Caucasians in the UK was mixed. Several studies observed higher rates of obesity among South Asian and black children compared to Caucasians, whereas other studies observed either lower rates or no differences. The existing literature is limited by a lack of studies using UK representative samples, as well as the failure to consider differences in SES by ethnic group (ethnic minorities in the UK have lower SES than Caucasians). Also, categorising Bangladeshis, Indians and Pakistanis as 'South Asians' may mask the differences in obesity prevalence between these groups and the problems defining obesity using BMI cut-offs in some ethnic minority groups (at the same BMI level, children from some ethnic minority groups have higher fat mass) [35]. Despite these limitations, obesity prevalence appeared to be higher in South Asian boys and lower in South Asian girls relative to their Caucasian counterparts, whereas girls from black subgroups appeared to have higher risk, and boys from black subgroups lower risk, compared to Caucasians. The reasons for possible ethnic differences in obesity rates are not entirely clear, but may be *partly* explained by SES differences [35].

In developed countries, children from families with low SES are at greater risk of obesity [2,30,36–38]. A recent systematic review of cross-sectional studies published between 1990 and 2005 concluded that there is an inverse association between SES (using parental education as the SES indicator) and obesity risk in children from developed countries [36]. The evidence suggested that children from all SES groups have been affected by the obesity epidemic; however, children whose parents (particularly mothers) have a low level of education were at greater risk. Stamatakis et al. [37] examined trends in obesity prevalence by SES in UK children aged 5–10 years using nationally representative cross-sectional data collected over several time periods to 2002–2003. A rapid increase in obesity prevalence was observed in all children, particularly from 1994 onwards; however,

prevalence had increased at a faster rate among children from lower SES groups [37]. A further study by Stamatakis et al. [38] showed that obesity rates had levelled off between 2002–2003 and 2006/2007 among UK children (aged 5–10 years), whereas obesity prevalence had continued to increase among children from lower socioeconomic groups, suggesting that the existing socioeconomic gap in childhood obesity in the UK may be expanding. Similarly, a study examining obesity trends between 2000 and 2006 in Australia reported that prevalence was only increasing in children attending low-SES schools [20]. Reasons for SES differences in obesity rates are complex and require further study, although poor diet and limited opportunities for physical activity may be important factors.

There is no obvious international trend towards systematic differences in obesity rates with age or between the sexes [30]. Although some studies have observed higher rates of obesity among older children (e.g. see prevalence figures in previous section 1.2.2), that may be due to greater exposure to the obesogenic environment with increasing age [30]. Apparent differences in obesity prevalence by gender may be a result of the method used to define obesity; the IOTF method underestimates prevalence in boys more than girls [1]. Thus, several studies have observed higher obesity rates in girls than boys when using the IOTF method, and no gender difference when national reference standards are used [1,2,18,30]. The plateau in prevalence described previously has been observed in all age groups and both genders [19,20,23,26], but this has not been shown in all studies [16].

1.2.3 Conclusion

The prevalence of childhood obesity is high and has increased rapidly over the past few decades in developed countries. Children of all ages, ethnic groups, socioeconomic backgrounds and both genders have been affected, although children from some ethnic minorities and lower socioeconomic groups are particularly at risk. Reasons for ethnic and SES differences are not entirely clear and require further study, although differences in dietary intake and physical activity may be important. Recent data indicate that prevalence of childhood obesity may have stabilised or levelled off in some developed countries in recent years, although it is too soon to be certain if this change is long-term, and obesity rates have not appeared to stabilise among children from lower socioeconomic groups. Possible reasons for the stabilisation are unknown at present, although public health campaigns to improve dietary and physical activity habits may be at least partly responsible [20,26]. However, prevalence remains unacceptably high, and therefore obesity prevention and treatment strategies are needed for all children and should also target children and families from specific groups. Developing countries have also experienced rising obesity rates among children in recent years, particularly among wealthier groups and urban populations, and recent data suggest that these rates are not levelling off. Overall, childhood obesity is a serious global public health problem, and interventions to prevent and reduce obesity among children are needed worldwide.

1.2.4 Summary box

Key points

- Childhood obesity prevalence is high and has increased rapidly over the decades in developed countries.
- Children from some ethnic minorities and lower socioeconomic groups are particularly at risk. Reasons for ethnic and SES differences are unclear, although differences in dietary intake and physical activity may be important.
- Recent prevalence of childhood obesity has levelled off in developed countries, although obesity rates have not among children from lower socioeconomic groups.
- Prevalence remains unacceptably high; obesity prevention and treatment strategies are needed for all children, and should target children and families from specific at-risk groups.
- Prevalence of childhood obesity in developing countries reflects a rise in obesity among children, particularly among wealthier groups and urban populations.
- Childhood obesity remains a serious global public health problem, and interventions to prevent and reduce obesity among the young are required internationally.

References

1. Reilly JJ, Kelly J, Wilson DC. Accuracy of simple clinical and epidemiological definitions of childhood obesity: systematic review and evidence appraisal. *Obesity Reviews* 2010; **11**: 645–655.
2. Lobstein T, Baur L, Uauy R. Obesity in children and young people: a crisis in public health. *Obesity Reviews* 2004; **5**: 4–85.
3. Reilly JJ, Wilson ML, Summerbell CD, Wilson DC. Obesity: diagnosis, prevention, and treatment; evidence based answers to common questions. *Archives of Disease in Childhood* 2002; **86**: 392–394.
4. Cole TJ, Freeman JV, Preece MA. Body mass index reference curves for the UK, 1990. *Archives of Disease in Childhood* 1995; **73**: 25–29.
5. SIGN. Management of obesity: A national clinical guideline. SIGN publication no. 115. 2010. Edinburgh, SIGN [Internet]. Available from: http://www.sign.ac.uk/pdf/sign115.pdf, accessed September 2011.
6. NHS National Institute for Health and Clinical Excellence (NICE). Guidance on the prevention, identification, assessment and management of overweight and obesity in adults and children. 2006. Clinical Guideline 43 [Internet]. Available from: http://guidance.nice.org.uk/CG43, accessed September 2011.
7. Barlow SE. Expert Committee recommendations regarding the prevention, assessment, and treatment of child and adolescent overweight and obesity: summary report. *Pediatrics* 2007; **120**: s124–s192.
8. Reilly JJ, Dorosty AR, Emmett PM. Identification of the obese child: adequacy of the BMI for clinical practice and epidemiology. *International Journal of Obesity* 2000; **24**: 1623–1627.
9. Baker JL, Olsen LW, Sorensen TI. Childhood body-mass index and the risk of coronary heart disease in adulthood. *New England Journal of Medicine* 2007; **357**: 2329–2337.
10. Reilly JJ, Methven E, McDowell ZC, et al. Health consequences of obesity. *Archives of Disease in Childhood* 2003; **88**: 748–752.
11. Kuczmarski RL, Ogden CL, Grummer-Strawn LM, et al. CDC Growth Charts: United States. *Advance Data* 2000; **314**: 1–28.
12. Cole TJ, Bellizzi MC, Flegal KM, Dietz WH. Establishing a standard definition for child overweight and obesity worldwide. *BMJ* 2000; **320**: 1240–1245.
13. Reilly JJ. Assessment of childhood obesity: National reference data or international approach? *Obesity Research* 2002; **10**: 838–840.
14. Wang Y, Lobstein T. Worldwide trends in childhood overweight and obesity. *International Journal of Pediatric Obesity* 2006; **1**: 11–25.
15. Janssen I, Katzmarzyk PT, Boyce WF, et al. Comparison of overweight and obesity prevalence in school-aged youth from 34 countries and their relationships with physical activity and dietary patterns. *Obesity Reviews* 2005; **6**: 123–132.
16. Olds TS, Maher CA. Evidence that the prevalence of childhood overweight is plateauing: data from nine countries. *International Journal of Pediatric Obesity* 2011; early online publication.
17. Lobstein T, Frelut ML. Prevalence of overweight among children in Europe. *Obesity Reviews* 2003; **4**: 195–200.

18. Cattaneo A, Monasta L, Stamatakis E, et al. Overweight and obesity in infants and pre-school children in the European Union: a review of existing data. *Obesity Reviews* 2010; **11**: 389–398.

19. Olds TS, Tomkinson GR, Ferrar KE, Maher CA. Trends in the prevalence of childhood overweight and obesity in Australia between 1985 and 2008. *International Journal of Obesity* 2010; **34**: 57–66.

20. Rokholm B, Baker JL, Sorensen TIA. The levelling off of the obesity epidemic since the year 1999 – a review of evidence and perspectives. *Obesity Reviews* 2010; **11**: 835–846.

21. National Centre for Health Statistics. National Health and Nutrition Examination Survey. Prevalence of obesity among children and adolescents: United States, Trends 1963–1965 Through 2007–2008 [Internet]. Available from: http://www.cdc.gov/nchs/data/hestat/obesity_child_07_08/obesity_child_07_08.htm, accessed September 2011.

22. Ogden CL, Carroll MD, Curtin LS, McDowell MA, Tabak CJ, Flegal KM. Prevalence of Overweight and Obesity in the United States, 1999–2004. *JAMA* 2006; **295**: 1549–1555.

23. Ogden CL, Carroll MD, Curtin LS, Lamb MM, Flegal KM. Prevalence of High Body Mass Index in US Children and Adolescents, 2007–2008. *JAMA* 2010; **303**: 242–249.

24. Chinn S, Rona R. Prevalence and trends in overweight and obesity in three cross sectional studies of British children, 1974–94. *BMJ* 2001; **322**: 24–26.

25. Reilly JJ, Dorosty AR. Epidemic of obesity in UK children. *Lancet* 1999; **354**: 1874–1875.

26. Stamatakis E, Zaninotto P, Falascheti E, Mindell J, Head J. Time trends in childhood and adolescent obesity in England from 1995 to 2007 and projections of prevalence to 2015. *Journal of Epidemiology and Community Health* 2010; **64**: 167–174.

27. The NHS information centre. Health Survey for England: Revised version of the Children Table 4, Children's overweight and obesity prevalence, by survey year, age-group and sex 1995–2007. November 2009 [Internet]. Available from: http://www.ic.nhs.uk/statistics-and-data-collections/health-and-lifestyles-related-surveys/health-survey-for-england, accessed September 2011.

28. The NHS information centre. Health Survey for England 2009: Volume 1 Health and Lifestyles. December 2010 [Internet]. Available from: http://www.ic.nhs.uk/statistics-and-data-collections/health-and-lifestyles-related-surveys/health-survey-for-england, accessed September 2011.

29. McCarthy HD, Ellis SM, Cole TJ. Central overweight and obesity in British youth aged 11–16 years: cross-sectional surveys of waist circumference. *BMJ* 2003; **326**: 624–628.

30. Reilly JJ. Descriptive epidemiology and health consequences of childhood obesity. *Best Practice & Research: Clinical Endocrinology & Metabolism* 2005; **19**: 327–341.

31. McCarthy HD, Jarrett KV, Crawley HF. The development of waist circumference percentiles in British children aged 5.0–16.9 y. *European Journal of Clinical Nutrition* 2001; **55**: 902–907.

32. Olds TS. One million skinfolds: secular trends in the fatness of young people 1951–2004. *European Journal of Clinical Nutrition* 2009; **63**: 934–946.

33. Freedman DS, Khan LK, Serdula MK, Ogden CL, Dietz WH. Racial and ethnic differences in secular trends for childhood BMI, weight, and height. *Obesity* 2006; **14**: 301–308.

34. Hedley AA, Ogden CL, Johnson CL, Carroll MD, Curtin LS, Flegal KM. Prevalence of overweight and obesity among US children, adolescents, and adults, 1999–2002. *JAMA* 2004; **291**: 2847–2850.

35. El-Sayed AM, Scarborough P, Galea S. Ethnic inequalities in obesity among children and adults in the UK: a systematic review of the literature. *Obesity Reviews* 2011; **12**: e516–e534.

36. Shrewsbury V, Wardle J. Socioeconomic status and adiposity in childhood: a systematic review of cross-sectional studies 1990–2005. *Obesity* 2008; **16**: 275–283.

37. Stamatakis E, Primatesta P, Chinn S, Rona R, Falascheti E. Overweight and obesity trends from 1974 to 2003 in English children: what is the role of socio-economic factors? *Archives of Disease in Childhood* 2005; **90**: 999–1004.

38. Stamatakis E, Wardle J, Cole TJ. Childhood obesity and overweight prevalence trends in England: evidence for growing socioeconomic disparities. *International Journal of Obesity* 2010; **34**: 41–47.

Chapter 1.3

Development of overweight and obesity across the life course

Catherine Hankey
University of Glasgow, Glasgow, UK

Obesity and overweight are persistent conditions and are compounded by the gradual age-dependant involuntary weight gain that occurs in adulthood (approximately 0.5 kg per year). In order to understand this unconscious weight gain, this chapter will address each of the key risk periods across the life course.

1.3.1 Childhood: birth to early school age

Childhood and adolescence are risk periods for excess weight gain. The Early Bird study identified the period from birth to 5 years of age as the stage when the majority of excess weight gain occurs, prior to puberty [1]. More recently, a considerable increase in weight gain has also been shown between children after 5 years of age, when formal schooling begins (school year one), and towards the end of primary/elementary school (school year six). The data in Figure 1.3.1 use information collected from the National Child Measurement programme in the UK to report the changes in school children's body mass index (BMI) [2]. For this report, the years 2006–2007 and 2014–2015 were considered [2]. Figure 1.3.1 highlights the recent trends in terms of obesity and overweight, and within that the trends evident in different subgroups of children. These changes in weight and growth rates reflect substantial changes in the environment and in the way children grow and live. Furthermore, weight gain may be occurring in children who are overweight and

moving towards obesity, but these changes are often known to be frequently overlooked by their parents [3]. This 'normalisation' of obesity and overweight may hamper approaches to challenge excess weight gain.

1.3.2 Adolescence and young adulthood

Weight gain is rapid in the translational period spanning adolescence to young adulthood [4]. Birth cohorts for surveys completed in 1998, 2003 and 2008 were used to examine weight and BMI changes over time in different age groups. Results highlighted the temporal increases in obesity rates between different age groups. Most cohorts were heavier during the period spanning 1998–2003 than in the 2003–2008 surveys. Overall increases between 1998 and 2003 were 1–1.5 kg/m^2 units in BMI and 2–7 cm in waist circumference, greater in the younger age cohorts. Famously, the Freshman 15 study in the USA highlighted relocation – in particular, a move away from home for education – as a key driver for weight gain. This included an average weight gain in the first semester ranging from 3.5 to 7.8 lbs (1.6 kg–3.5 kg) [5]. It may be that the additional freedom of food choice, lack of accountability and the opportunity to explore alternative dietary and lifestyle choices favours weight gain.

Inactivity has also been suggested as an important factor in weight gain at this developmental stage. A number of studies have explored possible

Advanced Nutrition and Dietetics in Obesity, First Edition. Edited by Catherine Hankey.
© 2018 John Wiley & Sons Ltd. Published 2018 by John Wiley & Sons Ltd.

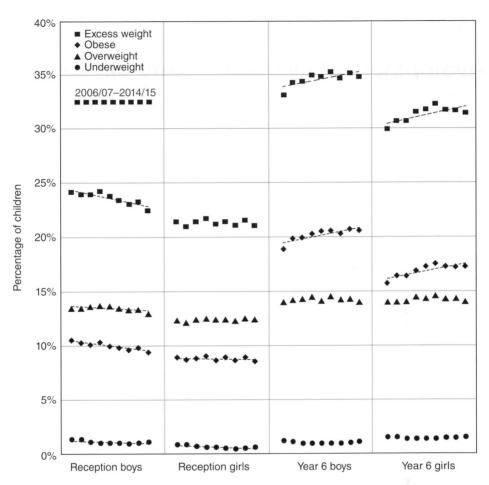

Figure 1.3.1 Prevalence of obesity, excess weight, overweight and underweight by year of measurement, school year and sex. NCMP 2006–2007 to 2014–2015. Significant upward or downward linear trends are shown with a dashed line [2]. Published with acknowledgment to Public Health England.

links with computer gaming/screen time as a proxy for inactivity. Cross-sectional and prospective associations between computer gaming and overweight (BMI ≥ 25 kg/m²) have been observed in women, with adjustment for age, job and amount of activity, among other factors. For men, only cross-sectional associations could be seen [6]. The impact of screen time on weight gain has also been reported by the findings of a Swedish study. This impact is likely to persist across the life-course, given the habitual nature of the use of games or mobile devices.

1.3.3 Marriage or cohabitation and body weight

The formalisation of a relationship via marriage or as cohabitating partners, with or without financial commitment, may lead to changes in lifestyle patterns and behaviour. Being part of a settled relationship favours contentment, a situation that itself encourages weight gain [7]. Married respondents were usually heavier than both never-married and divorced respondents [8]. Observations have suggested that food becomes central to a relationship as couples may have more time together to share mealtimes and make food purchases. Perhaps contentment and security reduce the importance of appearance or awareness of body weight, either subconsciously or otherwise.

Given that marriage and in fact parenthood are associated with weight gain in general, the US CARDIA study data were used to try to understand the impact of marriage in differing environmental settings [9]. Data on neighbourhoods compared married adults living in more affluent areas – with lower population density, better environments for food purchasing and more public facilities for sport and activity – with their unmarried neighbours exposed to the same environment. There was a positive association between weight gain and marriage in white, affluent couples, in comparison to their unmarried neighbours. Marriage showed no such associations with the same comparisons made in less affluent couples, living in poorer settings [9].

Given the recognised variation in marriage duration, a review investigated the associations between marital transitions, BMI and body weight [10]. Fourteen studies described transitions both in and out of marriage. The positive association between marriage and weight gain was supported, while dissolving a marriage was associated with weight loss. The range of weight changes vary according to the duration of the study period [10]. A short-term study suggested a weight gain of around 1.5 kg after 3 months of cohabitation [11]. Although the lack of any comparator in this study meant that the impact of moving in together was unclear, more certainty was seen in analyses of national survey data, which allowed comparison between newly married adult couples and those already married. The newly wedded adults had gained an additional 2 kg after a year [12].

For a range of possible reasons, the impact of leaving a marital relationship was associated with weight loss, although the impact of divorce has been considered as only 'temporary' [8]. Using data from men who either divorced or remained married, the impact on BMI in each category after more than 20 years was limited. Both groups of men gained weight, and the BMI rose from a healthy weight to an overweight category. This mirrors the weight gain seen across most Western populations.

Despite being a complex setting, with many compounding factors, marriage or cohabitation, but not ceasing of a marriage, may in certain circumstances offer opportunities for interventions to promote healthy weight programmes.

1.3.4 Pregnancy

Pregnancy is often a time of great anticipation, especially for healthy mothers without any specific concerns about the health of their unborn child. Anecdotally, many pregnant women regard pregnancy as an opportunity to bloom, disregarding any restrictions they usually apply to the energy they consume. Pregnancy is probably the only period across the life course when positive encouragement for weight gain is given by many. Eating for two, although widely known to be a myth, appears attractive to many who choose to believe it. Increasingly, given the worldwide epidemic of obesity, excessive weight gain in pregnancy has been less widely accepted, but it does still have a cross-cultural impact. Excessive gestational weight gain is associated with adverse infant, childhood and maternal outcomes, and research to develop interventions to address this issue is ongoing [13].

In the UK, there are no data to assess how many pregnant women are obese or overweight. The Centre for Maternal and Child Enquiries [14] conducted a UK-wide audit of obesity during pregnancy for a 2-month period during 2009. The results disclosed that 5% of all women who had given birth (≥24 weeks' gestation) were identified as having a BMI of ≥35 kg/m² at any time during pregnancy. Even more concerning was that the median BMI for these women was >35 kg/m². This was 39.1 kg/m², and 2% had a BMI of ≥40 (morbid obesity). Moreover, 0.2% of pregnant women reported having a BMI of ≥50, categorized as super-morbid obese.

Recognizing the issue of obesity and excessive weight gain in pregnancy, the United States Institute of Medicine [15] produced some guidance material for weight gain, which differed according to individuals' initial BMI. This issue was judged as important, given the demographic changes that had taken place in those women who were becoming pregnant. They were older at conception, tended to gain more weight than in the past, were more likely to have a twin or triplet birth, and were more likely to be overweight or obese at conception. A recent pilot observational study aimed to determine the feasibility of implementing a programme within the UK National Health Service to limit maternal weight gain [16]. The findings demonstrated the difficulties in actually measuring body weight in women across their pregnancy, implying an unwillingness in the women or their health professionals in make weighing a routine practice. This has been demonstrated in other studies [17] involving the measurement of body weight. This highlighted the positive association between higher weight gain and adverse perinatal outcomes. Currently, UK clinical guidelines do not advocate regular weighing during pregnancy [18].

Awareness of the risks of excess maternal weight gain appears to be surprisingly low. The views of women on their gestational weight gain were sought in a survey of almost 500 pregnant women. Weight measurements were made at their 12th-week clinic appointment, and their opinions of weight gain were sought [19]. Over half of all respondents were obese, and 62% were living in areas of mild to moderate deprivation. Over three-quarters of participants felt dissatisfied with their current weight, although a majority (60%) expressed limited concern about potential weight gain. Also, 39% were unconcerned about weight gain during their pregnancy, including 34 (19%) who reported having retained the weight gained in earlier pregnancies. These data suggest a lack of awareness among obese women regarding excessive gestational weight gain. A pilot study in pregnant women of low socioeconomic status suggested the ability of health professionals to reach and engage successfully with these women was poor. Despite them recognising the importance of the issue of obesity and excess gestational weight gain [20].

It is clear that opportunities exist to challenge the excessive weight gain observed in pregnancy. To date, the various approaches attempted have met with only limited success. While an opportunity is present, it remains unclear how best to reduce the

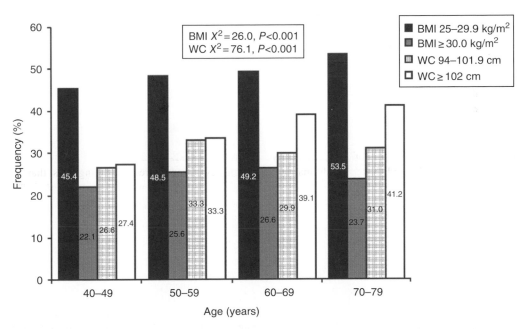

Figure 1.3.2 Distribution of subjects with high BMI (25–29.9 kg/m^2 or ≥30 kg/m^2) or high waist circumference (94–101.9 cm or ≥102 cm) by 10-year age groups. Source: Taken from Han et al. 2015 [21].

elevated weight gain associated with pregnancy without incurring a detrimental impact on infant and maternal health.

1.3.5 Retirement and aging

Obesity is increasing in older adults, a category where obesity was traditionally considered unusual. The European Male Aging Study noted an unremitting increase in BMI and waist circumference from middle age until the seventh and eighth decades [21] (Figure 1.3.2).

A large US study highlighted a positive relationship between childhood poverty and downward socioeconomic status across the life course and an increase in older-age obesity and overweight [21]. This study demonstrates that increased body mass in middle and late adulthood is a likely consequence of the complex interplay among individuals' genes, dynamic socioeconomic experiences and historical context in which they live. While BMI changes after 55–60 years of age, waist circumferences continue to increase, indicating increasing body fat with reduced muscle mass [4]. It has been speculated that the loss of occupational role/status, leading to a lack of structure to the day, limited empowerment, a reduction in social contact and financial concerned may lead to depression, which is strongly associated with obesity and weight gain [21].

Retirement involves adapting to multiple new demands (reduced income, social isolation, grandchildren responsibilities, bereavement, etc.), but few people currently make structured forward preparations for life or health after retirement. However, some responsible employers and national pre-retirement agencies already provide courses on financial planning, adult education and keeping fit. The potential to deliver a more structured approach for diet and lifestyle changes, to preserve function and physical and mental health, is important for this high-risk group. Reducing or retarding chronic disease, compressing morbidity and optimising physical and mental health would improve functional capacity, quality of life and cognitive function to favour prolonged independent living, and enable continued contribution to domestic and social life. This would benefit the individual, the family and the economy as a whole. To date, however, the opportunity has yet to be fully realised.

1.3.6 Conclusion

Weight change across particular phases of the life course are increasingly common. Many populations, both from the more economically developed and less economically developed nations, are becoming more affluent and therefore gaining weight. The epidemic of obesity, when considered in detail, appears to show that specific periods of life are particularly associated with weight gain. Opportunities for tailored and appropriate interventions to manage weight are available.

1.3.7 Summary box

> **Key points**
>
> - Specific key periods across the life course are often associated with weight gain.
> - Obesity prior to pregnancy and obesity during pregnancy are increasingly common.
> - Excess weight gain evident in young children is frequent but often goes unnoticed, or is not a concern to parents/carers.
> - Awareness of weight gain may be limited with an increasing acceptance and normalisation of obesity.
> - Obesity in older adults is increasingly common, bringing with it many of the comorbidities usually seen earlier in life.

References

1. Gardner DS, Hosking J, Metcalf BS, Jeffery AN, Voss LD, Wilkin TJ. Contribution of early weight gain to childhood overweight and metabolic health: a longitudinal study (EarlyBird 36). *Pediatrics* 2009; **123**(1): e67–e73.
2. Public Health England. National Child Measurement Programme. 2015. Changes in children's body mass index between 2006/7 and 2014/15. Figure 2. Available from: http://www.bhfactive.org.uk/userfiles/Documents/ncmp_chnages_in_bmi.pdf, accessed 20 December 2016.

3. Jeffery AN, Metcalf BS, Hosking J, Mostazir MB, Voss LD, Wilkin TJ. Awareness of body weight by mothers and their children: repeated measures in a single cohort (EarlyBird 64). *Child Care Health and Development* 2015; **41**(3): 434–442.

4. Lean ME, Katsarou C, McLoone P, Morrison D. Changes in BMI and waist circumference in Scottish adults: repeated use of cross sectional surveys to explore multiple age groups and birth-cohorts. *International Journal of Obesity* 2013; **37**: 800–808.

5. Lowe MR, Annunziato RA, Markowitz JT, Didie E, Bellace DL, Riddell L, et al. Multiple types of dieting prospectively predict weight gain during the freshman year of college. *Appetite* 2006; **47**: 83–90.

6. Thomée S, Lissner L, Hagberg M, Grimby-Ekman A. Leisure time computer use and overweight development in young adults – a prospective study. *BMC Public Health* 2015; **15**: 839–852.

7. Meltzer AL, Novak SA, McNulty JK, Butler EA, Karney BR. Marital satisfaction predicts weight gain in early marriage. *Health Psychology* 2013; **32**(7): 824–827.

8. Teachman J. Body weight, marital status, and changes in marital status. *Journal of Family Issues* 2016; **37**(1): 74–96.

9. Boone-Heinonen J, Howard AG, Meyer K, Lewis CE, Kiefe CI, Laroche HH, Gunderson EP, Gordon-Larsen P. Marriage and parenthood in relation to obesogenic neighborhood trajectories: The CARDIA study. *Health & Place* 2015; **34**: 229–240.

10. Dinour L, Leung MM, Tripicchio G, Khan S, Yeh MC. The association between marital transitions, body mass index, and weight: a review of the literature. *Journal of Obesity* 2012; **2012**: 294974.

11. Anderson AS, Marshall DW, Lea EJ. Shared lives-an opportunity for obesity prevention? *Appetite* 2004; **43**(3): 327–329.

12. Rauschenbach B, Sobal J, Frongillo EA. The influence of change in marital status on weight change over one year. *Obesity Research* 1995; **3**(4): 319–327.

13. Hankey CR. Obesity and maternal weight gain. *Current Obesity Reports* 2015; **4**(1): 60–4.

14. Centre for child and maternal enquiries CMACE. Maternal obesity in the UK findings from a national project. 2010. Available from: http://www.publichealth.hscni.net/sites/default/files/Maternal%20Obesity%20in%20the%20UK.pdf, last accessed 8 September 2016.

15. Institute of Medicine. Weight gain: re-examining the guidelines. 2009. Available from: http://www.nationalacademies.org/hmd/Reports/2009/Weight-Gain-During-Pregnancy-Reexamining-the-Guidelines.aspx.

16. Craigie AM, Macleod M, Barton KL, Treweek S, Anderson AS, WeighWell team. Supporting postpartum weight loss in women living in deprived communities: design implications for a randomised control trial. *European Journal of Clinical Nutrition* 2011; **65**(8): 952–958.

17. Narayanan RP, Weeks AD, Quenby S, Rycroft D, Hart A, Longworth H, Charnley M, Abayomi J, Topping J, Turner MA, Wilding JP. Fit for birth – the effect of weight changes in obese pregnant women on maternal and neonatal outcomes: a pilot prospective cohort study. *Clinical Obesity* 2016; **6**(1, Feb): 79–88. Last accessed 19 August 2016.

18. Hasted T, Stapleton H, Beckmann MM, Wilkinson SA. Clinician's attitudes to the introduction of routine weighing in pregnancy. *Journal of Pregnancy* 2016; **2016**: 2049673.

19. NICE Clinical guideline 189. Obesity: identification, assessment and management. 2014. Available from: https://www.nice.org.uk/guidance/cg189?unlid=74409180520165793347, accessed 8 September 2016.

20. Leslie WS, Gibson A, Hankey CR. Prevention and management of excessive gestational weight gain: a survey of overweight and obese pregnant women. *BMC Pregnancy and Childbirth* 2013; **13**: 10.

21. Han TS, Lee DM, Lean ME, Finn JD, O'Neill TW, Bartfai G, Forti G, Giwercman A, Kula K, Pendleton N, Punab M, Rutter MK, Vanderschueren D, Huhtaniemi IT, Wu FC, Casanueva FF, EMAS Study Group. Associations of obesity with socio-economic and lifestyle factors in middle-aged and elderly men: European Male Aging Study (EMAS). *European Journal of Endocrinology* 2015; **172**(1): 59–67.

Chapter 1.4

Diagnostic criteria and assessment of obesity in adults

Mike Lean

University of Glasgow, Glasgow, UK

Obesity is defined as a disease by the World Health Organisation. Its International Classification of Diseases code has subcategories of some historical interest, which do not correspond well to the clinical or public health concerns about obesity, or to management strategies. Most people think they know what is meant by 'obesity' in principle, but different criteria may be applied in relation to different intervention or treatment strategies, and between different populations or subgroups. The diagnostic criteria for other diseases such as hypertension or hyperlipidaemia similarly vary between genders and racial groups, or between children and adults, so different diagnostic criteria are used at different ages to initiate and assess treatment.

Modern obesity research has revealed complex genetic–environment interactions in its aetiology, and the interacting neural and endocrine components that modulate appetite and eating. New management packages, with better-defined goals and success criteria, have emerged, and so diagnostic criteria have come under new scrutiny. Importantly, in order to establish diagnostic criteria, a robust definition of obesity is required, to characterise the disease. In principle, obesity is obviously a disease of having too much body fat, but measuring body fat is not simple. Furthermore, any diagnosis based on measuring body fat, which is a component of both normal and obese individuals, will inevitably have to rely on arbitrary criteria. Body fat can only accumulate over time in people who are (for genetic and/or environmental reasons) predisposed. The

2010 Scottish Intercollegiate Guidelines Network (SIGN) guideline on obesity [1] took the important step of defining obesity as a disease process: 'Obesity is defined as a disease process, characterised by excessive body fat accumulation, with multiple organ-specific consequences'. Accepting that there is a disease process operating, it becomes possible, if we have reliable markers of the process, to diagnose it before its full clinical manifestation becomes apparent.

1.4.1 Indicators of rising body fat content

Direct measures of body fat include computer tomography, magnetic resonance imaging, bioelectrical impedance analysis or dual-energy X-ray absorptiometry scan. These tools are primarily used in obesity research, whereas in routine clinical practice other anthropometric measures are used as a proxy measure of body fat.

1.4.2 Weight and body mass index (BMI)

The simplest indicator of obesity, or body fat content, is of course body weight. For monitoring patients over time, weight is the most reliable measure. However, body weight varies with stature as well as fatness. Many mathematical corrections have

Advanced Nutrition and Dietetics in Obesity, First Edition. Edited by Catherine Hankey.
© 2018 John Wiley & Sons Ltd. Published 2018 by John Wiley & Sons Ltd.

Table 1.4.1   International classifications and sub-categories for BMI (adapted from references [2–4])

Classification	BMI (kg/m^2)	
	Principal cut-off points	Additional cut-off points
Underweight	**<18.50**	**<18.50**
Severe thinness	<16.00	<16.00
Moderate thinness	16.00–16.99	16.00–16.99
Mild thinness	17.00–18.49	17.00–18.49
Normal range	**18.50–24.99**	**18.50–22.99**
		23.00–24.99
Overweight	**≥25.00**	**≥25.00**
Pre-obese	25.00–29.99	25.00–27.49
		27.50–29.99
Obese	**≥30.00**	**≥30.00**
Obese class I	30.00–34.99	30.00–32.49
		32.50–34.99
Obese class II	35.00–39.99	35.00–37.49
		37.50–39.99
Obese class III	≥40.00	≥40.00

been applied to eliminate the influence of stature. The BMI (kg/m^2) is not the best of the many indices proposed, but for adults it does eliminate most of the effects of stature, and it is simple enough for wide use in epidemiology. Women have more fat and less muscle than men at any given weight or BMI, so the sexes should always be separated in any analysis.

WHO adopted the now-conventional BMI categories for overweight and obesity in 1995, 2000 and 2004 (Table 1.4.1) for health monitoring in populations, and to establish associations between diet and lifestyle and health outcomes [2–4]. These are arbitrary BMI cut-offs, and the detailed health–outcome associations of BMI, or BMI categories, vary between genders, with age, and between social and racial groups. The conventional BMI categories were not intended for clinical diagnosis of individuals. They are not completely accurate in classifying individuals' body fat contents, so some people such as sportsmen, classified as 'obese' with BMI > 30 kg/m^2, actually have low body fat, but have expanded muscle masses. Muscle is more dense than fat, so variations in muscle mass introduce rather large errors in BMI classification.

It remains true that *most* people with BMI >30 kg/m^2 in a population survey do in fact have excess body fat, to a degree that it is likely to affect health adversely. Almost nobody with BMI >35 kg/m^2 has an acceptable amount of body fat. In the category with a BMI of 25–30 kg/m^2, a relatively large number are en route to, or at risk of, a BMI of >30 kg/m^2. Hence, these conventional BMI categories are still useful in epidemiology. They were designed with European adult populations in mind and do need to be interpreted carefully when applied to groups with unusual features. Thus, a mean BMI of 27 kg/m^2 is of concern for the whole adult population of UK, with mean age about 45 years. However, a mean BMI of 27 kg/m^2 for a group of young people in their 20s would be of much greater concern. South Asian adults generally have more body fat, and less muscle, than Europeans at any given BMI, so a mean BMI of 27 kg/m^2 would also be of greater concern in a group of South Asians, implying more frequent attributable health problems [4]. Older BMI criteria had different cut-offs for men and women. This makes sense if the concern is the *absolute* level of risk attached to high body fat content: women can clearly tolerate great fat masses more than men (being smaller, they need a greater proportion of body fat than men to survive long famines). The same BMI cut-offs are now applied to men and women to indicate similar *relative* excess of health impairment for both sexes.

The BMI is likely to remain a key indicator of body fat and obesity for surveys in the foreseeable future. It is essential for the measurements of weight and height to be made as reliably, accurately and precisely as possible. Equipment must be calibrated regularly, particularly stadiometers used to measure height, since squaring height to compute BMI also squares any errors and biases in its measurement.

1.4.3 Waist circumference

The waist circumference was introduced into public health thinking very specifically in 1996, in the SIGN obesity guideline, not as a diagnostic criterion, but as a tool for health promotion [5]. The BMI was too complex and conceptually problematic for health promotion among the general public, even with the weight vs. height charts to compute it. Research found that waist circumference was in fact a marginally better indicator of both total body fat and associated health risks than BMI, in addition to being simpler.

As with BMI, cut-offs are arbitrary. The waist cut-offs that prevailed, and which have now entered both public health and clinical guidelines worldwide, emerged from a pragmatic risk analysis of a large Dutch database to incorporate both BMI and the older marker 'waist/hip ratio', supported by correlations with risks of diabetes and cardiovascular risk factors. Waist >102 cm for men and >88 cm for women form 'Action Level 2' (broadly equivalent to BMI 30, obesity), above which risks are high and professional help is required for weight loss. The lower 'Action Level 1', of waist circumference >94 cm for men and >80 cm for women (similar to BMI 25 kg/m^2), indicates a rising risk and the need for individuals to take personal action against weight gain [6]. Subsequent research has confirmed that waist circumference is at least as good as BMI, and in some cases marginally better, to predict obesity-related health risks, particularly type 2 diabetes.

The earlier term 'waist–hip ratio' (WHR) proved to be less accurate than waist alone, but does relate to type 2 diabetes in cross-sectional surveys [7], because the onset of diabetes incurs a loss of muscle mass, and hence a drop in hip circumference. (Subsequent research showed that hip circumference relates more to muscle mass than to fat.) For all practical purposes, it is unnecessary to adjust waist circumference for height.

There is potential for observer-error in measuring the waist, but this is not a major concern if it is done carefully. It should be measured according to the WHO guidelines – with the subject standing, using an inelastic tape, horizontal, between the iliac crest and lowest rib (which can be felt with a finger even in the most obese) [8]. An error of 1–2 cm in this position makes very little difference. Most people categorised as 'obese' on the strength of a waist greater than 88 or 102 cm would have excess body fat, even with relatively inexpert measurement. In extreme obesity, the belly becomes pendulous, hanging towards the ground, and so variations in body fat will no longer be detectable. Waist only correlates accurately with body fat content in people with BMI below about 40. However, this is not an obstacle to categorising, or diagnosing, people as obese.

At lower levels of total body fat, waist circumference might misclassify people as being overweight or obese, because it is specifically increased in people with larger-than-usual amounts of intra-abdominal fat. In large population surveys with a wide range of BMI, etc., most of the variance in waist circumference relates to variations in total body fat content: waist is primarily a marker of total body fat, and a little better than BMI for this purpose. In groups with similar BMI, variance in waist circumference is driven more by variations in intra-abdominal fat mass. In a group of individuals with exactly the same total body fat, different waist circumferences would indicate differences in intra-abdominal fat.

There are important differences in waist circumferences and fat distribution among different races (more so than ethnic differences). Thus, South Asian people generally have larger waists, with more intra-abdominal fat than Europeans, at the same

Table 1.4.2 Comorbidities risk associated with different levels of BMI and suggested waist circumference in adult South Asians (adapted from IDF-WPR and IOTF 2002)

| | | Risk of comorbidities | |
| | | Waist circumference | |
Classification	BMI (kg/m²)	<90 cm (men) <80 cm (women)	≥90 cm (men) ≥80 cm (women)
Underweight	<18.5	Low (but risk of other clinical problems)	Average
Normal range	18.5–22.9	Average	Increased
Overweight	≥23		
At risk	23–24.9	Increased	Moderate
Obese I	25–29.9	Moderate	Severe
Obese II	≥30	Severe	Very severe

height and weight. For this reason, South Asians are at greater risk of metabolic complications from obesity at lower levels of waist circumference. In an attempt to equalise the level of risk at which intervention is indicated, a table of modified waist cut-offs has been produced (Table 1.4.2).

'Waist-deniers'

Confusion about the associations of waist circumference has dissuaded some guideline-writers from accepting it as an alternative, or equivalent, to BMI for predicting body fat and health risks. Its major advantage – its very simplicity – may have engendered suspicion, and tables have been constructed combining cut-offs of BMI and waist. This approach valuably identifies people at risk despite a low BMI; however, risk assessment is most accurate using continuous variables without categorisation. This is not the same as diagnosis, and is unhelpful for health promotion.

Several large surveys have suggested that WHR is better than waist circumference. The Interheart study is one. However, the waist measurement methods did not use the standard WHO method; data came from a large number of different countries, so different methods were used (shortest circumference) [9]. Others have suggested introducing ratios of waist with height to generate an index. This tends to eliminate differences between the sexes, but

at the expense of a more complicated, less immediate message.

1.4.4 Diagnosis of obesity by genetic markers

All disease arises through a conjunction of genetic and environmental factors, many mediated, as with obesity, by the behavioural patterns of individuals. To become obese, an individual must consume more energy that he or she expends. An increase in BMI from 23 to 30 kg/m² requires the accumulation of about 160,000 kcal of excess fat. This has to be consumed over a period of time as energy above the need for energy balance. There are large numbers of physiological mediators of appetite and eating, and of energy expenditure, all of which may be disrupted by genetic factors, either at the level of a gene mutation or through altered expression of a gene. It has long been recognised that there are familial, and probably genetic, factors responsible for obesity, and very large numbers of gene variants have been shown over the years to have weak associations with greater BMI, and effect sizes are generally very small. Evolutionary success has depended on the body weight and appetite being under complex physiological and ultimately genetic control, such that weight loss is opposed by a range of mechanisms all directed at increasing food consumption and limiting non-essential energy expenditure. Obesity is usually considered to be polygenic, that is, there need to be 'defects', or altered expression, in several regulatory systems simultaneously. These 'defects' can be considered simply exaggerated normal mechanisms for evolutionary survival. None of the genetic variants so far identified, or even combinations, are sufficient to explain the obesity epidemic. The main influence is environmental, but there is growing interest in the role of epigenetics, for example, by studying the effects of diet and stresses in pregnancy to program the expression of genes related to appetite and energy balance (refer to Chapter 3.1). Susceptibility to weight gain can be exaggerated, or unmarked, by treatment with various obesogenic drugs [10].

1.4.5 Obesity diagnosis with clinical staging

A more functional diagnosis of obesity, based not solely on criteria from BMI or other static measure of body fat, includes criteria of clinical staging. This approach is used routinely in cancer diagnosis, where the staged diagnosis defines treatment. The Edmonton system combines conventional BMI categories with a descriptive term to denote the degree of functional impairment. This system was loosely directed towards treatment, and importantly drew attention that there could be an 'end-stage' in obesity – for example, with severe arthritis – in which even successful weight loss would not improve function significantly, and so only symptomatic palliative care is indicated [11] (Figure 1.4.1).

A simplified diagnostic staging was adopted in the 2010 SIGN clinical guideline, more overtly linked to the very limited range of evidence-based treatments available.[1] It again recognised that, for some patients, only symptomatic palliative care would be indicated. Within the SIGN 2010 guideline, the concept and diagnostic category of 'severe and complicated obesity' was recognised. In the past, the term 'morbid obesity' was used by WHO and others for use in epidemiology, to denote the category with BMI >35 kg/m². The word *morbid*

(latin, *morbus* = disease) was used in recognition that many people with BMI >35 kg/m² were functionally affected and unwell because of their obesity, but many are not, so this is clearly inadequate for diagnostic staging. The term 'severe and complicated obesity' has thus been introduced to identify individuals who require more aggressive intervention, either because their obesity has progressed to an extreme level (e.g. BMI >35 kg/m²), or because, at a lower level of BMI, they already have serious secondary medical and functional complications, such as diabetes or arthritis. 'Complicated obesity' (which points to clinical complications and treatment indications) is preferable to 'complex obesity' (which can be misinterpreted as referring to aetiology).

The principle of clinical and functional staging for the diagnosis of obesity is a valuable advance, both for epidemiological classification and to determine clinical action. Adding clinical staging for diagnosis makes it less necessary to modify the BMI or waist categories for different races or ethnic groups, which can be difficult to define in mixed populations.

1.4.6 Summary box

> **Key points**
>
> - Obesity is a disease, defined as the disease process of excess body fat accumulation, with multiple organ-specific clinical and public health consequences.
> - A BMI of 30 kg/m² is the most widely used criterion for the classification of obesity, in epidemiology, but not for clinical or diagnostic use in individuals.
> - For health promotion, waist circumference is the simplest and most robust criterion: >80 cm (women) or >94 cm (men) marks a need for self-determined action to avoid further gain; >88 cm (women) or >102 cm (men) indicates high health risks and a need for professional support for sustained weight loss.
> - For clinical decision-making, clinical assessment of co-morbid conditions must be added to BMI or waist level to determine the appropriate intervention.

EOSS: EDMONTON OBESITY STAGING SYSTEM - *Staging Tool*

WHO CLASSIFICATION OF WEIGHT STATUS (**BMI kg/m²**)
Obese Class I .... 30 - 34.9
Obese Class II .... 35 - 39.9
Obese Class III .... ≥40

STAGE 0

- **NO** sign of obesity-related risk factors
- **NO** physical symptoms
- **NO** psychological symptoms
- **NO** functional limitations.

Case Example:
Physically active female with a BMI of 32 kg/m², no risk factors, no physical symptoms, no self-esteem issues, and no functional limitations.

Class I, Stage 0 Obesity

EOSS Score

WHO Obesity Classfication

STAGE 1

- Patient has obesity-related **SUBCLINICAL** risk factors
  (borderline hypertension, impaired fasting glucose, elevated liver enzymes, etc.)
  - *OR* -
- **MILD** physical symptoms - patient currently not requiring medical treatment for comorbidities - *OR* -
  (dyspnea on moderate exertion, occasional aches/pains, fatigue, etc.)
- **MILD** obesity-related psychological symptoms and/or mild impairment of well-being
  (quality of life not impacted)

Case Example:
38 year old female with a BMI of 59.2 kg/m², borderline hypertension, mild lower back pain, and knee pain. Patient does not require any medical intervention.

Class III, Stage 1 Obesity

Stage 0 / Stage 1 Obesity

Patient *does not meet clinical criteria for admission* at this time.
Please refer to primary care for further preventative treatment options.

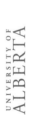

STAGE 2

- Patient has **ESTABLISHED** obesity-related comorbidities requiring medical intervention
  (HTN, Type 2 Diabetes, sleep apnea, PCOS, osteoarthritis, reflux disease) - *OR* -
- **MODERATE** obesity-related psychological symptoms - *OR* -
  (depression, eating disorders, anxiety disorder)
- **MODERATE** functional limitations in daily activities
  (quality of life is beginning to be impacted)

Case Example:
32 year old male with a BMI of 36 kg/m² who has primary hypertension and obstructive sleep apnea.

Class II, Stage 2 Obesity

STAGE 3

- Patient has **significant** obesity-related end-organ damage (myocardial infarction, heart failure, diabetic complications, incapacitating osteoarthritis) - *OR* -
- **SIGNIFICANT** obesity-related psychological symptoms - *OR* -
  (major depression, suicide ideation)
- **SIGNIFICANT** functional limitations
  (eg: unable to work or complete routine activities, reduced mobility)
- **SIGNIFICANT** impairment of well-being
  (quality of life is significantly impacted)

Case Example:
49 year old female with a BMI of 67 kg/m² diagnosed with sleep apnea, CV disease, GERD, and suffered from stroke. Patient's mobility is significantly limited due to osteoarthritis and gout.

Class III, Stage 3 Obesity

STAGE 4

- **SEVERE** (potential end stage) from obesity-related comorbidities - *OR* -
- **SEVERELY** disabling psychological symptoms - *OR* -
- **SEVERE** functional limitations

Case Example:
45 year old female with a BMI of 54 kg/m² who is in a wheel chair because of disabling arthritis, severe hyperpnea, and anxiety disorder.

Class III, Stage 4 Obesity

Sharma AM & Kushner RF, *Int J Obes* 2009

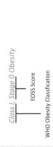
Alberta Health Services

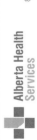
UNIVERSITY OF ALBERTA

Figure 1.4.1 Edmonton clinical staging. From IJO (ref [11]).

References

1. SIGN No 115. Management of obesity: A national clinical guideline. 2010. Available from: http://www.sign.ac.uk/pdf/sign115.pdf.
2. World Health Organisation. Physical status: the use and interpretation of anthropometry. WHO Technical Report. WHO: Geneva 1995.
3. World Health Organisation. Obesity: preventing and managing the global epidemic. WHO Technical Report Series 894. WHO: 2000.
4. World Health Organisation Expert Consultation. Appropriate body-mass index for Asian populations and its implication for policy and intervention strategies. *Lancet* 2004; **363**: 157–163.
5. SIGN 8. Management of obesity: a national clinical guideline. 1996.
6. Han TS, Van Leer EM, Seidell JC, Lean MEJ. Waist circumference action levels in the identification of cardiovascular risk factors: prevalence study in a random sample. *BMJ* 1995; **311**: 1401–1405.
7. Carey VJ, Walter EE, Colditz GA, et al. Body fat distribution and risk of non-insulin-dependent diabetes mellitus in women. The Nurses' Health Study. *American Journal of Epidemiology* 1997; **145**: 614–619.
8. Yusuf S, Hawken S, Ounpuu S, et al. Effect of potentially modifiable risk factors associated with myocardial infarction in 52 countries (the INTERHEART study): case-control study. *Lancet* 2004; **364**: 937–952.
9. World Health Organisation. Measuring obesity: classification and description of anthropometric data. Copenhagen WHO: 1989.
10. Leslie WS, Hankey CR, Lean ME. Weight gain as an adverse effect of some commonly prescribed drugs: a systematic review. *QJM* 2007; **100**: 395–404.
11. Sharma AM, Kushner RF. A proposed clinical staging system for obesity. *International Journal of Obesity* 2009; **33**: 289–295.

Chapter 1.5

Diagnostic criteria and assessment of obesity in children

Alison Gahagan[1] and Laura Stewart[2]
[1] NHS South West London, London, UK
[2] Perth Royal Infirmary, Perth, UK

1.5.1 Introduction

The effective management of childhood obesity is dependent on accurately identifying and assessing the weight status of a child or young person [1]. In addition to the need to tackle the lack of parental awareness and their inability to recognise their child's overweight status results in low levels of weight concern [2]. A health professional is tasked with the role of ensuring that the issue of excess weight is raised in a sensitive manner, in order to help parents understand the potential health risks of their child carrying excessive weight but also motivate them to engage in treatment [3,4]. This chapter provides key aspects of accurately assessing childhood overweight and obesity [3–6]. While there is a constant need to ensure dietetic and medical treatments are clinically and cost-wise effective, it is also important to consider what clinical outcomes are most useful to measure and judge treatment effectiveness.

1.5.2 Diagnosis of overweight and obesity in children and young people

The importance of overweight and obesity lies in the association of excess body fat with ill health. Therefore, the diagnosis of overweight and obesity requires the measurement of body fat. Direct methods of measuring body fat include computer

tomography (CT), magnetic resonance imaging (MRI), bio-electrical impedance analysis (BIA) and dual-energy X-ray absorptiometry (DEXA) scan [1,7–9]. These tools are primarily of greater use in research and occasionally tertiary care centres due to their high costs. In routine practice, body mass index (BMI) is the recommended 'easy-to-use' proxy measure of body fat [1,3–7,9].

Body mass index

BMI [weight (kg)/height (m)^2] has been widely used to define and diagnose obesity in adults [3,6,9]. There is widespread national and international support for the use of BMI to clinically diagnose obesity and overweight in children and adolescents [3–7]. However, BMI has well-documented limitations as an absolute measure of body fat, such as that it does not distinguish abdominal fat and visceral fat, it does not take into account excess muscle mass [1,3,9]. However, BMI is the most practical measure to estimate excess body fat in children [1,10].

BMI for age centiles in clinical practice

Child BMI varies throughout growth and differs between sexes, which means that both age and gender needs to be taken into account when interpreting BMI status [10]. Child BMI is classified using thresholds that are derived from a reference population, known as the *child growth reference*. In the

Advanced Nutrition and Dietetics in Obesity, First Edition. Edited by Catherine Hankey.

UK, the 1990 population-based BMI centile charts (UK 1990) [11] are recommended for use for those 4 years and above, and WHO data for those under 4 years, available to order from Harlow Healthcare (www.healthforallchildren.co.uk).

In practice, BMI should be calculated and plotted on a centile chart for children above the age of 2 [3–4,6–7]. A cut-off with high specificity (a positive result from a test with high specificity means there is a high probability of presence of the disease) has generally been regarded as more important for clinical applications than high sensitivity (a test with high sensitivity means a high probability of a negative result) to avoid diagnosis of non-obese children as obese [1,3–6,10]. The 91st and 98th centiles on the WHO/UK 1990 charts for age and sex are recommended as the clinical cut-offs to diagnose overweight and obesity, respectively. Table 1.5.1 summarises the clinical centile cut-off points used to diagnose overweight and

obesity in the UK based on systematic reviews [1,10] and evidence-based guidelines [3,6]. International Obesity Task Force (IOTF) cut-off points are also available [12]. A systematic review by Reilly et al. [10] concluded that evidence was lacking for BMI using the IOTF approach in preference to national BMI percentiles for identifying children and adolescents with excess body fat and cardiometabolic risk factors.

Table 1.5.2 demonstrates that BMI can indicate very different weight states in children and adolescents of different ages. For example, a BMI of 19.5 would categorise a 5-year-old girl as obese, a 10-year-old boy as overweight and a 15-year-old boy or girl as being of healthy weight. It is essential that a child's BMI is plotted on a centile chart, or height and weight added to a child BMI calculator that is adjusted for age and sex (see Section 1.5.6, titled 'Useful tools and websites').

BMI for age standard deviation scores (SDSs) or z-scores

BMI can also be defined in terms of a BMI standard deviation score (SDS) or BMI z-score (BMI at 50th centile for age and sex is an SDS of 0) [13]. Software (LMS Growth) is available to convert BMI measurements into BMI SD scores [13]. Expressing the degree of overweight or obesity as an SD score is useful for statistical purposes but also provides more details for children and adolescents at the extremes of BMI, that is, those above the 98th centile. BMI SDSs are now included in WHO/UK 1990 BMI management charts; see Table 1.5.1 for its relation to clinical diagnosis.

There is a need to distinguish those with 'severe' to 'extreme' obesity [14]. Experts have suggested

Table 1.5.1 Clinical diagnostic criteria for overweight and obese children and young people (aged <18) in the UK

Clinical terminology	BMI centiles*	SDS or z-score*
Overweight	≥91st centile	≥+1.33 SDS
Obesity	≥98th centile	≥+2 SDS
Severe obesity	≥99.6th centile	≥+2.67 SDS
Very severe obesity		≥+3.33 SDS
Extreme obesity		≥+4 SDS

*Defined relative to the WHO/UK 1990 reference chart for age and sex.

Table 1.5.2 Absolute BMIs for boys and girls aged 5, 10 and 15 to classify as clinically overweight or obese (UK 1990 cut-offs)

		Male		Female	
Age	BMI centile	91st (overweight)	98th (obese)	91st (overweight)	98th (obese)
5 years		17.4	18.6	17.7	19.1
10 years		19.5	21.7	20.4	22.9
15 years		23.1	26.0	24.2	27.2

that the 'severely obese' (≥99.6th centile) are in greater need of clinical assessment and treatment [4–6,15]. In the UK, the ≥99.6th (+2.67 SDS) centile line is included on the charts along with centiles for +3.0 SDS, +3.33 SDS, +3.66 SDS and +4 SDS (extreme obesity). In the USA, the 97th centile is the highest curve available on the growth charts; hence, cut-offs points for the 99th centile are provided for reference in clinical guidelines [4,16]. Thus, a child with a BMI ≥3.33 SD above the mean at age 18 years is the equivalent of the adult definition of morbid obesity (BMI ≥40 kg/m^2) [17].

Waist measurements

It is recommended that the waist be taken as the midway between the lowest rib and the iliac crest, and that the child be asked to bend to one side to locate this point. Several studies agree that waist circumference is a useful tool to provide information on central adiposity, which is associated with high blood pressure, dyslipidaemia and insulin resistance in children and adolescents [19,20]. It is not yet clear what the universal cut-off points should be to assess risk [5,6,10]. Evidence-based clinical guidelines recommend that waist circumference not be used to diagnose overweight and obesity in children [3,4,6,17,18], but that it may be used to give additional information on the risk of developing other long-term health problems and for clinical monitoring purposes [3,7].

1.5.3 Assessment

Once a child has been diagnosed as overweight (above the 91st centile), a key aim of assessment is to build a rapport with the parent and/or child, as many parents have had negative experiences around weight-related issues or be completely unaware of the condition [2,21]. This is discussed further in Chapter 6.1 (weight management in children).

Anthropometric measurements

Accurate measurements of both weight and height are needed to calculate BMI. These should be taken with the child in light clothes and with no shoes. When measuring height, care should be taken to ensure that the child's head is positioned such that the Frankfurt plane is horizontal (lining up the ear hole with the bottom of the eye socket) [22]. Self-reported weight and height should never be considered appropriate, as this will lead to inaccurate data collection and BMI outcomes.

Waist measurements can be a useful tool in the clinical setting to help children monitor their outcomes; however, care must be taken to ensure that it is measured in a consistent manner – most importantly, following the same technique.

Talking about body weight

Research tells us that more than half of parents cannot recognise when their child is overweight [2], and thus care should be taken when raising the issue of weight with children and parents [23]. Health professionals need to talk openly, but sensitively, about children's weight [24]. It is important to help educate parents about BMI and to explain the associated health risks at different BMI levels. Although guidelines recommend the clinical terms 'overweight' and 'obese', these should be maintained for diagnostic purposes only. Weight can be a sensitive and emotive issue, so it would be helpful for health professionals to think carefully about how they approach the subject matter. To avoid parents feeling blamed or judged, using more neutral terms such as 'weight', 'excess weight', carrying extra weight' or 'BMI for age' (if explained) can be useful [4,24]. Preliminary research shows that weight feedback provided in a factual and non-emotive way by a healthcare professional can significantly influence a parent's readiness to initiate lifestyle changes [25]. Other factors indicating when a parent may be more likely to be ready to address their child's weight issues include: the child being aged 8 years or above, and a belief that their child's weight is a health problem [21,24,26]. Talking about weight at an early stage of assessment can help in exploring the understanding of the parents/family about referral and their possible expectations of treatment.

Clinical factors

At the initial child weight management assessment, it is useful to obtain additional clinical information to build a fuller picture of the child's obesity and risk of future obesity-related comorbidities. In some child weight management services, this may be completed as part of a multi-disciplinary team assessment or as part of the criteria required on referral into the service. Clinical obesity guidelines outline a number of areas that are useful to include during assessment [3–7]:

- BMI – plot a growth chart and discuss growth patterns (look out for short stature, as obese children are generally tall) [6,17].
- Weight history patterns, including any previous attempts at weight control
- Family history of overweight/obesity and co-morbidities (e.g. type 2 diabetes, prediabetes, hypertension, dyslipidaemia in first-degree relatives)
- Associated comorbidities (such as hypertension, hyperinsulinaemia, dyslipidaemia, type 2 diabetes, and exacerbation of conditions such as asthma) and risk factors
- Level of family support and family setup – that is, who is important at home, who the child spends time with and any other significant carers, such as, for example, grandparents
- Level of emotional/psychosocial distress – for example, low self-esteem, bullying, teasing
- Explore school and social history – this provides an opportunity to engage with the child by exploring his or her world
- Other weight-related signs and symptoms – for example, exercise intolerance, hip/knee/foot pain, shortness of breath, acanthosis nigricans (thickened velvety darkened skin usually around the neck) [6,17]

When to consider a medical referral?

In clinical practice, most children managed in the community will have obesity with no underlying medical cause and no comorbidity [6]. If medical input is required or further investigation is needed to assess risk factors for comorbidities, this can be done in primary care by following recommendations from a range of specialist bodies [27,28]. Some children showing signs of psychological distress or disordered eating should be considered for referral to psychological assessment and treatment [3,6].

Referral to secondary care or paediatric specialists should only be considered for children or adolescents with very severe to extreme obesity; those who are obese with a serious obesity-related comorbidity that requires weight loss. Another group are those having complex needs such as significant learning difficulties (see OSCA guidance for assessing obesity in secondary paediatric practice in the UK); or as per NICE C43 and SIGN 115 [3,6,17]. Referral to a paediatric endocrinologist should be made for any obese child who is short in stature, as this may be an indication of an underlying endocrine cause of their obesity, such as hypothyroidism, growth hormone deficiency or Cushing's syndrome [6,17].

1.5.4 Treatment success criteria

It is becoming common practice for childhood weight management interventions to be commissioned at a local, regional or national level. The National Obesity Observatory published a Standard Evaluation Framework [29,30] to aid the evaluation of child obesity programmes in the UK. While it does recommend measuring the change in a child's BMI using the BMI SDS rather than the BMI centile, it does not assist in providing guidance on the extent of weight or BMI change required to be clinically efficacious in reducing disease risk.

Due to lack of data, expert clinical opinion collectively agrees that the primary goal of obesity treatment for children who are overweight and most children who are obese ought to be weight maintenance. This is an acceptable target that will create a reduction in BMI because of ongoing linear growth [3–4,6–7]. Table 1.5.3 shows a case study demonstrating this. It is recommended that, in older children and those diagnosed as severely obese, small amounts of weight loss be considered acceptable, up to 0.5–1 kg per month, under clinical supervision [3–4,6].

It is important to note that there is a limited but growing evidence base on the impact of improving

Table 1.5.3   Case study example of a 10-year-old girl and treatment effect

Age (years) at each appointment	Weight (kg)	Height (m)	Weight change (kg)	BMI	BMI SDS
10	50	1.3	–	29.6	3.14
10.5	50.5	1.325	+0.5	28.8	2.95
11	50.5	1.36	0	27.3	2.63
		Change +0.06	**Change +0.5**	**Change −2.3**	**Change of −0.51***

*SDS is a clinically effective change in adiposity indicator to reduce cardiovascular disease risk.

BMI SDS and on reducing cardiovascular disease risk factors. The small number of studies published suggest that a reduction of 0.1–0.5 BMI SDS after a 1–2-year follow-up is sufficient to show changes in cardiometabolic risk factors, such as improvements in insulin sensitivity, some lipid profiles, blood pressure and body composition [31–36]. This is a promising area for future research, to provide a better understanding of the effects that child weight management interventions have on improving weight status and health.

1.5.5 Conclusion

There is widespread international support for the use of BMI to clinically diagnose obesity in children [3–6]. Despite its well-documented limitations, it is the most practical measure of defining excess body fat in children, provided values are interpreted using relative national child growth references, taking into account age and sex [1,10]. When a child is classified as *overweight* or *obese* (≥91st or ≥98th centile using the WHO/UK 1990 reference [11]), this should be integrated with a comprehensive assessment, including raising awareness of the child's overweight in a sensitive, non-judgemental manner to encourage parents (and adolescents) to help bring their weight under control. Following this, a comprehensive assessment is crucial before deciding upon appropriate treatment options and discussing weight maintenance as a likely clinically effective outcome of the treatment. Further research and guidance is required to help define additional clinical outcomes in order to demonstrate treatment success.

1.5.6 Summary box

Key points

- BMI should be calculated for children.
- BMI needs to be plotted on age- and sex-appropriate charts for each country.
- BMI SDS should be reported for programme outcomes.
- Waist measurement is useful for measuring clinical progress.

1.5.7 Useful tools and websites

BMI management charts and LMS growth (free to download)

Order from Harlow Healthcare,
 www.healthforallchildren.co.uk

Online child BMI calculators (adjusted for age and sex)

NHS Choices Healthy weight BMI calculator,
 www.nhs.uk/Tools/Pages/Healthyweightcalculator.
 aspx
Weight Concern child and young person's BMI calculator, www.weightconcern.com/node/9

Talking about weight

Raising the issue of weight in children (download tool), Department of Health (2006), www.dh.gov.
 uk/prod_consum_dh/groups/dh_digitalassets/
 documents/digitalasset/dh_096580.pdf

Weight Concern leaflet, www.weightconcern.com/node/134

Online toolkit preventing weight bias, Rudd Center for food policy and obesity, www.yaleruddcenter.org/resources/bias_toolkit/index.html

References

1. Reilly JJ. Assessment of obesity in children and adolescents: synthesis of recent systematic reviews and clinical guidelines. *Journal of Human Nutrition and Dietetics* 2010; **23**: 205–211.
2. Parry LL, Netuveli G, Parry J, Saxena S. A systematic review of parental perception of overweight status in children. *The Journal of Ambulatory Care Management* 2008; **31**: 253–268.
3. National Institute for Health and Clinical Excellence (NICE). Obesity: guidance on the prevention, identification, assessment and management of overweight and obesity in adults and children. Clinical guideline 43. London: NICE; 2006.
4. Barlow SE. Expert committee recommendations regarding the prevention, assessment, and treatment of child and adolescent overweight and obesity: summary report. *Pediatrics* 2007; **120**(4): S164–S192.
5. Krebs NF, Himes JH, Jacobson D, Nicklas TA, Guilday P, Styne D. Assessment of child and adolescent overweight and obesity. *Pediatrics* 2007; **120**(4): 192–227.
6. Scottish Intercollegiate Guidelines Network (SIGN). Management of obesity in children and young people. SIGN publication no. 115. Edinburgh: SIGN; 2010.
7. National Health and Medical Research Council (NHMRC). Clinical practice guidelines for the management of overweight and obesity in children and adolescents. Canberra: NHMRC; 2006.
8. Dinsdale H, Ridler C, Ells LJ. A simple guide to classifying body mass index in children. Oxford: National Obesity Observatory, 2011.
9. National Obesity Observatory (NOO). Body mass index as a measure of obesity, 2009.
10. Reilly JJ, Kelly J, Wilson DC. Accuracy of simple clinical and epidemiological definitions of childhood obesity: systematic review and evidence appraisal. *Obesity Reviews* 2010; **11**(9): 645–655.
11. Cole TJ, Freeman JV, Preece MA. Body mass index reference curves for the UK, 1990. *Archives of Disease in Childhood* 1995; **73**: 25–29.
12. Cole TJ, Bellizzi MC, Flegal KM, Dietz WH. Establishing a standard definition for child overweight and obesity worldwide: international survey. *BMJ* 2000; **320**: 1240–1243.
13. Pan H, Cole TJ. LMS growth, a Microsoft Excel add-in to access growth references based on the LMS method. Version 2.74. 2011. Available from: http://www.healthforallchildren.co.uk/.
14. Freedman DS, Mei Z, Srinivasan SR, Berenson GS, Dietz WH. Cardiovascular risk factors and excess adiposity among overweight children and adolescents: the Bogalusa Heart Study. *Journal of Pediatrics* 2007; **150**: 12–17.

15. Whitlock EP, O'Connor EA, Williams SB, Beil TL, Lutz KW. Effectiveness of weight management programs in children and adolescents. Evidence report number. 170. Agency for Healthcare Research and Quality. Publication No. 08-E014. Rockville, MD, Agency for Healthcare Research and Quality. 2008.
16. Center for Disease Control and Prevention. 2000. CDC Growth Charts: United States.
17. Obesity Services for Children and Adolescents (OSCA) Network Group. OSCA consensus statement on the assessment of obese children & adolescents for paediatricians. London: Royal College of Paediatrics and Child Health (RCPCH). 2010.
18. McCarthy HD, Jarrett KV, Crawley HF. The development of waist circumference percentiles in British children aged 5.0–16.9 y. *European Journal of Clinical Nutrition* 2001; **55**: 902–907.
19. Reilly JJ, Methven E, McDowell ZC, Hacking B, Alexander D, Stewart L, Kelnar CJH. Health consequences of obesity. *Archives of Disease in Childhood* 2003; **88**: 748–752.
20. Katzmarzyk PT, Srinivasan SR, Chen, W, Malina RM, Bouchard C, Berenson GS. Disease risk factors in a biracial sample of children and adolescents body mass index, waist circumference, and clustering of cardiovascular. *Pediatrics* 2004; **114**: 198–205.
21. Stewart L, Chapple J, Hughes, AR. Parents journey through treatment for their child's obesity: a qualitative study. *Archives of Disease in Childhood* 2008; **93**: 35–39.
22. Cross government obesity unit, Department of Health. The National Child Measurement Programme Guidance for PCTs 2010/11.
23. Stewart L. Recognizing childhood obesity: the role of the school nurse. *British Journal of School Nursing* 2008; **3**(7): 323–326.
24. Chadwick P, Sacher P, Swain C. Talking to families about overweight children. *British Journal of School Nursing* 2008; **3**(6): 271–276.
25. Jeffery AN, Voss LD, Metcalf BS, Alba S, Wilkin TJ. Parents' awareness of overweight in themselves and their children: cross sectional study within a cohort. *BMJ* 2005; **330**: 23–24.
26. Rhee KE, De Lago CW, Arscott-Mills T, Mehta SD, Davis RK. Factors associated with parental readiness to make changes for overweight children. *Pediatrics* 2005; **116**: 94–101.
27. Gibson P, Edmunds L, Haslam DW, Poskitt E. An approach to weight management in children and adolescents (2–18 years) in primary care. *The Journal of Family Health Care* 2002; **12**(4):108–109.
28. Map of medicine for overweight and obese children – initial assessment in primary care. Map of Medicine (MoM) Clinical Editorial team and Fellows. London: MoM; 2011.
29. The National Obesity Observatory. National standard evaluation framework for weight management interventions. 2009.
30. Roberts K, Cavill N, Rutter H. The National Obesity Observatory. Measuring diet and physical activity in weight management interventions. 2011.
31. Reinehr T, Andler W. Changes in the atherogenic risk factor profile according to degree of weight loss. *Archives of Disease in Childhood* 2004; **89**: 419–422.

32. Reinehr T, Kiess W, Kapellen T, et al. Insulin sensitivity among obese children and adolescents, according to degree of weight loss. *Pediatrics* 2004; **114**: 1569–1573.

33. Reinehr T, de Sousa G, Toschke AM, et al. Long-term follow-up of cardiovascular disease risk factors in children after an obesity intervention. *American Journal of Clinical Nutrition* 2006; **84**: 490–496.

34. Sabin MA, Ford A, Hunt L, et al. Which factors are associated with a successful outcome in a weight management programme for obese children? *Journal of Evaluation in Clinical Practice* 2007; **13**: 364–368.

35. Ford AL, Hunt LP, Cooper A, et al. What reduction in BMI SDS is required in obese adolescents to improve body composition and cardiometabolic health? *Archives of Disease in Childhood* 2010; **95**: 256–261.

36. Kolsgaard MP, et al. Reduction in BMI z-score and improvement in cardiometabolic risk factors in obese children and adolescents. The Oslo Adiposity Intervention Study – a hospital/public health nurse combined treatment. *BMC Pediatrics* 2011; **11**: 47.

Consequences and comorbidities associated with obesity

Chapter 2.1

Obesity in the development of type 2 diabetes

Nazim Ghouri
University of Glasgow, Glasgow, UK

2.1.1 Introduction

The burden of obesity in relation to the quality of health and development of illness and disease is of increasing concern. For healthcare professionals, arguably the first disease that comes to mind when asked about the complications of obesity is type 2 diabetes. With type 2 diabetes also on the rise globally, more and more healthcare professionals are being involved in the management of obese people with this disease and the clinical sequelae that follow for an individual with diabetes.

This chapter reviews the importance of diabetes as a major complication of obesity, starting with examining the epidemiological relationship between diabetes and obesity. The role of physical activity influencing the risk of diabetes will also be considered, given the importance given to regular and frequent physical activity in the obese with type 2 diabetes. The pathophysiological role of obesity in diabetes, including the association of ectopic fat states, such as non-alcoholic fatty liver disease (NAFLD), will be examined. Finally, the influence of ethnicity in relation to obesity and risk of type 2 diabetes will be addressed, before summarising the natural history of type 2 diabetes, to highlight the complications and impact on healthcare systems.

2.1.2 Diabetes and obesity, the epidemiological relationship

Worldwide, the prevalence of diabetes is estimated at around 285 million people [1]. In 2012, the prevalence of diabetes (both type 1 diabetes and type 2 diabetes) in the UK was estimated to be 4.6%, which translates to 3 million people [2]. However, nearly 20% of people with diabetes are unaware that they have the disease [3]. Around 85% of people (90% of adults) with diabetes have type 2 diabetes [4]. Both the prevalence (proportion of population found to have a condition) and incidence (the risk of developing a new condition within a specified period) of type 2 diabetes have been increasing the UK, with prevalence doubling from 2.3% in 1996 to 4.6% in 2012 [2,5], and incidence increasing from 2.71/1000 person-years to 4.42/1000 person-years between 1996 and 2005 [5]. Furthermore, the projected figures for the increasing global prevalence of diabetes are in agreement with UK estimates – in 2004, the predicted global prevalence of diabetes in 2030 was 4.4% (366 million people) [6]; however, in 2010, the prevalence was predicted at 6.4% (430 million) [1].

The growing incidence of diabetes is nearly all type 2 diabetes – the incidence increasing from 2.60/1000 person-years in 1996 to 4.31/1000

Advanced Nutrition and Dietetics in Obesity, First Edition. Edited by Catherine Hankey.
© 2018 John Wiley & Sons Ltd. Published 2018 by John Wiley & Sons Ltd.

person-years in 2005 – whereas the incidence of type 1 diabetes remained relatively constant [5]. This growing incidence and prevalence of type 2 diabetes is being linked to the increasing prevalence of obesity – the proportion of individuals newly diagnosed with type 2 diabetes who were obese increased from 46% to 56% over the 10-year period [5].

This adverse effect of obesity is not surprising, as it is recognised that weight gain is an important proven risk factor in developing type 2 diabetes [7–9]. A 5-year follow-up of over 50,000 healthy men aged 40–75 years found that men with a BMI of >35 kg/m^2 were at 42-fold higher risk of developing type 2 diabetes than men with a BMI of <23 kg/m^2 [8]. Moreover, the landmark data from Hillier and colleagues illustrated how the severity of obesity lowered the age of onset of type 2 diabetes in the USA. Defining early onset of type 2 diabetes as a diagnosis before the age of 45, they calculated the mean BMI in this group to be 39 kg/m^2; however, the usual group (age>45) had a mean BMI of 33 [10]. There was also a significant inverse linear relationship between BMI and age at diagnosis of type 2 diabetes ($P < 0.0001$) (Table 2.1.1). Research is also confirming the belief that, with growing numbers of younger people becoming obese, the number of younger adults being diagnosed with type 2 diabetes is also on the rise [11]. Thus, it can be safely

concluded that obesity is a key driver, if not *the* main driver, for the growing (and premature) development of type 2 diabetes.

2.1.3 Epidemiological evidence for both obesity and reduced physical activity

While it is recognised that undertaking less physical activity is associated with an increased risk of diabetes [9,12], are the adverse effects of being less active greater than the adverse effects of being obese? It has been shown that a high BMI (>30 kg/m^2) is a more important risk factor for the development of type 2 diabetes than physical inactivity in women, with active obese women having a diabetes hazard ratio of 11.5 compared to 1.15 for inactive women who are of a healthy BMI, and 1 for active, normal-weight women [12]. Similar data has been shown in a smaller study that included men and women, which also categorised subjects according to normal or impaired glucose regulation (impaired fasting glucose or impaired glucose tolerance) at baseline (Table 2.1.2) [9]. This latter study shows

Table 2.1.1 Relationship between age at diagnosis of type 2 diabetes and BMI

Age at diagnosis type 2 diabetes (years)	Average BMI (kg/m^2)
<30	38.3
31–35	37.1
36–40	38.3
41–45	36.3
46–50	35.9
51–55	35
56–60	33.9
61–65	31.7
66–70	31.1
>70	28.8

Source: Adapted from reference [10].

Table 2.1.2 Relative risk of type 2 diabetes according to joint levels of physical activity, BMI (adjusted for age, sex, study year, systolic blood pressure, smoking status and education)

	BMI (kg/m^2)	
	<30	>30
Physical activity	**Relative risk (subjects with normal glucose regulation)**	
Low	1.10	13.2
Medium	2.22	7.32
High	1	3.79
Physical activity	**Relative risk (subjects with impaired glucose regulation)**	
Low	15.5	19
Medium	12.7	30.1
High	5.5	30.2

that increasing body mass, reduced physical activity and impaired glucose regulation all independently contribute to the risk of developing type 2 diabetes. An obese individual with impaired glucose regulation who undertakes low physical activity has a 30-fold increased risk of developing type 2 diabetes compared with a person who has a normal BMI, normal glucose regulation and is physically active. While being obese is a stronger risk factor than being inactive in relation to the risk of developing type 2 diabetes, novel data suggests that cardiorespiratory fitness is almost as important as body fatness in increasing risk [13], and as fitness can only be increased by undertaking more physical activity, the importance of undertaking regular physical activity when trying to reduce the risk of developing type 2 diabetes cannot be underestimated.

2.1.4 Pathophysiological processes linking obesity and type 2 diabetes

It is clear from the epidemiological data reported that obesity is strongly associated with onset and, in particular, the premature onset, of type 2 diabetes. The pivotal pathophysiological process that results in obesity causing type 2 diabetes appears to be the development of insulin resistance [14]. *Insulin resistance* can be defined as 'the inability of a known quantity of exogenous or endogenous (i.e. from the pancreatic beta cells) insulin to increase glucose uptake and utilisation in an individual as much as it does in a normal population' [15]. In other words, an individual with insulin resistance requires more insulin to have the same effect in controlling glycaemia, and ultimately the body cannot produce enough insulin to maintain normoglycaemia, leading to states of impaired glucose control (including states such as impaired fasting glucose and impaired glucose tolerance), and ultimately type 2 diabetes. Impaired glucose tolerance is an important intermediate pathological state in the pathway to type 2 diabetes, as individuals in this state have lost around 80% of pancreatic beta cell function [16].

The connection between obesity and increased levels of circulating insulin was first described in the 1960s [17], with research showing that, in systemic insulin resistance, there was compensatory activity by insulin-secreting beta cells. It has also been recognised that obese individuals have increased circulating free fatty acids, and this is associated with insulin resistance and dysglycaemia [18]. Finally, it is known that obese normoglycaemic individuals have both increased beta cell mass and function [17,19]. Thus, obesity-induced glucose intolerance appears to reflect the failure of beta cell activity [14].

Several mechanisms have been suggested in trying to explain why obesity causes insulin resistance and, subsequently, type 2 diabetes. These include increased production of adipokines/cytokines that contribute to insulin resistance [20]; ectopic fat deposition mainly in the liver but also in skeletal muscle and the resulting effect on glucose/insulin homeostasis [21]; and impaired mitochondrial activity [22]. Impaired mitochondrial activity, reflected by reduced mass and/or function, could be one of the many important pathologies connecting obesity to diabetes, both by decreasing insulin sensitivity and by compromising beta cell function.

Ectopic fat deposition in the liver can contribute to insulin resistance, with ongoing deposition exacerbating the insulin-resistant state [21]. It is not surprising, therefore, that liver fat has a strong association with obesity and type 2 diabetes. Obesity is a common feature of people with NAFLD – a condition when a person has more than 5% fat in their liver [23]. Up to 93% of people with NAFLD are thought to be obese [24]. Likewise, 75% of people with obesity have NAFLD, compared to a prevalence of 16% in people with a normal BMI [25].

The most compelling information describing the associations between NAFLD, obesity/adiposity and type 2 diabetes comes from the pilot data from bariatric surgery outcomes and reduced-energy diets in obese patients with type 2 diabetes. By applying the concept of 'tracing the reverse route from cure to cause' for the pathogenesis of type 2 diabetes [26], it can be hypothesised that, if a reduction in adiposity (particularly liver fat content) is associated with a significant improvement in the dysglycaemic state in type 2 diabetes [27,28], then the presence of liver fat is a reflection of a relatively increased adiposity state, with both liver fat and excess adiposity contributing to the development of type 2 diabetes. One study clearly demonstrates that, in a group of obese subjects, weight loss from a strict moderately hypocaloric very-low-fat diet (liquid diet formula with 50% carbohydrate, 43% protein, 3% fat, 12 g dietary fibre, supplemented with raw fruit and vegetables, totalling ~ 1,200 kcal/day), followed by a period of weight stabilisation, resulted in an 8% weight loss over a mean of 7 weeks. This was associated with an 81% reduction in liver fat, with the reduction in overall body adiposity only falling 1.9% over the same period [27]. Mean fasting plasma glucose improved from 8.8 mmol/l to 6.4 mmol/l in these subjects. Therefore, in an obese state, the relatively small quantity of fat deposited in the liver has the key influence in glycaemic control.

Interestingly, despite these pathophysiological mechanisms described in the preceding text, it is recognised that not every obese individual develops diabetes, for reasons remaining as yet unknown, and even genetic factors fail to fully explain the discrepancy [14]. Consequently, a recently published consensus report, cosponsored by the American Diabetic Association, the Endocrine Society and the European Association for the Study of Diabetes, on obesity, insulin resistance and type 2 diabetes,

highlights the need for further research for identifying why all patients with obesity do not develop type 2 diabetes, and the mechanisms by which obesity and insulin resistance contribute to beta cell decompensation [14]. Nevertheless, given the current body of evidence, one can conclude that, for many individuals, obesity drives insulin resistance and increases the chances of ectopic fat deposition, chiefly in the liver, which appears to have a significant influence on the progression of insulin resistance that culminates in the onset of type 2 diabetes (Figure 2.1.1).

2.1.5 Influence of ethnicity on obesity and risk of type 2 diabetes

Much of the data in the preceding text in relation to obesity and risk of type 2 diabetes come mainly from populations of white European extraction. However, much of the projected increase in the global prevalence of diabetes is attributable to Asia – namely, the Indian subcontinent, China and the Middle East [1]. The prevalence of diabetes is expected to rise 54% between 2010 and 2030;

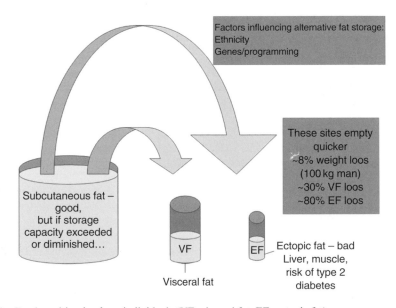

Figure 2.1.1 Fat deposition in obese individuals (VF: visceral fat; EF: ectopic fat).

however, the prevalence is expected to rise by 72% in South Asian countries, and by 94% in countries from the Middle East. Interestingly the prevalence in Europe is only expected to rise by 20% concurrently. In terms of absolute numbers, India, China and Pakistan will provide 63 million of the 145 million extra people who will have diabetes by 2030, with India alone contributing 37 million people.

In light of this epidemiological data, is it possible that obesity, or indeed weight gain in general, has a stronger association with the onset of type 2 diabetes in such high-risk populations? A recent review plotted the relative risk of type 2 diabetes against BMI for people of South Asian and white European origin (Figure 2.1.2) [29]. The graph illustrates clearly that the BMI threshold associated with the exponential increase in diabetes risk occurs at 22–23 kg/m² (in the 'normal' BMI range of 18.5–25) for South Asians, whereas in white Europeans the increase occurs at a BMI in excess of 30 kg/m². Similarly, a study from Canada investigating multi-ethnic populations (South Asian, Chinese, Aboriginal and Europeans) calculated the ethnicity-specific BMIs

for an equivalent risk of impaired glucose control akin to the risk of diabetes [30]. They calculated the risk for a European with a BMI of 30 kg/m², and subsequently calculated the equivalent BMI that would give the same risk in the other ethnic groups. The equivalent BMIs in the South Asian, Chinese and Aboriginal populations were 21, 20.6 and 21.8 kg/m², respectively.

Perhaps one explanation for the relationship between BMI thresholds and the risk of type 2 diabetes is that the current BMI categories for weight are not as useful or sensitive in other ethnicity groups in relation to metabolic risk. For example, BMI-matched South Asians and Europeans have more body fat for the same BMI [13,31]. Or equally, in South Asians, the fat appears to be relatively more distributed around the abdomen as compared to Europeans, as indicated by an increased waist–hip ratio [13,32], which is recognised as a stronger predictor of the risk of type 2 diabetes than BMI in South Asians [33]. Regardless of the underlying reason(s), one thing is clear – people of ethnicities such as South Asian or Chinese who are overweight are more at risk of developing diabetes as compared

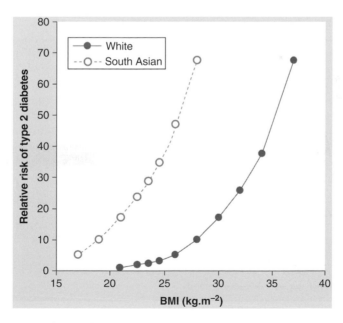

Figure 2.1.2 Relative risk of type 2 diabetes according to BMI for whites and South Asians. Source: Reproduced from [29], with permission from Future Medicine Ltd.

to their European counterparts. Thus, consensual international opinion and guidelines have suggested ethnicity-specific BMI and waist circumference (a surrogate for waist–hip ratio) cut-offs that are lower than those for white populations to reflect this increased risk [34].

2.1.6 Diabetes – the impact of the disease

Recent data from a study involving 1 million people showed that having a diagnosis of diabetes causes premature death – a 40-year-old male with diabetes will lose 6–7 years of life due to the disease [35].

The main complications from type 2 diabetes are vascular in nature, falling into two main categories – *macrovascular* complications such as ischaemic heart disease, cerebrovascular disease and peripheral vascular disease; and *microvascular* complications such as retinopathy, nephropathy and neuropathy [36]. Retinopathy is the leading cause of blindness in the working population in the USA [37]. Further, many patients with type 2 diabetes often experience more than one type of complication. For example, many patients experience problems with their feet, including deformity and ulceration, which are often multifactorial in aetiology [38]. Moreover, the lifetime risk for a patient with type 2 diabetes for developing a foot ulcer is 25% [39], with type 2 diabetes accounting for up to 80% of non-traumatic amputations (of which 85% is preceded by a foot ulcer) [40]. Ultimately, complications such as retinopathy are linked to the level of dysglycaemia [41]. Optimising glycaemic control, particularly in the early years, has a positive influence on complications [42], but this requires concerted and sustained effort in the management of patients – by both healthcare professionals and the patients themselves.

The direct drug costs of managing patients with type 2 diabetes have been disproportionately increasing over the past 10–15 years. While prevalence in the UK has increased by 50%, the drug costs have doubled over the same period [43].

Therefore, while the cost of obesity in itself burdens health resources financially, the subsequent effects of type 2 diabetes only add to the financial drain. Moreover, patients with diabetes are more likely to be admitted to hospital. Recent data from 219 hospitals in the UK, in the 2009 National Audit of Inpatient Diabetes Care, suggested that a little over 15% of patients with diabetes are admitted, of which 94% have type 2 diabetes [44]. Although having type 2 diabetes increases the chances of hospital admissions, only around 12% of admissions are diabetes related [45]. Thus, patients with diabetes are a high-risk group, growing in number.

2.1.7 Conclusions

Having reviewed the association between obesity and type 2 diabetes, it is clear that these two conditions have a close relationship. The epidemiological trends showing the worldwide increase in obesity are being mirrored in type 2 diabetes. Of growing concern is the manner in which obesity adversely influences the age of onset of type 2 diabetes, and, with greater numbers of children and younger adults becoming obese and people becoming more sedentary, it is unsurprising that more and more younger people are being diagnosed with type 2 diabetes.

Substantial evidence suggests that obesity causes the body to become insulin resistant, which is worsened by liver fat deposition. Ultimately, the pancreatic beta cells fail, and type 2 diabetes ensues. Moreover, some ethnic groups such as South Asians appear to be more sensitive to the adverse effects of weight gain, with type 2 diabetes occurring in people with normal BMIs for this group, indicating the probable need for ethnicity-specific BMI classification. Once a diagnosis of type 2 diabetes is made, the combined efforts of the patient and healthcare professionals are required to control glycaemia (through lifestyle changes and, where necessary, medication) in order to minimise the development and progression of complications that can cause significant morbidity and premature mortality.

2.1.8 Summary box

Key points

- The UK and worldwide prevalence of diabetes is increasing, and it is nearly all type 2 diabetes in aetiology.
- The increasing numbers of people developing type 2 diabetes is driven by the worsening obesity epidemic.
- Obesity drives insulin resistance, increasing the chances of liver fat deposition, which can significantly influence the development of type 2 diabetes.
- Ethnicity can negatively influence the adverse metabolic effects of weight gain – South Asian and Chinese people have greater risk of diabetes at any given BMI.
- People with diabetes are at increased risk of premature death and multiple complications including blindness, limb amputations and renal impairment.

References

1. Shaw JE, Sicree RA, Zimmet PZ. Global estimates of the prevalence of diabetes for 2010 and 2030. *Diabetes Research and Clinical Practice* 2010; **87**(1): 4–14.
2. Diabetes UK. Diabetes prevalence 2012. 2013. 29-7-2013.
3. Holt TA, Stables D, Hippisley-Cox J, O'Hanlon S, Majeed A. Identifying undiagnosed diabetes: cross-sectional survey of 3.6 million patients' electronic records. *British Journal of General Practice* 2008; **58**(548): 192–196.
4. Diabetes UK. Diabetes in the UK 2012: Key statistics in diabetes. 1-4-2013, 29-7-2013.
5. Gonzalez ELM, Johansson S, Wallander MA, Rodriguez LAG. Trends in the prevalence and incidence of diabetes in the UK: 1996–2005. *Journal of Epidemiology and Community Health* 2009; **63**(4, Apr): 332–336.
6. Wild S, Roglic G, Green A, Sicree R, King H. Global prevalence of diabetes: estimates for the year 2000 and projections for 2030. *Diabetes Care* 2004; **27**(5, May): 1047–1053.
7. Colditz GA, Willett WC, Rodnitzky A, Manson JE. Weight gain as a risk factor for clinical diabetes mellitus in women. *Annals of Internal Medicine* 1995; **122**: 481–486.
8. Chan JM, Rimm EB, Colditz GA, Stampfer MJ, Willett WC. Obesity, fat distribution, and weight gain as risk factors for clinical diabetes in men. *Diabetes Care* 1994; **17**(9): 961–969.
9. Hu G, Lindstrom J, Valle TT, Eriksson JG, Jousilahti P, Silventoinen K, et al. Physical activity, body mass index, and risk of type 2 diabetes in patients with normal or impaired glucose regulation. *Archives of Internal Medicine* 2004; **164**(8): 892–896.
10. Hillier TA, Pedula KL. Characteristics of an adult population with newly diagnosed type 2 diabetes: the relation of obesity and age of onset. *Diabetes Care* 2001; **24**(9): 1522–1527.
11. Wilmot EG, Davies MJ, Yates T, Benhalima K, Lawrence IG, Khunti K. Type 2 diabetes in younger adults: the emerging UK epidemic. *Postgraduate Medical Journal* 2010; **86**(1022): 711–718.
12. Weinstein AR, Sesso HD, Lee IM, Cook NR, Manson JE, Buring JE, et al. Relationship of physical activity vs. body mass index with type 2 diabetes in women. *JAMA* 2004; **292**(10): 1188–1194.
13. Ghouri N, Purves D, McConnachie A, Wilson J, Gill JM, Sattar N. Lower cardiorespiratory fitness contributes to increased insulin resistance and fasting glycaemia in middle-aged South Asian compared with European men living in the UK. *Diabetologia* 2013; **56**(10): 2238–2249.
14. Eckel RH, Kahn SE, Ferrannini E, Goldfine AB, Nathan DM, Schwartz MW, et al. Obesity and type 2 diabetes: what can be unified and what needs to be individualized? *Journal of Clinical Endocrinology and Metabolism* 2011; **96**(6): 1654–1663.
15. Lebovitz HE. Insulin resistance: definition and consequences. *Experimental and Clinical Endocrinology & Diabetes* 2001; **109**(2): S135–S148.
16. DeFronzo RA. Banting lecture. From the triumvirate to the ominous octet: a new paradigm for the treatment of type 2 diabetes mellitus. *Diabetes* 2009; **58**(4): 773–795.
17. Bagdade JD, Bierman EL, Porte D, Jr. The significance of basal insulin levels in the evaluation of the insulin response to glucose in diabetic and nondiabetic subjects. *Journal of Clinical Investigation* 1967; **46**(10): 1549–1557.
18. Boden G. Free fatty acids, insulin resistance, and type 2 diabetes mellitus. *Proceedings of the Association of American Physicians* 1999; **111**(3): 241–248.
19. Ferrannini E, Camastra S, Gastaldelli A, Maria SA, Natali A, Muscelli E, et al. Beta-cell function in obesity: effects of weight loss. *Diabetes* 2004; **53**(3): S26–S33.
20. Deng Y, Scherer PE. Adipokines as novel biomarkers and regulators of the metabolic syndrome. *Annals of the New York Academy of Sciences* 2010; **1212**: E1–E19.
21. Preiss D, Sattar N. Non-alcoholic fatty liver disease: an overview of prevalence, diagnosis, pathogenesis and treatment considerations. *Clinical Science (London)* 2008; **115**(5): 141–150.
22. Bournat JC, Brown CW. Mitochondrial dysfunction in obesity. *Current Opinion in Endocrinology Diabetes and Obesity* 2010; **17**(5): 446–452.
23. Byrne CD, Olufadi R, Bruce KD, Cagampang FR, Ahmed MH. Metabolic disturbances in non-alcoholic fatty liver disease. *Clinical Science (London)* 2009; **116**(7): 539–564.
24. McCullough AJ. Update on nonalcoholic fatty liver disease. *Journal of Clinical Gastroenterology* 2002; **34**(3): 255–262.
25. Bellentani S, Saccoccio G, Masutti F, Croce LS, Brandi G, Sasso F, et al. Prevalence of and risk factors for hepatic steatosis in Northern Italy. *Annals of Internal Medicine* 2000; **132**(2): 112–117.
26. Taylor R. Pathogenesis of type 2 diabetes: tracing the reverse route from cure to cause. *Diabetologia* 2008; **51**(10): 1781–1789.

27. Petersen KF, Dufour S, Befroy D, Lehrke M, Hendler RE, Shulman GI. Reversal of nonalcoholic hepatic steatosis, hepatic insulin resistance, and hyperglycemia by moderate weight reduction in patients with type 2 diabetes. *Diabetes* 2005; **54**(3): 603–608.

28. Hollingsworth KG, Abubacker MZ, Joubert I, Allison ME, Lomas DJ. Low-carbohydrate diet induced reduction of hepatic lipid content observed with a rapid non-invasive MRI technique. *British Journal of Radiology* 2006; **79**(945): 712–715.

29. Hall LML, Sattar N, Gill JMR. Risk of metabolic and vascular disease in South Asians: potential mechanisms for increased insulin resistance. *Future Lipidology* 2008; **3**(4): 411–424.

30. Razak F, Anand SS, Shannon H, Vuksan V, Davis B, Jacobs R, et al. Defining obesity cut points in a multiethnic population. *Circulation* 2007; **115**(16): 2111–2118.

31. Hall LM, Moran CN, Milne GR, Wilson J, MacFarlane NG, Forouhi NG, et al. Fat oxidation, fitness and skeletal muscle expression of oxidative/lipid metabolism genes in South Asians: implications for insulin resistance? *PLoS ONE* 2010; **5**(12): e14197.

32. McKeigue PM, Shah B, Marmot MG. Relation of central obesity and insulin resistance with high diabetes prevalence and cardiovascular risk in South Asians. *Lancet* 1991; **337**(8738): 382–386.

33. World Health Organisation – EC. Waist Circumference and Waist–Hip Ratio. 11-12-2008. 29-7-2013.

34. Alberti KG, Eckel RH, Grundy SM, Zimmet PZ, Cleeman JI, Donato KA, et al. Harmonizing the metabolic syndrome: a joint interim statement of the International Diabetes Federation Task Force on Epidemiology and Prevention; National Heart, Lung, and Blood Institute; American Heart Association; World Heart Federation; International Atherosclerosis Society; and International Association for the Study of Obesity. *Circulation* 2009; **120**(16): 1640–1645.

35. Seshasai SR, Kaptoge S, Thompson A, Di AE, Gao P, Sarwar N, et al. Diabetes mellitus, fasting glucose, and risk of cause-specific death. *The New England Journal of Medicine* 2011; **364**(9): 829–841.

36. Klein R. Hyperglycemia and microvascular and macrovascular disease in diabetes. *Diabetes Care* 1995; **18**(2): 258–268.

37. Zhang X, Saaddine JB, Chou CF, Cotch MF, Cheng YJ, Geiss LS, et al. Prevalence of diabetic retinopathy in the United States, 2005–2008. *JAMA* 2010; **304**(6): 649–656.

38. Bowering CK. Diabetic foot ulcers. Pathophysiology, assessment, and therapy. *Canadian Family Physician* 2001;**47**: 1007–1016.

39. Singh N, Armstrong DG, Lipsky BA. Preventing foot ulcers in patients with diabetes. *JAMA* 2005; **293**(2): 217–228.

40. Trautner C, Haastert B, Giani G, Berger M. Incidence of lower limb amputations and diabetes. *Diabetes Care* 1996; **19**(9): 1006–1009.

41. Colagiuri S, Lee CM, Wong TY, Balkau B, Shaw JE, Borch-Johnsen K. Glycemic thresholds for diabetes-specific retinopathy: implications for diagnostic criteria for diabetes. *Diabetes Care* 2011; **34**(1): 145–150.

42. Kohner EM. Microvascular disease: what does the UKPDS tell us about diabetic retinopathy? *Diabetic Medicine* 2008; **25**(2): 20–24.

43. Gray AM. Diabetes: costs and cost-effectiveness. *Diabetic Medicine* 2010; **27**(9): 971–972.

44. Rayman G. Diabetes update – inpatient audit. 2013. 30-7-2013.

45. Wallymahmed ME, Dawes S, Clarke G, Saunders S, Younis N, MacFarlane IA. Hospital in-patients with diabetes: increasing prevalence and management problems. *Diabetic Medicine* 2005; **22**(1): 107–109.

Chapter 2.2

Obesity in the development of cardiovascular disease

Peter Clifton

University of South Australia, Adelaide, Australia

2.2.1 Relationship between BMI and cardiovascular mortality

In a large meta-analysis in nearly 900,000 subjects from 57 prospective cohorts, including smokers and non-smokers, it was found that ischemic heart disease deaths increased linearly from 2.7 in 1000 per year at a BMI of 22.5 kg/m^2 to 7.8 in 1000 per year at a BMI of 40 kg/m^2. In non-smokers, the rates were 1.68–6.52 in 1000 per year. Stroke deaths increased from 1.2 to 1.3 between a BMI of 22 to 30 kg/m^2, and then rose more steeply up to 2.9 at a BMI of 45, and, in non-smokers, 0.96–1.86 in 1000 per year [1].

In males (smokers and non-smokers), the total vascular death rate increased from 4.8 to 12.9 in 1000 per year across the BMI range (22.5 to >40 kg/m^2), while in females the rate was about half that, increasing from 2.4 to 6.1 in 1000 per year over the same BMI range. Smoking increases death rates by 2 in 1000 per year in men and 1 in 1000 per year in women between the ages of 35 and 69, and is additive across the BMI range.

A more recent study has investigated BMI and all-cause mortality in a pooled analysis of 19 prospective studies from the National Cancer Institute Cohort Consortium, which included 1.46 million white (non-Hispanic) adults and 160,087 deaths, and, as in the preceding study, the age-standardised rate of death from any cause in non-smokers was generally lowest among participants with a BMI of 22.5–24.9 kg/m^2 [2].

2.2.2 Causes of increased cardiovascular mortality

Obesity increases blood pressure; increases the risk of sleep apnoea that can also increase blood pressure; enhances sympathetic activity and elevates insulin resistance, blood glucose and blood triglycerides; and lowers high-density lipoprotein (HDL) cholesterol. It is not clear as to which of these is the most important factor(s), and also whether obesity – independently of all these risk factors – is still associated with cardiovascular disease (CVD). Obesity is associated with increased inflammation, impaired endothelial function, lower adiponectin, increased liver fat, increased fibrinogen and other clotting factors, and increased PAI-I (which impairs fibrinolysis). However, in established heart disease and heart failure, obesity is associated with lower mortality. All of these factors will be discussed briefly.

Fat distribution and association with cardiovascular events

Central fat distribution as assessed by increased waist circumference (WC) and waist-to-hip ratio (WHR) is associated with increased numbers of CVD events, but how much additional information it adds to BMI is dependent on age and population. In a meta-analysis of more than 258,000 participants and 4300 CVD events, a 1 cm increase in WC increased the risk of a cardiovascular event by

2%, while a 0.01 unit increase in WHR increased the risk by 5%, with similar effects in men and women [3]. In the Norfolk cohort of the EPIC study, coronary events increased by 50–90% from the first to the fifth quintile of WHR after adjustment for BMI [4]. In a meta-analysis of nine studies in the UK, a 1 standard deviation (SD) increase in WHR or WC increased mortality by 15%, but they were not significantly more discriminatory than BMI [5]. In the USA, NHANES III waist-to-thigh ratio (WTR) in both sexes ($P < 0.01$ for both) and WHR in women ($P < 0.001$) were positively associated with total mortality in middle-aged adults (30–64 years), while BMI and WC exhibited U- or J-shaped associations. In older adults (65–102 years), a higher BMI in both sexes ($P < 0.05$) and higher WC in men ($P = 0.001$) were associated with increased survival, while the remaining measures of body fat distribution exhibited either no association or an inverse relation with mortality [6].

Visceral fat

Visceral fat is intra-abdominal fat that is found in the greater omentum, around the intra-abdominal organs and blood vessels, and fatty acids from visceral fat go directly to the liver via the portal circulation.

If fat is measured directly with computed tomography scan, as in the 3001 subjects in the Framingham Heart Study [7], both subcutaneous adipose tissue (SAT) and visceral adipose tissue (VAT) are significantly associated with blood pressure, fasting plasma glucose, triglycerides and high-density lipoprotein cholesterol, and with increased odds of hypertension, impaired fasting glucose, diabetes, and metabolic syndrome (P range < 0.01). However, VAT is more strongly correlated with most metabolic risk factors than SAT. In women, the odds ratio of metabolic syndrome per 1 SD increase in VAT (4.7) was stronger than that for SAT (3; P for difference between SAT and VAT < 0.0001); similar differences were noted for men (OR for VAT, 4.2; OR for SAT, 2.5). Furthermore, VAT but not SAT contributed significantly to risk factor variation after adjustment for BMI and waist circumference ($P \leq 0.01$).

2.2.3 Changes in cardiovascular risk associated with obesity

Changes in risk over time

From NHANES1 (1971–1975) to NHANES II and NHANES 111 (1988–1994), the enhanced mortality risk with obesity has been reducing (and overall mortality has reduced by 63% or more), and overweight was not associated with excess mortality in NHANES 111 [8]. It was suggested that better treatment of obesity, particularly blood pressure control and treatment with statins, has accounted for the mortality reduction in this group. In addition, cardiovascular risk factors have declined at all BMI levels (particularly blood pressure >140/90, which had fallen from 42% to 24%), and, with the exception of type 2 diabetes, the falls were greater in the higher-BMI category [9].

Changes in risk in heart disease and heart failure – the obesity paradox

In a meta-analysis of nine studies with 28,090 participants with heart failure, overweight and obesity were associated with lower all-cause and CVD mortality by 16–33% and 19–40%, respectively [10]. In patients undergoing percutaneous coronary intervention, obese patients had a 35–37% lower short-term and long-term (5-year) mortality, while in patients undergoing a CABG, short-term mortality was reduced, but long-term mortality was similar [11]. In patients having no procedures, overweight and obesity was still associated with reduced mortality. Patients with obesity may be presenting earlier and receiving more aggressive treatment compared to those with normal BMI. In patients undergoing CABG, lowest mortality was seen with a BMI of 30–35 [12].

2.2.4 Obesity and cardiovascular risk factors

Hypertension

A meta-analysis of 19 cross-sectional studies in the Asia-Pacific region, which examined BMI in comparison to WC and WHR as predictors of hypertension, WHR was the most consistent risk factor between regions in both men and women, but no measure of obesity was systematically better [13].

Sympathetic function

Enhanced sympathetic function increases blood vessel contraction and improves sodium reabsorption in the kidney, and can increase circulating adrenalin and noradrenalin. In normotensive obesity, renal sympathetic tone is doubled, while sympathetic activity in the heart is only 50% of normal. In obesity-related hypertension, there is a similar elevation of renal noradrenalin spillover, but cardiac noradrenalin spillover is more than double that of normotensive obese, and 25% higher than in healthy volunteers. The obese who develop hypertension appear to lose the suppression of cardiac sympathetic outflow seen in the normotensive obese [14]. Excess body weight in young individuals is associated with increased sympathetic activity and impaired endothelial function even in the absence of hypertension, and the increased sympathetic activity may initiate hypertension [15].

Endothelin

Endothelin is a potent vasoconstrictor released from the endothelium. A high plasma endothelin predicts the development of hypertension in normotensive subjects over 7 years with a 79% increase in the highest quartile [16].

Sleep apnoea and blood pressure

In a cardiovascular health study of nearly 6000 older participants, daytime sleepiness (and not snoring) was the only sleep symptom that was significantly associated with mortality in women (and not in men after age adjustment). The age hazard ratio was 1.82 in women [17]. This means the death rate per 1000 women per year with daytime sleepiness was nearly double the death rate in women of a similar age but who did not have daytime sleepiness. Sleep apnoea and intermittent hypoxia lead to sympathetic activation, oxidative stress, inflammation and neurohumoral changes [18]. Metabolic syndrome is 9.1

times more likely to be present in subjects with obstructive sleep apnoea [19], and sleep apnoea is an independent risk factor for hypertension [20] and insulin resistance [21]. Sleep apnoeic men have higher plasma concentrations of leptin, tumour necrosis factor (TNF) alpha and interleukin-6 (both pro inflammatory cytokines) than non-apnoeic obese men. Indexes of sleep-disordered breathing are positively correlated with visceral fat, but not with BMI or total/subcutaneous fat [22].

Dyslipidaemia

Obesity increases fasting and postprandial triglyceride levels, probably by increased delivery of free fatty acids (FFA) to the liver [23,24], although enhanced cholesterol synthesis in the liver too may play a role [25]. Increased very-low-density lipoprotein (VLDL) secretion precedes impaired control of endogenous glucose production in obese men with impaired suppression by insulin [26]. Elevated fasting triglyceride is invariably associated with lower-HDL cholesterol [27]. Metabolic syndrome is a cluster of abnormalities associated with central obesity and insulin resistance, and includes elevated glucose, elevated triglyceride and low-HDL cholesterol and elevated blood pressure [28]. The greater the number of abnormal factors, the greater the CVD risk [29].

Endothelial dysfunction

Endothelial dysfunction as assessed by flow-mediated dilatation, plethysmography, endothelin responsiveness [30] and increased levels of endothelial-derived molecules, such as endothelin [31] and adhesion molecules [32], is associated with obesity and an increased risk of coronary events [33] in a wide spectrum of health and diseased populations, including children and adolescents [34]. In obesity-discordant monozygotic twins, a lower adiponectin level was associated with greater endothelial dysfunction [35].

Coagulation and fibrinolysis

In monozygotic twins, the levels of most coagulation factors are similar within all twin pairs, with the intra-class correlations ranging from 0.73 to 0.97 ($P<0.03$). In obese twin pairs, fibrinogen and factor IX, factor XI, and factor XII, and plasminogen activator inhibitor-1 (PAI-1) were increased. Intra-pair differences in fibrinogen and PAI-1 correlated with those in BMI, adiposity and fasting insulin levels ($r=0.40$–0.58) [36].

2.2.5 Pathophysiological processes linking obesity and cardiovascular disease

Inflammation, FFA, adiponectin and insulin resistance

Adipocyte expansion is associated with a wide array of changes, and it is currently not clear which the fundamental disease-causing mechanism is. Low-grade chronic inflammation in adipose tissue, as expressed by enhanced numbers of macrophages, monocytes and lymphocytes, is a common observation, but the initiating factor has not been identified. Possibilities include necrosis or apoptosis of adipocytes; hypoxia of adipocytes from inadequate blood supply and resulting endoplasmic reticulum stress and finally mitochondrial dysfunction from excessive FFAs and glucose, which can then switch on a wide array of chemokines and cytokines [37–41].

Macrophage accumulation has been observed in human adipose tissue. The extent of accumulation has strong positive correlations with BMI and adipocyte area, and is negatively related to insulin sensitivity [42]. Visceral fat of obese humans contains more macrophages than subcutaneous fat, and the visceral fat macrophage number correlates with fasting glucose and insulin and liver lesions in obese patients [43]. Obese subjects with impaired glucose homeostasis have preferential visceral fat macrophage infiltration [44].

Along with adipose tissue inflammation, plasma acute-phase markers such as fibrinogen, sialic acid, C-reactive protein (CRP) and serum amyloid A are chronically elevated to a moderate level in obesity [45,46], along with IL6, TNF-alpha, TNF-alpha receptor and circulating adhesion molecules.

FFAs

FFAs inhibit insulin-stimulated glucose uptake and glycogen synthesis. FFAs also cause hepatic insulin resistance by inhibiting insulin-mediated suppression of glycogenolysis, and have been shown to activate inflammatory pathways [47].

Insulin sensitivity/adiponectin

Adiponectin inhibits liver gluconeogenesis and promotes fatty acid oxidation in skeletal muscle. In addition, adiponectin counteracts the pro-inflammatory effects of TNF-alpha on the arterial wall by reducing ceramide production, and probably protects against the development of arteriosclerosis. It is not clear whether low adiponectin is the primary cause of IR and endothelial dysfunction in obesity, or whether inflammation is required [48].

Leptin resistance

Leptin has been found to have a role in the regulation of whole-body metabolism by stimulating energy expenditure, inhibiting food intake and restoring euglycaemia. However, in most cases of obesity, leptin resistance limits its biological efficacy [40]. Adiponectin resistance is also seen in obesity. Adiponectin and leptin increase the rates of fatty acid oxidation and decrease muscle lipid content, which may in part be the underlying mechanism in their insulin-sensitising effect.

2.2.6 Research requirements

It is not clear if those obese individuals without CVD risk factors achieve this state by limiting adipocyte hypertrophy and increasing adipocyte numbers and thus limiting adipocyte stress and death, or whether they have a muted inflammatory response to adipocyte hypertrophy [49]. It may be possible to have a large fat mass, have a minimal inflammatory response and retain insulin sensitivity of the adipocyte, and control FFA release and thus the accumulation of fat in liver and muscle [50]. These individuals may also have good clearance mechanisms in fat tissue, thus ensuring that plasma triglycerides and apo B remains low [51]. Although metabolically healthy obese people do not have an increased risk of heart attacks, they do have an enhanced risk of heart failure [52].

2.2.7 Summary box

Key points

- Central fat distribution as assessed by increased WC and WHR is associated with increased numbers of CVD events. The additional information that it adds to BMI is dependent on age and population of interest.
- Leptin has a role in whole-body metabolism regulation by stimulating energy expenditure, inhibiting food intake and restoring euglycaemia. In obesity, leptin resistance limits biological efficacy.
- It is unclear if low adiponectin concentrations are the primary cause of IR and endothelial dysfunction in obesity, or whether inflammation is required.
- Metabolically healthy obese people do not have an increased risk of heart attacks, but their risk of heart failure is enhanced.

References

1. Prospective Studies Collaboration, Whitlock G, Lewington S, Sherliker P, Clarke R, Emberson J, Halsey J, Qizilbash N, et al. Body-mass index and cause-specific mortality in 900000 adults: collaborative analyses of 57 prospective studies. *Lancet* 2009; **373**(9669): 1083–1096.
2. Berrington de Gonzalez A, Hartge P, Cerhan JR, Flint AJ, Hannan L, MacInnis RJ, et al. Body-mass index and mortality among 1.46 million white adults. *The New England Journal of Medicine* 2010; **363**(23): 2211–2219.
3. de Koning L, Merchant AT, Pogue J, Anand SS. Waist circumference and waist-to-hip ratio as predictors of cardiovascular events: meta-regression analysis of prospective studies. *European Heart Journal* 2007; **28**(7): 850–856.
4. Canoy D, Boekholdt SM, Wareham N, Luben R, Welch A, Bingham S, et al. Body fat distribution and risk of coronary heart disease in men and women in the European Prospective Investigation into Cancer and Nutrition in Norfolk cohort: a population-based prospective study. *Obesity (Silver Spring)* 2009; **17**(6): 1232–1239.
5. Czernichow S, Kengne AP, Stamatakis E, Hamer M, Batty GD. Body mass index, waist circumference and waist–hip ratio: which is the better discriminator of cardiovascular disease mortality risk? Evidence from an individual-participant meta-analysis of 82,864 participants from nine cohort studies. *Obesity Reviews* 2011; **12**(9): 680–687.
6. Reis JP, Macera CA, Araneta MR, Lindsay SP, Marshall SJ, Wingard DL. Comparison of overall obesity and body fat distribution in predicting risk of mortality. *Circulation* 2007; **116**(25): 2933–2943.
7. Fox CS, Massaro JM, Hoffmann U, Pou KM, Maurovich-Horvat P, Liu CY, et al. Abdominal visceral and subcutaneous adipose tissue compartments: association with metabolic risk factors in the Framingham Heart Study. *Circulation* 2007; **116**(1): 39–48.
8. Flegal KM, Graubard BI, Williamson DF, Gail MH. Excess deaths associated with underweight, overweight, and obesity. *JAMA* 2005; **293**(15): 1861–1867.
9. Gregg EW, Cheng YJ, Cadwell BL, et al. Secular trends in cardiovascular disease risk factors according to body mass index in US adults. *JAMA* 2005; **293**: 1868–1874.
10. Oreopoulos A, Padwal R, Kalantar-Zadeh K, Fonarow GC, Norris CM, McAlister FA. Body mass index and mortality in heart failure: a meta-analysis. *American Heart Journal* 2008; **156**(1): 13–22.
11. Oreopoulos A, Padwal R, Norris CM, Mullen JC, Pretorius V, Kalantar-Zadeh K. Effect of obesity on short- and long-term mortality postcoronary revascularization: a meta-analysis. *Obesity (Silver Spring)* 2008; **16**(2): 442–450.
12. Oreopoulos A, McAlister FA, Kalantar-Zadeh K, Padwal R, Ezekowitz JA, Sharma AM, et al. The relationship between body mass index, treatment, and mortality in patients with established coronary artery disease: a report from APPROACH. *European Heart Journal* 2009; **30**(21): 2584–2592.
13. Obesity in Asia Collaboration. Is central obesity a better discriminator of the risk of hypertension than body mass index in ethnically diverse populations? *Journal of Hypertension* 2008; **26**(2): 169–177.
14. Esler M. The sympathetic system and hypertension. *American Journal of Hypertension* 2000; **13**(6Pt2): 99S–105S.
15. Lambert E, Sari CI, Dawood T, Nguyen J, McGrane M, Eikelis N, et al. Sympathetic nervous system activity is associated with obesity-induced subclinical organ damage in young adults. *Hypertension* 2010; **56**(3): 351–358.
16. Kumagae S, Adachi H, Jacobs DR Jr, Hirai Y, Enomoto M, Fukami A, et al. High level of plasma endothelin-1 predicts development of hypertension in normotensive subjects. *American Journal of Hypertension* 2010; **23**(10): 1103–1107.
17. Newman AB, Spiekerman CF, Enright P, Lefkowitz D, Manolio T, Reynolds CF, et al. Daytime sleepiness predicts mortality and cardiovascular disease in older adults. The Cardiovascular Health Study Research Group. *Journal of the American Geriatrics Society* 2000; **48**(2): 115–123.
18. Lam JC, Mak JC, Ip MS. Obesity, obstructive sleep apnea and metabolic syndrome. *Respirology* 2011; doi: 10.1111/j.1440-1843.2011.02081.x.

19. Coughlin SR, Mawdsley L, Mugarza JA, Calverley PM, Wilding P. Obstructive sleep apnoea is independently associated with an increased prevalence of metabolic syndrome. *European Heart Journal* 2004; **25**(9): 735–741.

20. Nieto FJ, Young TB, Lind BK, Shahar E, Samet JM, Redline S, et al. Association of sleep-disordered breathing, sleep apnea, and hypertension in a large community-based study. Sleep Heart Health Study. *JAMA* 2000; **283**(14): 1829–1836.

21. Ip MS, Lam B, Ng MM, Lam WK, Tsang KW, Lam KS. Obstructive sleep apnea is independently associated with insulin resistance. *American Journal of Respiratory and Critical Care Medicine* 2002; **165**(5): 670–676.

22. Vgontzas AN, Papanicolaou DA, Bixler EO, Hopper K, Lotsikas A, Lin HM, et al. Sleep apnea and daytime sleepiness and fatigue: relation to visceral obesity, insulin resistance, and hypercytokinemia. *Journal of Clinical Endocrinology and Metabolism* 2000; **85**(3): 1151–1158.

23. Lewis GF, Uffelman KD, Szeto LW, Weller B, Steiner G. Interaction between free fatty acids and insulin in the acute control of very low density lipoprotein production in humans. *Journal of Clinical Investigation* 1995; **95**(1): 158–166.

24. Julius U. Influence of plasma free fatty acids on lipoprotein synthesis and diabetic dyslipidemia. *Experimental and Clinical Endocrinology & Diabetes* 2003; **111**(5): 246–250.

25. Prinsen BH, Romijn JA, Bisschop PH, de Barse MM, Barrett PH, Ackermans M, et al. Endogenous cholesterol synthesis is associated with VLDL-2 apoB-100 production in healthy humans. *Journal of Lipid Research* 2003; **44**(7): 1341–1348.

26. Sørensen LP, Søndergaard E, Nellemann B, Christiansen JS, Gormsen LC, Nielsen S. Increased VLDL-triglyceride secretion precedes impaired control of endogenous glucose production in obese, normoglycemic men. *Diabetes* 2011; **60**(9): 2257–2264.

27. Sacks FM; Expert Group on HDL Cholesterol. The role of high-density lipoprotein (HDL) cholesterol in the prevention and treatment of coronary heart disease: expert group recommendations. *American Journal of Cardiology* 2002; **90**(2): 139–143.

28. Expert panel on detection, evaluation, and treatment of high blood cholesterol in adults. 'Executive summary of the third report of the National Cholesterol Education Program (NCEP). Expert panel on detection, evaluation, and treatment of high blood cholesterol in adults (Adult Treatment Panel III)'. *JAMA* 2001; **285** (19, May): 2486–2497.

29. Knuiman MW, Hung J, Divitini ML, Davis TM, Beilby JP. Utility of the metabolic syndrome and its components in the prediction of incident cardiovascular disease: a prospective cohort study. *European Journal of Cardiovascular Prevention & Rehabilitation* 2009; **16**(2): 235–241.

30. Weil BR, Westby CM, Van Guilder GP, Greiner JJ, Stauffer BL, DeSouza CA. Enhanced endothelin-1 system activity with overweight and obesity. *American Journal of Physiology-Heart and Circulatory Physiology* 2011; **301**(3): H689–H695.

31. Ferri C, Bellini C, Desideri G, Di Francesco L, Baldoncini R, Santucci A, et al. Plasma endothelin-1 levels in obese hypertensive and normotensive men. Diabetes 1995; **44**(4): 431–436.

32. Ferri C, Desideri G, Valenti M, Bellini C, Pasin M, Santucci A, De Mattia G. Early upregulation of endothelial adhesion molecules in obese hypertensive men. *Hypertension* 1999; **34**(4 Pt 1): 568–573.

33. Meyers MR, Gokce N. Endothelial dysfunction in obesity: etiological role in atherosclerosis. *Current Opinion in Endocrinology Diabetes and Obesity* 2007; **14**(5): 365–369.

34. Woo KS, Chook P, Yu CW, Sung RY, Qiao M, Leung SS, et al. Overweight in children is associated with arterial endothelial dysfunction and intima-media thickening. *International Journal of Obesity and Related Metabolic Disorders* 2004; **28**: 852–857.

35. Pietiläinen KH, Bergholm R, Rissanen A, Kaprio J, Häkkinen AM, Sattar N, et al. Effects of acquired obesity on endothelial function in monozygotic twins. *Obesity (Silver Spring)* 2006; **14**(5): 826–837.

36. Kaye SM, Pietiläinen KH, Kotronen A, Joutsi-Korhonen L, Kaprio J, Yki-Järvinen H, et al. Obesity-related derangements of coagulation and fibrinolysis: a study of obesity-discordant monozygotic twin pairs. *Obesity (Silver Spring)* 2011; **20**(1): 88–94.

37. Bastard JP, Maachi M, Lagathu C, Kim MJ, Caron M, Vidal H, et al. Recent advances in the relationship between obesity, inflammation, and insulin resistance. *European Cytokine Network* 2006; **17**(1): 4–12.

38. de Ferranti S, Mozaffarian D. The perfect storm: obesity, adipocyte dysfunction, and metabolic consequences. *Clinical Chemistry* 2008; **54**(6): 945–955.

39. Lionetti L, Mollica MP, Lombardi A, Cavaliere G, Gifuni G, Barletta A. From chronic overnutrition to insulin resistance: the role of fat-storing capacity and inflammation. *Nutrition Metabolism and Cardiovascular Diseases* 2009; **19**(2): 146–152.

40. Galic S, Oakhill JS, Steinberg GR. Adipose tissue as an endocrine organ. *Molecular and Cellular Endocrinology* 2010; **316**(2): 129–139.

41. Dyck DJ. Adipokines as regulators of muscle metabolism and insulin sensitivity. *Applied Physiology Nutrition and Metabolism* 2009; **34**(3): 396–402.

42. Weisberg SP, McCann D, Desai M, Rosenbaum M, Leibel RL, Ferrante AW Jr. Obesity is associated with macrophage accumulation in adipose tissue. *Journal of Clinical Investigation* 2003; **112**(12): 1796–1808.

43. Cancello R, Tordjman J, Poitou C, Guilhem G, Bouillot JL, Hugol D, et al. Increased infiltration of macrophages in omental adipose tissue is associated with marked hepatic lesions in morbid human obesity. *Diabetes* 2006; **55**(6): 1554–1561.

44. Harman-Boehm I, Blüher M, Redel H, Sion-Vardy N, Ovadia S, Avinoach E, et al. Macrophage infiltration into omental versus subcutaneous fat across different populations: effect of regional adiposity and the comorbidities of obesity. *Journal of Clinical Endocrinology and Metabolism* 2007; **92**(6): 2240–2247.

45. Browning LM, Krebs JD, Jebb SA. Discrimination ratio analysis of inflammatory markers: implications for the study of inflammation in chronic disease. *Metabolism* 2004; **53**(7): 899–903.

46. Zhao Y, He X, Shi X, Huang C, Liu J, Zhou S, et al. Association between serum amyloid A and obesity: a meta-analysis and systematic review. *Inflammation Research* 2010; **59**(5): 323–334.

47. Boden G. Effects of free fatty acids (FFA) on glucose metabolism: significance for insulin resistance and type 2 diabetes. *Experimental and Clinical Endocrinology & Diabetes* 2003; **111**(3): 121–124.

48. Lumeng CN, Saltiel AR. Inflammatory links between obesity and metabolic disease. *Journal of Clinical Investigation* 2011; **121**(6): 2111–2117.

49. Karelis AD, Faraj M, Bastard JP, St-Pierre DH, Brochu M, Prud'homme D, Rabasa-Lhoret R. The metabolically healthy but obese individual presents a favorable inflammation profile. *Journal of Clinical Endocrinology and Metabolism* 2005; **90**(7): 4145–4150.

50. Primeau V, Coderre L, Karelis AD, Brochu M, Lavoie ME, Messier V, et al. Characterizing the profile of obese patients who are metabolically healthy. *International Journal of Obesity (London)* 2011; **35**(7): 971–981.

51. Sniderman AD, Faraj M. Apolipoprotein B, apolipoprotein A-I, insulin resistance and the metabolic syndrome. *Current Opinion in Lipidology* 2007; **18**(6): 633–637.

52. Mørkedal B, Vatten LJ, Romundstad PR, Laugsand LE, Janszky I. Risk of myocardial infarction and heart failure among metabolically healthy but obese individuals. The HUNT Study, Norway. *Journal of the American College of Cardiology* 2014; **63**(11): 1071–1078.

Chapter 2.3

Obesity as a risk factor in the development of cancer

Angela M Craigie and Annie S Anderson

University of Dundee, Dundee, UK

2.3.1 Introduction

Obesity has been described as the most important avoidable cause of cancer in non-smokers, and it is predicted that it will eventually become the main risk factor. This chapter considers the epidemiological evidence linking adiposity with the development of cancer, and describes the proposed mechanisms by which excess body fat may impact on cancer risk. Using evidence from several large-scale studies, some evidence on whether weight loss can reduce cancer incidence and cancer recurrence is presented, along with an overview of the established guidelines for cancer risk reduction and cancer survivorship.

2.3.2 Obesity and the development of cancer: the epidemiological evidence

Global estimates for cancer show that there were around 12.7 million cancer cases and 7.6 million cancer deaths in 2008, most of which occurred in the developing world [1]. It is predicted that, by 2030, the number of cancers worldwide will double due to population growth, ageing and lifestyle factors (including smoking, obesity, physical inactivity, diet, alcohol intake and sun exposure) [2], and that, in the UK, increases in obesity will account for about 87000–130000 of cancer cases [3]. Indeed,

obesity has been described as far and away the most important avoidable cause of cancer in non-smokers, with predictions that it will eventually become the main risk factor [4].

It is recognised that weight gain, overweight and obesity are associated with increased occurrence, morbidity and mortality in several cancer sites. In their 2007 review of food, nutrition, physical activity and the prevention of cancer, the World Cancer Research Fund (WCRF) [5] graded the evidence for an association between obesity and cancer of the breast (postmenopausal), colorectum, endometrium, kidney, pancreas and oesophagus as 'convincing', and gall bladder cancer as 'probable'. It is estimated that obese individuals have approximately a 1.5–3.5-fold increased risk of developing these cancers, as compared to non-obese individuals [6]. Current estimates suggest that significant proportions of these cancers can be reduced through decreases in excess body fat. For example, it is estimated that, in the UK, 38% of endometrial cancer, 31% of oesophageal, 16% of postmenopausal breast cancer and 14% of colorectal cancer can be attributed to excess body fat [7]. Links with other cancers have also been reported in the Million Women Study in the UK, which associated high BMI with increased risk for multiple myeloma, leukaemia, non-Hodgkin's lymphoma and ovarian cancer [8].

Gender and ethnic differences in the relationship between BMI and specific cancers have been reported in a systematic review and meta-analysis of prospective observational studies [9]. Significantly

Advanced Nutrition and Dietetics in Obesity, First Edition. Edited by Catherine Hankey.

stronger associations were found between BMI and colon cancer risk for men than women, and between BMI and breast cancers in the Asia-Pacific region as compared to North America, Europe and Australia [9]. For cancers of the female reproductive organs, the effect of BMI on risk is greatest after the menopause [10]. In premenopausal women, obesity may protect against breast cancer [5].

In addition to overall body size, adult weight gain (since age 18 years and since menopause) is thought to be a risk factor for the development of postmenopausal breast [10] and possibly colon [11] cancer. It is notable that, at any BMI, weight gain in adulthood is associated with a greater risk of breast cancer [10], and that, after age 50 years, weight gain of 2–10 kg has been associated with a 30% increase in risk [12]. In addition to BMI, waist size has also been demonstrated to be strongly associated with cancers of the colon, pancreas, breast and endometrium.

Current evidence has prompted researchers to question whether obesity management might be an opportunity for cancer prevention [13].

2.3.3 Pathophysiological processes linking obesity and cancer

A number of metabolic and hormonal abnormalities arising from excess fat storage are implicated in cancer causation, such as those involving insulin and leptin, cell growth factors (insulin-like growth factor (IGF-1) and IGF-binding proteins) and steroids [14].

Insulin and growth factors

Of increasing interest is the interaction between growth factors (such as insulin and IGF-1) and oestrogen signalling, and the impact of both obesity and physical activity on insulin resistance, insulin presence in the peripheral tissue and hyperinsulinaemia. Increased blood insulin levels result in lower levels of IGF-binding protein 1, which can in turn lead to an increase in free IGF-1 levels. Metabolic syndrome (the clustering of risk factors for cardiovascular disease and type 2 diabetes) and type 2 diabetes have also been associated with increased prevalence of colon cancer [15]. Metabolic syndrome may also increase cancer risk, suggesting that the metabolic disturbances associated with this disorder promote genetic instability.

Raised oestrogens

These are likely to contribute to the greater risk of breast and endometrial cancers in obese patients. Exposure to increased oestrogen levels (especially in postmenopausal women), whether from endogenous production or exogenous when taken as hormone replacement therapy, is a well-established risk factor for breast and uterus cancers [16].

In addition, cancer-site-specific mechanisms have been postulated in relation to tissue damage caused by obesity. For example, increasing gall stones has been implicated as a factor in gallbladder cancer, and increased gastro-oesophageal reflux in patients with abdominal obesity has been implicated in the development of oesophageal cancer [17]. The relationship between colorectal cancer and obesity is thought to be related primarily to the effect of obesity in increased inflammation that might account for why the disease risk is reduced with anti-inflammatory agents such as aspirin [18].

2.3.4 Weight loss and cancer risk reduction

There have been no long-term trials of intentional weight loss on cancer end points (incidence or recurrence), but results from several observational studies suggest that weight reduction may be associated with cancer risk reduction [17,19].

Observational studies of weight loss and cancer risk

Two prospective cohorts have examined the association between intentional weight loss and cancer incidence (the Iowa Women's Health Study, IWHS) or mortality (the American Cancer Society's Cancer Prevention Study I, CPS-I).

The IWHS followed up 21,707 postmenopausal women and reported decreased cancer incidence rates of 11% for any cancer (RR=0.91, 95% CI 0.79–1) in women who had experienced intentional weight loss in adulthood (of ≥9.1 kg) [20]. Those in the lowest breast cancer risk group were women who maintained or lost weight from age 18–30 years and then lost weight (>5% body weight) from age 30 years to menopause (RR 0.36, 95% CI 0.22–0.60), indicating important effects of relatively small amounts of weight loss [21].

The CPS-I study results were less consistent and depended on whether the participants had obesity-related pre-existing illnesses and how much weight had been lost. In women, mortality from all cancers was again reduced, but only in those who had obesity-related illnesses: by 37% if they lost 0.5–9 kg (RR=0.63, 95% CI 0.43–0.93) or 29% if they lost ≥9 kg (RR=0.71, 95% CI 0.52–0.97) [22]. In those without obesity-related illnesses, the associations with mortality were only significant for those who had obesity-related cancers and had lost less than 9 kg, whereby their mortality risk had increased (RR=1.62, 95% CI 1.10–2.58). It is notable, however, that this was based on a small sample of only 10 deaths. In men, no significant associations were found [23].

Several others have considered associations regardless of intentionality of weight loss [19], including the US Nurses' Health Study that followed up a cohort of 49,514 postmenopausal women for 24 years. They demonstrated that women who (a) had never used postmenopausal hormones, (b) had lost 10 kg or more since menopause and (c) kept the weight off for at least two consecutive questionnaire cycles (around 4 years) were at a significantly lower risk of developing breast cancer than those who maintained weight (RR 0.43, 95% CI 0.21–0.86) [10].

Intervention studies of weight loss and cancer risk

The Women's Health Initiative [24] tested the impact of a low-fat diet (20% energy goal) versus control in 48,835 postmenopausal women. Most women were either overweight (36%) or obese (38%). Although the trial was not designed to assess the effects of weight loss, in comparison to the control arm, the low-fat group did experience a modest weight loss (−2.2 kg) in year 1, and they maintained this greater weight reduction throughout the remainder of the trial (−0.8 kg at year 6). After 8 years, there was a 9% difference between intervention and control groups in breast cancer incidence.

Two major trials of diet have been undertaken in women with breast cancer. The Women's Healthy Eating and Living (WHEL) trial [25] tested a diet low in fat (15–20% energy), high in fibre (30 g) and high in fruits and vegetables (three servings of fruits, five servings of vegetables, plus 16 oz of vegetable juice) in 3088 women. No difference in body weight was detected after 7.3 years, and no difference in breast cancer occurrence. These findings are in contrast to the findings of the Women's Intervention Nutrition Study (WINS) [26], which aimed to test the hypothesis that a dietary intervention targeting diet composition (reduction in fat to a goal of 15% energy) would prolong relapse-free survival in 2437 women with resected breast cancer. Body weight was not an intervention target; however, after 5 years follow-up, those who received the dietary intervention weighed a statistically significant 2.7 kg (3.7%) less than the control group (P=0.005). This modest difference was associated with a 24% lower risk of relapse than found in the control group (HR=0.76, 95% CI=0.60–0.98).

Modest weight loss is associated with cancer risk reduction (which would be considered highly desirable if a drug was being tested), and there appears to be a dose–response relationship, with higher weight loss associated with greater risk reduction.

Bariatric surgery studies of weight loss and cancer risk

A number of studies have now reported reduced cancer incidence following bariatric surgery. In the Swedish Obesity Subjects (SOS) study, Sjöström et al. [27] studied cancer incidence in 2010 obese adults undergoing bariatric surgery and 2037 matched controls after a 10.9-year follow-up. In women, they reported a marked 42% reduction in cancer risk (79 vs. 130 new cases in the surgery vs. control groups, respectively). There was a negligible impact on men, suggesting a higher impact on endocrine cancers, although data was not specific to any one cancer site. Similar findings were reported in the Utah Obesity Study, where total cancer incidence was 27% lower after gastric bypass in women, with little impact on men [28]. A Canadian cohort study reported a reduction of 78% cancer risk over 5-year follow-up, with a notable 83% reduction for breast cancer [29]. However, Ostund et al. [30] examined a total of 13,123 obese surgery patients and found no overall decrease in standardised incidence ratios and no decreases in breast, endometrial or kidney cancer.

Collectively, these studies suggest some inconsistency in outcomes. Where positive effects have been reported, these suggest that significant weight loss can reduce cancer risk within a relatively short time period, with marked differences by gender. Longer-term follow-up and the impact of weight gain on risk remain to be assessed.

Studies of weight loss and cancer-related biomarkers

Byers and Sedjo's [17] review of studies designed to examine the impact of weight loss on cancer-related biomarkers shows considerable promise, although there are few long-term trials, and these have not included cancer end points. Biomarkers studied include cancer-related hormonal factors (oestradiol, sex hormone–binding globulin), inflammation-related biomarkers (C-reactive protein, TNF-alpha and interleukin 6 (IL-6), and growth factors (IGF-1 and IGF-binding proteins)). Oestradiol is considered a causal mediator for postmenopausal breast and endometrial cancers, and the authors conclude that even modest weight loss could have substantial and fairly immediate effects on risk. They suggest that a 10% weight loss is associated with a reduction of free oestradiol levels by about one-third. Inflammatory markers have been associated with BMI and cancer risk, and a similar magnitude of reduction in C-reactive protein is found with weight loss, with smaller effects on TNF-alpha and IL-6. Weight loss studies have shown inconsistent results on IGF-1 and IGF-binding proteins, although insulin does show significant reductions with a decrease in body weight.

2.3.5 Development of weight loss regimens for cancer risk reduction

At a public health level, in the absence of surgery, effective weight loss programmes based on current national guidelines on obesity management including diet, physical activity and behaviour change are crucial tools. It is important within such studies to focus on weight loss (shown to be effective) rather than diet or physical activity alone. Imayama et al. [30] tested the impact of diet, exercise or both on inflammatory biomarkers (C-reactive protein, serum amyloid, interleukin-6, leukocyte) and weight loss and demonstrated that an energy-restricted diet with or without exercise reduced biomarkers of inflammation [31].

Both components are likely to have significant effects on cancer risk, but the combined effect is greater. The addition of physical activity may be important in cancer risk reduction due to an independent effect on relevant metabolic pathways (notably insulin), although Byers and Sedjo [17] suggest that 'the relationship between physical activity and both obesity and cancer risk is largely inextricable in the context of intentional weight loss'.

Fundamental to the design of weight loss trials (and prior to the investment in expensive, long-term follow-up trials) is the development and feasibility testing of robust and acceptable interventions that can demonstrate weight reduction in people at risk of developing cancer. In the UK, Harvie et al. [32] have tested a novel dietary approach comparing 25% energy restriction via intermittent energy restriction (IER) (~2266 kJ/day for 2 days/week, plus the energy required for weight maintenance for the remaining 5 days) or continuous energy restriction (CER) (~6276 kJ/day for 7 days/week) in 107 overweight or obese premenopausal women over 6 months. Subjects were recruited from a breast cancer family history clinic and from the general population. All participants received fortnightly motivational phone calls, received feedback on weight at monthly clinic appointments and were encouraged to use behavioural techniques such as self-monitoring and social and stimulus control to maintain diets. All participants were advised to maintain their current activity levels throughout the trial and did not receive specific advice on physical activity. The authors reported similar results for biomarkers and weight losses in both groups (weight change for IER was −6.4 kg vs. −5.6 kg for CER ($P = 0.4$ for difference between groups). The impact of this magnitude of weight loss is unclear, given the scarcity of evidence, but observational studies of weight loss suggest significant cancer risk reduction [21]. Long-term trials of weight loss interventions and cancer outcomes may not be feasible, given the numbers required and the length of follow-up. However, weight loss trials in patients with cancer (notably breast cancer) are underway [33].

Anderson et al. [34] undertook an acceptability and feasibility study of a 3-month personalised lifestyle (diet, exercise and weight management) intervention in overweight adults who had completed curative treatment for colorectal cancer. Weight change was −1.2 (±4.4) kg overall and −4.1 (±3.7) kg in only those who had lost weight. Quality of life, measured using a patient-generated index questionnaire [35], also improved in 14 of the 17 patients (82%). Participants reported adherence related to tailored advice, personalised feedback and family support. Reported barriers included time following surgery, fatigue, having a stoma or chronic diarrhoea and conflicting instructions from clinicians who had advised patients 'to build themselves up', which was interpreted as promoting weight gain.

An ongoing weight loss trial ('BeWEL') for people who have had colorectal adenomas (identified through the national colorectal screening programme) aims to achieve 7% body weight loss after 12 months, using personal counsellors to promote changes in diet and physical activity, with emphasis on self-monitoring (provision of self-monitoring tools including body weight scales) [36]. Consultant endorsement of the trial has also been added to the protocol following formative work, indicating that many people are unaware of the relationship between lifestyle and colorectal cancer [37]. This trial has highlighted the opportunity for building lifestyle interventions into cancer screening settings.

2.3.6 Recommendations for cancer risk reduction and cancer survivorship

The WCRF has produced guidelines on diet, physical activity and body weight and the prevention of cancer [5]. With respect to body fatness, they stress that people should be as lean as possible within the normal range (noting that this range will vary by race). It was noted that cancer risk starts to increase below the BMI threshold of 25 kg/m², overwhich an individual is classified as 'overweight'. Data from US data reported an increased risk of deaths from a BMI of >21 kg/m² for cancer, and >23 kg/m² for cardiovascular disease and all other causes [5]. Allowing for variations in this relationship between populations, the public health message is therefore that adults should attain a median BMI of 21–23 kg/ m², and there should be no increase in the proportion of the population in the overweight/obese category [5]. At the individual level, they recommend that (a) body weight through childhood and adolescent growth should project towards the lower end of the normal BMI range at age 21, and (b) adults should maintain their body weight within the normal range from age 21 (i.e. avoiding increases in weight and waist circumference).

For cancer survivors, WCRF recommends that 'if able to do so' and unless otherwise advised, they should aim to follow the recommendations for diet, healthy weight and physical activity. They note that there is growing evidence that physical activity and other measures that control weight may help to prevent cancer recurrence, particularly breast cancer.

In their paper on nutrition and physical activity during and after cancer treatment [38], the American Cancer Society (ACS) advises that, throughout the cancer continuum, individuals should aim to achieve and maintain a healthy weight. Noting that people can become malnourished and underweight at diagnosis or after treatments, interventions for these people should aim to increase food intake and regain a positive energy balance. For cancer survivors who are overweight or obese, ACS recommends that modest weight loss (up to 2 lb/week) can be encouraged during treatment: 'as long as the treating oncologists approve, weight loss is monitored closely, and weight loss does not interfere with treatment'. After cancer treatment, weight gain or loss should be managed with a combination of dietary and physical activity strategies. Modest weight loss (5–10%) is encouraged even if ideal weight is not achieved.

2.3.7 Conclusion

There is now considerable evidence that associates excess body weight with the development of cancer at several sites. The mechanisms involved vary by cancer site, although hormonal, inflammatory and metabolic factors are implicated. As yet, there is no trial evidence on weight loss and reduction of cancer rates. However, observational evidence, notably from cohorts of people who have undergone bariatric surgery, suggests a significant effect on overall cancer reduction, especially in women over a relatively short time frame. Even modest weight loss has been observed to be associated with cancer risk reduction, although there is insufficient data to analyse this reduction by cancer site, and the effects are likely to be modest in men. There is some evidence that weight loss can be achieved by people with known cancer risk, but full-scale trials would confirm these observations. Current advice for patients with cancer should take into account weight status, with the aim of weight gain in the malnourished, and modest weight loss for the overweight and obese, achieved through a nutrient-dense diet, increased physical activity and behavioural techniques.

2.3.8 Summary box

Key points

- Weight gain, overweight and obesity are associated with increased occurrence, morbidity and mortality in several cancer sites: the breast (postmenopausal), colorectum, endometrium, kidney, pancreas, oesophagus and gall bladder.
- The mechanisms for these associations vary by site, but may be explained by metabolic and hormonal abnormalities arising from excess

fat storage. There is evidence that levels of biomarkers – for example, oestradiol, inflammatory markers and sex hormone–binding globulin – are altered by weight loss.
- Intentional weight loss is associated with a reduced incidence of cancer in women, but not in men. Such associations are particularly evident in obesity-related cancers, primarily postmenopausal breast cancer and endometrial cancer.
- Bariatric surgery trials have reported conflicting outcomes, with three of four trials reporting substantial reductions in cancer incidence. Two of these trials noted marked differences in gender, with positive effects found only in women.
- The impact of behavioural weight loss interventions on cancer incidence and recurrence is as yet unknown. Modest weight losses in intervention trials targeting dietary intake have been associated with reductions in breast cancer incidence and recurrence. However, weight loss intervention trials are dependent on the development of robust and acceptable interventions for people at risk of developing cancer.
- Current cancer prevention guidelines recommend being 'as lean as possible within the normal range of body weight', noting that cancer risk starts to increase below the BMI threshold of $25 \, kg/m^2$ for overweight.
- Cancer patients and cancer survivors are advised to maintain a healthy body weight, provided that any weight loss (if overweight or obese) is approved by the treating oncologist, monitored closely and does not interfere with treatment.

References

1. World Health Organization. GLOBOCAN 2008: Estimated cancer incidence, mortality, prevalence and disability-adjusted life years (DALYs) worldwide in 2008 [Internet]. Available from: http://globocan.iarc.fr/, accessed 7 January 2016.
2. Jemel A, Bray F, Center MM, Ferlay J, Ward E, Forman D. Global cancer statistics. *CA: A Cancer Journal for Clinicians* 2011; **61**: 69–90.
3. Wang YC, McPherson K, Marsh T, Gortmaker SL, Brown M. Health and economic burden of the projected obesity trends in the USA and the UK. *Lancet* 2011; **378**(9793): 815–825.
4. House of Commons Select Committee on Health. Third Report of Session 2003–2004: Obesity. London: The Stationary Office; 2004 [Internet]. Available from: http://www.parliament.the-stationery-office.co.uk/pa/cm200304/cmselect/cmhealth/23/23.pdf, accessed 7 January 2016.

5. World Cancer Research Fund / American Institute of Cancer Research. Food, nutrition, physical activity and the prevention of cancer: a global perspective 2007 [Internet]. Available from: http://www.dietandcancerreport.org/, accessed 7 January 2016.

6. Pischon T, Nothlings U, Boeing H. Obesity and cancer. *Proceedings of the Nutrition Society* 2008; **67**(2): 128–145.

7. World Cancer Research Fund (WCRF) / American Institute for Cancer Research. Cancer preventability estimates for body fatness [updated] 2013 [Internet]. Available from: http://www.wcrf.org/int/cancer-facts-figures/preventability-estimates/cancer-preventability-estimates-body-fatness, accessed 7 January 2016.

8. Reeves GK, Pirie K, Beral V, Green J, Spencer E, Bull D. Cancer incidence and mortality in relation to body mass index in the Million Women Study: cohort study. *BMJ* 2007; **335**(7630): 1134.

9. Renehan AG, Tyson M, Egger M, Heller RF, Zwahlen M. Body mass index and incidence of cancer: a systematic review and meta-analysis of prospective observational studies. *Lancet* 2008; **371**(9612): 536–578.

10. Eliasson AH, Colditz G, Rosner B, Willett W, Hankinson SE. Adult weight change and risk of postmenopausal breast cancer. *JAMA* 2006; **296**(2): 193–201.

11. Thygesen LC, Gronbaek M, Johansen C, Fuchs CS, Willett WC, Giovannucci E. Prospective weight change and colon cancer risk in male US health professionals. *International Journal of Cancer* 2008; **123**(5): 1160–1165.

12. Ahn J, Schatzkin A, Lacey JV Jr, Albanes D, Ballard-Barbash R, Adams KF, et al. Adiposity, adult weight change and postmenopausal breast cancer risk. *Archives of Internal Medicine* 2007; **167**(19): 2091–2102.

13. Anderson AS, Caswell S. Obesity management – an opportunity for cancer prevention. *Surgeon* 2009; **7**(5): 282–285.

14. Vigneri P, Frasca F, Sciacca L, Frittitta L, Vigneri R. Obesity and cancer. *Nutrition Metabolism and Cardiovascular Diseases* 2006; **16**(1): 1–7.

15. Giovannucci E. Metabolic syndrome, hyperinsulinemia and colon cancer: a review. *American Journal of Clinical Nutrition* 2007; **86**(3): s836–s842.

16. Travis RC, Key TJ. Oestrogen exposure and breast cancer risk. *Breast Cancer Research* 2003; **5**(5): 239–247.

17. Byers T, Sedjo RL. Does intentional weight loss reduce cancer risk? *Diabetes Obesity & Metabolism* 2011; **13**(12): 1063–1072.

18. Rothwell PM, Wilson M, Elwin CE, Norrving B, Algra A, Warlow CP, et al. Long-term effect of aspirin on colorectal cancer incidence and mortality: 20-year follow-up of five randomised trials. *Lancet* 2010; **376**(9754): 1741–1750.

19. Birks S, Peeters A, Backholer K, O'Brien P, Brown W. A systematic review of the impact of weight loss on cancer incidence and mortality. *Obesity Reviews* 2012; **13**(10): 868–891.

20. Parker ED, Folsom AR. Intentional weight loss and incidence of obesity-related cancers: the Iowa Women's Health Study. *International Journal of Obesity and Related Metabolic Disorders* 2003; **27**(12): 1447–1452.

21. Harvie M, Howell A, Vierkant RA, Kumar N, Cerhan JR, Kelemen LE, et al. Association of gain and loss of weight before and after menopause with risk of postmenopausal breast cancer in the Iowa women's health study. *Cancer Epidemiology Biomarkers & Prevention* 2005; **14**(3): 656–661.

22. Williamson D, Pamuk E, Thun M, et al. Prospective study of intentional weight loss and mortality in never-smoking overweight US white women aged 40–64 years. *American Journal of Epidemiology* 1995; **141**: 1128–1141.

23. Williamson D, Pamuk E, Thun M, et al. Prospective study of intentional weight loss and mortality in overweight white men aged 40–64 years. *American Journal of Epidemiology* 1999; **149**: 491–503.

24. Prentice R, Caan B, Chlebowski RT. Low-fat dietary pattern and risk of invasive breast cancer: The Women's Health Initiative Randomized Controlled Dietary Modification Trial. *JAMA* 2006; **295**(6): 629–642.

25. Pierce JP, Natarajan L, Caan BJ. Influence of a diet very high in vegetables, fruit, and fiber and low in fat on prognosis following treatment for breast cancer: The Women's Healthy Eating and Living (WHEL) randomized trial. *JAMA* 2007; **298**(3): 289–298.

26. Chlebowski RT, Blackburn GL, Thomson CA, Nixon DW, Shapiro A, Hoy MK, et al. Dietary fat reduction and breast cancer outcome: interim efficacy results from the Women's Intervention Nutrition Study. *Journal of the National Cancer Institute* 2006; **98**(24): 1767–1776.

27. Sjöström L, Gummesson A, Sjöström CD, Narbro K, Peltonen M, Wedel H, et al. Effects of bariatric surgery on cancer incidence in obese patients in Sweden (Swedish Obese Subjects Study): a prospective, controlled intervention trial. *The Lancet Oncology* 2009; **10**(7): 653–662.

28. Adams TD, Stroup AM, Gress RE, Adams KF, Calle EE, Smith SC, et al. Cancer incidence and mortality after gastric bypass surgery. *Obesity* 2009; **17**(4): 796–802.

29. Christou NV, Lieberman M, Sampalis F, Sampalis JS. Bariatric surgery reduces cancer risk in morbidly obese patients. *Surgery for Obesity and Related Diseases* 2008; **4**(6): 691–695.

30. Ostlund MP, Lu Y, Lagergren J. Risk of obesity-related cancer after obesity surgery in a population-based cohort study. *Annals of Surgery* 2010; **252**(6): 972–976.

31. Imayama I, Ulrich CM, Alfano CM, et al. Effects of a caloric restriction weight loss diet and exercise on inflammatory biomarkers in overweight/obese postmenopausal women: a randomised trial. *Cancer Research* 2012; **72**(9): 2314–2326.

32. Harvie MN, Pegington M, Mattson MP, Frystyk J, Dillon B, Evans G, et al. The effects of intermittent or continuous energy restriction on weight loss and metabolic disease risk markers: a randomized trial in young overweight women. *International Journal of Obesity* 2011; **35**(5): 714–727.

33. Rock CL, Byers TE, Colditz GA, et al. Reducing breast cancer recurrence with weight loss, a vanguard trial: the exercise and Nutrition to Enhance recovery and Good Health for You (ENERGY) trial. *Contemporary Clinical Trials* 2012; **34**(2): 282–295.

34. Anderson AS, Caswell S, Wells M, Steele RJ, Macaskill S. 'It makes you feel so full of life' LiveWell, a feasibility study of a

personalised lifestyle programme for colorectal cancer survivors. *Supportive Care in Cancer* 2010; **18**(4): 409–415.

35. Ruta DA, Garratt AM, Leng M, Russell IT, MacDonald LM. A new approach to measurement of quality of life: The Patient-Generated Index. *Medical Care* 1994; **3**(11): 1109–1126.

36. Craigie AM, Caswell S, Paterson C, Treweek S, Belch JJ, Daly F, et al. Study protocol for BeWEL: the impact of a BodyWEight and physicaL activity intervention on adults at risk of developing colorectal adenomas. *BMC Public Health* 2011; **11**: 184.

37. Stead M, Caswell S, Craigie AM, Eadie D, Anderson AS, the BeWEL team. Understanding the potential and challenges of adenoma treatment as a prevention opportunity. *Preventive Medicine* 2011; **54**(1): 97–103.

38. Doyle C, Kushi LH, Byers T, Courneya KS, Demark-Wahnefried W, Grant B, et al. for the 2006 Nutrition, Physical Activity and Cancer Survivorship Advisory Committee. Nutrition and physical activity during and after cancer treatment: an American Cancer Society guide for informed choices. *CA: A Cancer Journal for Clinicians* 2006; **56**(6): 323–353.

Chapter 2.4

Obesity as a risk factor in osteoarthritis and pulmonary disease

Pia Christensen

University of Copenhagen, Copenhagen, Denmark

2.4.1 Osteoarthritis – disease pathogenesis and consequences

Osteoarthritis (OA) is a common chronic, progressive musculoskeletal disorder characterised by gradual loss of articular cartilage. The disease most commonly affects the middle-aged and elderly, although it may begin earlier in life as a result of injury or limb overuse. It often manifests more acutely and over the longer term in weight-bearing joints such as the knee, hip and spine than in the wrist, elbow, and shoulder joints. All joints may be more affected if they are used extensively in work or sports, or if they have been damaged from fractures or other injuries. OA is a multifactorial disease with obesity as one of the main risk factors. It is a common disorder of synovial joints, and the whole joint is involved. It is a leading cause of chronic disability and has a significant impact on health-related quality of life [1]. The global prevalence of OA continues to rise, both because of an ageing population as well as because of the current obesity epidemic, with obesity in the elderly becoming an increasing problem [2].

OA can occur in any synovial joint in the body, but it is most common in the hands, knees, hips and spine. OA is pathologically characterised by areas of damage to the articular cartilage, centred on load-bearing areas, associated with new bone formation at the joint margins (osteophytes), changes in subchondral bone, variable degrees of mild synovitis and thickening of the joint capsule [3]. OA is regarded as a complex disease whose cause is not completely understood. The diagnosis is based on clinical presentation supported by radiography. Knee OA is the most common form of joint disease in people aged 50 years or more, and the prevalence of knee pain and symptomatic knee OA has increased substantially over the last 20 years [4]. Women have higher prevalence than men [5], and, in addition to sex, the main risk factors for radiographic changes include age, family history, joint injuries, selected activities and obesity [3].

Pain is the most prominent and disabling symptom of OA. The pain of OA is activity-related, with pain generally only coming on when a person carries out specific activities that induce the pain. For example, in persons with knee OA, walking up and down stairs often produces pain, whereas lying in bed most frequently does not. In more advanced disease, it is painful at rest and at night. OA accounts for more mobility disability in the elderly than any other disease. In the 1986 diagnostic criteria, recommended by the Diagnostic and Therapeutic Criteria Committee of the American Rheumatism Association, the presence of knee pain is required for the clinical diagnosis of knee OA [6]. Consequently, pain is the target for most treatment modalities, and their influence on pain is the key factor when evaluating the effect of a treatment [7]. Other clinical features of knee OA include joint stiffness, swelling and deformation [8] (Figure 2.4.1).

Advanced Nutrition and Dietetics in Obesity, First Edition. Edited by Catherine Hankey.
© 2018 John Wiley & Sons Ltd. Published 2018 by John Wiley & Sons Ltd.

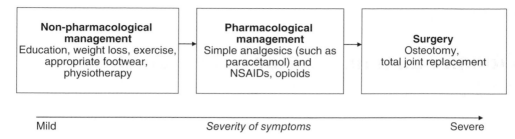

Figure 2.4.1 The spectrum of OA and its management. Source: Adapted from reference [8].

OA: clinical management

OA should be managed on an individual level and will, in most cases, consist of a combination of treatment options. The initial treatment of OA focuses primarily on assisting patients in changing their lifestyles (Figure 2.4.1). Treatment involves alleviating pain, and the aim of disease management is to educate the patients about how to handle living with the disease: how to control pain, improve function, and alter the disease process and its consequences. The hierarchy of management is recommended to consist of non-pharmacological treatments at first, then drugs, and then, if necessary, surgery [8,9].

In the newest guidelines for non-pharmacological treatment of knee OA from the American College of Rheumatology (ACR), the strongest recommendations focus on modifying lifestyle: the patients should participate in specialised exercise (cardiovascular and/or resistance land-based exercise plus aquatic exercise), and overweight patients should lose weight. A list of 10 other non-pharmacological approaches are conditionally recommended, such as participating in self-management programmes, wearing insoles, using walking aids as needed and participating in tai chi programmes [10]. Whereas the ACR guidelines point out approaches to be undertaken, they are very general and not very specific about content, timing, intensity, duration and mode of delivery. In the current European guidelines from the European League Against Rheumatism (EULAR), the aim is to produce detailed recommendations for patient care, and the end-result is 11 propositions, all with very detailed descriptions [11].

The pharmacological management of OA involves mostly oral analgesics [12]. Glucosamine compounds have also been debated, as they may have structure-modifying effects. However, the latest recommendation from the ACR is not to use glucosamine [10]. Intra-articular steroids and hyaluronan are other pharmacological treatment options, but both have very short lasting effects [13].

Surgery should be avoided if symptoms can be managed with other treatment options, and is therefore only recommended for patients with severe symptoms [8,10]. Surgical treatment is generally reserved for failed medical management, with functional disability affecting a patient's quality of life. Obese individuals with OA are more likely to require surgery, as shown by a case–control study involving >7000 individuals, which demonstrated a strong association between increasing BMI and total hip and knee replacements [14].

Obesity and weight loss in OA

The coexistence of OA and obesity has been recognised by epidemiologists for decades [15,16]. Obesity and OA share pathogenic features, and the development of one disease increases the risk of the other and may therefore be the onset of a vicious circle [17]. Excess weight may act through two different mechanisms to cause OA. One, which is the most obvious, is that the increased weight in itself increases the joint loading. This could induce stress on the cartilage, which may lead to trauma and breakdown, which would then lead to OA. The second mechanism involves a systemic factor. This could work as a growth factor that accelerates cartilage breakdown or affect the bone underneath the cartilage, and thereby lead to OA. Adipose tissue is metabolically active, especially in postmenopausal women, who have the highest risk of knee OA. Load, therefore, almost certainly plays a role in triggering the disease in many cases, but will probably be aided by a systemic factor [16]. This systemic factor or several factors may on their own also stimulate the development of OA, since part of the OA population are not obese [18].

OA has traditionally been regarded as non-inflammatory arthritis, but improved detection methods show that the inflammatory pathways are upregulated. These and other clinical and laboratory data suggest that there is a role for inflammation in OA, at least in some patients and in some phases of the disease. Several of the environmental risk factors mentioned (obesity, joint injury, joint overload) are mechanical.

Relative loss of muscle mass and strength over time also contributes to the onset of OA in obese individuals. Although muscle as well as fat mass increases with weight gain, overall, the volume of muscle mass remains relatively low and inadequate to match the loads placed upon it [19].

Furthermore, recent evidence from the Intensive Diet and Exercise for Arthritis study suggests that weight loss may have anti-inflammatory as well as biomechanical benefits in obese subjects with concomitant knee OA, as evidenced by reduced levels of IL-6 [20]. Intriguingly, although a definite association exists between obesity and OA in weight-bearing joints such as the knee and hip, obesity is also associated with the development of OA in non-weight-bearing joints, such as those in the hand. This suggests that non-mechanical risk factors must also play a part [21].

Also worthy of note is the association of obesity and OA with metabolic abnormalities, such as hyperinsulinaemia and other cardiometabolic defects. OA of the knee is associated with hyperinsulinaemia, which may play a role in OA in overweight patients, possibly via changes in insulin-like growth factor-1 [22].

Weight loss is recommended as a treatment option for overweight and obese patients with knee OA [10,23,24]. The immediate effect of weight loss will be an improvement in the joint symptoms [17,25]. One systematic review and meta-analysis has assessed changes in pain and function from randomised controlled trials applying weight loss strategies in obese patients with knee OA. The major finding was the association between improvements in physical disability and weight reduction, and that disability reduction could be predicted from weight loss. The patient's weight loss has to be at least 5% within a 20-week period to experience symptomatic relief, with greater weight loss leading to a larger effect [26].

While loss of approximately 5% of body weight has been shown to provide some relief in obese patients with OA, several studies have indicated that the ultimate goal should be an initial decrease in body weight of at least 10%, in order to provide significant reductions in pain [27,28]. Importantly, concomitant with OA pain reduction comes increased mobility and physical function [28,29].

Weight loss can be particularly difficult to achieve for an OA patient, since the limited physical function most certainly will lead to a limited physical activity level, leading to a decline in energy expenditure. This means that the average OA patient will have difficulty in losing weight based on the general dietetic advice and guidelines for weight loss (i.e. eat less sugar, less fat etc.). This is because their change in energy intake according to such guidelines will not be sufficient to induce weight loss of a magnitude that will motivate and encourage the patient to continue the effort.

In the CAROT study from Copenhagen [30,31], 192 participants with OA were included in a randomised trial in order to lose weight with a formula diet intervention lasting 16 weeks. The participants lost on average 12% of their initial body weight and experienced a highly significant improvement in symptoms [25]. They were followed up for a further 52 weeks, and randomised to one of three interventions aiming to find the optimal treatment to maintain the symptomatic effect of weight loss. The group of participants who followed the control and diet intervention had maintained a significantly larger proportion of the weight loss when combined with the participants randomised to follow specialised knee exercise [31]. The symptomatic responses were similar in all three groups and were successful in about 50% of the participants at the end of the trial visit [32] (Figure 2.4.2).

Quality of life is also improved following weight loss in patients with OA, as evidenced by

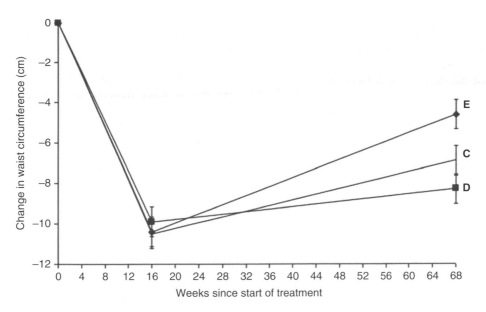

Figure 2.4.2 Adjusted changes in waist circumference by different weight loss interventions (error bars indicate standard error). D diet; E exercise; C control. Source: Taken from reference [31].

improvements in the composite physical health score in the Short Form-36 Health Survey, as well as improvements in satisfaction with body function and appearance [33].

For all obese patients with OA, weight loss should be advocated as a first-line management approach, with a goal of rapid initial weight loss of approximately 10% of body weight. The challenge of maintaining the weight loss and the question of whether weight loss can alter the progression of OA remain key areas of ongoing research. At present, clinicians should manage patients with OA using a combination of methods.

2.4.2 Chronic obstructive pulmonary disease

Chronic obstructive pulmonary disease (COPD) is the third leading cause of death globally. COPD is characterised by airflow obstruction and is associated with severe morbidity and mortality. COPD is the umbrella term for two conditions: chronic bronchitis and emphysema, both of which are related to similar aetiologies and may coexist [34]. The relationship between COPD and body composition has

been extensively studied. Underweight and low BMI are independent risk factors for mortality in patients with COPD [35]. A relationship between COPD and obesity is increasingly recognised, although the nature of this association remains unknown [36]. There is an inverse relationship between a person's BMI and the forced expiratory volume in the first second (FEV1). Increases in body weight lead to worsening of pulmonary function. The role of BMI relative to the risk of impaired lung function has also been investigated. Obesity is known to contribute to other respiratory illnesses, including asthma and sleep apnoea, making it logical to investigate obesity as a risk factor for loss of lung function [37].

A recent meta-analysis concluded that, for patients with COPD, being overweight or obese had a protective effect against mortality. However, the relationship between BMI and mortality in different classes of obesity needed further clarification in well-designed clinical studies [38].

In considering treatment options for COPD, clinicians should consider the possible protective effects of BMI before implementing weight-loss programmes in patients, especially in those with severe lung function impairment. In patients who are overweight or obese, fat-free mass index has been shown

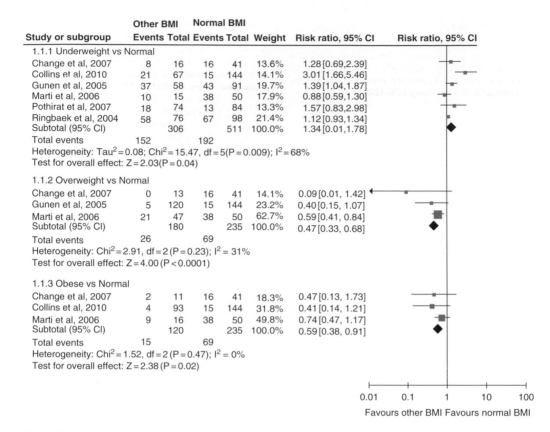

Figure 2.4.3   Relative risks of mortality with BMI among patients with COPD. Source: Taken from reference [38].

to be associated with higher exercise capacity; therefore, therapies that promote weight loss without the loss of lean body mass should be considered [36] (Figure 2.4.3).

2.4.3 Summary box

Key points

• Osteoarthritis is a common chronic, progressive musculoskeletal disorder, regarded as a complex disease whose cause is not completely understood. Pain is the most prominent and disabling symptom of osteoarthritis.

• Osteoarthritis should be managed on an individual level and will, in most cases, consist of a combination of treatment options.

• Weight loss is recommended as a treatment option for overweight and obese patients with knee OA. The immediate effect of weight loss will be an improvement in the joint problems.

• Chronic obstructive pulmonary disease (COPD) is characterised by airflow obstruction and is associated with severe morbidity and mortality. Nutritional issues not only impact patients physically but also psychologically, and clinicians should consider the possible protective effects of BMI before implementing weight-loss programmes in COPD patients.

References

1. Pereira D, Peleteiro B, Araujo J, Branco J, Santos RA, Ramos E. The effect of osteoarthritis definition on prevalence and incidence estimates: a systematic review. *Osteoarthritis and Cartilage* 2011; **19**(11, Nov): 1270–1285.

2. Mathus-Vliegen EM. Prevalence, pathophysiology, health consequences and treatment options of obesity in the elderly: a guideline. *Obesity Facts* 2012; **5**(3): 460–483.

3. Dieppe PA, Lohmander LS. Pathogenesis and management of pain in osteoarthritis. *Lancet* 2005; **365**(9463, Mar): 965–973.

4. Nguyen US, Zhang Y, Zhu Y, Niu J, Zhang B, Felson DT. Increasing prevalence of knee pain and symptomatic knee osteoarthritis: survey and cohort data. *Annals of Internal Medicine* 2011; **155**(11, Dec): 725–732.

5. Srikanth VK, Fryer JL, Zhai G, Winzenberg TM, Hosmer D, Jones G. A meta-analysis of sex differences prevalence, incidence and severity of osteoarthritis. *Osteoarthritis and Cartilage* 2005; **13**(9, Sep): 769–781.

6. Altman R, Asch E, Bloch D, Bole G, Borenstein D, Brandt K, et al. Development of criteria for the classification and reporting of osteoarthritis. Classification of osteoarthritis of the knee. Diagnostic and Therapeutic Criteria Committee of the American Rheumatism Association. *Arthritis and Rheumatism* 1986; **29**(8, Aug): 1039–1049.

7. Pham T, van der Heijde D, Altman RD, Anderson JJ, Bellamy N, Hochberg M, et al. OMERACT-OARSI initiative: Osteoarthritis Research Society International set of responder criteria for osteoarthritis clinical trials revisited. *Osteoarthritis and Cartilage* 2004; **12**(5, May): 389–399.

8. Hunter DJ, Felson DT. Osteoarthritis. *BMJ* 2006; **332**(7542, Mar 18): 639–642.

9. Felson DT. Clinical practice. Osteoarthritis of the knee. *The New England Journal of Medicine* 2006; **354**(8, Feb 23): 841–848.

10. Hochberg MC, Altman RD, April KT, Benkhalti M, Guyatt G, McGowan J, et al. American College of Rheumatology 2012 recommendations for the use of nonpharmacologic and pharmacologic therapies in osteoarthritis of the hand, hip, and knee. *Arthritis Care & Research (Hoboken)* 2012; **64**(4, Apr): 465–474.

11. Fernandes L, Hagen KB, Bijlsma JW, Andreassen O, Christensen P, Conaghan PG, et al. EULAR recommendations for the non-pharmacological core management of hip and knee osteoarthritis. *Annals of the Rheumatic Diseases* 2013; **72**(7, Jul): 1125–1135.

12. Bennell KL, Hunter DJ, Hinman RS. Management of osteoarthritis of the knee. *BMJ* 2012; **345**: e4934.

13. Bellamy N, Campbell J, Robinson V, Gee T, Bourne R, Wells G. Intraarticular corticosteroid for treatment of osteoarthritis of the knee. *Cochrane Database of Systematic Reviews* 2005; **(2)**: CD005328.

14. Wendelboe AM, Hegmann KT, Biggs JJ, Cox CM, Portmann AJ, Gildea JH, et al. Relationships between body mass indices and surgical replacements of knee and hip joints. *American Journal of Preventive Medicine* 2003; **25**(4, Nov): 290–295.

15. van Saase JL, Vandenbroucke JP, van Romunde LK, Valkenburg HA. Osteoarthritis and obesity in the general population. A relationship calling for an explanation. *Journal of Rheumatology* 1988; **15**(7, Jul): 1152–1158.

16. Felson DT. Weight and osteoarthritis. *American Journal of Clinical Nutrition* 1996; **63**(3, Mar): 430S–432S.

17. Bliddal H, Christensen R. The management of osteoarthritis in the obese patient: practical considerations and guidelines for therapy. *Obesity Reviews* 2006; **7**(4, Nov): 323–331.

18. Felson DT, Lawrence RC, Dieppe PA, Hirsch R, Helmick CG, Jordan JM, et al. Osteoarthritis: new insights. Part 1: the disease and its risk factors. *Annals of Internal Medicine* 2000; **133**(8, Oct 17): 635–646.

19. Vincent HK, Heywood K, Connelly J, Hurley RW. Obesity and weight loss in the treatment and prevention of osteoarthritis. *PM & R: The Journal of Injury, Function, and Rehabilitation* 2012; **4**(5, May): S59–S67.

20. Messier SP, Mihalko SL, Legault C, Miller GD, Nicklas BJ, DeVita P, et al. Effects of intensive diet and exercise on knee joint loads, inflammation, and clinical outcomes among overweight and obese adults with knee osteoarthritis: the IDEA randomized clinical trial. *JAMA* 2013; **310**(12, Sep 25): 1263–1273.

21. Yusuf E, Nelissen RG, Ioan-Facsinay A, Stojanovic-Susulic V, DeGroot J, van OG, et al. Association between weight or body mass index and hand osteoarthritis: a systematic review. *Annals of the Rheumatic Diseases* 2010; **69**(4, Apr): 761–765.

22. Silveri F, Brecciaroli D, Argentati F, Cervini C. Serum levels of insulin in overweight patients with osteoarthritis of the knee. *Journal of Rheumatology* 1994; **21**(10, Oct): 1899–1902.

23. Bliddal H, Christensen R. The treatment and prevention of knee osteoarthritis: a tool for clinical decision-making. *Expert Opinion on Pharmacotherapy* 2009; **10**(11, Aug): 1793–1804.

24. Zhang W, Nuki G, Moskowitz RW, Abramson S, Altman RD, Arden NK, et al. OARSI recommendations for the management of hip and knee osteoarthritis: part III: Changes in evidence following systematic cumulative update of research published through January 2009. *Osteoarthritis and Cartilage* 2010; **18**(4, Apr): 476–499.

25. Riecke BF, Christensen R, Christensen P, Leeds AR, Boesen M, Lohmander LS, et al. Comparing two low-energy diets for the treatment of knee osteoarthritis symptoms in obese patients: a pragmatic randomized clinical trial. *Osteoarthritis and Cartilage* 2010; **18**(6, Jun): 746–754.

26. Christensen R, Bartels EM, Astrup A, Bliddal H. Effect of weight reduction in obese patients diagnosed with knee osteoarthritis: a systematic review and meta-analysis. *Annals of the Rheumatic Diseases* 2007; **66**(4, Apr): 433–439.

27. Riddle DL, Stratford PW. Body weight changes and corresponding changes in pain and function in persons with symptomatic knee osteoarthritis: a cohort study. *Arthritis Care & Research (Hoboken)* 2013; **65**(1, Jan): 15–22.

28. Christensen R, Astrup A, Bliddal H. Weight loss: the treatment of choice for knee osteoarthritis? A randomized trial. *Osteoarthritis and Cartilage* 2005; **13**(1, Jan): 20–27.

29. Messier SP, Loeser RF, Miller GD, Morgan TM, Rejeski WJ, Sevick MA, et al. Exercise and dietary weight loss in overweight and obese older adults with knee osteoarthritis: the Arthritis, Diet, and Activity Promotion Trial. *Arthritis and Rheumatism* 2004; **50**(5, May): 1501–1510.

30. Christensen P, Bliddal H, Riecke BF, Leeds AR, Astrup A, Christensen R. Comparison of a low-energy diet and a very low-energy diet in sedentary obese individuals: a pragmatic randomized controlled trial. *Clinical Obesity* 2011; **1**: 31–40.

31. Christensen P, Frederiksen R, Bliddal H, Riecke BF, Bartels EM, Henriksen M, et al. Comparison of three weight maintenance programs on cardiovascular risk, bone and vitamins in sedentary older adults. *Obesity (Silver Spring)* 2013; **21**(10, Oct): 1982–1990.

32. Christensen R, Henriksen M, Leeds AR, Gudbergsen H, Christensen P, Sorensen TJ, et al. The effect of weight maintenance on symptoms of knee osteoarthritis in obese patients: 12 month randomized controlled trial. *Arthritis Care & Research (Hoboken)* 2015; **67**(5, May): 640–650.

33. Rejeski WJ, Focht BC, Messier SP, Morgan T, Pahor M, Penninx B. Obese, older adults with knee osteoarthritis: weight loss, exercise, and quality of life. *Health Psychology* 2002; **21**(5, Sep): 419–426.

34. Hanson C, Rutten EP, Wouters EF, Rennard S. Influence of diet and obesity on COPD development and outcomes. *International Journal of Chronic Obstructive Pulmonary Disease* 2014; **9**: 723–733.

35. Landbo C, Prescott E, Lange P, Vestbo J, Almdal TP. Prognostic value of nutritional status in chronic obstructive pulmonary disease. *American Journal of Respiratory and Critical Care Medicine* 1999; **160**(6, Dec): 1856–1861.

36. Franssen FM, O'Donnell DE, Goossens GH, Blaak EE, Schols AM. Obesity and the lung: 5. Obesity and COPD. *Thorax* 2008; **63**(12, Dec): 1110–1117.

37. McClean KM, Kee F, Young IS, Elborn JS. Obesity and the lung: 1. Epidemiology. *Thorax* 2008; **63**(7, Jul): 649–654.

38. Cao C, Wang R, Wang J, Bunjhoo H, Xu Y, Xiong W. Body mass index and mortality in chronic obstructive pulmonary disease: a meta-analysis. *PLoS One* 2012; **7**(8): e43892.

Chapter 2.5

Psychology and mental health issues in obesity

Louise Waters and Chris Williams
University of Glasgow, Glasgow, UK

Obesity research to date has focused on understanding the physical-health-related outcomes linked to overweight and obesity (e.g. increased risk of diabetes, myocardial infarction, osteoarthritis) [1]. More recent studies have investigated the links between psychosocial well-being and obesity.

From a bio-psychosocial perspective, obesity is multifactorial in cause, and as such the answers are also multifactorial. This provides an individualised understanding of obesity, but also sees the occurrence of obesity within the wider societal context that shapes these individual responses.

2.5.1 Attitudes towards shape and weight vary with time and place

Particularly within Western society, a premium is currently placed on beauty, with concepts of the 'ideal' body shape being viewed as ultra-slim and athletic [2]. Thinness is seen as safe, attractive and controlled. Fatness is associated with labels such as lazy, unattractive and uncontrolled. Consequently, overweight and obese individuals are often stigmatised [3], with obese individuals (particularly children and adolescents) being more likely to experience verbal abuse [4], social isolation and low self-esteem [5].

These 'ideals' are represented in many types of advertising and media. This includes the routine touching up of images to remove skin blemishes, enhance figures or stretch legs that are not thought to reflect the right sort of image. It has been suggested that up to 38% of women are on a weight loss diet at any one time [6]. These pressures apply to both men and women – with an increased emphasis on men needing to appear athletic and fit in shaving and other male-grooming adverts.

These pressures are in contrast to the consistent increases in population average weight over the last 20 years [7]. However, these values are socially driven and fluid. The notion of attractiveness and its prerequisites have changed greatly in recent centuries, and this may have had an influence on body image and the emergence of a dieting culture [8]. For example, in the sixteenth century, voluptuous women who appeared fertile and physically able to bear children were considered highly attractive, featuring in many examples of fine art from this era [8]. Sumo wrestlers in Japan are large and weighty – yet are feted as supreme sportsmen. Similarly, the Inuit tribes see obesity in women as being sexually attractive.

Such values change with time and place, and have become more extreme quite quickly in Westernised societies. A study of adult magazine centrefolds from between the 1970s and 1990s found an increasing discrepancy between the shape and weight (vital statistics) of the models, and this increasingly diverged from the 'real' weight of women as outlined in actuarial figures [9]. Similarly, the number of dietary articles in women's magazines has increased, and are often juxtaposed with articles

Advanced Nutrition and Dietetics in Obesity, First Edition. Edited by Catherine Hankey.
© 2018 John Wiley & Sons Ltd. Published 2018 by John Wiley & Sons Ltd.

such as to 'Be your own woman' and 'how to cook the perfect chocolate cake'. These changes have occurred in spite of studies finding that many men do not find thin, waif-like women attractive [10]. These pressures are not limited to the Western world. The rates of occurrence of eating disorders, once thought to be Western-only diseases, have now increased significantly in Asian communities, as Westernised values are being adopted across the world [11].

These different messages from society and from families shape attitudes towards food. Food is no longer seen just as food and a source of nutrition and health. It is seen as branded (Michelin-starred restaurants, celebrity chefs) and aspirational (with special, more expensively prepared ranges of foods in supermarkets). The end result is that value judgements in terms of weight are often made in society, and people start to negatively judge themselves in terms of their shape and weight.

Some additional aspects regarding peoples' relationships with food and psychology will help us understand the psychosocial factors that may promote obesity (Box 2.5.1).

2.5.2 Mental health issues and obesity

Among obese adults, low self-esteem has been associated with increased sadness and loneliness. A link between obesity and the likelihood of engaging in behaviours such as smoking and alcohol abuse has been demonstrated [19]. However, despite the purported links between obesity and psychosocial factors, many weight management interventions still primarily focus on physical health outcomes, paying little attention to the wider psychosocial outcomes [20]. An individual's psychosocial well-being may play an important role in increasing his or her motivation to participate in weight management interventions. However, such conditions are also important in their own right as low mood and anxiety are distressing, and may contribute to inactivity, poorer diet, alcohol misuse and comfort eating. Hence, research suggests that there may be an association between obesity and certain psychopathologies, in particular, anxiety and depression [21]. Thus, understanding

psychosocial factors and their associations with obesity seems an essential part of increasing the efficacy of weight management programmes.

Obesity and depression

According to the World Health Organization (WHO), depression affects approximately 350 million people globally and is among the leading causes of disability [22]. The high prevalence of both obesity and depression may be an indication of an association between the two disorders [23], with a considerable number of population-based studies being conducted to examine these potential associations.

From a psychiatric view point, such an association might be expected, since, as per the *Diagnostic and Statistical Manual of Mental Disorders* (fifth edition) [24], symptoms of depression include both an increase in food intake and a decrease in physical activity, two symptoms also associated with weight gain [25]. In addition, other psychosocial variables such as negative body image and stigmatisation of obese individuals can lead to low self-esteem and other symptoms of depression and psychological distress [26]. However, such a relationship has yet to be ascertained in community-based samples [23]. Nevertheless, even if rates of depression are no higher than normal in patients with obesity, the prevalence in society is so high that, even at average prevalence rates, it is a significant issue. It matters clinically because of the known association between comfort eating and depression, reduced activity (meaning less energy is used) and lack of motivation – all of which make decisions to make sustained weight change more difficult.

There are, however, a number of limitations that need to be considered when reviewing this area of research. Friedman and Brownell (1995) [27] point out in their extensive review of literature that the variability of findings in areas such as psychopathology and obesity is unsurprising, given the various methodologies and outcome measures used, together with the heterogeneity of the obese population and lack of focus on moderators of the obesity/mental health relationship. In addition, the range of mental health disorders explored has been limited, mainly focusing on major depressive disorders [28].

Box 2.5.1   Psychosocial factors that may promote obesity

(a) *Food is enjoyable to eat*

There is increased likelihood of a behaviour occurring if it is associated with reward. For eating, these rewards are twofold – first, negative reinforcement of eating by a reduction in aversive feelings (hunger); and second, the enjoyment of the taste itself. In animal studies, rats and others can be encouraged to do tasks for food rewards. Certain foods specifically stimulate the brain's reward centres, especially those rich in fat, carbohydrate and salt. It has been argued that junk foods (which are highly marketed and available) are designed to maximise these tastes.

(b) *Food as a source of comfort (comfort eating)*

When a child falls over and cries, many parents give them sweets to help them settle. It has been argued that this action associates soothing and hugs with the carbohydrate taste. Later in life, that pattern is repeated by using food to self-sooth/self-medicate against a range of aversive emotional states such as anger, anxiety, depression/sadness, guilt or shame, as well as during times of high stress [12,13].

(c) *Food as a medium for communication*

Most people can identify with times when they visited a relative or friend for a meal, and felt some pressure to say they enjoyed the food and to accept additional servings. Declining or saying that you did not enjoy what was offered would be rude and rejecting to the host. The key point is that people can feel pressure to eat when eating with others, and to act like they enjoy it, even if they do not. Social facilitation studies have also shown that eating with friends and family can increase food intake as engaging with others can draw attention away from the eaten food, thus stimulating food intake [14].

(d) *Food as a means of control or rejection of control*

Characteristic of *bulimia nervosa* and *binge eating disorder* is a sense of loss of control over eating. In contrast, in *anorexia nervosa*, control is paramount. People with anorexia often talk about feeling that the rigid control they exert over their appetite, weight and shape is one of the few areas in their lives they feel they can control. Mealtimes become a source of high emotion, with concerned parents sometimes wrapping their daughter or son in cotton wool, or shouting and threatening them unless they eat. These examples of so-called high expressed emotion are understandable, but are known to worsen outcomes [15].

(e) *Eating, shame and avoidance*

Eating can be enjoyable, yet for some it becomes very shameful. Many people with obesity feel embarrassed about how they look [16]. A proportion of overweight men and women also binge on food, and can go onto develop binge eating disorder or bulimia nervosa, when they act to reverse the binge eating by vomiting, missing meals or using laxatives or exercise to lose energy. People with binge eating disorder and bulimia often fail to present because of embarrassment and stigma [17], and may avoid eating in public or with those they know. People who binge often describe self-regret, self-loathing and low mood post-bingeing. All in all, obesity is associated with significant emotional impacts, whether it be in childhood or adulthood [18].

Anxiety and obesity

Anxiety disorders represent the most prevalent mental health disorders in the Western world, with 25% of individuals being affected by some variant of anxiety disorder at some point in their life [29]. Anxiety disorders are marked by a range of psychological symptoms that include excessive worry, fear and apprehension, alongside physical symptoms such as fatigue, palpitations, shortness of breath and difficulty sleeping.

Obesity may be a risk factor for anxiety disorders [30], with other research also suggesting a reverse relationship – that is, anxiety disorders acting as a risk factor for obesity [31]. A range of pathways through which obesity and anxiety disorders may be linked have been suggested. For example, similar to the links with depression, weight-related stigmatisation and discrimination may be distressing to individuals, leading to feelings of anxiety and strategies such as avoidance/staying at home in order to not encounter the discrimination [32]. This in turn may lead to increased energy intake and a decrease in physical and social activities, which may lead to further weight gain. Additionally, it has been suggested that the negative effects that obesity may have on physical health and quality of life may be particularly stressful and isolating [33], thus increasing the likelihood of anxiety. The less people do, the worse they feel. Then, the worse they feel, the less they do. Obese individuals may feel increased pressure from others around them to gain control over their weight; this can be distressing, particularly if they have experienced repeated failure at losing weight. Such preoccupation with dieting and weight loss has been shown to be correlated with anxiety [34]. Anxiety is also documented as representing a trigger for emotional eating, with experimental evidence suggesting that anxiety increases food consumption in obese individuals [35].

However, overall, research suggesting a link between obesity and anxiety remains equivocal, with some studies identifying strong relationships between the two disorders, while others have failed to find a significant relationship [36]. A potential reason for the mixed findings is the heterogeneous nature of both obesity and anxiety disorders, with the relationship between the two disorders potentially differing between the different sub-groups of society who have different socio-demographic, biological and behavioural characteristics. Hence, values of what is seen as attractive and normal may vary between individuals and also groups in society. For example, Puhl and Heuer (2009) [37] suggest that, because of the greater social pressure on women to conform to an 'ideal' body shape and the resulting discrimination that is seen towards obese women, obesity may be more strongly related to anxiety disorders in females compared to males. Although a review of all the relevant studies is beyond the scope of this chapter, a recent systematic review and meta-analysis by Gariepy, Nitka and Schmitz (2010) provides a good overview of the findings in this area [36].

2.5.3 Addressing the mixed messages

Cognitive behavioural therapy (CBT) [38] provides a means of making sense of these discrepant results. It argues that what people think affects how they feel and what they do. Hence, if two people are overweight, one might feel entirely comfortable about his/her shape and weight, and see himself/herself as big and beautiful. In contrast, the other might hate how he/she looks, feel his/her eating is out of control and have an eating pattern characterised by avoidance and swinging between every new diet, and then failure, which may lead to his/her feeling he/she has crashed back with significant depression. As how the person feels also can affect behaviour, the worsening of anxiety and depression can lead to additional behaviours such as withdrawal, avoidance, drinking too much, comfort eating or acting in ways that confirm to themselves how bad and unattractive they are (such as by eating too much). This vicious circle [39] is summarised in Figure 2.5.1.

A vicious circle can arise where changes in any of the five areas can create or worsen problems in any of the others. However, the implication is that making changes in any of the areas can also lead to improvements in the other aspects of life. CBT provides a framework for helping people work out why they feel as they do, identify problems relevant to them and then work on making changes using a planned step-by-step plan. The individualised summary is jointly shared, and problems worked on with support from a practitioner. This assessment has various possible targets for change – around assertiveness and saying no, dealing with upsetting thoughts, stabilising eating and more. Help could be offered by specialist CBT workers, but more likely be gained from using CBT self-help resources such as books that have a proven evidence base and are recommended for anxiety and depression [40–42]. These books, with support from a practitioner, can provide a useful framework for change that can tackle the important comorbidities of depression and anxiety.

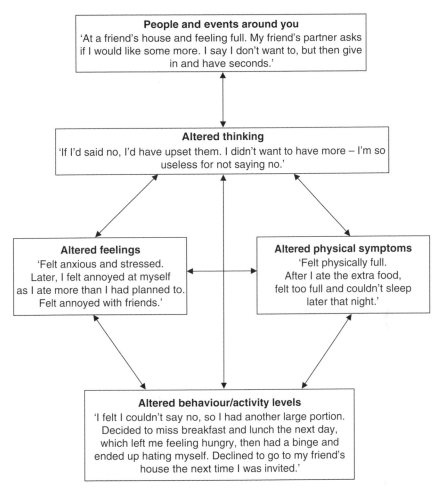

People and events around you
'At a friend's house and feeling full. My friend's partner asks if I would like some more. I say I don't want to, but then give in and have seconds.'

Altered thinking
'If I'd said no, I'd have upset them. I didn't want to have more – I'm so useless for not saying no.'

Altered feelings
'Felt anxious and stressed. Later, I felt annoyed at myself as I ate more than I had planned to. Felt annoyed with friends.'

Altered physical symptoms
'Felt physically full. After I ate the extra food, felt too full and couldn't sleep later that night.'

Altered behaviour/activity levels
'I felt I couldn't say no, so I had another large portion. Decided to miss breakfast and lunch the next day, which left me feeling hungry, then had a binge and ended up hating myself. Declined to go to my friend's house the next time I was invited.'

Figure 2.5.1 The Five Areas assessment model showing vicious circles to understand how the person feels (Williams 2009).

2.5.4 Conclusion

Obesity poses a significant challenge for individuals, families and society. Although seen predominantly as a physical condition associated with additional physical comorbidities, there is a significant personal cost in terms of low confidence, depression, anxiety and associated eating disorders such as bulimia nervosa and binge eating disorder. This chapter brings together these individual psychosocial factors and views them as part of a vicious circle, including personal beliefs. It discusses the impacts of others/wider society and the physical aspects, and finally also the impacts on behaviour/activity level that occur as part of obesity. These crucial 'five areas' provide a CBT formulation that can help individuals and clinicians identify maintaining factors for obesity, and also define key areas to target when planning change. It also encourages seeing the person within a social/systemic situation where the reactions of others also have a key role in affecting longer-term outcomes.

2.5.5 Summary box

Key points

- Attitudes to obesity vary with different cultures. In Western societies, a premium is the 'ideal' body shape – as ultra-slim and athletic. Other cultures regard obesity more positively.
- Adult relationships with food are complex – offering comfort and opportunities for communication, among other things. Food can be associated with binging and a loss of control.
- Many psychological conditions are associated with obesity – such as depression and anxiety.
- Poor psychological health frequently impairs the individual's motivation to participate in weight management interventions.
- Understanding psychosocial factors and studying their associations with obesity seem essential for increasing the effectiveness of weight management programmes.

References

1. Field AE, Coakley EH, Must A, Spadano JL, Laird N, Dietz WH, et al. Impact of overweight on the risk of developing common chronic diseases during a 10-year period. *Archives of Internal Medicine* 2001; **161**: 1581–1586.
2. Brownell K. Dieting and the search for the perfect body: where physiology and culture collide. *Behavior Therapy* 1991; **22**: 1–12.
3. Latner J, Stunkard AJ. Getting worse: the stigmatization of obese children. *Obesity Research* 2003; **11**: 452–456.
4. Falkner NH, Neumark-Sztainer D, Story M, Jeffery RW, Beuhring T, Resnick MD. Social, educational, and psychological correlates of weight status in adolescents. *Obesity Research* 2001; **9**: 32–42.
5. Porter JS, Bean MK, Gerke CK, Stern M. Psychosocial factors and perspectives on weight gain and barriers to weight loss among adolescents enrolled in obesity treatment. *Journal of Clinical Psychology in Medical Settings* 2010; **17**: 98–102.
6. Biener L, Heaton A. Women dieters of normal weight: their motives, goals, and risks. *American Journal of Public Health* 1995; **85**: 714–717.
7. Hill J, Wyatt HR, Reed GW, Peters JC. Obesity and the environment: where do we go from here? *Science* 2003; **299**: 853–855.
8. Vandereycken W. History of anorexia nervosa and bulimia nervosa. In: Fairburn CG, Brownell KD (eds) *Eating Disorders and Obesity*. New York: Guildford Press, 2002, pp. 151–155.
9. Katzmarzyk PT, Davis C. Thinness and body shape of playboy centrefolds from 1978–1998. *International Journal of Obesity and Related Metabolic Disorders* 2001; **25**: 590–592.
10. Rantala MJ, Coetzee V, Moore FR, Skrinda I, Kecko S, Krama T, et al. Facial attractiveness is related to women's cortisol and body fat, but not with immune responsiveness. *Biology Letters* 2013; **9**(4): 20130255.
11. Makino M, Tsuboi K, Dennerstein L. Prevalence of eating disorders: a comparison of Western and non-Western countries. *Medscape General Medicine* 2004; **6**: 49.
12. Adam TC, Epel ES. Stress, eating and the reward system. *Physiology & Behavior* 2007; **91**: 449–458.
13. Dallman MF, Pecoraro NC, la Fleur SE. Chronic stress and comfort foods: self-medication and abdominal obesity. *Brain Behavior and Immunity* 2005; **19**: 275–280.
14. Hetherington MM, Anderson AS, Norton GNM, Newson L. Situational effects on meal intake: A comparison of eating alone and eating with others. *Physiology & Behavior* 2006; **88**: 498–505.
15. Kyriacou O, Treasure J, Schmidt U. Expressed emotion in eating disorders assessed via self-report: an examination of factors associated with expressed emotion in carers of people with anorexia nervosa in comparison to control families. *International Journal of Eating Disorders* 2008; **41**: 37–36.
16. Goodman E, Whitaker RC. A prospective study of the role of depression in the development and persistence of adolescent obesity. *Pediatrics* 2002; **110**: 497–504.
17. Sánchez-Ortiz VC, Munro C, Startup H, Treasure J, Schmidt U. The role of email guidance in Internet-based cognitive-behavioural self-care treatment for bulimia nervosa. *European Eating Disorders Review* 2011; **19**: 342–348.
18. Cornette R. The emotional impact of obesity on children. *Worldviews on Evidence-Based Nursing* 2008; **5**: 136–141.
19. Strauss RS. Childhood obesity and self-esteem. *Pediatrics* 2000; **115**: e15–e19.
20. Barlow SE. Expert committee recommendations regarding the prevention, assessment and treatment of child and adolescent overweight and obesity. *Pediatrics* 2007; **120**(4): 5164–5192.
21. Strine TW, Mokdad AH, Dube SR, Balluz LS, Gonzalez O, Berry JT, et al. The association of depression and anxiety with obesity and unhealthy behaviors among community-dwelling US adults. *General Hospital Psychiatry* 2008; **30**: 127–137.
22. World Health Organization. Fact Sheet 369 – Depression, Geneva. 2012. Available from: http://www.who.int/mediacentre/factsheets/fs369/en/, viewed 7 January 2016.
23. Stunkard AJ, Faith MS, Allison KC. Depression and obesity. *Biological Psychiatry* 2003; **54**: 330–337.
24. American Psychiatric Association. *Diagnostic and Statistical Manual of Mental Disorders*, 5th edn. Washington, DC: APA, 2013.
25. de Wit L, Luppinob F, van Straten A, Penninx B, Zitman F, Cuijpers. Depression and obesity: a meta-analysis of community-based studies. *Psychiatry Research* 2010; **178**: 230–235.
26. Ross CE. Overweight and Depression. *Journal of Health and Social Behavior* 1994; **35**: 63–79.
27. Friedman MA. Brownell KD. Psychological correlates of obesity: moving to the next research generation. *Psychological Bulletin* 1995; **117**: 3–20.
28. Scott KM, McGee MA, Wells JE, Oakley Browne MA. Obesity and mental disorders in the adult general population. *Journal of Psychosomatic Research* 2008; **64**: 97–105.

29. Kessler RC, Wang PS. The descriptive epidemiology of commonly occurring mental disorders in the United States. *Annual Review of Public Health* 2008; **29**: 115–129.

30. Parikh NI, Pencina MJ, Wang TJ, Lanier KJ, Fox CS, D'Agostino RB, et al. Increasing trends in incidence of overweight and obesity over 5 decades. *The American Journal of Medicine* 2007; **120**: 242–250.

31. Canetti L, Bachar E, Berry EM. Food and emotion. *Behavioural Processes* 2002; **60**: 157–164.

32. Ashmore JA, Friedman KE, Reichmann SK, Musante GJ. Weight-based stigmatization, psychological distress, and binge eating behavior among obese treatment-seeking adults. *Eating Behaviors* 2008; **9**: 203–209.

33. Sareen J, Jacobi F, Cox BJ, Belik S-L, Clara I, Stein MB. Disability and poor quality of life associated with comorbid anxiety disorders and physical conditions. *Archives of Internal Medicine* 2006; **166**: 2109–2116.

34. Horner TN, Utermohlen V. A multivariate analysis of psychological factors related to body mass index and eating preoccupation in female college students. *Journal of the American College of Nutrition* 1993; **12**: 459–465.

35. Ganley RM. Emotion and eating in obesity: a review of the literature. *International Journal of Eating Disorders* 1989; **8**: 343–361.

36. Gariepy G, Nitka D, Schmitz N. The association between obesity and anxiety disorders in the population: a systematic review and meta-analysis. *International Journal of Obesity* 2010; **34**: 407–419.

37. Puhl RM, Heuer CA. The stigma of obesity: a review and update. *Obesity* 2009; **17**: 941–964.

38. Beck AT, Rush AJ, Shaw BP, Emery G. *Cognitive Therapy of Depression*. New York: Guilford Press, 1979.

39. Williams CJ. *Overcoming Depression and Low Mood: A Five Areas Approach*. Hodder Arnold: London, 2009.

40. Ridgway N, Williams CJ. Cognitive behavioural therapy self-help for depression: an overview. *Journal of Mental Health* 2011; **20**: 593–603.

41. National Institute for Health and Care Excellence. Generalised anxiety disorder and panic disorder (with or without agoraphobia) in adults. CG113. London: National Institute for Health and Care Excellence, 2007.

42. National Institute for Health and Care Excellence. Depression in adults (update). CG90. London: National Institute for Health and Care Excellence, 2009.

Chapter 2.6

Binge eating and obesity

Gianluca Lo Coco[1] and Lina A Ricciardelli[2]
[1] University of Palermo, Palermo, Italy
[2] Deakin University, Melbourne, Australia

2.6.1 Binge eating and obesity

Despite there being several pathways leading to obesity [1], there is evidence that binge eating may be an important contributor to its development [2]. Excessive food consumption without compensation increases the risk for the development of obesity, which in turn is associated with numerous complications [3]. Obesity has been found to develop several years after the onset of binge eating, and individuals who were overweight prior to the onset of binge eating tend to gain even more weight during adulthood [4].

Binge eating is defined as eating a larger amount of food than normal during a short period of time (within any 2-hour period) and, during this time, experiencing a loss of control over eating. Since the publication of research criteria for binge eating disorder (BED) in the *Diagnostic and Statistical Manual of Mental Disorders* (DSM-IV), substantial research has happened on the various aspects of BED, leading to its inclusion in the recently published DSM-5. BED, which is defined as engaging in frequent binge eating episodes without the concomitant use of compensatory behaviours, was first recognised in DSM-IV as a disorder in need of further study. It is now considered a distinct diagnosis in DSM-5, as there is evidence that affected individuals experience considerable distress and functional impairment associated with frequent binge eating episodes [5] (Box 2.6.1). The lifetime prevalence estimate of BED is 3% among adults and 1.6% among adolescents.

Box 2.6.1 The diagnosis of BED

The chapter titled *Feeding and Eating Disorders* in DSM-5 describes the diagnosis of BED as:

'… recurring episodes of eating significantly more food in a short period of time than most people would eat under similar circumstances, with episodes marked by feelings of lack of control. Someone with binge eating disorder may eat too quickly, even when he or she is not hungry. The person may have feelings of guilt, embarrassment, or disgust and may binge eat alone to hide the behaviour. This disorder is associated with marked distress and occurs, on average, at least once a week over three months'.

Although BED and obesity represent distinct phenomena, BED is the most common eating disorder found in obesity. Nearly 70% of individuals who binge eat have a BMI of $30\,kg/m^2$ and above, whereas slightly fewer than 30% of individuals who do not binge eat report comparable BMIs. It is also estimated that 10% of the obese population [6] and 30% of obese participants in weight reduction programmes have BED [7,8]. BED also occurs in normal-weight persons, but less frequently, and it may predispose individuals towards overweight and obesity. Some studies also show that, among both community and clinic studies, many individuals who meet the criteria for BED are not obese [9].

Binge eating has also been identified to be a main contributing factor to overweight and obesity among

Advanced Nutrition and Dietetics in Obesity, First Edition. Edited by Catherine Hankey.
© 2018 John Wiley & Sons Ltd. Published 2018 by John Wiley & Sons Ltd.

children and adolescents [10]. Other studies have shown that binge eating predicts overweight status in adolescents who were not initially overweight [11,12]. In addition, the prevalence of sub-clinical binge eating among overweight-treatment-seeking adolescents has been found to be similar to the levels reported among adults. Estimates of sub-clinical binge eating among adolescents and children range from 20% to 30%, and severe binge eating is estimated to be approximately 10% [10]. However, it is interesting to note that, in a large study of adolescent girls and boys from Norway, BMI was found to be significantly higher among those who engaged in binge eating with compensatory behaviours in comparison to those who only reported binge eating [13].

Regardless of weight status, it does appear that increased binge eating is associated with a significant amount of distress and dysfunction. Research has shown no differences in overall psychological distress, depressive symptoms as well as concerns about eating and shape between normal/overweight, obese and severely obese men and women diagnosed with BED [14,15]. Overall, distress commonly reported among individuals who binge eat seems not a consequence of weight gain, but most of these studies are based on cross-sectional data only. Further research is warranted to examine the causal relationships between binge eating and BMI.

2.6.2 Characteristics of binge eating in obese individuals

BED is a prevalent problem associated with obesity and is associated with an increased number of medical and psychiatric comorbidities. Furthermore, there is often psychosocial impairment relative to obese persons without BED [16] and hence with an increased healthcare utilisation, particularly in generalist medical settings [17]. Moreover, adults with concurrent binge eating and obesity are typically older, have a longer duration of illness, eat more meals and snacks throughout the day and exercise less than non-obese binge eaters [18]. Similarly, compared to obese adults who do not binge eat, adults with concurrent obesity and binge eating report more psychopathology [19], engage in more overeating episodes [20] and consume more energy

during both meals and binges [21]. Empirical studies also show that obese adults with BED have much more impairment in the psychosocial aspects of quality of life (e.g. work, sex life, self-esteem) than obese individuals without binge eating problems [22]. These findings suggest that, although binge eating and obesity are each associated with physiological and psychological consequences, the combination of BED and obesity may be particularly problematic with regard to comorbidity and risk.

Similar to adults, adolescents with BED are characterised by more eating-related psychopathological features, high levels of body image concerns, higher depressive symptoms, higher social anxiety and poorer self-esteem [10,23]. Binge eating has also been found to be related to impaired quality of life among obese adolescents [10,24]. However, it has been found to have a greater impact on the quality of life for girls than boys. Obese girls who engaged in binge eating showed more impairment in the areas of mobility, self-esteem, activities of daily living, fatigue and sleep, social functioning and work/school [10,24].

One of the reasons why binge eating may have less of a negative impact for adolescent boys is because binge eating is more socially sanctioned for males [25,26]. The nature of binge eating is also different among males, and it may simply reflect overeating. Although a greater number of men report eating large quantities of food at times other than at meals, they are less likely to call this pattern 'binge eating' [27]. Men are also less likely to be troubled by their binge eating and to feel depressed about it, and they also report less guilt [25]. In addition, men are less likely to report a sense of being out of control during binge eating in comparison to women [28]. In one study, Snow and Harris found that adolescent boys (in comparison to girls) thought that binge eating episodes were normal [29].

It is also important to distinguish problem from non-problem binge eating [30]. For many individuals, binge eating is distressing as it affects their physical and emotional health. However, for others, binge eating has no effect on their quality of life. In one of our early studies, we found only problem binge eating among adolescent girls [31]. However, among boys, we found support for both problem and non-problem binge eating. That is, many boys engaged in binge eating without experiencing any negative emotional outcomes such as distress, worry, anxiety or guilt.

Another reason why binge eating may be viewed more positively by boys than girls is because binge eating is one of the strategies that boys may use to attain physical bulk. Specifically, adolescent boys may use binge eating/overeating in combination with weight-loss strategies and the use of food supplements to improve their muscular build [26,32]. However, further studies are needed to more fully evaluate whether this is in fact the case, and whether these strategies may lead to weight gain and obesity later in life.

Interestingly, only a few reports have documented the overlap between BED and night eating syndrome (NES) among obese persons. Although individuals with BED and NES share a feeling of loss of control over their eating, the amount of food they consume during binges and nocturnal eating episodes is quantitatively different. BED individuals eat more frequently during the day than both the NES and only-obese individuals, whereas only 7% of individuals with BED described nocturnal snacking in at least half of the nights [33].

Clinical studies have also shown that binge eating is highly prevalent among obese individuals presenting for bariatric surgery [34]. However, systematic reviews examining pre-surgical binge eating as a predictor of post-surgical weight loss have concluded that most evidence does not support this relationship [35]. Nevertheless, it is noteworthy that pre-surgery binge eating and disordered eating are related to an increased risk of post-surgical uncontrolled eating and 'grazing' [36], and the presence of binge eating post-operatively seems associated with less weight loss or more weight regain. Overall, the factors contributing to successful outcomes after surgery are multiple, and the importance of single-predictive variables (such as binge eating) should not be over-emphasised [37].

2.6.3 Factors to consider in the development and treatment of binge eating and obesity

It has been argued that binge eating behaviour is an emotion regulation strategy for coping with negative feelings such as frustration, and even the depressive symptoms associated with body dissatisfaction [38]. Specifically, binge eating may be used to cope with negative affect by providing immediate distraction or comfort [39].

More recent research, using experience sampling methodologies in the form of ecological momentary assessment, has examined associations between mood and binging behaviours in naturalistic settings. Ecological momentary assessment collects information about target behaviour(s) and relevant experiences, including antecedents and consequences, as they occur naturally during the day. Studies using ecological momentary assessment support that increases in negative affect often precede binge episodes in individuals with BED and bulimia nervosa [40,41]. In addition, these studies have demonstrated that loss-of-control eating episodes among obese individuals are associated with both increased stress and increased negative affect, regardless of whether the episodes were characterised by overeating [42]. Moreover, individuals with BED seem vulnerable to engaging in emotional overeating because they lack adaptive emotion regulation strategies and skills, including being able to identify and cope with emotional states [43].

In summary, research supports a negative affect regulation model for binge eating, which posits that overweight individuals overeat as an attempt to regulate the emotions they are feeling. The increase in negative feelings and mood (i.e. 'I'm feeling sad') triggers binge episodes, and binge eating functions to alleviate negative emotions by using food for comfort and distraction. Binge eating in response to negative emotions becomes a conditioned response that is maintained through negative reinforcement.

It is also noteworthy that a considerable number of studies have documented the pervasiveness of negative weight bias across areas including education, workplace and even healthcare settings [44]. *Weight bias* is defined as the negative attitudes and beliefs attributed to an individual based on his or her body weight. Weight bias leads to stigmatisation of persons with obesity through the attribution of stereotypes such as being lazy, being less intelligent compared to persons without obesity or having no willpower. Moreover, individuals with obesity who internalise this bias also attribute these negative stereotypes to themselves and base their self-evaluation on these stigmatising attitudes. Such widespread stigma is related to a number of negative psycho-logical outcomes, such as more severe depression, body image dissatisfaction, poorer self-esteem, dis-turbed and binge eating [45]. Treatment-seeking obese patients with BED demonstrate high levels of internalised weight bias, which in turn is associated with greater eating psychopathology, depression and lower self-esteem [46].

In addition to negative affect and the stigma associ-ated with obesity, another factor to also consider in both the development and treatment of binge eating among obese individuals is body dissatisfaction. Several studies have demonstrated a strong relation-ship between body dissatisfaction and binge eating [47,19], and there is also evidence in support of binge eating as a mediator of the link between body dissat-isfaction and psychological distress, especially for obese people who seek both dietary and psychologi-cal support [48]. Overweight and obese individuals, including adolescents, who are more dissatisfied with their bodies are more likely to gain weight and com-mence binge eating than those who are more satisfied with their bodies [47]. In addition, a weight control trial of overweight and obese women has shown that improved body satisfaction was associated with a greater reduction in binge eating [49]. This suggests that body satisfaction may protect overweight and obese individuals against excessive weight gain and binge eating. Individuals who are more satisfied with their bodies are likely to feel more positive about themselves in other areas of their lives, have higher levels of self-esteem and also engage in more positive lifestyle behaviours. Thus, body dissatisfaction is an important factor to target in both prevention and treat-ment programmes. Effective programme components for adolescents and adults include increasing resist-ance to sociocultural pressures for thinness, develop-ing healthy weight management skills, developing stress and coping skills and self-esteem training [50]. In addition, media literacy training has also been found to be effective for adolescents [51].

Interestingly, weight reduction programmes that include behavioural and pharmacological compo-nents, on the whole, have shown similar levels of effectiveness in terms of reductions in BMI for obese individuals with or without BED [23]. In addition, although individuals who binge eat dem-onstrate higher loss of control in eating and greater hunger levels.

Despite these challenges, it has been established that weight reduction programmes can be effective at reducing loss of control in eating and hunger lev-els, and also at reducing binge eating. In one pro-gramme with adolescents, binge eating declined from 24% at baseline to 8% at the 6-month follow-up, and to 3% at the 12-month follow-up [23]. The adolescents participated in 24 weeks of group behavioural counselling that addressed lifestyle management, and received the weight loss medica-tion, sibutramine.

Well-controlled studies have demonstrated that cognitive behavioural therapy (CBT) and interper-sonal psychotherapy (IPT) are effective in reducing binge eating and the associated psychological dis-tress, but do not produce clinically significant weight loss [52]. Binge eating recovery rates were equivalent for CBT and IPT at post-treatment (79% vs. 73%) and at 1-year follow-up (59% vs. 62%). It is also noteworthy that, among individuals who recovered from BED post-treatment, those who remained recovered at the 12-month follow-up had lost weight during the course of follow-up (−5.3 lb or −2.4 kg), whereas those who were no longer recovered from BED at the end of the follow-up had gained weight (+4.6 lb or +2.1 kg).

Guided self-help based on CBT is effective in the short term. It has been shown to reduce binge eating without compromising compliance with behavioural weight loss treatments, an approach widely used to treat obesity (and binge eating) [53]. A randomised trial that compared the short- and longer-term outcomes of IPT, CBT self-help and behavioural weight loss treatment for BED found no differences among the three interventions at post-treatment for binge eating and specific eating disorder psychopathology. However, both IPT and CBT self-help were more effective than behavioural weight loss treatment in eliminating binge eating at the 2-year follow-up [54]. In summary, 'the opti-mal approach to treating obese BED patients may be a combination of behavioural weight management to address weight loss and psychosocial interventions that specifically target disordered eating symptoms' [55, p. 124].

In conclusion, BED is a fluctuating and persisting disorder that is commonly associated with obesity, particularly among obese adults who seek treat-ment. A careful assessment of binge eating among obese patients can guide the choice of treatment to reduce such dysfunctional eating behaviours. However, further research is necessary to determine the aetiology of this problematic eating pattern and to improve strategies for clinical management.

2.6.4 Summary box

Key points

- Binge eating is defined as eating a larger amount of food than normal during a short period of time and, during this time, experiencing a loss of control over eating.
- Binge eating has been identified to be a main contributing factor to overweight and obesity among children, adolescents and adults.
- The combination of binge eating and obesity is particularly problematic with regard to comorbidity and risk.
- BED is the most common eating disorder found in obese patients.
- Adults and adolescents with BED are characterised by more eating-related psychopathological features and higher depressive symptoms.
- Research supports a negative affect regulation model for binge eating.
- Overweight individuals overeat as an attempt to regulate the emotions that they are feeling.
- Psychosocial interventions that specifically target disordered eating symptoms are effective in reducing BED symptoms.

References

1. Ogden CL, Yanovski SZ, Carroll MD, Flegal KM. The epidemiology of obesity. *Gastroenterology* 2007; **132**: 2087–2102.
2. Yanovski SZ, Nelson JE, Dubbert BK, Spitzer RL. Association of binge eating disorder and psychiatric comorbidity in obese subjects. *American Journal of Psychiatry* 1993; **150**: 1472–1479.
3. Eckel RH. Nonsurgical management of obesity in adults. *The New England Journal of Medicine* 2008; **358**: 1941–1950.
4. Reas DL, Grilo CM. Timing and sequence of the onset of overweight, dieting, and binge eating in overweight patients with binge eating disorder. *International Journal of Eating Disorders* 2007; **40**: 165.
5. Striegel-Moore RH, Franko DL. Should binge eating disorder be included in the DSM-V? A critical review of the state of the evidence. *Annual Review of Clinical Psychology* 2008; **4**: 305–324.
6. Bruce B, Agras WS. Binge eating in females: a population based investigation. *International Journal of Eating Disorders* 1992; **12**: 365–373.
7. de Zwann M, Mitchell JE, Seim HC, Specker S, Pyle RL, Raymond N, et al. Eating related and general psychopathology in obese females with binge-eating disorder. *International Journal of Eating Disorders* 1994; **15**: 43–52.
8. Spitzer RL, Devlin M, Walsh BT, Hasin D, Wing R, Marcus M, et al. Binge eating disorder: A multisite field trial of the diagnostic criteria. *International Journal of Eating Disorders* 1992; **11**: 191–203.
9. Grilo CM. Binge eating disorder. In: Fairburn CG, Brownell KD (eds) *Eating Disorder and Obesity*, 2nd edn. New York: Guildford Press, 2002, pp. 178–182.
10. Pasold TL, McCracken A, Ward-Begnoche WL. Binge eating in obese adolescents: emotional and behavioral characteristics and impact on health-related quality of life. *Clinical Child Psychology and Psychiatry* 2014; **19**: 299–312.
11. Swallen KC, Reither EN, Haas SA, Meier AM. Overweight, obesity, and health-related quality of life among adolescents: the National Longitudinal Study of Adolescent Health. *Pediatrics* 2005; **115**: 340–347.
12. Wardle J, Cooke L. The impact of obesity on psychological well-being. *Best Practice & Research Clinical Endocrinology & Metabolism* 2005; **19**: 421–440.
13. Abebe DS, Lien L, Torgersen L, von Soest T. Binge eating, purging and non-purging compensatory behaviours decrease from adolescence to adulthood: a population-based, longitudinal study. *BMC Public Health* 2012; **12**: 32.
14. Didie ER, Fitzgibbon M. Binge eating and psychological distress: is the degree of obesity a factor? *Eating Behaviors* 2005; **6**: 35–41.
15. Dingemans AE, Van Furth EF. Binge eating psychopathology in normal weight and obese individuals. *International Journal of Eating Disorders* 2012; **45**: 135–138.
16. Grilo CM, White MA, Masheb RM. DSM-IV psychiatric disorder comorbidity and its correlates in binge eating disorder. *International Journal of Eating Disorders* 2009; **42**: 228–234.
17. Marques L, Alegria M, Becker AE, Chen C, Fang A, Chosak A, et al. Comparative prevalence, correlates of impairment, and service utilization for eating disorders across U.S. ethnic groups: implications for reducing ethnic disparities in health care access for eating disorders. *International Journal of Eating Disorders* 2011; **44**: 412–420.
18. Goldschmidt AB, Le Grange D, Powers P, Crow SJ, Hill LL, Peterson CB, et al. Eating disorder symptomatology in normal-weight vs. obese individuals with binge eating disorder. *Obesity* 2011; **19**: 1515–1518.
19. Striegel-Moore RH, Wilson GT, Wilfley DE, Elder KA, Brownell KD. Binge eating in an obese community sample. *International Journal of Eating Disorders* 1998; **23**: 27–37.
20. Engel SG, Kahler KA, Lystad CM, Crosby RD, Simonich HK, Wonderlich SA, et al. Eating behavior in obese BED, obese

non-BED, and non-obese control participants: a naturalistic study. *Behaviour Research and Therapy* 2009; **47**: 897–900.

21. Hsu LKG, Mulliken B, McDonagh B, Krupa Das S, Rand W, Fairburn CG, et al. Binge eating disorder in extreme obesity. *International Journal of Obesity* 2002; **26**: 1398–1403.

22. Rieger E, Wilfley DE, Stein RI, Marino V, Crow SJ. A comparison of quality of life in obese individuals with and without binge eating disorder. *International Journal of Eating Disorders* 2005; **37**: 234–240.

23. Bishop-Gilyard CT, Berkowitz RI, Thomas A. Wadden TA, Gehrman CA, Cronquist JL, et al. Weight reduction in obese adolescents with and without binge eating. *Obesity* 2011; **19**: 982–987.

24. Ranzenhofer LM, Columbo KM, Tanofsky-Kraff M, Shomaker LB, Cassidy O, Matheson BE, et al. Binge eating and weight-related quality of life in obese adolescents. *Nutrients* 2012; **4**: 167–180.

25. Carlat DJ, Camargo CA. Review of bulimia nervosa in males. *American Journal of Psychiatry* 1991; **148**: 831–843.

26. Ricciardelli LA, McCabe MP. A biopsychosocial model of disordered eating and the pursuit of muscularity in adolescent boys. *Psychological Bulletin* 2004; **130**: 179–205.

27. Katzman MA, Wolchik SA, Braver SL. The prevalence of frequent binge eating and bulimia in a nonclinical college sample. *International Journal of Eating Disorders* 1984; **3**: 53–62.

28. Norris ML, Apsimon M, Harrison M, Obeid N, Buchhilz A, Henderson KA, et al. An examination of medical and psychological morbidity in adolescent males with eating disorders. *Eating Disorders: The Journal of Treatment & Prevention* 2012; **20**: 405–415.

29. Snow JT, Harris MB. Disordered eating in South-western Pueblo Indians and Hispanics. *Journal of Adolescence* 1989; **12**: 329–336.

30. Fairburn CG. *Overcoming Binge Eating.* New York: The Guilford Press, 2005.

31. Ricciardelli LA, Williams RJ, Kiernan MJ. Bulimic symptoms in adolescent girls and boys. *International Journal of Eating Disorders* 1999; **26**: 217–221.

32. McCabe MP, Ricciardelli LA. A longitudinal study of body change strategies among adolescent males. *Journal of Youth and Adolescence* 2003; **32**: 105–133.

33. Allison KC, Grilo CM, Masheb RM, Stunkard AJ. Binge eating disorder and night eating syndrome: a comparative study of disordered eating. *Journal of Consulting and Clinical Psychology* 2005; **73**: 1107–1115.

34. Niego SH, Kofman MD, Weiss JJ, Geliebter A. Binge eating in the bariatric surgery population: a review of the literature. *International Journal of Eating Disorders* 2007; **40**: 349–359.

35. Livhits M, Mercado C, Yermilov I, Parikh JA, Dutson E, Mehran A, et al. Preoperative predictors of weight loss following bariatric surgery: a systematic review. *Obesity Surgery* 2012; **22**: 70–89.

36. Colles SL, Dixon JB, O'Brien PE. Grazing and loss of control related to eating: two high-risk factors following bariatric surgery. *Obesity* 2008; **16**: 615–622.

37. Meany G, Coinceicao E, Mitchell JE. Binge eating, binge eating disorder and loss of control eating: effects on weight

outcomes after bariatric surgery. *European Eating Disorders Review* 2014; **22**: 87–91.

38. Stein RI, Kenardy J, Wiseman CV, Dounchis JZ, Arnow BA, Wilfley DE. What's driving the binge in binge eating disorder? A prospective examination of precursors and consequences. *International Journal of Eating Disorders* 2007; **40**: 195–203.

39. Wild B, Eichler M, Feiler S, Friedrich HC, Hartmann M, Herzog W, et al. Dynamic analysis of electronic diary data of obese patients with and without binge eating disorder. *Psychotherapy and Psychosomatics* 2007; **76**: 250–252.

40. Engelberg MJ, Steiger H, Gauvin L, Wonderlich SA. Binge antecedents in bulimic syndromes: An examination of dissociation and negative affect. *International Journal of Eating Disorders* 2007; **40**: 531–536.

41. Haedt-Matt A, Keel P. Revisiting the affect model of regulation of binge eating: a meta-analysis of studies using ecological momentary assessment. *Psychological Bulletin* 2011; **137**: 660–681.

42. Goldschmidt AB, Engel SG, Wonderlich SA, Crosby RD, Peterson CB, Le Grange D, et al. Momentary affect surrounding loss of control and overeating in obese adults with and without binge eating disorder. *Obesity* 2012; **20**: 1206–1211.

43. Gianini LM, White MA, Masheb RM. Eating pathology, emotion regulation, and emotional overeating in obese adults with binge eating disorder. *Eating Behaviors* 2013; **14**: 309–313.

44. Puhl RM, Heuer CA. The stigma of obesity: a review and update. *Obesity* 2009, **17**: 941–964.

45. Friedman KE, Reichmann SK, Costanzo PR, Zelli A, Ashmore JA, Musante GJ. Weight stigmatization and ideological beliefs: relation to psychological functioning in obese adults. *Obesity Research* 2005; **13**: 907–916.

46. Durso LE, Latner JD, White MA, Masheb RM, Blomquist KK, Morgan PT, et al. Internalized weight bias in obese patients with binge eating disorder: associations with eating disturbances and psychological functioning. *International Journal of Eating Disorders* 2012; **45**: 423–427.

47. Sonneville KR, Calzo JP, Horton NJ, Haines J, Austin SB, Field AE. Body satisfaction, weight gain and binge eating among overweight adolescent girls. *International Journal of Obesity* 2012; **36**: 944–949.

48. Lo Coco G, Salerno L, Bruno V, Caltabiano ML, Ricciardelli LA. Binge eating partially mediates the relationship between body image dissatisfaction and psychological distress in obese treatment seeking individuals. *Eating Behaviors* 2014; **15**: 45–48.

49. Wardle J, Waller J, Rapoport L. Body dissatisfaction and binge eating in obese women: the role of restraint and depression. *Obesity Research* 2001; **9**: 778–787.

50. Stice E, Shaw H. Eating disorder prevention programs: a meta-analytic review. *Psychological Bulletin* 2004; **130**: 206–227.

51. Yager Z, Diedrichs PC, Ricciardelli LA, Halliwell E. What works in secondary schools? A systematic review of classroom body image programs. *Body Image* 2013; **10**: 271–281.

52. Wilfley DE, Welch RR, Stein RI, Spurrell EB, Cohen LR, Saelens BE, et al. A randomized comparison of group

cognitive-behavioral therapy and group interpersonal psycho-therapy for the treatment of overweight individuals with binge eating disorder. *Archives of General Psychiatry* 2002; **59**: 713–721.

53. Wilson GT, Grilo C, Vitousek K. Psychological treatment of eating disorders. *American Psychologist* 2007; **62**: 199–216.

54. Wilson GT, Wilfley DE, Agras WS, Bryson SW. Psychological treatments of binge eating disorder. *Archives of General Psychiatry* 2010; **67**: 94–101.

55. Marcus MD, Wildes JE. Binge eating. In: Caballero B. Allen L, Prentice A. (eds) *Encyclopedia of Human Nutrition*, 3rd edn. Elsevier: Academic Press, 2013, pp. 120–125.

SECTION 3

Aetiology of obesity in adults

Chapter 3.1

Genetics and epigenetics in the aetiology of obesity

Panagiotis Balaskas and Maria E Jackson
University of Glasgow, Glasgow, UK

3.1.1 Introduction

The heritability of obesity is estimated at between 40% and 70% [1], with evidence implicating mutations and variants in many genes. Much of the variation that is obesogenic in the modern environment may have been advantageous during historical periods of food scarcity, with the most energy-efficient individuals being more likely to survive and reproduce [2]. Some ethnic groups, for example, Polynesians, have a greater tendency to overweight [2]. As expected, the genes implicated include many involved in the regulation of metabolism, satiety and appetite, but also include variants associated with addiction and motivation to engage in physical exercise [3]. Additional complexity comes from *epigenetics* – modifications, often in response to environment, that alter the way in which genes are used. The majority of obesity has a complex multifactorial / polygenic aetiology (see Table 3.1.1); but, in a small proportion of cases, obesity can be explained by rare mutations in single genes (monogenic obesity) or rare chromosomal rearrangements such as those causing syndromic obesity. Study of these rare disorders provides insight into the genes and pathways that are likely to play a role in common obesity.

3.1.2 Monogenic forms of obesity

Very rare, severe and early-onset forms of obesity are caused by mutations in genes involved in the leptin–melanocortin pathway (LMCP), which regulates food intake and appetite (Figure 3.1.1). The hormone leptin, produced by adipocytes, binds to a cell surface protein, the leptin receptor (LEPR), present on cells within the hypothalamus; this binding triggers a series of downstream events (Figure 3.1.1) that lead to a feeling of satiety [4]. Leptin is coded for by the *LEP* gene, of which we should have two working copies, one inherited from each parent. The absence of leptin, due to loss-of-function mutations in both copies of *LEP*, leads to severe obesity and hyperphagia [4–7]. Carriers, who have loss-of-function mutations in only one copy of *LEP*, have increased body mass index (BMI) but do not show severe obesity. It is not clear whether leptin levels differ in these carriers as compared to controls [8]. Mutations affecting other components of the LMCP can also cause severe obesity, the most important being LEPR and the melanocortin 4 receptor (MC4R) (Figure 3.1.1). It has been estimated that approximately 3% of severely obese adults and children have loss-of-function mutations

Advanced Nutrition and Dietetics in Obesity, First Edition. Edited by Catherine Hankey.
© 2018 John Wiley & Sons Ltd. Published 2018 by John Wiley & Sons Ltd.

Table 3.1.1 Monogenic, polygenic and multifactorial obesity. Note that 'variants' can denote gene alterations of minor functional effects, whereas pathogenic mutations are those variants that are known to have serious consequences

Monogenic obesity	Pathogenic mutation in one particular gene has a major effect, leading to obesity; the effect may be dominant or recessive. Other genes or environmental factors may still influence the severity of the condition.	**Recessive:** requires that *both* copies (maternal AND paternal) of the gene have mutations present. **Dominant:** requires a pathogenic mutation to be present in *one* of the two copies (maternal OR paternal) of the gene.
Polygenic obesity	Obesity is the cumulative result of variants in many different genes; individually, the gene variants are not pathogenic, but in combination can lead to obesity.	
Multifactorial obesity	Obesity is the cumulative result of both environmental factors plus variants in a number of different genes.	
Syndromic obesity	Obesity is present as part of a characteristic group of signs and symptoms that are seen together in a particular condition – for example, Prader–Willi syndrome, which is characterised by short stature, learning difficulties, weak muscle tone in infancy, delayed or incomplete puberty and hyperphagia leading to obesity. The underlying genetic cause may be the deletion or duplication of a section of a particular chromosome, which may include several adjacent genes.	

in both copies of *LEPR* [9], such that feelings of satiety are not generated even when leptin is present at normal levels. However, the most prevalent form of monogenic obesity is the one caused by mutations in *MC4R*, which codes another receptor required in the LMCP (Figure 3.1.1). Mutation of only one copy of *MC4R* can result in severe obesity [7], although 40% of carriers of such mutations do not become obese [10]. Loss-of-function of both copies of *MC4R* leads to obesity in all cases [10] with greater severity [11]. In a healthy German population, the frequency of *MC4R* mutant alleles that impaired protein function was 0.07%, though none of the carriers were obese [11]. Nevertheless, it has been estimated that up to 6% of early-onset obesity and around 2.5% of adult-onset obesity cases are caused by *MC4R* mutations [7,10,12]. The age of onset might depend on the degree to which *MC4R* mutations impair functionality [12]. In contrast, rare variants of *MC4R* reported to be associated with enhanced function may have a protective effect against obesity [13]. Mutations affecting genes encoding downstream elements of the LMCP have also been reported [7] (Figure 3.1.1).

Monogenic forms of obesity account for a minority (about 5–10%) [14,15] of obese individuals, but demonstrate the clear role of genes. However, the data for *MC4R* indicates that other genetic and/or environmental factors may play a significant role even with 'monogenic' disease.

3.1.3 Syndromic obesity

Obesity occurs as part of the spectrum of characteristics present in approximately 30 syndromes, together with other distinct features, such as developmental delay, dysmorphism and abnormal behaviour. Prader–Willi syndrome (PWS) and Bardet–Biedl syndrome (BBS) are the most well-known and studied obesity-related syndromes [1].

Roughly 1 in 25,000 births are affected by PWS, which is characterised by neonatal hypotonia, intellectual disability, behavioural problems and hyperphagia leading to severe obesity [16,17]. PWS is an imprinting-related disorder (imprinted genes are differentially expressed dependent upon parent of origin) that is associated with a region of

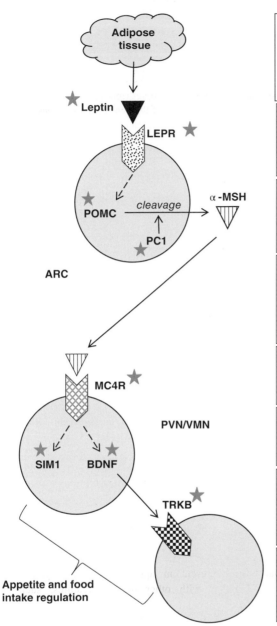

LEP gene: leptin

AR mutations: SEO+H, hypogonadotropic hypogonadism with late-onset puberty, hypothyroidism, immune dysfunction, respiratory infections

LEPR gene: leptin receptor

AR mutations: SEO+H, hypogonadotropic hypogonadism with late-onset puberty, leptin resistance

POMC gene: proopiomelanocortin

AR mutations: SEO+H, hypoadrenalism due to ACTH deficiency, decreased blood glucose, icterus, pale skin, red hair

PCSK1 gene: PC1 proprotein convertase

AR mutations: SEO+H, decreased blood glucose, diarrhoea, hypogonadotropic hypogonadism

MC4R gene: melanocortin 4 receptor

CD mutations: SEO+H, increased lean mass, increased bone density, increased height

SIM1 gene: regulatory protein

AD mutations: SEO+H, developmental delay, behavioural problems

BDNF gene: brain-derived neurotrophic factor

AD mutations: SEO+H, cognitive and memory impairment

NTRK2 gene: TRKB neurotrophic tyrosine kinase receptor type 2

AD mutations: SEO+H, developmental delay, memory and speech impairment

Figure 3.1.1 Mutations in the LMCP are associated with severe early-onset obesity with hyperphagia (SEO+H). The hormone leptin produced by adipose tissue binds its receptor (LEPR) in the hypothalamus, leading to cleavage of proopiomelanocortin (POMC) by PC1 proprotein convertase to generate α-melanocyte-stimulating hormone- (α-MSH); α-MSH binds to the MC4R receptor, leading to further signalling via components including SIM1, BDNF and TRKB; this signalling leads to feelings of satiety and regulation of food intake. Components of the pathway associated with SEO+H when mutated are indicated by a star, with information relating to additional phenotypes seen in monogenic obesity shown on the right. Gene variants in some of these components (e.g. *MC4R* and *BDNF*) have already been shown to be associated with common obesity, and, given the interplay of multiple elements within the pathway, it is likely that variants of additional LMCP genes will be found to be associated with polygenic obesity. AR: autosomal recessive (mutations required in both copies of the gene); CD: codominant (mutation only required in one copy of the gene, but the condition is more severe if both copies are mutated); AD: autosomal dominant (mutation only required in one copy of the gene); ARC: arcuate nucleus; PVN/VMN: paraventricular nucleus/ventromedial nucleus; *SIM1*: single-minded, homolog, *Drosphila*, homolog of, 1.

chromosome 15 (15q11–13) which, in healthy people, is only expressed from the paternal copy. The maternal copy of 15q11–13 is silenced during oogenesis by a process involving DNA methylation (addition of methyl-groups to the cytosine of specific CG dinucleotides). Most PWS patients have a deletion affecting the paternal 15q11–13, and recent evidence suggests that loss of only the small nucleolar RNA (snoRNA) gene cluster *SNORD116* is sufficient for patients to show typical PWS features [17]. Studies in mice demonstrate high expression of *SNORD116* in regions of the hypothalamus that control food intake and regulate energy balance [18]. The actual roles of the *SNORD116* products are still not clear, but potential roles in gene regulation and/or modification of other RNAs seem likely [18].

Another imprinting disorder associated with obesity is Albright's hereditary osteodystrophy (AHO), which is caused by mutation of the maternal copy of the *GNAS* (guanine nucleotide-binding protein, alpha-stimulating activity polypeptide 1) gene. Only the maternal *GNAS* appears to be expressed in the hypothalamus, and GNAS defects affect signal transduction via MC4R, thus providing insight on obesity aetiology in these patients [19].

BBS is caused by mutation of both copies of any one of a group of at least 18 genes (*BBS1–18*) [20]. These genes are involved in the formation and function of primary cilia, mainly through the BBSome, a complex responsible for the proper localisation of transmembrane proteins, including receptors. Obesity in BBS appears to result from BBSome failure to deliver key receptors such as LEPR to the membrane of hypothalamic neurons. This is supported by the fact the BBS patients show leptin resistance, a feature seen in people with LEPR deficiency [20]. Interestingly, in some cases, individuals with pathogenic mutations in both copies of one BBS gene are healthy, whereas siblings carrying a third mutation, in another BBS gene, are affected [20].

3.1.4 Copy number variations

Copy number variants (CNVs) represent chromosome segments, usually longer than one kilobase (kb) of DNA, that, as a consequence of deletions or duplications of DNA, vary in copy number between individuals [21]. Common CNVs (frequency ≥ 5%) are usually benign, but rare CNVs (frequency ≤ 1%) have been implicated in various diseases, including obesity. CNVs larger than two megabases occur in 1.3% of obese patients but not in controls, and smaller CNVs are overrepresented in the obese population [5]. Several CNVs have been associated with obesity, but one of the best characterised is deletion of a 220 kb region of chromosome 16 (16p11.2), which accounts for about 0.5% of severe early-onset obesity cases [22]. The region deleted includes a number of genes, including SH2B adaptor protein 1 (*SH2B1*), in which mutations have also been shown to cause severe obesity. Not all carriers of this deletion are obese, but adults of normal weight who carry the 16p11.2 deletion have transmitted the deletion to their obese children [22], indicating that other genetic and environmental factors contribute to the pathogenic effect [22]. A separate 600 kb deletion in 16p11.2 is also associated with obesity, and, interestingly, individuals with the reciprocal 16p11.2 duplication have increased risk of being underweight as adults [21].

3.1.5 Polygenic / multifactorial or common obesity

Monogenic and syndromic forms of obesity are rare, but they illustrate the profound impact on weight that can result from loss of function in any one of a large number of genes. However, there is a massive level of variation between human genomes [23], and although individual variants may have only minor effects on the function of genes or their products, the cumulative effect of many different low-risk variants may predispose to obesity [24]. The simplest type of variant is the single nucleotide variant or single nucleotide polymorphism (SNP; a *polymorphism* is defined as a variant with a frequency of greater than 1%). Genetic recombination during the production of eggs and sperm allows reshuffling of variants in our DNA, but large chunks of DNA, known as 'haplotype blocks', tend to be inherited as intact blocks through many generations, and thus certain combinations of variants within particular blocks tend to stay together (linkage). Genome-wide association studies (GWAS) take advantage of this in order to identify common variants of small effect, by assaying for millions of SNPs across the genomes of thousands of obese and lean people [24,25]. However, the SNPs identified by GWAS may not be the causal or functional variants responsible for increasing the risk – they might be benign variants present in the same haplotype block as the actual causal ones.

To date, GWAS has identified approximately 60 different genes to be associated with obesity [5,24–27] (Figure 3.1.2). The strongest association in many different populations, for both adults and children, comes from SNPs within non-coding sequences of the fat mass and obesity–associated (*FTO*) gene. *FTO* codes for a nucleic acid demethylase that is highly expressed in the hypothalamus [24], and *FTO*-deficient mice are lean, whereas *FTO*-overexpressing mice are obese. However, recent evidence suggests that the *FTO* risk alleles identified by GWAS associate with increased expression of the adjacent *IRX3* (Iroquois homeobox protein 3) gene in human brain rather than with *FTO* expression levels [28]. *IRX3* encodes a regulatory protein known to play a role in neural development; *IRX3*-deficient mice are 25–30% lighter than control litter-mates and are resistant to weight gain when fed a high-fat diet [28]. Both *FTO* and *IRX3* may be important, but these data highlight one of the issues related to GWAS – that functional studies are required in order to validate GWAS associations.

Other genes consistently found to be associated with obesity by GWAS in various populations include: *SH2B1*, neuronal growth regulator 1 (*NEGR1*), glucosamine-6-phosphate deaminase 2 (*GNPDA2*), *MC4R* and brain-derived neurotrophic factor (*BDNF*) [24,25]. Food choices also appear to have a genetic component: GWAS demonstrated a variant in the opioid receptor mu-1 gene (*OPRM1*) to influence fat intake in adolescents [29]. While the *FTO/IRX3* association has been replicated in many populations, some associations are more prominent in particular subsets of populations [26], indicating that the genetic factors underlying obesity may vary considerably depending on ethnic origin (Figure 3.1.2).

From GWAS, it is clear that some genes involved in monogenic obesity are also implicated in the common form. However, in monogenic obesity, rare DNA changes almost completely disrupt the normal function of the gene, whereas in polygenic obesity the variants are common but individually of small effect (Figure 3.1.3). It is the additive effect of many such common variants that predisposes to obesity. Although heritability of obesity is estimated at 40–70% and GWAS have led to the discovery of many potential obesity-related loci, these loci are able to explain only a small proportion, less than 2%, of the heritability of BMI [1]. The strongest association, that of *FTO/IRX3*, explains only 0.34% of BMI variance [1,27].

3.1.6 Epigenetic modifications and obesity

For imprinted genes, such as those associated with PWS and AHO, the epigenetic marks are established during gametogenesis and maintained after fertilisation throughout the life of the individual. However, epigenetic modifications are also used in a more dynamic way to regulate gene expression in response to environmental signals. The best-characterised epigenetic modification is DNA methylation, and genes that have been found to have abnormal methylation pattern in obese people include *LEP*, with decreased methylation, and *POMC* (proopiomelanocortin; Figure 3.1.1), with increased methylation [30]. However, it is less clear whether the abnormal methylation is the cause or the result of obesity, and increased methylation of the hypoxia inducible factor 3A gene (*HIF3A*) in the adipose tissue of obese individuals was found to be the consequence of increased BMI [31]. Abnormal methylation has been linked with *in utero* factors that affect the offspring's susceptibility to adult obesity, and, perhaps surprisingly, both foetal malnutrition and maternal overweight confer an increased risk of later obesity in the offspring [2,32]. One of the effects of increased maternal weight is decreased foetal methylation in the insulin-like growth factor 2 gene (*IGF2*) with increased plasma IGF2, which is a risk factor for obesity [32]. Other factors that can affect DNA methylation patterns in the offspring are the diet of the mother and contact with xenobiotic obesogens, such as pesticides or antipsychotic drugs, during pregnancy, all associated with

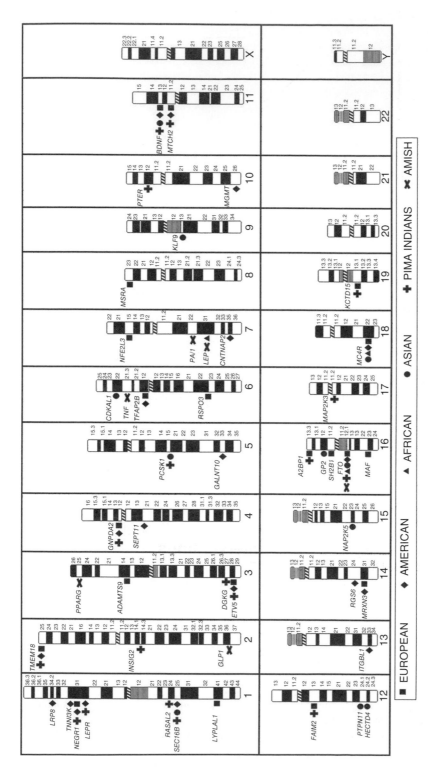

Figure 3.1.2 Significant obesity-related loci identified by GWAS in different populations. Genes are shown in their positions on chromosomes 1–22; some chromosomes (X,Y,21,22) have no significant loci. Some genes, such as *FTO/IRX3*, have been linked to obesity in all populations studied; others, such as *MC4R* and *BDNF*, are reported in a subset of populations only; and some are only reported as significant in one population [26,41–53]. Most GWAS have been done in European and American populations, making comparison biased. Nonetheless, it can be observed that Americans and Europeans share more common loci compared to other groups (such as Asians, who seem to differ substantially), suggesting a degree of common genetic background. Pima Indians and Amish represent ethnic groups with high and low prevalence of obesity, respectively. Note: BMI was used as the major measurement of obesity, along with other anthropometric traits such as waist circumference, waist-to-hip ratio and fat percentage. In most studies, participants were adults, although a few included children or adolescents as well.

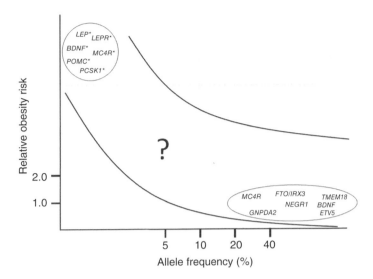

Figure 3.1.3 Allele frequency of obesity-associated variants is inversely correlated to relative risk. Loss of function (*) mutations leading to monogenic obesity are very rare, whereas genetic variants (sometimes in the same genes) associated with polygenic obesity are common. The most significant mutations and variants are expected to lie between the two curves; rare variants of minor effect will prove difficult to characterise, and common variants of major effect are unlikely. There may also exist variants of low frequency that carry moderate risk (indicated by '?'). Note that the figure is illustrative and does not attempt to show all genes / variants.

increased risk of obesity [33]. Measurement of the neonatal methylation status of relevant genes, using tissues such as placenta or umbilical cord, could act as future biomarkers of obesity risk [32].

A 6-month exercise programme resulted in increased methylation of several metabolism-associated genes in the adipose tissue, with reduced gene expression in some [34]. This, along with the fact that the methylation pattern in obese patients after weight loss surgery resembles more that of lean individuals, is an additional argument that some epigenetic modifications may be the result of obesity, rather than the cause [30].

Histone modifications, including methylation and acetylation, can have a profound effect on gene expression, and obesity with hyperlipidaemia has been shown to develop in mice deficient in one of the histone methylases [3]. Furthermore, microRNAs (miRNAs) have been linked to obesity; these are small non-coding RNAs that play an important role in the regulation of gene expression in many biological processes, including adipogenesis [35]. Many miR-NAs have been found to be deregulated in adipose tissue in obese patients compared to controls [35].

Again, whether this is the cause or the result of obesity needs to be considered; however, genetic variants in DNA/histone-modifying enzymes, or in miRNAs or their target sequences, may influence gene expression changes in response to an obesogenic environment, both during development and during adult life.

3.1.7 Genetic factors affecting response to weight loss interventions

Genetic variation affects not only the predisposition to obesity but also the ability to successfully lose weight. Variants of genes associated with addictive behaviours have been implicated in obesity and the ability to resist food temptation [36]. Many studies have demonstrated an association between variants of genes, including beta-3 adrenergic receptor (*ADRB3*) and *LEPR*, and the degree of weight loss following energy restriction [37]. Furthermore, variants in circadian rhythm genes have been shown to affect dietary adherence as well as weight loss [37], and may influence energy expenditure in response to dieting [38]. The degree of weight loss following bariatric surgery is influenced by genetic variants, including those in *FTO/IRX3* and *MC4R* [39]. Also, interestingly, maternal weight loss as a result of bariatric surgery leads to decreased risk of obesity in offspring, associated with epigenetic changes [2]. Although it is currently premature to implement such findings in clinical practice, it does provide hope for more effective future interventions tailored to personal genetic make-up.

3.1.8 Genetic testing in obesity

Although obesity is a growing health problem worldwide, there are no formal guidelines regarding genetic testing [16]. In cases of extreme early-onset obesity, it may be useful to use any additional clinical features seen (Figure 3.1.1) in order to direct testing to the likeliest candidate genes or regions in each case [16]. However, even in apparently monogenic obesity, the situation may be more complex. Conventional clinical molecular laboratory investigations tend to focus on individual genes, but recent innovations in technologies for investigating DNA sequence – the so-called 'next-generation DNA sequencing (NGS)' – allows the simultaneous analysis of large numbers of genes. Using such technology, one extremely obese patient was shown to possess two *BBS1* mutations and one melanocortin 3 receptor (*MC3R*) mutation, which were all predicted to be damaging, in addition to several other variants of obesity-related genes [40]. An NGS approach analysing the coding sequences of 43 genes involved in obesity and diabetes has been developed as a potential diagnostic test [41]. Validation of this assay in obese patients successfully identified the previously reported mutations, but additional damaging mutations in different obesity genes were also found in some cases [41]. Such NGS analyses should allow more effective diagnosis in monogenic obesity, and will be helpful in elucidating other genetic variants that contribute to severity.

Genetic testing in common obesity is more complicated. Some online companies are already offering direct-to-consumer genetic testing, with prediction on common obesity risk. However, each of the gene variants identified by GWAS explain only a small proportion of obesity heritability, and therefore testing for such variants in clinical practice is not currently helpful for providing advice on the risk of obesity [27].

3.1.9 Perspectives

Despite the characterisation of many genetic loci involved in obesity, far more than it has been possible to discuss here, only a proportion of the heritability of obesity can be explained. More research is needed to discover the 'missing heritability' and to investigate gene–environment interactions – the easy availability of energy-dense foods and more sedentary lifestyles are key factors. There do not appear to be separate genes influencing childhood-onset versus adult-onset obesity [5]; instead, it is the severity of the mutations, in conjunction with other genetic variants and lifestyle, that determines the age of onset. Whole genome sequencing by NGS is likely to facilitate identification of new genes responsible for monogenic obesity [14] as well as the variants that influence the likelihood and severity of obesity. This will allow improved genetic diagnostics in relation to obesity, in addition to providing potential targets for generating new therapies. A personalised medicine approach to obesity is likely to be developed: identifying relevant causal mutations/variants in patients may lead to specific drug and/or dietary therapeutic approaches, leading to optimum results for individuals based on their personal set of genetic variants [14].

Obesity-linked genetic variants have been identified in many genes associated with a variety of traits, including satiety [4–7], food choice [29], addiction [36], physical activity [3] and circadian rhythm [37]. When epigenetic responses to the environment, together with variants in the genes encoding components of the epigenetic machinery, are added into the mix, it is clear that we require not only an understanding of the effects of individual variants, but an appreciation of how the (potentially) hundreds of relevant variants that may be present in a single individual interact together, and with the environment, to generate the overall obesity risk.

3.1.10 Summary box

Key points

- Pathogenic (or highly deleterious) gene mutations inherited from parents are responsible for about 5–10% of severe obesity.
- The majority of severe obesity has a complex aetiology, with contributions from both the environment and the cumulative effects of multiple gene variants that are individually of very small effect.
- Genetic variants that influence obesity can affect many aspects of not only our physiology and metabolism but also our personality traits, such as food preference and motivation to exercise.
- Genetic variants can influence response to weight loss interventions such as dieting and surgery.
- The latest DNA technologies will facilitate both our understanding of the genetic basis of obesity and, subsequently, our ability to provide personalised advice based on individual genetic make-up.

References

1. Waalen J. The genetics of human obesity. *Translational Research* 2014; doi:10.1016/j.trsl.2014.05.010 [Epub ahead of print].
2. O'Rourke RW. Metabolic thrift and the genetic basis of human obesity. *Annals of Surgery* 2014; **259**: 642–648.
3. Palou A, Bonet ML. Challenges in obesity research. *Nutricion Hospitalaria* 2013; **28**(5): 144–153.
4. Oswal A, Yeo GS. The leptin melanocortin pathway and the control of body weight: lessons from human and murine genetics. *Obesity Reviews* 2007; **8**: 293–306.
5. Choquet H, Meyre D. Molecular basis of obesity: current status and future prospects. *Current Genomics* 2011; **12**: 154–168.
6. Zhao Y, Hong N, Liu X, Wu B, Tang S, Yang J, et al. A novel mutation in leptin gene is associated with severe obesity in Chinese individuals. *Biomed Research International* 2014; 912052.
7. Farooqi IS, O'Rahilly S. Mutations in ligands and receptors of the leptin-melanocortin pathway that lead to obesity. *Nature Clinical Practice Endocrinology & Metabolism* 2008; **4**: 569–577.
8. Saeed S, Bech PR, Hafeez T, Alam R, Falchi M, Ghatei M, et al. Changes in levels of peripheral hormones controlling appetite are inconsistent with hyperphagia in leptin-deficient subjects. *Endocrine* 2014; **45**: 401–408.
9. Farooqi IS, Wangensteen T, Collins S, Kimber W, Matarese G, Keogh JM, et al. Clinical and molecular genetic spectrum of congenital deficiency of the leptin receptor. *The New England Journal of Medicine* 2007; **356**: 237–247.

10. Stutzmann F, Tan K, Vatin V, Dina C, Jouret B, Tichet J, et al. Prevalence of melanocortin-4 receptor deficiency in Europeans and their age-dependent penetrance in multigenerational pedigrees. *Diabetes* 2008; **57**: 2511–2518.
11. Hinney A, Bettecken T, Tarnow P, Brumm H, Reichwald K, Lichtner P, et al. Prevalence, spectrum, and functional characterization of melanocortin-4 receptor gene mutations in a representative population-based sample and obese adults from Germany. *Journal of Clinical Endocrinology and Metabolism* 2006; **91**: 1761–1769.
12. Lubrano-Berthelier C, Dubern B, Lacorte JM, Picard F, Shapiro A, Zhang S, et al. Melanocortin 4 receptor mutations in a large cohort of severely obese adults: prevalence, functional classification, genotype-phenotype relationship, and lack of association with binge eating. *Journal of Clinical Endocrinology and Metabolism* 2006; **91**: 1811–1818.
13. Stutzmann F, Vatin V, Cauchi S, Morandi A, Jouret B, Landt O, et al. Non-synonymous polymorphisms in melanocortin-4 receptor protect against obesity: the two facets of a Janus obesity gene. *Human Molecular Genetics* 2007; **16**(15): 1837–1844.
14. Blakemore AI, Froguel P. Investigation of Mendelian forms of obesity holds out the prospect of personalized medicine. *Annals of the New York Academy of Sciences* 2010; **1214**: 180–189.
15. Choquet H, Meyre D. Genomic insights into early-onset obesity. *Genome Medicine* 2010; **2**: 36.
16. Phan-Hug F, Beckmann JS, Jacquemont S. Genetic testing in patients with obesity. *Best Practice & Research Clinical Endocrinology & Metabolism* 2012; **26**: 133–143.
17. Bieth E, Eddiry S, Gaston V, Lorenzini F, Buffet A, Conte Auriol F, et al. Highly restricted deletion of the SNORD116 region is implicated in Prader–Willi Syndrome. *European Journal of Human Genetics* 2014; doi:10.1038/ejhg.2014.103 [Epub ahead of print].
18. Zhang Q, Bouma GJ, McClellan J, Tobet S. Hypothalamic expression of snoRNA Snord116 is consistent with a link to the hyperphagia and obesity symptoms of Prader–Willi syndrome. *International Journal of Developmental Neuroscience* 2012; **30**: 479–485.
19. Linglart A, Maupetit-Mehouas S, Silve C. GNAS-related loss-of-function disorders and the role of imprinting. *Hormone Research in Paediatrics* 2013; **79**: 119–129.
20. M'Hamdi O, Ouertani I, Chaabouni-Bouhamed H. Update on the genetics of Bardet-Biedl syndrome. *Molecular Syndromology* 2014; **5**: 51–56.
21. D'Angelo CS, Koiffmann CP. Copy number variants in obesity-related syndromes: review and perspectives on novel molecular approaches. *Journal of Obesity* 2012; 845480.
22. Walters RG, Coin LJ, Ruokonen A, De Smith AJ, El-Sayed Moustafa JS, Jacquemont S, et al. Rare genomic structural variants in complex disease: lessons from the replication of associations with obesity. *PLoS One* 2013; **8**: e58048.
23. The 1000 Genomes Project Consortium. A map of human genome variation from population-scale sequencing. *Nature* 2010; **467**: 1061–1073.
24. Tan LJ, Zhu H, He H, Wu KH, Li J, Chen XD. Replication of 6 obesity genes in a meta-analysis of genome-wide association studies from diverse ancestries. *PLoS One* 2014; **9**: e96149.

25. Speliotes EK, Willer CJ, Berndt SI, Monda KL, Thorliefsson G, Jackson AU, et al. Association analyses of 249,796 individuals reveal 18 new loci associated with body mass index. *Nature Genetics* 2010; **42**: 937–948.

26. Fall T, Ingelsson E. Genome-wide association studies of obesity and metabolic syndrome. *Molecular and Cellular Endocrinology* 2014; **382**: 740–757.

27. Ng MC, Bowden DW. Is genetic testing of value in predicting and treating obesity? *North Carolina Medical Journal* 2013; **74**: 530–533.

28. Smemo S, Tena JJ, Kim KH, Gamazon ER, Sakabe NJ, Gomez-Marin C, et al. Obesity-associated variants within FTO form long-range functional connections with IRX3. *Nature* 2014; **507**: 371–375.

29. Haghighi A, Melka MG, Bernard M, Abrahamowicz M, Leonard GT, Richer L, et al. Opioid receptor mu 1 gene, fat intake and obesity in adolescence. *Molecular Psychiatry* 2014; **19**: 63–68.

30. Van Dijk SJ, Molloy PL, Varinli H, Morrison JL, Muhlhausler BS. Epigenetics and human obesity. *International Journal of Obesity* 2014; doi:10.1038/ijo.2014.34 [Epub ahead of print].

31. Dick KJ, Nelson CP, Tsaprouni L, Sandling JK, Aissi D, Wahl S, et al. DNA methylation and body-mass index: a genome-wide analysis. *Lancet* 2014; **383**: 1990–1998.

32. Reynolds RM, Jacobsen GH, Drake AJ. What is the evidence in humans that DNA methylation changes link events in utero and later life disease? *Clinical Endocrinology* 2013; **78**: 814–822.

33. Levian C, Ruiz E, Yang X. The pathogenesis of obesity from a genomic and systems biology perspective. *Yale Journal of Biology and Medicine* 2014; **87**: 113–126.

34. Ronn T, Volkov P, Davegardh C, Dayeh T, Hall E, Olsson AH, et al. A six months exercise intervention influences the genome-wide DNA methylation pattern in human adipose tissue. *PLoS Genetics* 2013; **9**: e1003572.

35. Alexander R, Lodish H, Sun L. MicroRNAs in adipogenesis and as therapeutic targets for obesity. *Expert Opinion on Therapeutic Targets* 2011; **15**: 623–636.

36. Volkow ND, Wang GJ, Tomasi D, Baler RD. The addictive dimensionality of obesity. *Biological Psychiatry* 2013; **73**: 811–818.

37. Rudkowska I, Perusse L. Individualized weight management: what can be learned from nutrigenomics and nutrigenetics? *Progress in Molecular Biology and Translational Science* 2012; **108**: 347–382.

38. Mirzaei K, Xu M, Qi Q, de Jonge L, Bray GA, Sacks F, et al. Variants in glucose- and circadian rhythm-related genes affect the response of energy expenditure to weight-loss diets: the POUNDS LOST Trial. *American Journal of Clinical Nutrition* 2014; **99**: 392–399.

39. Still CD, Wood GC, Chu X, Erdman R, Manney CH, Benotti PN, et al. High allelic burden of four obesity SNPs is associated with poorer weight loss outcomes following gastric bypass surgery. *Obesity* 2011; **19**: 1676–1683.

40. Gerhard GS, Chu X, Wood GC, Gerhard GM, Benotti P, Petrick AT, et al. Next-generation sequence analysis of genes associated with obesity and nonalcoholic fatty liver disease-related cirrhosis in extreme obesity. *Human Heredity* 2013; **75**: 144–151.

41. Bonnefond A, Philippe J, Durand E, Muller J, Saeed S, Arslan M, et al. Highly sensitive diagnosis of 43 monogenic forms of diabetes or obesity through one-step PCR-based enrichment in combination with next-generation sequencing. *Diabetes Care* 2014; **37**(2, Feb): 460–467.

42. Bian L, Traurig M, Hanson RL, Marinelarena A, Kobes S, Muller YL, et al. MAP2K3 is associated with body mass index in American Indians and Caucasians and may mediate hypothalamic inflammation. *Human Molecular Genetics* 2013; **22**: 4438–4449.

43. Fesinmeyer MD, North KE, Ritchie MD, Lim U, Franceschini N, Wilkens LR, et al. Genetic risk factors for BMI and obesity in an ethnically diverse population: results from the population architecture using genomics and epidemiology (PAGE) study. *Obesity (Silver Spring)* 2013; **21**: 835–846.

44. Hsueh WC, Mitchell BD, Schneider JL, St Jean PL, Pollin TI, Ehm MG, et al. Genome-wide scan of obesity in the Old Order Amish. *Journal of Clinical Endocrinology and Metabolism* 2001; **86**: 1199–1205.

45. Lombard Z, Crowther NJ, Ven der Merwe L, Pitamber P, Norris SA, Ramsay M. Appetite regulation genes are associated with body mass index in black South African adolescents: a genetic association study. *BMJ Open* 2012; **2**(3): e000873.

46. Malhotra KL, Kobes S, Knowler WC, Baier LJ, Bogardus C, Hanson RL. A genome-wide association study of BMI in American Indians. *Obesity (Silver Spring)* 2011; **19**: 2102–2106.

47. Monda KL, Chen GK, Taylor KC, Palmer C, Edwards TL, Lange LA, et al. A meta-analysis identifies new loci associated with body mass index in individuals of African ancestry. *Nature Genetics* 2013; **45**: 690–696.

48. Rampersaud E, Mitchell BD, Pollin TI, Fu M, Shen H, O'Connell JR, et al. Physical activity and the association of common FTO gene variants with body mass index and obesity. *Archives of Internal Medicine* 2008; **168**: 1791–1797.

49. Sibbel SP, Talbert ME, Bowden DW, Haffner SM, Taylor KD, Chen YD, et al. RGS6 variants are associated with dietary fat intake in Hispanics: the IRAS Family Study. *Obesity (Silver Spring)* 2011; **19**: 1433–1438.

50. Steinle NI, Hsueh WC, Snitker S, Pollin TI, Sakul H, St Jean PL, et al. Eating behavior in the Old Order Amish: heritability analysis and a genome-wide linkage analysis. *American Journal of Clinical Nutrition* 2002; **75**: 1098–1106.

51. Traurig MT, Perez JM, Ma L, Bian L, Kobes S, Hanson RL, et al. Variants in the LEPR gene are nominally associated with higher BMI and lower 24-h energy expenditure in Pima Indians. *Obesity (Silver Spring)* 2012; **20**: 2426–2430.

52. Velez Edwards DR, Naj AC, Monda K, North KE, Neuhouser M, Magvanjav O, et al. Gene-environment interactions and obesity traits among postmenopausal African-American and Hispanic women in the Women's Health Initiative SHARe Study. *Human Genetics* 2013; **132**: 323–336.

53. Zhao J, Bradfield JP, Zhang H, Sleiman PM, Kim CE, Glessner JT, et al. Role of BMI-associated loci identified in GWAS meta-analyses in the context of common childhood obesity in European Americans. *Obesity (Silver Spring)* 2011; **19**: 2436–2439.

Chapter 3.2

Food intake and appetite in the aetiology of obesity

John E Blundell, Michelle Dalton and Catherine Gibbons
University of Leeds, Leeds, UK

3.2.1 Introduction

There are strong logical reasons why food consumption is important for obesity. For many health professionals, it is obvious that overconsumption of food is responsible for the rise in the prevalence of obesity over the last 25 years – a phenomenon often referred to as 'the obesity epidemic'. Advocates of this view have drawn attention to data from the USA in which the increase in the average body weight of the population between 1970 and 2000 is mirrored by the increase in the availability of food produced – and, presumably, consumed [1]. It was argued that the increase in energy intake was more than sufficient to account for the rise in obesity. However, other researchers have argued that a decline in energy expenditure (through changing working practices) over a 50-year period could also be more than sufficient to account for the level of obesity [2]. This polarisation can be referred to as 'the energy balance wars'. This antagonism (or healthy academic competition) is detracting from useful scientific analysis, but it does draw attention to the need to justify and prove the impact of food intake on obesity, rather than assume that it occurs. In passing, it can be noted that the present writers has argued that obesity arises from a combination of increased energy intake (EI) and a decrease in energy expenditure (EE). Such states may operate separately in different individuals or – perhaps more frequently – coexist in the same person. Therefore,

we should not seek to defend the position that obesity is entirely dependent on an overconsumption of food, although obesity does arise from a positive energy balance ($EI > EE$).

Two fundamental questions about food intake in humans are: 'What to eat?' and 'How much to eat?' Two subsidiary questions are, where and with whom to eat – neither of which is trivial, but these will not be the focus of this chapter. In addition, it should be recognised that food consumption (or energy intake) is a behavioural act, and therefore eating is a phenomenon that is subject to laws of behaviour rather than just rules of physiology. Some key terms that are useful to identify are 'appetite', 'hunger', 'satiation' and 'satiety' (see Box 3.2.1).

3.2.2 Food intake: biology or culture?

Food intake is viewed by different groups of researchers as an exclusively biological or cultural phenomenon. On the one hand, for some theorists, eating is a way of getting food into the body to provide the energy and nutrients required for maintenance and growth. This implies a biological purpose; other features of food intake – such as opportunities for personal interaction or social discourse – are regarded as mere embellishments, not related to the true purpose. In contrast, other

---

Box 3.2.1 Glossary of terms relating to appetite, hunger, satiation and satiety

Appetite
There are two definitions in circulation:
(a) Covers the whole field of food intake, selection, motivation and preference;
(b) Refers specifically to the qualitative aspects of eating, its sensory aspects or responsiveness to environmental stimulation, which can be contrasted with the *homeostatic view*, based on eating in response to physiological stimuli, such as an energy deficit.

Hunger
(a) Construct or intervening variable that indicates the drive to eat. Not directly measurable, but can be inferred from objective conditions.
(b) Conscious sensation reflecting a mental urge to eat. Can be traced to changes in physical sensations in parts of the body – stomach, limbs or head. In its strong form, may include feelings of light-headedness, weakness or emptiness in stomach. Hunger will be used in this sense throughout this chapter.

Satiation
Process that leads to the termination of eating; therefore, controls the meal size. Influenced by sensory qualities, palatability, energy density, density (weight and volume) and portion size. Also known as intra-meal satiety.

Satiety
Process that leads to inhibition of further eating, decline in hunger and increase in fullness after a meal has finished. Influenced by total energy, macronutrient composition, types of fibres, carbohydrates, proteins and fats. Also known as post-ingestive satiety or inter-meal satiety.

---

groups of researchers, such as anthropologists or sociologists, construe eating as a means of fulfilling social obligations, embodying rituals and influencing personal relations [3]; any physiological consequences are regarded as a side effect. These opposing positions create a conflict, which can be resolved by viewing biological and cultural determinism as incomplete explanations. While eating has its origins in biological obligations, the integrated patterns of eating are shaped and given values though the influence of culture. Part of the framework for understanding food intake is to see eating as a bio-cultural interaction, as depicted in Figure 3.2.1. Since normal eating is 100% behaviour, it can be seen as a bio-behavioural bridge through which eating expresses biological needs in a social landscape.

Humans are omnivores

One of the most salient features of appetite in humans depends on the fact that humans are omnivores. Unlike herbivores or carnivores whose feeding habits are biologically programmed for restricted types of foods, omnivores have a much greater range of potentially edible items. One consequence of this has been that humans are able to colonise and exploit many different types of environments that sustain quite distinctive nutritional repertoires. It follows that, for humans, the type of food that is put into the mouth is not heavily programmed biologically, but depends on the local culture, geography, climate, religion, ethnic principle and social forces. This means that the processes of food intake control have to be geared to a variety of dietary scenarios, and the control mechanisms have to be sufficiently adaptable to deal with a wide range of food types. Although food is basically comprised of fats, proteins and carbohydrates, it is put into the mouth in a large number of forms that are associated with a multitude of tastes and textures. The behavioural act of putting a selected type of food into the mouth is a precursor of eating. This means that food choice depends on the environment. In certain circumstances, rational food choice can be undermined by an environment in which the nutritional value (and therefore the biological value) of specific food items can be concealed or confused. This can easily

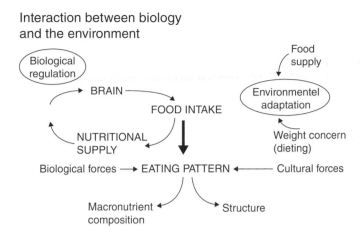

Figure 3.2.1 Model to illustrate that the behavioural act of food consumption reflects an interaction between biological and cultural influences.

happen in technologically advanced societies in which synthetic foods, which contain arbitrary and unlikely combinations of composition, texture and tastes, can be readily manufactured. This can lead to quantitatively (eating too much) and qualitatively (making poor, unhealthy choices) inappropriate eating habits.

Food intake, obesity and the obesogenic environment

The human omnivorous habit, together with the huge variety of manufactured foods available, may be responsible for the epidemic of obesity. It is claimed that the epidemic is maintained (and possibly initiated) by an 'obesogenic environment' that encourages overconsumption [4,5]. In turn, it has been argued that overconsumption is 'passive' and depends on the energy density of the diet [6]. This overconsumption is permitted because of the asymmetry of the appetite control system in which excess food intake is readily allowed, whereas under-consumption (biological deficit) is strongly resisted. In other words, in an obesogenic environment, overeating is easy but undereating is difficult.

Does this mean that the food industry (through its contribution to the obesogenic environment) is responsible for obesity? Before reaching such a conclusion, it should be considered that overconsumption of food is just one example of the more widespread practice of acquiring material objects well beyond any limit defined by personal need [7]. People in industrialised societies are encouraged to purchase more clothes, shoes, TVs, motorcars, refrigerators, furniture and palatable foods; only the last of these is blamed for obesity. The prevailing socioeconomic system encourages the materialistic self-interest and unnecessary consumption (and purchasing) deemed essential for economic growth. Thus, overconsumption takes place in a climate of abundance, aggressive advertising and easy accessibility in which food purchase is strongly promoted. Overconsumption is legitimised, not prohibited, by prevailing cultural values [8]. Consequently, the argument for the role of food in excessive energy intake is economic and political, but made possible by the biological asymmetry of the appetite system and the presence of a persistent biological drive.

3.2.3 Food intake, obesity and energy balance

It is widely considered that weight gain can only be achieved with a surfeit of energy intake over expenditure, and this draws attention to the concept of energy balance. This concept is often depicted as a set of kitchen scales with food on one side and physical activity on the other; whichever has the greatest value causes either an energy surfeit or deficit.

However, it has been recognised for some years that this simple mechanistic model gives a false representation [9]. The balance mechanism is not a simple physical device but an active, physiologically regulated system. This means that food intake not only influences the energy intake side of the equation, but also has an effect on energy expenditure [10]. In turn, physical activity not only influences energy expenditure, but also has an effect on energy intake [11]. This picture has been referred to as 'dynamic' rather than 'static' energy balance [12] and is consistent with new ways of viewing appetite control [13].

What is the driver of food intake?

Over 50 years ago, animal research gave rise to the idea that the drive to eat originated in an excitatory centre of the hypothalamus. This idea generated considerable research activity but made the source of the drive to eat rather inaccessible – particularly for dealing with human food intake. Around the same time (but in a completely separate domain of science), a group of physiologists working in the field of human nutrition developed the idea that energy expenditure was the main driver of appetite. It was proposed that 'the intakes of foods [of individuals] must originate in the differences in energy expenditure' [14]. This idea was ignored for over 50 years, during which time the discovery of leptin led to an upsurge of research on fat and, consequently, to the belief that adipose tissue was the main controller of food intake. However, although adipose tissue stores define the state of obesity, there is little evidence that they influence normal eating behaviour. Indeed, it has been demonstrated that, in overweight and obese people, the size of individual meals and the total daily energy consumed are associated not with the amount of fat in the body, or BMI, but with the fat-free mass (FFM) or lean tissue [15,16]. This makes logical sense since it proposes that the source of the drive for food arises from the energy needed to maintain physical integrity and to provide the power for adaptive behaviour (eating and foraging). This means that the drive for food is generated by the energy requirements to run the body. In turn, approximately 60% of the body's energy requirement is contributed to by the resting metabolic rate (RMR). Consequently, RMR can provide the basis for the appetite drive [17], and this resonates with an older concept of needs translated into drives. The RMR in turn is mainly influenced by the amount of lean tissue (FFM) and much less by the amount of adipose tissue (fat mass, FM). Therefore, the activity of this FFM is an important determinant of meal size and daily energy intake [15]. This process can account for what appears to be a rather mundane observation: that, in general, men eat more than women. This is because men have a greater FFM than women, and therefore a greater energy requirement.

This explanation can also account for the fact that obese people eat more (on average) than lean individuals, and also why they continue to feel hungry and eat more in the absence of any energy deficit or food restriction. Even in the resting state, most obese people show considerable hunger (contrary to some popular commentaries) and eat in accordance with this [18]. Although obese people are characterised – by definition – as having larger amounts of adipose tissue (FM), they also have larger amounts of FFM (needed to support the larger tissue bulk) and therefore higher RMRs than lean people (again, contrary to much speculation) [19].

The role of body composition (FM and FFM) in the determination of food intake helps to explain how the drive to eat arises from physiological requirements for energy (as Edholm proposed more than 50 years ago). Both FFM and RMR are associated with the size of individual meals and the total daily energy intake. This has produced a new formulation for appetite control [13], illustrated in Figure 3.2.2.

Adipose tissue and food intake

Given the association between food intake (overconsumption) and obesity, it seems logical that fat tissue should be involved in appetite control. This idea is incorporated in the lipostatic hypothesis, which was an early example of this suggestion. The discovery of leptin, deemed to be the dominant signal informing the brain about fat stores in the

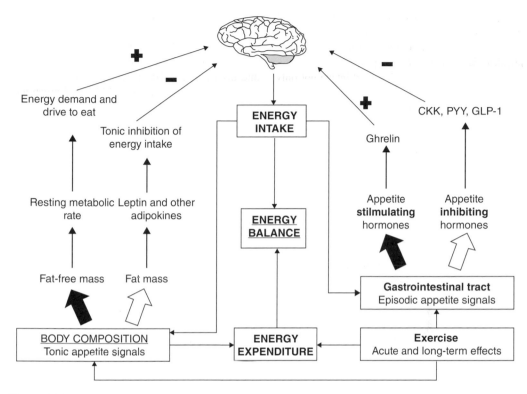

Figure 3.2.2   Formulation to show the separate effects of FFM and FM on the tonic drive to eat. Through a major influence on RMR, FFM reflects the energy requirements of the body and is a driver of eating. FM reflecting the store of energy in the body can modulate this drive, but this is weakened as FM increases. Episodic influences on food intake arise, partly from the action of food in the stomach and the periodic release of peptides from the gut after eating.

body [20], seemed to confirm the central role of adipose tissue as a controller of food intake. Indeed, it has been proposed that there is an intimate and reciprocal relationship between the control of adipose tissue and the control of food intake [21]. However, careful studies in humans (see the subsection titled 'Satiation and Satiety') have shown that the situation is not so simple, and that there is no obvious relationship between the amount of fat in the body and the control of food intake. Indeed, for obese people, the large amount of adipose tissue in the body does not help, but rather hinders, the control of appetite. Why is this? One plausible proposal is that, for lean, normal-weight people, fat exerts a regulatory role and inhibits food intake according to the amount of energy stored in the body (in the fat stores). Leptin is probably a mediator in this action. However, as people gain fat and leptin levels increase, the phenomenon of leptin resistance occurs (this is widely agreed), together with insulin resistance. These actions lead to a weakening of the inhibitory control (or 'disinhibition') of appetite by fat. Therefore, the greater the amount of body fat, the less help a person gets from the fat stores to control eating [22]. In addition, it is well documented that a larger amount of body fat is associated with unhelpful dispositions such as the tendency for binge eating, food craving and with a trait called 'disinhibition' (measured by questionnaires). Together, these tendencies make people more vulnerable to 'opportunistic eating' and further serve to increase food intake [23].

3.2.4 The 'satiety cascade' – episodic control of food intake

In the theoretical treatment of food intake control (in relation to body weight), it is conventional to refer to long-term and short-term processes – also referred to as 'tonic' and 'episodic', respectively. The tonic controllers change gradually over time and reflect enduring and slowly changing mechanisms (such as FFM and RMR). In contrast, the episodic controllers fluctuate markedly during the course of a day in relation to the episodes of eating; these mechanisms are considered to be responsible for controlling the size of meals and the period of inhibition against eating that follows a meal (postprandial period). The 'satiety cascade' was developed to account for the episodic control of eating and to provide a framework for thinking about the different mechanisms involved: nutritional, physiological and psychological. The satiety cascade reflects the fact that eating itself is influenced by a number of factors – including the sight, taste, texture and smell of food; thoughts and beliefs about food; as well as the actual nutritional composition and the environmental factors surrounding eating [24]. Figure 3.2.3 shows a model of the satiety cascade, illustrating that the influence of overlapping variables such as sensory and cognitive processes are integrated with physiological

consequences – all generated by the act of food consumption. Acting conjointly, these factors influence the expression of eating behaviour, and therefore determine – in part – the amount of food consumed and the willingness to eat.

Satiation and satiety

Two fundamental components of the satiety cascade are satiation and satiety. Satiation represents the effects of those processes that occur while a person is in contact with food during the eating process itself. The processes of satiation influence the duration and then the termination of an episode of eating, and therefore control meal size. Along with the composition of the food being eaten, these determine the amount of food energy put into the mouth. Following the termination of a meal (or other eating episode), the effects of ingested food exert a control over the processes of satiety, which reflects the suppression of the motivation to eat and an inhibition against eating behaviour for a measurable period of time. Satiety is often best indicated by changes in subjective appetite sensations such as hunger and fullness, which provide valid markers of the intensity and rate of change of satiety [25]. Satiety is also influenced by the physiological actions of the consumed food, especially the effects in the stomach and the hormones released from the gastrointestinal tract during the digestion and absorption of foods [26].

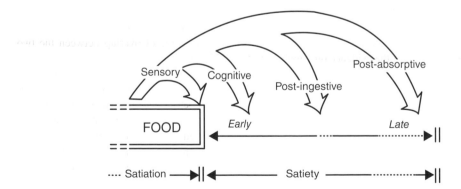

Figure 3.2.3 The satiety cascade, which conceptualises the episodic control of eating. It shows the relation between satiation and satiety in controlling the pattern of eating, and illustrates how food intake is influenced by psychological, nutritional and physiological factors. These factors act conjointly to determine the intensity and duration of the periods of eating and non-eating [13].

Although there is a view that satiety is encoded in specific peptide hormones such as CCK or GLP-1, recent studies suggest that there is no single peptide, nor any unique peptide profile, that is responsible for satiety [27]. We can envisage that different peptide combinations – reflecting the varying physiological actions of different foods – can all deliver the same sensations and the same degree of satiety.

Foods and the satiety cascade

It has been noted earlier that satiation and satiety are quite complex states constructed from a series of overlapping and interacting factors. Having identified some of the key processes involved in the satiety cascade, one natural and important question is: how do different foods impact on these processes? Do some foods possess nutritional properties that allow them to have a stronger effect than others, and therefore a better profile for controlling appetite? This is a key research area, and much attention has been directed to the macronutrients and to the issue of whether fats, proteins or carbohydrates have equally potent actions. In addition, what are the effects of volume, dietary fibre and the glycaemic index? Do solid foods and beverages have equivalent effects? In short, how are the properties of foods related to their capacity to influence satiation, satiety or both, and therefore to influence the amount and type of energy ingested? One currently significant issue is whether it is possible to technologically engineer functional foods that will help people manage their appetites, and therefore their body weight [28]. In Europe, the European Food Safety Authority (EFSA) has been established, in part, to assess the strength of the evidence on which such satiety claims for foods are based. This is a huge and complex issue that cannot be adequately summarised in this short chapter. However, details can be found elsewhere [29], and there is an agreed methodology available to examine the effects of foods on the satiety cascade [30]. Moreover, it is safe to conclude that not all foods produce equivalent effects, and it is possible to construct a diet (or meal) from foods that will deliver the most potent control over satiation and satiety [31]. However, it is a separate issue whether people can be motivated to eat such a judicious diet. In an obesogenic environment, in which there is a strong promotion of purchasing and eating, many cultural forces oppose (and often undermine) an individual's intention to gain control over his or her own eating behaviour. The range of the obesogenic culture means that it will be very difficult for any single food to exert an effect on the satiety cascade that is sufficient to have an effect on the whole diet and on daily energy intake – in the absence of additional behavioural control procedures.

Homeostatic and hedonic aspects

The control of food intake is often conceived as being influenced by homeostatic and hedonic processes. Homeostatic regulation is usually used to explain the quantitative changes in eating and food intake, such as those that occur in relation to energy expenditure (see the subsection titled 'Satiation and satiety') or during the operations of the satiety cascade (see subsection titled 'The "satiety cascade" – episodic control of food intake"). The homeostatic system comprises a network of brain neurotransmitters, peripheral signals and hormonal inputs that indicate the strength of physiological signalling. In contrast, hedonic processes are concerned with the influence of pleasure and palatability in eating. This system is coordinated by the brain's reward circuitry and reflects the degree of attractiveness (positive or negative) of foods and the sensitivity of the response to foods. There is considerable debate about whether overconsumption and obesity are due to defects in the homeostatic or hedonic systems [32]. However, it is becoming clear that there is a degree of overlap between the two systems [33]. Just as the homeostatic system can be subdivided into components (e.g. tonic vs. episodic; drive to eat vs. satiety), the hedonic system comprises distinct entities. One important division is between the processes of liking and wanting [34]. Liking is defined as the subjective state of perceiving pleasure (of food), whereas wanting represents a directional component in the tendency to approach food (usually a specific class of foods – such as sweet and fatty items). Although liking and wanting can be dissociated and certainly do not invariably occur together, in those foods for which liking and wanting are generated simultaneously, there is a strong stimulus to consume. The identification of such foods is currently a matter of great interest since they carry a high risk of being overconsumed. The existence of a responsive hedonic system, together with the presence of highly palatable foods in the food supply, creates a potent scenario for the promotion of eating. In addition, it gives rise to the 'palatability dilemma'. Is it possible to raise the palatability of a food (so that it will be attractive to consume) while at the same time introducing attributes into the food that will induce satiety and inhibit eating? This is one of the fascinating technological challenges facing the development of functional foods.

3.2.5 Conclusions

Food intake is influenced by both biology and culture; the role that each plays depends on the aspect of food intake under consideration. The amount of energy that food brings into the body depends on the foods selected for consumption and the patterns of eating across a day (this means the number of meals and snacks). The huge range of foods eaten by humans in different habitats across the world indicates that the choice of foods that people consume is largely a cultural and environmental phenomenon. Biology determines the intensity of an individual's drive to eat and the strength of inhibition of the processes of satiation and satiety. Also, the biological system operates asymmetrically – permitting overconsumption, but strongly resisting under-eating. These processes should be interpreted in relation to the existence of an obesogenic environment that encourages overconsumption. The proposed framework suggests ways of thinking about the control of food intake in relation to weight gain and obesity in the first decades of the twenty-first century.

3.2.6 Acknowledgements

Research reported in this chapter has been supported by Biotechnology and Biological Sciences Research Council (BBSRC grant numbers BBS/B/05079 and BB/G005524/1) and by the European Union's Seventh Framework Programme for research, technological development and demonstration under grant agreement No. 266408 (SATIN).

3.2.7 Summary box

Key points

- The role of food in excessive energy intake is economic and political, but facilitated by biological irregularity of appetite structure and a persistent biological drive to eat.
- Around 60% of the body's energy requirement is from RMR, providing a basis for appetite drive.
- A greater quantity of body fat is associated with unhelpful outlooks such as the tendency for binge eating, food cravings and 'disinhibition'. People can become vulnerable to 'opportunistic eating', favouring increased energy intakes.
- Satiety is affected by many things, including peptide hormones, although no particular profiles are thought responsible. Different peptide combinations – reflecting the varying physiological actions of different foods – can all deliver the same sensations and degree of satiety.
- Not all foods produce equivalent effects, and it is possible to construct a diet (or meal) from foods that will deliver the most potent control over satiation and satiety.
- The hedonic system, and the presence of highly palatable foods in the food supply, can promote eating.
- It is uncertain whether the palatability of a food can be increased, making it more attractive to consume, while introducing traits to induce satiety and inhibit eating.

References

1. Swinburn B, Sacks G, Ravussin E. Increased food energy supply is more than sufficient to explain the US epidemic of obesity. *American Journal of Clinical Nutrition* 2009; **90**(6): 1453–1456.
2. Church TS, Thomas DM, Tudor-Locke C, Katzmarzyk PT, Earnest CP, Rodarte RQ, et al. Trends over 5 decades in US occupation-related physical activity and their associations with obesity. *PloS One* 2011; **6**(5): e19657.
3. Fischler C. *L'Homnivore*. Paris: Odile Jacob, 1990.
4. Egger G, Swinburn B. An 'ecological' approach to the obesity pandemic. *BMJ* 1997; **315**(7106): 477.
5. Swinburn B, Sacks G, Hall KD, McPherson K, Finegood DT, Moodie ML, et al. The global obesity pandemic: shaped by global drivers and local environments. *Lancet* 2011; **378**(9793): 804–814.
6. Blundell JE, Macdiarmid JI. Fat as a risk factor for overconsumption. *Journal of the American Dietetic Association* 1997; **97**(7): S63–S69.

7. Judt T. *Ill Fares the Land*. London: Allen Lane Penguin, 2010.
8. Bauman Z. *Liquid Times – Living in an Age of Uncertainty*. Cambridge UK: Polity Press, 2007.
9. Speakman JR, O'Rahilly S. Fat: an evolving issue. *Disease Models & Mechanisms* 2012; **5**(5): 569–573.
10. Stubbs R, Tolkamp B. Control of energy balance in relation to energy intake and energy expenditure in animals and man: an ecological perspective. *British Journal of Nutrition* 2006; **95**(04): 657–676.
11. Blundell JE. Physical activity and appetite control: can we close the energy gap? *Nutrition Bulletin* 2011; **36**: 356–366.
12. Hall KD, Sacks G, Chandramohan D, Chow CC, Wang YC, Gortmaker SL, et al. Quantification of the effect of energy imbalance on bodyweight. *Lancet* 2011; **378**(9793): 826–837.
13. Blundell JE, Caudwell P, Gibbons C, Hopkins M, Naslund E, King N, et al. Role of resting metabolic rate and energy expenditure in hunger and appetite control: a new formulation. *Disease Models & Mechanisms* 2012; **5**(5): 608–613.
14. Edholm O, Fletcher J, Widdowson EM, McCance R. The energy expenditure and food intake of individual men. *British Journal of Nutrition* 1955; **9**(03): 286–300.
15. Blundell JE, Caudwell P, Gibbons C, Hopkins M, Naslund E, King NA, et al. Body composition and appetite: fat-free mass (but not fat mass or BMI) is positively associated with self-determined meal size and daily energy intake in humans (Research Support, Non-US Gov't). *British Journal of Nutrition* 2011; **107**(3): 445–449.
16. Weise C, Hohenadel M, Krakoff J, Votruba S. Body composition and energy expenditure predict ad-libitum food and macronutrient intake in humans. *IJO* 2014; **38**(2): 243–251.
17. Caudwell P, Finlayson G, Gibbons C, Hopkins M, King N, Näslund E, et al. Resting metabolic rate is associated with hunger, self-determined meal size, and daily energy intake and may represent a marker for appetite. *American Journal of Clinical Nutrition* 2013; **97**(1): 7–14.
18. Barkeling B, King NA, Näslund E, Blundel JE. Characterization of obese individuals who claim to detect no relationship between their eating pattern and sensations of hunger or fullness. *IJO* 2006; **31**(3): 435–439.
19. Prentice AM, Black A, Coward W, Davies H, Goldberg G, Murgatroyd P, et al. High levels of energy expenditure in obese women. *BMJ* 1986; **292**(6526): 983.
20. Zhang Y, Proenca R, Maffei M, Barone M, Leopold L, Friedman JM. Positional cloning of the mouse obese gene and its human homologue. *Nature* 1994; **372**(6505): 425–432.
21. Woods SC, Ramsay DS. Food intake, metabolism and homeostasis. *Physiology & Behavior* 2011; **104**(1): 4–7.
22. Blundell JE, Gillett A. Control of food intake in the obese. *Obesity Research* 2001; **9**(4): 263S–270S.
23. Bryant EJ, King NA, Blundell JE. Disinhibition: its effects on appetite and weight regulation. *Obesity Reviews* 2008; **9**(5): 409–419.
24. Blundell JE, Rogers PJ, Hill AJ. Evaluating the satiating power of foods: implications for acceptance and consumption. In: Solms J, et al. (ed) *Food Acceptance and Nutrition*. London: Academic Press, 1987, pp. 205–19.
25. Flint A, Raben A, Blundell JE, Astrup A. Reproducibility, power and validity of visual analogue scales in the assessment of appetite sensations in single test meal studies. *IJO* 2000; **24**: 38–48.
26. Murphy K, Dhillo W, Bloom S. Gut peptides in the regulation of food intake and energy homeostasis. *Endocrine Reviews* 2006; **27**(7): 719.
27. Gibbons C, Caudwell P, Finlayson G, Webb DL, Hellström PM, Näslund E, et al. Comparison of postprandial profiles of ghrelin, active GLP-1, and total PYY to meals varying in fat and carbohydrate and their association with hunger and the phases of satiety. *The Journal of Clinical Endocrinology & Metabolism* 2013; **98**(5): E847–E855.
28. Blundell JE. Making Claims: functional foods for managing appetite and weight. *Nature Reviews Endocrinology* 2010; **6**: 53–56.
29. Blundell J, Bellisle F. *Satiation, Satiety and the Control of Food Intake: Theory and Practice*. Oxford: Woodhead Publishing Limited, 2013.
30. Blundell JE, De Graaf C, Hulshof T, Jebb S, Livingstone B, Lluch A, et al. Appetite control: methodological aspects of the evaluation of foods. *Obesity Reviews* 2010; **11**(3): 251–270.
31. Poortvliet PC, Berube-Parent S, Drapeau V, Lamarche B, Blundell JE, Tremblay A. Effects of a healthy meal course on spontaneous intake, satiety and palatability. *British Journal of Nutrition* 2007; **97**: 584–90.
32. Saper CB, Chou TC, Elmquist JK. The need to feed: homeostatic and hedonic control of eating. *Neuron* 2002; **36**(2): 199–211.
33. Finlayson G, King NA, Blundell JE. Liking vs. wanting food: importance for human appetite control and weight regulation. *Neuroscience & Biobehavioral Reviews* 2007; **31**(7): 987–1002.
34. Dalton M, Finlayson G. Psychobiological examination of liking and wanting for fat and sweet taste in trait binge eating females. *Physiology & Behavior* 2014; **136**: 128–134.

Chapter 3.3

Physiological control of appetite and food intake

Carel W le Roux and Werd Al-Najim
University College Dublin, Dublin, Ireland

3.3.1 Introduction

Energy from food intake will be stored as fat if more energy is consumed than expended, as stated in the first law of thermodynamics states. The major organ involved in this process is the brain, although many physiological systems, including the endocrine, gastrointestinal, central nervous, peripheral nervous and cardiovascular systems, are involved in this homeostasis process. Figure 3.3.1 shows how peripheral signals from different body organs are integrated to control energy homeostasis. Small changes in any of these determinants can, over time, result in substantial changes in body weight. This chapter will focus on the physiology of obesity and the key peripheral and central signals involved in the regulation of body weight.

3.3.2 Central homeostatic regulation

Homeostatic regulation of body weight occurs primarily in the hypothalamus, which is a small structure in the brain located above the brainstem. The hypothalamus integrates peripheral signals that indicate satiety levels and energy stores, as well as higher cortical factors, such as emotional and reward factors, to regulate food intake and maintain energy homeostasis.

In the hypothalamus, the arcuate nucleus (ARC) is the main region involved in the homeostatic control of food intake. Within the ARC, two groups of neurons are prominently implicated in the regulation of feeding. One group, localised more medially in the ARC, co-expresses orexigenic (appetite-stimulant) neuropeptides – that is, neuropeptide Y (NPY) and Agouti-related protein (AgRP). The second group of neurons tends to cluster more laterally in the ARC and co-expresses anorexigenic (appetite suppressant) neuropeptides – that is, cocaine- and amphetamine-related transcript (CART) and pro-opiomelanocortin (POMC). Neuronal projections from the ARC then communicate with other key hypothalamic regions, such as the paraventricular nucleus, dorsomedial nucleus, and ventromedial and lateral hypothalamic nuclei.

The blood–brain barrier surrounding the ARC is not complete, and this allows peripheral signals, secreted by the adipocytes and pancreas, to gain access to the signalling pathway in the ARC. In addition, the vagus nerve and the sympathetic fibres of the nervous system transmit peripheral signals produced in the gastrointestinal tract to the brainstem, where signals then integrate with those of the hypothalamus to control appetite (Table 3.3.1).

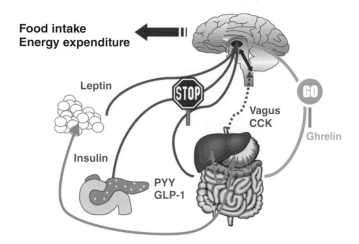

Food intake
Energy expenditure

Leptin

STOP

Vagus
CCK

GO

Ghrelin

Insulin

PYY
GLP-1

Figure 3.3.1 Integration of the key hormonal signals released from different body organs to control food intake and energy homeostasis. Leptin and insulin circulate in the blood at concentrations proportionate to body-fat mass; together with PYY-36, GLP-1 and CCK, which are released from the GI tract, they decrease appetite by inhibiting orexigenic neurons while stimulating anorexigenic neurons in the hypothalamus. The gastric hormone ghrelin has the opposite function.

Table 3.3.1 Central signals, peripheral signals and nutrients involved in the regulation of appetite and energy homeostasis

Location	Anorexigenic	Orexigenic
Hypothalamus	Pro-opiomelanocortin (POMC)	Neuropeptide Y (NPY)
	Cocaine- and amphetamine-related transcript (CART)	Agouti-related protein (AgRP)
Gastrointestinal tract	Cholecystokinin (CCK)	Ghrelin
	Glucagon-like peptide-1 (GLP-1)	
	Peptide tyrosine tyrosine (PYY)	
Pancreas	Insulin	
	Pancreatic polypeptide (PP)	
Adipocytes	Leptin	
Nutrients	Glucose	
	Non-esterified fatty acids (NEFAs)	

3.3.3 Peripheral homeostatic regulation of energy intake

Long- and short-term energy balance is regulated by a number of satiety signals. Afferent signals transmit via the bloodstream and vagus nerve to the hypothalamus and brainstem, to provide information about the state of the external and internal environments as related to energy balance. In turn, the central control systems transduce these messages into efferent signals governing the search for and acquisition of food, and also modulates the subsequent disposal of food once inside the body. Hormones such as leptin and insulin regulate long-term energy balance. Short-term energy balance requires several signals that send information to the brain on a meal-to-meal basis and include nutrients such as glucose, non-esterified fatty acids (NEFAs), hormones such as ghrelin, cholecystokinin (CCK), glucagon-like peptide-1 (GLP-1), pancreatic polypeptide (PP) and PYY (Table 3.3.2).

Table 3.3.2 Changes to the peripheral hormones in obese compared to normal-weight subjects

Factor	Obesity status
Leptin	Elevated
Insulin	Elevated
Ghrelin	Reduced
CCK	Unchanged
GLP-1	Reduced
PYY	Reduced/unchanged
PP	Reduced/unchanged

Long-term satiety signals

Leptin

Leptin is the best described afferent signal from fat to the brain. This 167–amino acid hormone, synthesised by adipose tissue, crosses the blood–brain barrier through a saturable transporter mechanism. Leptin acts in the ARC to reduce food intake and increase energy expenditure by increasing the expression of anorexigenic neuropeptides POMC and CART and decreasing the expression of the orexigenic neuropeptides AgRP and NPY. Congenital leptin deficiency in humans causes hyperphagia and obesity, and, in these patients, leptin treatment reduces food intake to normal amounts, and results in weight loss (98% represented by loss of fat) [1,2].

In normal subjects, the circulating levels of leptin are correlated with the level of body fat. However, women tend to have up to four times higher plasma leptin concentration than men, at a given body mass, even after correction for body fat percentage [3]. Although elevated levels of leptin should be representing reduced appetite and, consequently, weight maintenance or weight loss, the failure of leptin to prevent weight gain has been hypothesised to be a result of leptin resistance in the obese. Leptin resistance results in reduced leptin transport across the blood–brain barrier and impaired leptin signalling in the hypothalamus [4,5]. During weight and fat mass loss, leptin levels decrease quickly. This is a very powerful signal that leads to dramatic increases in hunger and modest decreases in energy expenditure.

Leptin levels that are reduced, therefore, result in increased hunger, thus promoting weight regain [6].

Insulin

Insulin is produced by the β cells of the pancreas to primarily maintain glucose homeostasis, and has been thought to be important in the long-term stability of body weight and fat mass. With a short plasma half-life of 3 minutes, insulin provides a minute-to-minute update of ongoing metabolic activity via a signal to the brain. Insulin rises in the blood following a meal in a concentration directly proportional to the total body fat [7], and reaches the ARC via the blood–brain barrier through a saturable transporter mechanism. Insulin administered directly into the brains of rodents causes a dose-dependent reduction of food intake [8]. Conversely, reducing the amount of insulin in the brain by using a brain-specific insulin receptor knockout in rats results in hyperphagia, increased food intake and increased adiposity [9].

Short-term satiety signals (e.g. satiety-inducing gut hormones)

Cholecystokinin

Cholecystokinin (CCK) was the first gut hormone described to signal nutrient intake from the gut to the brain and leading to the inhibition of further food intake [10]. CCK is released by endocrine cells (I cells) in the jejunum and duodenum in response to fat and protein ingestion. CCK does not change according to body weight or percentage body fat as both lean and obese subjects have similar fasting CCK concentrations [11]. Peripheral administration of CCK in humans reduces food intake and delays gastric emptying. In a study carried out on 12 non-obese subjects, food intake was approximately reduced by 362 g in those peripherally infused with CCK compared to saline infusion [12]. However, the effect of CCK is short-lived; when administered more than 30 minutes prior to the start of a meal, it does not alter food intake [12]. A short plasma half-life of a few minutes means that CCK only transiently decreases food intake, but also stimulates the release of digestive enzymes from the pancreas and gallbladder to increase intestinal motility and delay gastric emptying. The anorexigenic effects of CCK are mediated through CCK1 and CCK2 receptors within the gastrointestinal tract on the vagus nerve and in the hypothalamus and brainstem [13].

Peptide tyrosine tyrosine (PYY)

Peptide tyrosine tyrosine (also known as peptide YY, PYY) is a 36–amino acid peptide released from the L cells of the distal bowel in two forms, PYY_{1-36} and PYY_{3-36} (biologically active major form), and acts through the five hypothalamic G-protein-coupled receptors (Y1–Y5). Levels of PYY rise after a meal in proportion to the consumed energy, peaking at the second hour and remaining elevated for a number of hours. PYY_{3-36} acts on the Y2 receptor in the arcuate nucleus of the hypothalamus to decrease food intake by inhibiting the NPY and AgRP neuropeptides and disinhibiting the POMC neuropeptide [14]. Both PYY_{1-36} and PYY_{3-36} also have local effects on gut motility [15], inhibiting the secretion of gastric acid and pancreatic enzymes, and also inhibiting gallbladder emptying [16–18].

PYY_{3-36} has been shown to physiologically reduce food intake in rodents [14,19] as well as in lean and obese humans [20]. Intravenous infusion of PYY_{3-36} at a rate of 0.8 pmol kg^{-1} min^{-1} into lean humans increased mean plasma PYY_{3-36} levels from 8.3 to 43.5 pM. Plasma PYY_{3-36} returned to baseline concentrations within 30 minutes of the end of the infusion. Despite this, at a free-choice buffet meal 2 hours after the end of the infusion, there was a significant reduction in energy intake of approximately 36%, with no effect on fluid intake or on gastric emptying, as assessed by paracetamol absorption [21]. Despite lower basal levels of PYY_{3-36} in obese subjects, obesity does not appear to be associated with resistance to the effects of PYY_{3-36}. Infusion of PYY_{3-36} into a group of obese volunteers resulted in a comparable 30% reduction in energy intake when compared with lean controls [20]. Quantification of the dynamic postprandial response to energy consumed may shed light on the relationship between PYY, satiety and obesity. This may be important as obese individuals report decreased satiety and may consequently consume more energy,

thus sustaining body weight or perhaps favouring further weight gain.

Pancreatic polypeptide

Pancreatic polypeptide (PP) is a polypeptide secreted by PP cells of the pancreatic islets in response to the ingestion of food [24]. This release is proportional to the energy ingested, and postprandial levels remain elevated for up to 6 hours [22]. PP is thought to have arisen by gene duplication of the PYY gene as PP and PYY are structurally closely related [23]. Obese subjects have been shown to have low fasting plasma PP concentrations compared to lean subjects [24]. Peripheral administration of PP in humans increases satiety, with a consequent reduction in meal energy intake by 22%, and 24-hour cumulative energy intake reduced by 25%. The mechanisms by which PP reduces food intake have not been established, but it appears that PP acts through the NPY Y4 receptor. These Y4 receptors are expressed within the hypothalamus and brainstem, and thus are anatomically well placed to influence food intake.

Glucagon-like peptide-1

Glucagon-like peptide-1 (GLP-1) is a 30–amino acid peptide product of the cleavage of the proglucagon precursor, secreted by the L cells of the distal bowel together with PYY. GLP-1 is a potent incretin, stimulating insulin secretion from pancreatic islet B-cells in response to carbohydrate ingestion. GLP-1 also stimulates B-cell proliferation, and inhibits glugacon secretion, gastric acid secretion and gastric emptying [25].

GLP-1 receptors are located in the hypothalamus, among other areas of the brain [26]. GLP-1 is released in response to a meal, and leads to a reduction in food intake and appetite through actions on the hypothalamus, but also through the vagus and brainstem [27]. A meta-analysis of studies on GLP-1 infusion indicates a reduction in food intake of 11% in obese and lean subjects [28]. Administration of GLP-1 agonists in the form of exenatide and liraglutide decreases prospective energy consumption and hunger ratings, in addition to inducing a reduction in body weight [25]. Liraglutide (in 1.2 and 1.8 mg doses) has been used since 2012 for the treatment of type 2 diabetes (under the brand name *Victoza*). It has been approved by the FDA to be licensed for the treatment of obesity (in a 3 mg dose), as it has shown a result of 8% total-body weight loss, compared to 2.6% with placebo.

Ghrelin

Ghrelin is a 28–amino acid peptide synthesised in the endocrine cells of the stomach, and at much lower levels in the hypothalamus [29]. Ghrelin stimulates feeding by increasing NPY and AgRP levels in the ARC [30], increasing gastric acid secretion and motility, and reducing pancreatic insulin secretion. Infusion of ghrelin into subjects with appetite loss due to cancer increased energy intake by 31% [31]. This compares with an increase in energy intake of 28% when ghrelin was administered to healthy human volunteers [32]. Plasma ghrelin levels are highest when fasting; they fall after eating and correlate with a subjective rating of hunger, with carbohydrates having more of a suppressive effect compared to protein and lipids. The levels also rise through the day and fall overnight [33]. A state of negative energy balance increases fasting ghrelin concentrations [34], while levels reduce after food and exercise [35]. Distension of the stomach with water does not lead to ghrelin reduction [36,37]; however, ingestion of non-nutritive fibre does decrease ghrelin [38]. In humans, ghrelin levels are high in patients with anorexia nervosa and heart failure cachexia, and after diet-induced weight loss [39–41]. However, in obese individuals, ghrelin levels are low, falling after a meal [42], suggesting a role of ghrelin in longer-term energy balance as well as in meal initiation.

3.3.4 Conclusion

While individuals can and should take steps to control their weight, several physiological mechanisms could counteract the best of intentions. Adipose tissue is an active endocrine organ; it plays a key role in long-term energy and metabolism homeostasis by its secretion to a number of hormones that have a direct influence on the control of body weight.

On the other hand, the gastrointestinal tract contributes to the short-term energy and metabolism homeostasis by its secretion to several hormones that act as satiety enhancers. Nevertheless, these hormones work synergistically, and many clinical trials are currently investigating the combining of hormones to reduce body weight, and to development of safe and effective pharmacotherapeutic agents. Self-control through diet and lifestyle adjustments may be less powerful than pathophysiological factors, and hence understanding how the brain receives signals from the gut and adipose tissue may help us develop better interventions.

3.3.5 Summary box

Key points

- The hypothalamus is roughly the size of an almond and is responsible for the homeostatic regulation of body weight.
- Dieting is not usually successful in the long-term maintenance of reduced body weight, and most reduced-weight obese individuals eventually regain the lost weight.
- Leptin and insulin are hormones contributing to the long-term energy and metabolism homeostasis.
- Cholecystokinin, peptide tyrosine tyrosine, pancreatic polypeptide, glucagon-like peptide-1 and ghrelin are hormones contributing to the short-term energy and metabolism homeostasis, providing the brain with minute-to-minute information regarding satiety and energy stores.
- GLP-1 agonists in the form of exenatide and liraglutide are currently the only peripheral hormone agonists being licensed for the treatment of obesity.
- Self-control through diet and lifestyle adjustments may be less powerful than pathophysiological factors.

References

1. Farooqi IS, Bullmore E, Keogh J, Gillard J, O'Rahilly S, Fletcher PC. Leptin regulates striatal regions and human eating behavior. *Science* 2007; **317**(5843): 1355.

2. Farooqi IS, Matarasse G, Lord GM, Keogh JM, Lawrence E, Agwu C, et al. Beneficial effects of leptin on obesity, T cell hyporesponsiveness, and neuroendocrine/metabolic dysfunction of human congenital leptin deficiency. *Journal of Clinical Investigation* 2002; **110**(8): 1093–1103.

3. Havel PJ, Kasim-Karakas S, Mueller W, Johnson PR, Gingerich RL, Stern JS. Relationship of plasma leptin to plasma insulin and adiposity in normal weight and overweight women: effects of dietary fat content and sustained weight loss. *Journal of Clinical Endocrinology and Metabolism* 1996; **81**(12): 4406–4413.

4. Schwartz MW, Peskind E, Raskind M, Boyko EJ, Porte D Jr. Cerebrospinal fluid leptin levels: relationship to plasma levels and to adiposity in humans. *Nature Medicine* 1996; **2**(5): 589–593.

5. El-Haschimi K, Pierroz DD, Hileman SM, Biorbaek C, Flier JS. Two defects contribute to hypothalamic leptin resistance in mice with diet-induced obesity. *Journal of Clinical Investigation* 2000; **105**(12): 1827–1832.

6. Morton G, Cummings DE, Baskin DG, Barsh GS, Schwartz MW. Central nervous system control of food intake and body weight. *Nature* 2006; **443**(7109): 289–295.

7. Baura GD, Foster DM, Porte D Jr, Kahn SE, Bergman RN, Cobelli C, et al. Saturable transport of insulin from plasma into the central nervous system of dogs in vivo. A mechanism for regulated insulin delivery to the brain. *Journal of Clinical Investigation* 1993; **92**(4): 1824–1830.

8. Porte D Jr, Woods SC. Regulation of food intake and body weight by insulin. *Diabetologia* 1981; **20**(3): 274–280.

9. Obici S, Feng Z, Karkanias G, Baskin DG, Rossetti L. Decreasing hypothalamic insulin receptors causes hyperphagia and insulin resistance in rats. *Nature Neuroscience* 2002; **5**(6): 566–572.

10. Enriori PJ, Evans AE, Sinnayah P, Jobst EE, Tonelli-Lemos S, Billes SK, et al. Diet-induced obesity causes severe but reversible leptin resistance in arcuate melanocortin neurons. *Cell Metabolism* 2007; **5**(3): 181–194.

11. Milewicz A, Budzubsja B, Mikulski E, Demissie M, Tworowska U. Influence of obesity and menopausal status on serum leptin, cholecystokinin, galanin and neuropeptide Y levels. *Gynecological Endocrinology* 2000; **14**(3): 196–203.

12. Gibbs J, Young RC, Smith GP. Cholecystokinin decreases food intake in rats. *Journal of Comparative and Physiological Psychology* 1973; **84**(3): 488–495.

13. Wank SA. Cholecystokinin receptors. *American Journal of Physiology* 1995; **269**(5): G628–G646.

14. Batterham RL, Cowley MA, Small CJ, Herzog H, Cohen MA, Dakin CL, et al. Gut hormone PYY$_{3-36}$ physiologically inhibits food intake. *Nature* 2002; **418**(6898): 650–654.

15. Hagan MM. Peptide YY: a key mediator of orexigenic behavior. *Peptides* 2002; **23**(2): 377–382.

16. Adrian TE, Savage AP, Sagor GR, Allen JM, Bacarese-Hamilton AJ, Tatemoto K, et al. Effect of peptide YY on gastric, pancreatic, and biliary function in humans. *Gastroenterology* 1985; **89**(3): 494–499.

17. Hoentjen F, Hopman WP, Jansen JB. Effect of circulating peptide YY on gallbladder emptying in humans. *Scandinavian Journal of Gastroenterology* 2001; **36**(10): 1086–1091.

18. Hoentjen F, Hopman WP, Maas MI, Jansen JB. Role of circulating peptide YY in the inhibition of gastric acid secretion by dietary fat in humans. *Scandinavian Journal of Gastroenterology* 2000; **35**(2): 166–171.

19. Halatchev IG, Ellacott KL, Fan W, Cone RD. Peptide YY$_{3-36}$ inhibits food intake in mice through a melanocortin-4 receptor-independent mechanism. *Endocrinology* 2004; **145**(6): 2585–2590.

20. Batterham RL, Cohen MA, Ellis SM, Le Roux CW, Withers DJ, Frost GS, et al. Inhibition of food intake in obese subjects by peptide YY$_{3-36}$. *The New England Journal of Medicine* 2003; **349**(10): 941–948.

21. Batterham RL, Bloom SR. The gut hormone peptide YY regulates appetite. *Annals of the New York Academy of Sciences* 2003; **994**(1): 162–168.

22. Adrian TE, Bloom SR, Bryant MG, Polak JM, Heitz PH, Barnes AJ. Distribution and release of human pancreatic polypeptide. *Gut* 1976; **17**(12): 940–944.

23. Hort Y, Baker E, Sutherland GR, Shine J, Herzog H. Gene duplication of the human peptide YY gene (PYY) generated the pancreatic polypeptide gene (PPY) on chromosome 17q21. 1. *Genomics* 1995; **26**(1): 77–83.

24. Glaser B, Zoghlin G, Pienta K, Vinik Al. Pancreatic polypeptide response to secretin in obesity: effects of glucose intolerance. *Hormone and Metabolic Research* 1988; **20**(05): 288–292.

25. Russell-Jones D, Gough S. Recent advances in incretin-based therapies. *Clinical Endocrinology* 2012; **77**(4): 489–499.

26. Larsen PJ, Tang-Christensen M, Holst JJ, Orskov C. Distribution of glucagon-like peptide-1 and other preproglucagon-derived peptides in the rat hypothalamus and brainstem. *Neuroscience* 1997; **77**(1): 257–270.

27. Suzuki K, Jayasena CN, Bloom SR. Obesity and appetite control. *Experimental Diabetes Research* 2012; **2012**: 824305.

28. Verdich C, Flint A, Gutzwiller JP, Naslund E, Beglinger C, Hellstrom PM, et al. A meta-analysis of the effect of glucagon-like peptide-1 (7–36) amide on ad libitum energy intake in humans. *Journal of Clinical Endocrinology and Metabolism* 2001; **86**(9): 4382–4389.

29. Kojima M, Hosoda H, Date Y, Nakazato M, Matsuo H, Kangawa K. Ghrelin is a growth-hormone-releasing acylated peptide from stomach. *Nature* 1999; **402**(6762): 656–660.

30. Nakazato M, Murakami N, Date Y, Kojima M, Matsuo H, Kangawa K, et al. A role for ghrelin in the central regulation of feeding. *Nature* 2001; **409**(6817): 194–198.

31. Neary NM, Small CJ, Wren AM, Lee JL, Druce MR, Palmieri C, et al. Ghrelin increases energy intake in cancer patients with impaired appetite: acute, randomized, placebo-controlled trial. *Journal of Clinical Endocrinology and Metabolism* 2004; **89**(6): 2832–2836.

32. Wren AM, Seal LJ, Cohen MA, Brynes AE, Frost GS, Murphy KG, et al. Ghrelin enhances appetite and increases food intake in humans. *Journal of Clinical Endocrinology and Metabolism* 2001; **86**(12): 5992.

33. Cummings DE, Purnell JQ, Frayo RS, Schmidova K, Wisse BE, Weigle DS. A preprandial rise in plasma ghrelin levels suggests a role in meal initiation in humans. *Diabetes* 2001; **50**(8): 1714–1719.

34. Ariyasu H, Takaya K, Tagami T, Ogawa Y, Hosoda K, Akamizu T, et al. Stomach is a major source of circulating ghrelin, and feeding state determines plasma ghrelin-like immunoreactivity levels in humans. *Journal of Clinical Endocrinology and Metabolism* 2001; **86**(10): 4753–4758.

35. Ravussin E, Tschop M, Morales S, Bouchard C, Heiman ML. Plasma ghrelin concentration and energy balance: overfeeding and negative energy balance studies in twins. *Journal of Clinical Endocrinology and Metabolism* 2001; **86**(9): 4547–4551.

36. Tschöp M, Weyer C, Tataranni PA, Devanarayan V, Ravussin E, Heiman ML. Circulating ghrelin levels are decreased in human obesity. *Diabetes* 2001; **50**(4): 707–709.

37. Williams DL, Cummings DE, Grill HJ, Kaplan JM. Meal-related ghrelin suppression requires postgastric feedback. *Endocrinology* 2003; **144**(7): 2765–2767.

38. Nedvídková J, Krykorkova I, Bartak V, Papezova H, Gold PW, Alexci S, et al. Loss of meal-induced decrease in plasma ghrelin levels in patients with anorexia nervosa. *Journal of Clinical Endocrinology and Metabolism* 2003; **88**(4): 1678–1682.

39. Otto B, Cuntz U, Fruehauf E, Wawarta R, Folwaczny C, Riepl RL, Heiman ML, et al. Weight gain decreases elevated plasma ghrelin concentrations of patients with anorexia nervosa. *European Journal of Endocrinology* 2001; **145**(5): 669–673.

40. Cummings DE, Clement K, Purnell JQ, Vaisse C, Foster KE, Frayo RS, et al. Elevated plasma ghrelin levels in Prader–Willi syndrome. *Nature Medicine* 2002; **8**(7): 643–644.

41. Sumithran P, Prendergast LA, Delbridge E, Purcell K, Shulkes A, Kriketos A, et al. Long-term persistence of hormonal adaptations to weight loss. *The New England Journal of Medicine* 2011; **365**(17): 1597–1604.

42. Le Roux CW, Patterson M, Vincent RP, Hunt C, Ghatei MA, Bloom SR. Postprandial plasma ghrelin is suppressed proportional to meal calorie content in normal-weight but not obese subjects. *Journal of Clinical Endocrinology and Metabolism* 2005; **90**(2): 1068–1071.

Chapter 3.4

Obesogenic medication in the aetiology of obesity

Wilma S Leslie

University of Glasgow, Glasgow, UK

3.4.1 Introduction

The development of obesity is a long-term multifactorial process. While changes in diet and physical activity are considered key factors in terms of underpinning the obesity epidemic, other additional factors have been proposed that modify the likelihood or extent of weight gain [1,2]. In principle, this could be through influences on (1) food choice and intakes, (2) absorption/malabsorption, (3) physical activity, or (4) any of the biochemical pathways that contribute to energy expenditure [3].

There are many prescription drugs currently in use that are associated with weight gain, and this contributes to 'pharmaceutical iatrogenesis' [1,3]. Many are used in the treatment of chronic noncommunicable diseases, are consistently associated with weight gain and are considered obesogenic (Table 3.4.1) [4–7]. In some conditions (e.g. type 1 diabetes), weight gain is indicative of effective treatment, but weight gain as a result of drug treatment is an unwanted side effect for many. A survey carried out to elicit the perceived reasons for weight gain found that 8–10% of adults felt their weight gain was a consequence of drug treatment [8]. The use of many of the drugs associated with weight gain has increased significantly over the past 30 years [1]. However, evidence regarding the amount to which they can contribute to weight gain is not widely promoted.

3.4.2 Drugs associated with weight gain

Psychotropic medications are one group of drugs associated with weight gain. Antipsychotics, used to treat many psychiatric disorders including schizophrenia and other psychoses, have been long been acknowledged as being associated with weight gain, and several reviews have examined their effect on body weight [9–12]. Weight gain is reported as a consequence of most atypical antipsychotics; however, the magnitude of weight gain is dependent on the drug used (Table 3.4.1). Olanzapine and clozapine have been found to have the greatest effect on body weight. Weight gains ranging from 4.4 kg/10 weeks to 10 kg/~1 year [10,12] have been observed. Risperidone and ziprasidone are reported to have the least effect on body weight (−3 kg to +2.3 kg) [12]. Prescribing of atypical antipsychotics has increased since the recommendation – in particular, following the recommendation of the UK National Institute for Health and Clinical Excellence (NICE) that they be used as a first-line option in the treatment of schizophrenia [13]. In 2006–2007, prescriptions accounted for two-thirds of all antipsychotic prescriptions [14]. Half of these patients could therefore expect a weight gain of 3–10 kg.

Epilepsy affects around 500,000 (1:130) people in developed countries, and the drug valproate is one of the first-line treatments in its management [15].

Table 3.4.1 Summary of systematic review data on the effect of obesogenic drugs on body weight [12]

Drug (number of studies)	Conditions	Follow-up (weeks)	Range of weight change (kg)*
Psychotropic drugs			
Valproate (4)	Epilepsy, bipolar disorder	12–47	+1.2 to +5.8
Lithium (1)	Bipolar disorder	52	+4
Clozapine (2)	Schizo-affective disorder, schizophrenia	14–52	+4.2 to +9.9
Olanzapine (4)	Bipolar disorder, psychosis, schizophrenia	12–51	+2.8 to +7.1
Risperidone (2)	Schizo-affective disorder, schizophrenia	14–24	+2.1 to +2.3
Ziprasidone (1)	Schizophrenia	52	−2.7 to −3.2
Corticosteroids			
Prednisone (1)	Graves' ophthalmopathy	24	+2
Anti-hyperglycaemic drugs			
Insulin (6)	Type 2 diabetes	12 weeks–10 years	+1.8 to +6.6
Glipizide (5)	Type 2 diabetes	16–52	−0.3 to +3.8
Glimepiride (2)	Type 2 diabetes	14–52	+0.8 to +2.3
Glibenclamide (2)	Type 2 diabetes	24 weeks–10 years	+1.4 to ~+4
Chlorpropamide (1)	Type 2 diabetes	10 years	~+5
Troglitazone (1)	Type 2 diabetes	12	+0.06
Rosiglitazone (1)	Type 2 diabetes	12	−0.95 to +0.36
Pioglitazone (3)	Type 2 diabetes	12–52	+0.7 to +1.9
Tricyclic antidepressants			
Nortriptyline (1)	Depression	12	+3.7
Doxepin (1)	Depression	13	+2.7
Amitriptyline (1)	Depression	104	+1.7
Beta-adrenergic blocking agents			
Atenolol and/or metoprolol (4)	Hypertension	13 weeks–4 years	+0.5 to +1.5
Propranolol (2)	Post-myocardial infarction, hypertension	52 weeks–10 years	−0.6 to +2.3

* Greatest weight gain not always related to the longest follow-up period.

It is also used in the treatment of manic episodes associated with bipolar disorder, which affects around 1% of the population [16]. Weight gain is a common side effect of valproate, with the frequency of weight gain reported as ranging from 7 to 71% among adults [17]. In one study, 24% of patients who commenced treatment gained 5–10% body weight, and 47% gained more than 10% [18]. Data from randomised controlled trials (RCTs) that compared valproate therapy with an alternative drug and quantified the weight gain found mean increases in weight of 2.5–5.8 kg within 1 year of treatment (Table 3.4.1) [12,20].

Lithium has been used for many years in the treatment of people experiencing mania (bipolar disorder) [19], and weight gain is a notable side effect of treatment. Treatment is reported to cause an initial and often large weight gain, which then remains constant [19,20]. Around 75% of patients who were prescribed lithium experienced weight gain [20]. The average weight gain has been reported at around 4 kg within 2 years following initiation of treatment [12,20].

Tricyclic antidepressants are one of the oldest classes of antidepressant that, despite the introduction of selective serotonin reuptake inhibitors (SSRIs), are still used extensively [12]. Weight gain as a result of treatment has been found to be variable, but mean gains of 2–4 kg have been reported (Table 3.4.1) [12].

Prescription medications used in the treatment of non-communicable diseases associated with obesity, such as diabetes, heart disease and hypertension, are also associated with weight gain [4–7,21]. Increases in obesity over the past 30 years have been mirrored by a dramatic rise in the prevalence of diabetes. In the USA, the incidence of type 2 diabetes is reported as doubling, and much of the increase is observed in those who are obese (BMI $\geq$30 kg/m^2) [22]. In the UK, around 2.8 million people suffer from either type 1 or type 2 diabetes [23]. Drugs used in the treatment of type 2 diabetes include insulin, sulphonylureas and thiazolidinediones, and all are associated with weight gain, albeit to differing degrees.

Insulin therapy often has the greatest effect on body weight. Review of RCTs that compared insulin therapy only with either oral agents or with insulin plus oral agents showed increases in weight of 1.8 kg at 12 weeks, 5.2 kg at around 6 months and 6.6 kg at 1 year. Data from the United Kingdom Prevention of Diabetes study (UKPDS) showed that longer-term treatment can result in a mean weight gain of around 6.5 kg at 10 years.[12] Some correlation between dosage of insulin and weight gain is evident, with more intensive therapy associated with greater weight gain [11,12]. Treatment with insulin therapy in type 2 diabetes is often delayed, and weight gain is considered one factor contributing to this delay [24].

Weight gain of 0.8–3.6 kg within 1 year of treatment with sulphonylureas to around 4–5 kg at 10 years is reported in studies that compared treatment with an alternative oral hypoglycaemic, placebo or insulin. Thiazolidinediones appear to have less effect on body weight, with effects reported as ranging from weight loss to +1.9 kg at 1 year in one review [12], and around +2.9 kg in another [11].

Beta-blockers (unless contraindicated) have a prominent role in the management of coronary heart disease, which affects around 2.7 million people in

the UK [25]. Beta-blockers may also be used in the management of hypertension, although they are not recommended as an initial treatment [25]. The effect of beta-blocker therapy on body weight has been shown to be relatively small but more marked in those prescribed propranolol – around 2 kg at 1-year follow-up, and 3 kg at 2 years [12,21].

Corticosteroids have long been associated with weight gain. One RCT, in which weight gain as a result of treatment with prednisone was quantified, found an increase in body weight of 2 kg at 6 months post treatment [12].

3.4.3 Discussion

Not all drugs associated with weight gain are discussed here. However, the ones presented are those consistently reported in medical/scientific literature, many of which are used to treat chronic non-communicable diseases. The effects on body weight differ greatly among the different drug categories, but for all the drugs, weight gain is a result of treatment. Given the prevalence of the diseases/conditions for which obesogenic drugs are used, the number of individuals in the population receiving treatment with these drugs is potentially quite high. During adulthood, the average annual weight gain in the general population is around 0.5–1 kg [26,27]. The weight gain observed as a consequence of treatment with some of the drugs highlighted here, often over a shorter time period, is greater than this. Thus, pharmacotherapy has become a significant factor in the continually rising prevalence of obesity.

In many developed countries, up to two-thirds of men and women are considered either overweight or obese, with further increases predicted [28–30]. Those who are overweight or obese have been shown to be more likely than those of normal weight to be prescribed drugs associated with weight gain. Comparison of 1150 obese patients with 1150 age-and-sex-matched controls of normal weight showed that a higher percentage of the obese were prescribed drugs used to treat chronic non- communicable diseases, including those considered obesogenic [31]. This has the potential to trap individuals in a vicious cycle, as any existing weight problem may be exacerbated by drug therapy. Body mass index (BMI) may be shifted towards the obese category, and risks of developing obesity-related comorbid conditions are increased.

Many patients with chronic long-term conditions do not comply with treatment, and non-compliance has been reported as an issue with many of the drugs presented here [12]. The adverse effect of weight gain may be a significant factor in non-compliance. The potential for weight gain should be discussed with patients at the commencement of treatment using any drug that is associated with weight gain. The use of alternative drugs may be possible and should be considered. However, if this is not possible, then support should be made available to help patients minimise potential weight gain and the related non-communicable diseases associated with obesity. The recently published Scottish Intercollegiate Guideline Network guideline on obesity management highlights the drugs associated with weight gain, and recommends that weight management be discussed with patients at the commencement of treatment [32].

Treatment with obesogenic medications may impede, but not negate, the success of weight management interventions. The Lifestyle Challenge study recruited patients with obesity-related comorbid diseases, and they were prescribed a range of obesogenic drugs [33]. Individuals taking drugs associated with weight gain were heavier at baseline and achieved less weight loss after a 20-week behavioural weight management programme (3.7 kg vs. 5.8 kg). In patients with type 2 diabetes, treated with either insulin or oral hypoglycaemic drugs, an intensive lifestyle intervention was successful in achieving significant weight loss in comparison to those randomised to usual care (−6.15% vs. −0.88%; $P<0.001$) [34]. For those prescribed antipsychotic medications, an 18-month behavioural weight control programme resulted in significant weight loss in those allocated to the intervention in comparison to those allocated to usual care, in whom significant weight gain was observed (between-group difference of 6.7 kg, $P<0.01$) [35].

3.4.4 Conclusion

All factors that contribute to the rising tide of obesity should be recognised and addressed [36]. The weight gain potential of some commonly prescribed drugs is evident, and, given the current prevalence of obesity, is a pertinent adverse effect. Prescribers need to be aware of the potential effects of commonly used medications on body weight, and the use of alternative drugs, if available and known to be of equal efficacy, should be considered. Patients should also be made aware of the possibility of weight gain at the time of initial prescription. While the provision of effective advice and support to avoid or minimise weight gain would be the optimal approach for patients receiving treatment with obesogenic medications, weight loss is achievable, but may require intensive interventions. The potential effect of obesogenic medications should be taken into consideration when evaluating individuals presenting for weight management.

3.4.5 Summary box

Key points

- Many medications prescribed for the long term cause continued weight gain.
- Prescribers ought to be mindful to the impact of medications on body weight, and should mention this to patients when treatment is chosen.
- Comparable medications, where available, without weight gain as a side effect, ought to be considered by prescribers.
- Effective advice and support to avoid or minimise weight gain would be the optimal approach in patients receiving treatment with obesogenic medications.
- Weight loss is achievable, but may require intensive long-term interventions.

References

1. Bray GA, Champagne CM. Beyond energy balance: there is more to obesity than kilocalories. *Journal of the American Dietetic Association* 2005; **105**: S17–S23.
2. Keith SW, Redden DT, Katzmarzyk PT, Boggiano MM, Hanlon E, Benca RM, et al. Putative contributors to the secular increase in obesity: exploring the roads less travelled. *International Journal of Obesity* 2006; **30**: 1585–1594.
3. Kopelman P. Iatrogenisis and weight control: drug induced obesity. *Obesity Reviews* 2006; **7**(2): IS0082.

4. World Health Organisation. Obesity, preventing and managing the global epidemic. Report of a WHO consultation on obesity, 1998.

5. Lean MEJ. Management of obesity and overweight. *Medicine* 1998; **26**: 9–13.

6. Pijl H, Meinders AE. Bodyweight change as an adverse effect of drug treatment. *Drug Safety* 1998; **14**: 329–342.

7. Finer N. Clinical assessment, investigation and principles of management: realistic weight goals. In: Kopleman PG, Stock MJ (eds) *Clinical Obesity*. London: Blackwell Science, 1998, pp. 350–376.

8. Vossenaar M, Anderson A, Lean M, Ocke M. Perceived reasons for weight gain in adulthood. *International Journal of Obesity* 2004; **28**(S1): S67.

9. Malone M. Medications associated with weight gain. *The Annals of Pharmaco Therapy* 2005; **39**: 2046–2055.

10. Allison DB, Mentore JL, Moonseong H, Chandler LP, Cappelleri JC, Infante MC, et al. Antipsychotic-induced weight gain: a comprehensive research synthesis. *American Journal of Psychiatry* 1999; **156**: 1686–1696.

11. Abramof–Ness R, Apovian CM. Drug induced weight gain. *Drugs of Today* 2005; **8**: 547–555.

12. Leslie WS, Hankey CR, Lean MEJ. Weight gain as an adverse effect of some commonly prescribed drugs: a systematic review. *The Quarterly Journal of Medicine* 2007; **100**: 395–404.

13. NICE. Schizophrenia: core interventions in the treatment and management of schizophrenia in adults in primary and secondary care. 2009. Available from: http://www.nice.org.uk/nicemedia/live/11786/43608/43608.pdf.

14. NICE. Implementation uptake report: atypical antipsychotic drugs for the treatment of schizophrenia. 2008. Available from: http://www.nice.org.uk/media/410/E9/ImplUptakeReport AtypicalAntipsychotics.pdf.

15. NICE. The epilepsies: the diagnosis and management of the epilepsies in adults and children in primary and secondary care. 2004. Available from: http://www.nice.org.uk/nicemedia/live/10954/29532/29532.pdf.

16. NICE. Bipolar disorder: the management of bipolar disorder in adults, children and adolescents, in primary and secondary care. 2006. Available from: http://www.nice.org.uk/nicemedia/live/10990/30193/30193.pdf.

17. Jallon P, Picard F. Bodyweight gain and anticonvulsants. *Drug Safety* 2001; **24**: 969–978.

18. Corman CL, Leung NM, Guberman AH. Weight gain in epileptic patients during treatment with valproic acid: a retrospective study. *Canadian Journal of Neurological Sciences* 1997; **24**: 240–244.

19. Kerry RJ, Liebling LI, Owen G. Weight change in lithium responders. *Acta Psychiatrica Scandinavica* 1970; **46**: 238–243.

20. Vestergard P, Poulstrup I, Schou M. Prospective studies on a Lithium cohort. *Acta Psychiatrica Scandinavica* 1987; **78**: 434–441.

21. Sharma A, Pischon T, Hardt S, Kunz I, Luft FC. B-adrenergic receptor blockers and weight gain: a systematic analysis. *Hypertension* 2001; **37**: 250–254.

22. Fox CS, Pencina MJ, Meigs JB, Vasan RS, Levitzky YS, D'Agiostino RB Sr. Trends in the Incidence of Type 2 diabetes mellitus from the 1970s to the 1990s: the Framingham heart study. *Circulation* 2006; **113**: 2914–2918.

23. Diabetes UK. Reports and statistics. 2010. Available from: http://www.diabetes.org.uk/Professionals/Publications-reports-and-resources/Reports-statistics-and-case-studies/Reports/Diabetes-prevalence-2010/

24. Barnett A, Allsworth J, Jameson K, Mann R. A review of the effects of antihyperglycaemic agents on body weight: the potential of incretin targeted therapies. *Current Medical Research and Opinion* 2007; **23**: 1493–1507.

25. NICE. Management of stable angina. 2011. Available from: http://www.nice.org.uk/nicemedia/live/13549/55660/55660.pdf.

26. Heitmann BL, Garby L. Patterns of long-term weight changes in overweight developing Danish men and women aged between 30 and 60 years. *International Journal of Obesity* 1999; **23**: 1074–1078.

27. Norman JE, Bild D, Lewis CE, Liu K, West DS. The impact of weight change on cardiovascular disease risk factors in young black and white adults: the CARDIA study. *International Journal of Obesity* 2003; **27**: 369–376.

28. Wang CY, McPherson K, Marsh T, Steven L Gortmaker SL, Brown M. Health and economic burden of the projected obesity trends in the USA and the UK. *Lancet* 2011; **378**: 815–825.

29. Scottish Government. The Scottish health survey 2010. 2011. Available from: http://scotland.gov.uk/Publications/2011/09/22144303/3, accessed Oct 2016.

30. The NHS Information Centre. Health survey for England 2009. 2010. Available from: http://www.ic.nhs.uk/webfiles/publications/003_Health_Lifestyles/hse09report/HSE_09_Summary.pdf.

31. Counterweight Project Team. Impact of obesity on drug prescribing in primary care. *British Journal of Clinical Practice* 2005; **55**: 743–749.

32. Scottish Intercollegiate Guideline Network. Management of obesity. 2010.

33. Malone M, Alger-Mayer SA, Anderson DA. Medication associated with weight gain may influence outcome in a weight management programme. *The Annals of Pharmaco Therapy* 2005; **39**: 1204–1208.

34. The Look AHEAD Research Group. Long-term effects of a lifestyle intervention on weight and cardiovascular risk factors in individuals with type 2 diabetes mellitus: four-year results of the look AHEAD trial. *Archives of Internal Medicine* 2010; **170**: 1566–1575.

35. Poulin MJ, Chaput JP, Simard V, Vincent P, Bernier J, Gauthier Y, et al. Management of antipsychotic-induced weight gain: prospective naturalistic study of the effectiveness of a supervised exercise programme. *Australian and New Zealand Journal of Psychiatry* 2007; **41**: 980–989.

36. Foresight. Tackling obesities: future choices – project report. Government office for science. 2007. Available from: http://www.bis.gov.uk/foresight/our-work/projects/published-projects/tackling-obesities, accessed Oct 2016.

Chapter 3.5

Gut microbiome in obesity

Kevin Whelan
King's College London, London, UK

3.5.1 The gut microbiome

The gut microbiome comprises 100 trillion bacteria containing 100-fold more unique genes than the human genome [1]. It is estimated that 1000–1150 bacterial species are able to colonise the human gastrointestinal tract, with each individual harbouring 100–1000 of such species [1]. Approximately 90% of the gut microbiome belongs to the two main phyla: *Firmicutes* (e.g. *Lactobacillus, Clostridium*); and *Bacteroidetes* (e.g. *Bacteroides*) [2]. The gut microbiome is mostly strict anaerobes, predominately bacteroides, bifidobacteria, eubacteria, gram-positive cocci, clostridia, lactobacilli, methanogens and sulphate-reducing bacteria. Depending upon the species, these bacteria can exert a range of impacts on the host, some of which might be beneficial, and some, harmful.

An important and beneficial function of the gut microbiome is the suppression of enteropathogens (e.g. *Clostridium difficile*) through a process described as *colonisation inhibition*. This involves competition for nutrients and a geographic niche in the colonic lumen; the production of antimicrobial compounds that inhibit the growth of enteropathogens; and the production of lactate and short-chain fatty acids (SCFAs) that maintain an acidic colonic environment. In addition, SCFAs have other benefits, such as the stimulation of colonic water absorption and the provision of a metabolisable energy source to colonocytes that supports the maintenance of gut mucosal integrity. The gut microbiome also has important roles in both the development of the gastrointestinal immune system as well as the metabolism of non-digestible carbohydrates (e.g. fermentable fibres). Therefore, it is not only the presence/absence or numbers of specific bacterial groups in the gut microbiome that are important to human health, but also their functional and metabolic characteristics within the gut.

Only a minority of the bacteria in the gut can be grown using traditional culture techniques. However, advances in molecular microbiology (e.g. metagenomic sequencing) have enabled researchers to more completely characterise not only individual bacterial species in the gut but also their community structure and genomic function. For example, some studies have shown that bacteria populate the gut in discrete clusters, with some species frequently co-occurring together ('enterotypes') [3].

The large number of bacteria able to colonise the gastrointestinal tract allows for large inter-individual variability. The variability can be affected by a number of factors related to the environmental pressures that shape the microbial ecosystem. These include geographical location (e.g. Europe vs. rural Africa) [4], early diet (e.g. breastfeeding vs. formula milk) [5], antibiotics and disease [6].

Diet is clearly a major determinant of obesity through excess energy intake. However, both cross-sectional studies and intervention studies show that diet is also a primary determinant of the

Advanced Nutrition and Dietetics in Obesity, First Edition. Edited by Catherine Hankey.
© 2018 John Wiley & Sons Ltd. Published 2018 by John Wiley & Sons Ltd.

gut microbiome. One cross-sectional study of 98 healthy volunteers reported that *Bacteroides* were positively associated with dietary fat intake and negatively associated with fibre intake, whereas the opposite was true for *Firmicutes* and *Proteobacteria* [7]. More recently, a study of 1135 humans reported that 63 dietary factors were associated with variation in the gut microbiome, including intakes of energy and macronutrients, as well as specific food items such as bread, sugar-sweetened beverages, buttermilk, whole milk, alcoholic drinks, coffee and tea [8]. Meanwhile, an intervention study comparing animal-based diets with plant-based diets found that changes in microbial diversity occurred very rapidly following dietary manipulation [9]. Therefore, investigating relationships between the gut microbiome and obesity are challenging, since they are both influenced by diet.

3.5.2 Microbiome, obesity and weight loss

The association between obesity and the gut microbiome and the effect of weight loss on the gut microbiome have been investigated in a range of human studies, some of which are summarised in Table 3.5.1 [10–14].

A number of observational studies have reported higher *Firmicutes* and lower *Bacteroidetes* (and, therefore, a higher *Firmicutes–Bacteroidetes* ratio) in obese humans as compared to lean counterparts [11,15], although this is not consistently shown in all studies [10,16]. Lower microbiome diversity and richness (i.e. lower number of bacterial species) have also been reported in people with obesity [17,18]. Indeed, a systematic review of 10 observational studies found that three studies reported lower richness and two reported lower diversity of

Table 3.5.1 Examples of human studies investigating the interplay between diet, obesity, weight loss and the gastrointestinal microbiome (adapted from Graham et al., 2015) [14]

Author	Method	Result
Duncan et al. (2008) [10]	Major bacterial groups were measured in 33 obese and 14 controls (lean) during weight-maintaining conditions.	No evidence that the proportions of *Bacteroidetes* and *Firmicutes* were associated with human obesity.
Ley et al. (2006) [11]	12 obese adults randomised to fat- or carbohydrate-restricted weight loss diets. Stool samples analysed for microbiome using sequencing over 1 year.	Obese subjects had higher *Firmicutes*, lower *Bacteroidetes* and a higher *Firmicutes–Bacteroidetes* ratio. Weight loss resulted in reduction in *Firmicutes* and increase in *Bacteroidetes*, irrespective of diet type.
Cotillard et al. (2013) [12]	49 obese or overweight subjects underwent a 6-week high-protein weight loss diet, followed by a 6-week weight-maintenance diet. Stool samples were collected and food intake measured at baseline, 6 and 12 weeks.	18 individuals with a low gene count (microbiome with less genetic/functional capacity) and 27 with high gene count (microbiome with more genetic/functional capacity) were identified. Following an energy-restricted diet, gene richness increased significantly in the low-gene-count group.
Kong et al. (2013) [13]	30 obese women underwent gastric bypass surgery, resulting in significant weight loss. Stool and white adipose tissue samples were taken at baseline and 3 months post-operatively.	58 initially undetectable genera were detected post-operatively in all patients. Following weight loss surgery, there were more associations detectable between the gut microbiome and gene expression as compared to before the weight loss surgery.

microbiome among obese compared to lean counterparts [17]. Following meta-analysis of the data from all studies, obese individuals had 7.47% lower richness and 2.07% lower diversity, with the authors questioning the clinical significance of such small differences. No consistent differences in phyla were identified across the studies [17]. It is important to note that the gut microbiome within an individual is actually rather stable.

The findings from observational studies are also supported by a number of dietary intervention studies that have investigated the effect of energy restriction and subsequent weight loss on the gut microbiome in the obese. Some intervention studies report a reduction in *Firmicutes* and an increase in *Bacteroidetes* (and, therefore, lowering of the *Firmicutes–Bacteroidetes* ratio, which has been shown to be raised in some studies of obesity) during dietary energy restriction and weight loss [15], although others report no such change [10].

Studies of the gut microbiome in obesity are complicated by the mutually dependent interactions between diet, the microbiome and obesity. For example, observational studies on the association between obesity and the gut microbiome are confounded by the fact that people with obesity consume different diets compared to lean comparators, while intervention studies on the effect of weight loss on the gut microbiome are confounded by the fact that weight loss is often induced by dietary modification. Therefore, in both instances, dietary differences, rather than obesity or weight loss alone, are likely to be partly responsible for any observed differences in gut microbiome.

This has been elegantly overcome by using surgically induced weight loss based on an animal model. A study reported an increase in *Verrucomicrobia* and *Gammaproteobacteria* in mice following Roux-en-Y gastric bypass (RYGB) surgery, as compared with controls (without RYGB) [19]. When the microbiome from these mice was then transplanted into mice without an established gut microbiome (germ-free mice), those who received microbiome transplant from the RYGB donors experienced greater weight loss and decreased fat mass as compared to those who received microbiome transplant from controls.

The mice colonised with microbiome from the RYGB donors had lower energy harvest from the gut (i.e. lower caecal SCFAs) [19]. Interestingly, mice undergoing RYGB lost 29% of their initial body weight, whereas those that received microbiome transplant from RYGB donors only lost 5% body weight, suggesting that the gut microbiome is not the major contributor responsible for weight loss [19]. These findings are perhaps expected; the surgical intervention was always going to lead to enormous differences in energy consumption and absorption, but differences in the microbiome are affecting body weight (despite them not having surgery) as a result of receiving a microbiome from mice who have. The effect of surgically induced weight loss on the microbiome has also been investigated in humans. An increase in microbiome diversity was reported following RYGB in obese humans, with 58 previously undetectable genera subsequently added to the gut microbiome following surgery, many of which were *Proteobacteria* [13]. Higher microbiome diversity has been considered beneficial, as numerous studies have shown that those with gastrointestinal and metabolic disorders have lower diversity. However, the role of microbial diversity as a direct cause has not been confirmed. Changes in the expression of genes related to white adipose tissue (WAT) also occurred, and these were also associated with changes in bacterial genera, many of which were independent of the change in energy intake, thus suggesting a potential mechanism through which microbiome might impact body weight [13]. The mechanisms through which the microbiome impacts host gene expression, whether direct or indirect, are unknown and are the focus of much current research.

3.5.3 Metabolic mechanisms of the microbiome in obesity

In addition to studies indicating an association between obesity, weight loss and the gut microbiome, a range of evidence, mostly from animal studies, suggests plausible mechanisms through which the microbiome may exert such effects, and are summarised in Figure 3.5.1.

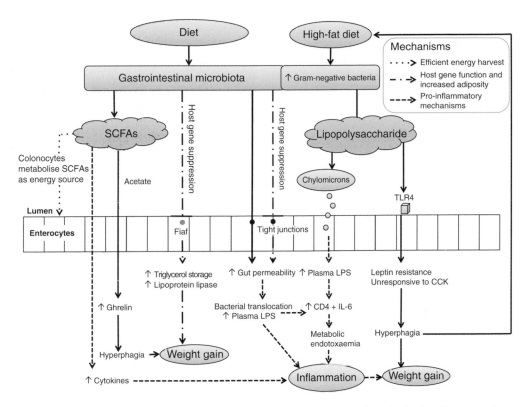

Figure 3.5.1 Potential mechanisms of the relationship between the gastrointestinal microbiota and obesity (adapted from reference [14]). Some animal studies and a small number of human studies demonstrate alterations in this metabolic balance that are hypothesised to be linked to obesity. For example, some studies show that a high-fat diet favours gram-negative bacteria, while others show that this may lead to raised serum lipopolysaccharide concentrations, which could lead to inflammation and weight gain. In contrast, some studies have shown that microbiome-derived SCFAs stimulate satiety hormones such as leptin and polypeptide YY (LPS, lipopolysaccharide; SCFAs, short-chain fatty acids).

Colonic energy harvest

Some dietary carbohydrates (especially polysaccharides) are not digested and absorbed in the small intestine and reach the colon, where they can be fermented to provide energy for microbial metabolism. A by-product of carbohydrate fermentation in the colon are the SCFAs, including acetate, propionate and butyrate, which are then absorbed and utilised as an energy source by the human colonocytes.

In one study, SCFAs were 20% higher in stools of obese compared to lean humans, therefore potentially acting as an additional energy source for the host – that is, the microbiome in the obese is more efficient at energy harvest from the diet [16].

However, the greater levels of colonic SCFAs may not be causal in obesity. For example, these may merely be the result of greater SCFA production from the already-described altered microbiome, or the greater levels in stool may not be due to greater production but owing to reduced absorption (as a mechanism to avoid additional energy harvest) [20].

SCFAs may have numerous independent effects on the development of obesity. A rodent study has shown that increased acetate production during a high-fat diet activates the parasympathetic nervous system, resulting in increased ghrelin and insulin secretion [21]. This generates a positive feedback loop, resulting in hyperphagia (due to increased ghrelin) and increased energy storage (due to increased insulin secretion), which, in an obesogenic environment characterised by exposure to energy-dense diets, promotes obesity and metabolic syndrome [21].

It is worth highlighting that SCFAs may also stimulate satiation through PYY and leptin production. Acetate has been shown to cause an anorectic effect by working directly on the hypothalamus [22]. Therefore, the role of SCFAs in body weight regulation involves a number of opposing mechanisms.

Host gene function and increased adiposity

Some components of the gut microbiome suppress the expression of genes for proteins, such as the fasting-induced adipose factor (Fiaf) and tight junction proteins expressed in the intestinal epithelia.

Fiaf plays a central role in triglyceride metabolism [23]. The suppression of Fiaf by specific components of the gut microbiome increases lipoprotein lipase activity in adipocytes and promotes triglycerol storage in host fat cells [24]. Mice that do not have any gut microbiome (germ-free mice) have higher levels of circulating Fiaf, resulting in lower LPL activity and, therefore, reduced fat storage. Therefore, aspects of the gut microbiome might stimulate host weight gain through the suppression of Fiaf, which results in impairing triglyceride metabolism and promoting fat storage [24].

The gut microbiome profile can also impact on the expression of genes encoding gut permeability (e.g. tight junction proteins), and can therefore influence permeability [25]. This is important because increased gut permeability can expose the systemic circulation to the gut microbiome, which in turn can drive inflammation and metabolic endotoxaemia.

Pro-inflammatory mechanisms

Some bacterial components are associated with inflammation, which itself is associated with obesity. For example, lipopolysaccharide (LPS), an endotoxin contained within the cell membrane of gram-negative bacteria (e.g. *Bacteroides*, *Prevotella*), triggers inflammation in the host as part of an innate immune response. In some studies, LPS has been shown to result in inflammation and weight gain, with one

study in mice showing similar weight gain after infusion with a low dose of LPS as that occurring during a high-fat diet [26]. The inflammation caused by microbiome-derived LPS has been linked to a variety of mediators, including toll-like receptor-4.

A variety of animal studies have established the connection between LPS, inflammation and weight gain. However, for this to occur, the microbiome-derived LPS from the gut lumen must enter the host bloodstream, which has been shown to occur through both the integration of LPS into chylomicrons, as well as increases in gut permeability allowing passive exposure.

Chylomicron formation increases following a high-fat meal, resulting in greater transport of LPS to the systemic circulation in humans [27]. Increases in plasma LPS concentrations are associated with greater inflammation, including CD14 and interleukin (IL)-6 [26]. Therefore, a high-fat diet (in addition to resulting in increased energy intake) also results in greater transport of microbiome-derived LPS into the circulation, and the subsequent inflammation and metabolic endotoxaemia.

Gut permeability is a key exposure regulator of the systemic circulation to the contents of the gut lumen, including the gut microbiome. The more permeable the gastrointestinal tract, the less effective it is as a barrier to LPS. When the gastrointestinal epithelium is compromised, whole bacteria and their products (such as LPS) may translocate and enter the blood stream. Bacterial translocation has been shown to be higher in mice fed a high-fat diet than those fed standard chow [28]. Therefore, in addition to increasing chylomicron production, a high-fat diet may also result in a microbiome profile that reduces the host expression of genes encoding tight junction proteins that maintain gut integrity and reduce gut permeability [25].

Raised serum levels of LPS are also associated with obesity through other mechanisms and can stimulate leptin resistance, which can lead to hyperphagia and weight gain [29].

However, the role of the gut microbiome in driving intestinal inflammation is not a simple relationship. First, although LPS is pro-inflammatory, some by-products of microbial metabolism (e.g. SCFAs such as butyrate) can be immuno-regulatory [30]. Second, the role of the gram-negative-bacteria-derived LPS in inflammation and obesity is in contrast to observations that obese humans have more *Firmicutes* (generally gram positive) and fewer *Bacteroidetes* (gram negative) than lean humans [11,15]. However, other bacterial groups such as *Prevotellaceae* have been shown to be higher in the obese, and are composed of LPS, which would stimulate the inflammation found in obesity [31].

3.5.4 Modifying the microbiome in the management of obesity

The finding that the gut microbiome is altered in obesity, together with plausible physiological mechanisms to suggest at least some causality, raises the possibility that interventions that modify the microbiome may be efficacious in the prevention or management of obesity.

A randomised controlled trial of a probiotic (*Lactobacillus rhamnosus* CGMC1.3724) compared with placebo in obese people undergoing moderate energy restriction found no differences in weight loss between the groups at 12 weeks, although there was a clinically and statistically significant greater weight loss among females in the probiotic group (−4.4 kg), as compared to those in the placebo group (−2.6 kg) [32]. More recently, a randomised controlled trial was undertaken of a commercially available probiotic yoghurt containing lactobacilli (*Lactobacillus acidophilus* LA5) and bifidobacteria (*Bifidobacterium lactis* BB12), compared to a control yoghurt in conjunction with an energy-restricted diet (dietary advice) in 89 overweight and obese women. Although significant weight loss occurred in both groups after 12 weeks, there was no significant difference in the weight loss between the probiotic yoghurt (−5.3 kg) and control yoghurt (−5 kg) groups [33].

A meta-analysis of randomised controlled trials of probiotics and their effect on body weight and body mass index (BMI) was recently published [34]. Probiotics were shown to significantly reduce body weight by 0.59 kg (95% CI, 0.30–0.87, data from 21 trials) and reduce BMI by 0.49 kg/m^2 (95% CI, 0.24–0.74, data from 19 trials), indicating a small but statistically significant effect. Trials were of varied durations (ranging from 3 weeks to 24 weeks) and used various probiotics; however, those of longer durations and those using multi-species probiotics were more effective. However, only four of the trials were specifically in people who were overweight or obese. Restricting the meta-analysis to trials where the mean baseline BMI was >25 kg/m^2 still showed a significant reduction in BMI of 0.58 kg/m^2 (95% CI, 0.28–0.88; $P < 0.01$) during probiotic supplementation [34].

Prebiotics are defined as selectively fermented ingredients that result in specific changes in the composition and/or activity of the gastrointestinal microbiome, thus conferring benefit(s) upon host health. They have also been investigated for their effect on body weight. A study in non-obese humans reported that inulin/oligofructose increased GLP-1 and peptide YY concentrations and suppressed appetite [35]. However, despite GLP-1 concentrations strongly correlating with markers of prebiotic fermentation, it has not been possible to demonstrate that changes in microbiome induced by prebiotics *per se* are the cause of the reductions in appetite (as opposed to the fibre-satiating properties) [35]. A meta-analysis of randomised controlled trials confirmed the effect of specific prebiotics on satiety; however, their impact on energy intake and body weight was found to be equivocal [36].

Finally, in a randomised controlled trial in obese males with metabolic syndrome (defined as either >30 kg/m^2 or waist circumference >102 cm, together with fasting plasma glucose >5.6 mmol/L), faecal microbiome transplant from lean donors did not result in significant weight loss. However, it did increase insulin sensitivity, with the median rate of glucose disappearance changing from 26.2 μmol/kg/min at baseline to 45.3 μmol/kg/min following the faecal microbiome transplant [37].

Further research is required to investigate whether interventions that modify the microbiome can impact on body weight, and therefore identify whether they have a role in obesity management.

3.5.5 Conclusion

There is now considerable evidence to suggest that the gut microbiome is altered in obesity. While diet wields a large influence on body weight, the gut microbiome is integral to the host metabolic response to diet. There is some evidence that the microbiome in the obese harvests energy more effectively, may manipulate host gene function and may drive systemic inflammation, which in some studies has been shown to be associated with increased body weight. The extent to which alterations in the microbiome are a cause or a consequence of weight gain or weight loss are difficult to elucidate in humans due to the complex multidirectional interactions between diet, the microbiome and obesity. However, if the microbiome plays even a minor role in influencing body weight, then it holds future potential for preventing or managing obesity through it's modulation. What remains clear, however, is that diet, and particularly its energy content, remains a central factor in obesity development.

3.5.6 Summary box

Key points

- There are key differences in the gut microbiome of people with obesity, as compared to lean controls.
- Animal studies suggest that altered gut microbiome could be involved in the aetiology of obesity, rather than merely being an epiphenomenon. This includes evidence that significant weight loss occurs when the microbiome from mice that have undergone bariatric surgery are transplanted into germ-free mice.
- The proposed mechanisms for the role of the microbiome in obesity include evidence that (1) they harvest colonic energy more effectively; (2) they may manipulate host gene function that increases adiposity; and (3) some components can propagate metabolic endotoxaemia.
- Research in this area is limited by the complex and multidirectional interplays between diet, obesity, weight change and the gut microbiome.
- Evidence in humans that the gut microbiome may be manipulated to reduce body weight is in its infancy, and initial findings indicate that any effect is likely to be small.

References

1. Qin J, Li R, Raes J, et al. A human gut microbial gene catalogue established by metagenomic sequencing. *Nature* 2010; **464**: 59–65.
2. Bajzer M, Seeley R. Obesity and gut flora. *Nature* 2006; **444**: 1009–1010.
3. Arumugam M, Raes J, Pelletier E, et al. Enterotypes of the human gut microbiome. *Nature* 2011; **473**: 174–180.
4. De Filippo C, Cavalieri D, Di Paola M, et al. Impact of diet in shaping gut microbiota revealed by a comparative study in children from Europe and rural Africa. *Proceedings of the National Academy of Sciences (USA)* 2010; **107**: 14691–14696.
5. Power SE, O'Toole PW, Stanton C, Ross RP, Fitzgerald GF. Intestinal microbiota, diet and health. *British Journal of Nutrition* 2014; **111**: 387–402.
6. Falony G, Joossens M, Vieira-Silva S, et al. Population-level analysis of gut microbiome variation. *Science* 2016; **352**(6285): 560–564.
7. Wu G, Chen J, Hoffman C, et al. Linking long-term dietary patterns with gut microbial enterotypes. *Science* 2011; **334**: 105–108.
8. Zhernakova A, Kurilshikov A, Bonder MJ, et al., Population-based metagenomics analysis reveals markers for gut microbiome composition and diversity. *Science* 2016; **352**(6285): 565–569.
9. David L, Maurice C, Carmody R, et al. Diet rapidly and reproducibly alters the human gut microbiome. *Nature* 2014; **505**: 559–563.
10. Duncan S, Lobley G, Holtrop G, et al. Human colonic microbiota associated with diet, obesity and weight loss. *International Journal of Obesity* 2008; **32**: 1720–1724.
11. Ley R, Turnbaugh P, Klein S, Gordon J. Human gut microbes associated with obesity. *Nature* 2006; **444**: 1022–1023.
12. Cotillard A, Kennedy S, Chun Kong L, et al. Dietary intervention impact on gut microbial gene richness. *Nature* 2013; **500**: 585–588.
13. Kong L, Tap J, Aron-Wisnewsky J, et al. Gut microbiota after gastric bypass in human obesity: Increased richness and associations of bacterial genera with adipose tissue genes. *American Journal of Clinical Nutrition* 2013; **98**: 16–24.
14. Graham C, Mullen A, Whelan K. Obesity and the gastrointestinal microbiota: a review of associations and mechanisms. *Nutrition Reviews* 2015; **73**(6): 376–385.
15. Turnbaugh PJ, Hamady M, Yatsunenko T, et al. A core gut microbiome in obese and lean twins. *Nature* 2009; **457**: 480–484.
16. Schwiertz A, Taras D, Schäfer K, et al. Microbiota and SCFA in lean and overweight healthy subjects. *Obesity* 2009; **18**: 190–195.
17. Sze MA, Schloss PD. Looking for a signal in the noise: revisiting obesity and the microbiome. *mBio* 2016; **7**(4): e01018–16.
18. Turnbaugh P, Gordon J. The core gut microbiome, energy balance and obesity. *The Journal of Physiology* 2009; **587**: 4153–4158.
19. Liou A, Paziuk M, Luevano J, Machineni S, Turnbaugh P, Kaplan L. Conserved shifts in the gut microbiota due to gastric

bypass reduce host weight and adiposity. *Science Translational Medicine* 2013; **5**: 178ra41.

20. Fava F, Gitau R, Griffin BA, Gibson GR, Tuohy KM, Lovegrove JA. The type and quantity of dietary fat and carbohydrate alter fecal microbiome and short-chain fatty acid excretion in a metabolic syndrome 'at-risk' population. *International Journal of Obesity* 2013; **37**: 216–223.
21. Perry RJ, Peng L, Barry NA, et al., Acetate mediates a microbiome-brain-β-cell axis to promote metabolic syndrome. *Nature* 2016; **534**(7606): 213–217.
22. Frost G, Sleeth M, Sahuri-Arisoylu M, et al. The short-chain fatty acid acetate reduces appetite via a central homeostatic mechanism. *Nature Communications* 2014; **5**: 3611.
23. Kim H, Youn B, Shin M, et al. Hypothalamic Angptl4/Fiaf is a novel regulator of food intake and body weight. *Diabetes* 2010; **59**: 2772–2780.
24. Bäckhed F, Ding H, Wang T, et al. The gut microbiota as an environmental factor that regulates fat storage. *Proceedings of the National Academy of Sciences (USA)* 2004; **101**: 15718–15723.
25. Macia L, Thorburn A, Binge L, et al. Microbial influences on epithelial integrity and immune function as a basis for inflammatory diseases. *Immunological Reviews* 2012; **245**: 164–176.
26. Cani P, Amar J, Iglesias MA, et al. Metabolic endotoxemia initiates obesity and insulin resistance. *Diabetes* 2007; **56**: 1761–1772.
27. Ghoshal S, Witta J, Zhong J, de Villiers W, Eckhardt E. Chylomicrons promote intestinal absorption of lipopolysaccharides. *Journal of Lipid Research* 2009; **50**: 90–97.
28. Amar J, Chabo C, Waget A, et al. Intestinal mucosal adherence and translocation of commensal bacteria at the early onset of type 2 diabetes: Molecular mechanisms and probiotic treatment. *EMBO Molecular Medicine* 2011; **3**: 559–572.
29. Raybould HE. Gut microbiota, epithelial function and derangements in obesity. *The Journal of Physiology* 2012; **590**: 441–446.
30. Cavaglieri C, Nishiyamab A, Fernandes L, Curic R, Miles E, Calder P. Differential effects of short-chain fatty acids on proliferation and production of pro- and anti-inflammatory cytokines by cultured lymphocytes. *Life Sciences* 2003; **73**: 1683–1690.
31. Zhang H, DiBaise J, Zuccolo A, et al. Human gut microbiota in obesity and after gastric bypass. *Proceedings of the National Academy of Sciences (USA)* 2009; **106**: 2365–2370.
32. Sanchez M, Darimont C, Drapeau V, et al. Effect of *Lactobacillus rhamnosus* CGMCC1.3724 supplementation on weight loss and maintenance in obese men and women. *British Journal of Nutrition* 2014; **111**: 1507–1519.
33. Madjd A, Taylor MA, Mousavi N, Delavari A, Malekzadeh R, Macdonald IA, Farshchi HR. Comparison of the effect of daily consumption of probiotic compared with low-fat conventional yogurt on weight loss in healthy obese women following an energy-restricted diet: a randomized controlled trial. *American Journal of Clinical Nutrition* 2016; **103**(2): 323–329.
34. Zhang Q, Wu Y, Fei X. Effect of probiotics on body weight and body-mass index: a systematic review and meta-analysis of randomized, controlled trials. *International Journal of Food Sciences and Nutrition* 2015; **67**(5): 571–580.
35. Cani PD, Lecourt E, Dewulf EM, et al. Gut microbiota fermentation of prebiotics increases satietogenic and incretin gut peptide production with consequences for appetite sensation and glucose response after a meal. *American Journal of Clinical Nutrition* 2009; **90**: 1236–1243.
36. Kellow NJ, Coughlan MT, Reid CM. Metabolic benefits of dietary prebiotics in human subjects: a systematic review of randomised controlled trials. *British Journal of Nutrition* 2014; **111**: 1147–1161.
37. Vrieze A, Van Nood E, Holleman F, et al. Transfer of intestinal microbiota from lean donors increases insulin sensitivity in individuals with metabolic syndrome. *Gastroenterology* 2012; **143**: 913–916.

Chapter 3.6

Physical activity and physical inactivity in the aetiology of obesity

Sjaan R Gomersall and Wendy J Brown
University of Queensland, Queensland, Australia

3.6.1 Introduction

Overweight and obesity are associated with increased risks of many poor health outcomes, including cardiovascular disease, type 2 diabetes, arthritis, depression and some cancers [1]. Overweight and obesity arise in adults as a result of accumulative weight gain, which occurs when there is a positive energy balance – that is, when energy intake exceeds energy expenditure, resulting in energy storage. Conversely, weight maintenance occurs when the body is in a state of energy balance, when energy intake and energy expenditure are balanced over a period of time, resulting in minimal energy storage [2]. Therefore, it can be hypothesised that energy expenditure is an important determinant of long-term energy balance and, consequently, weight change over time. Energy expenditure should be viewed as a continuum of behaviours, as energy is expended in all waking activities – including those performed lying and sitting down (commonly termed *sedentary behaviours*); light to moderate activities such as walking or household chores; and vigorous activities such as running or playing competitive sports.

The objective of this chapter is to describe the evidence for cross-sectional and longitudinal associations between physical activity, physical fitness and sedentary behaviour with overweight and obe-

sity in adults. Relationships between current physical activity guidelines and weight gain prevention are also discussed.

3.6.2 Physical activity and body weight: does physical inactivity lead to weight gain?

Many studies with a cross-sectional design have shown inverse relationships between physical activity and body weight or body mass index (BMI) [3,4]. One example is the Copenhagen City Heart Study of more than 3653 women and 2626 men. This study showed that both men and women are statistically less likely to be concurrently obese if they have moderate or high levels of leisure-time physical activity. The odds ratios (OR) (95% confidence interval [CI]) 0.70 (0.59–0.83) and 0.51 (0.40–0.64), respectively for women and 0.71 (0.58–0.85) and 0.65 (0.52–0.80) respectively for men [4]. However, the direction of this association cannot be confirmed by the results of this type of study, as high body weight may predispose people to inactivity.

Few large-cohort studies have examined the relationships between physical activity and weight gain. While there appears to be an inverse relationship, with increased or higher levels of physical activity resulting in less weight gain over time, the exact dose–response relationships are unclear. Reviews in this area are consistently limited by the large variations in study and analytical design, accuracy and reliability of the measures used to capture physical activity, and the concurrent inability to control for confounding factors, including changes in diet and energy intake.

Given that there is a high rate of weight gain in young adult women, it is surprising that few studies have examined the relationships between physical activity and weight gain at this life stage. Indeed, a review of the determinants of weight gain in young adult women found only one prospective cohort study that assessed both physical activity and weight change in young adult women [5]. In the Coronary Artery Risk Development in Young Adults (CARDIA) study [6], the researchers assessed changes in leisure-time physical activity and weight in a group of 1541 women at 2–5 years and 5–7 years of the 10-year study period. Women who increased and then maintained their activity levels had the smallest weight gain (0.8 lb/year, or 0.36 kg/year), as compared to those who either maintained or decreased their activity levels, who gained, on average, 2.4 lb/year (or 1.1 kg/year). These results are important because they support the notion that *increasing* activity levels may be important in disrupting the typical homeostatic mechanisms that tend to promote energy conservation and, therefore, weight gain over time [2].

Focusing on slightly older women, data from the Nurses' Health Study show an average weight gain of 5.7 kg in 8 years among 46,754 women who were aged 23–45 years in 1989 [7]. Those who maintained a 'high level' of physical activity (>30 min walking/day or >20 min jogging/day), or who *increased* their physical activity by at least 30 min/day, were less likely to gain weight (defined as >5% of initial weight). Overall, the researchers concluded that sustained physical activity for at least 30 min/day, particularly if more intense, was associated with a reduction in long-term weight gain. They also concluded that, for weight gain prevention, the type of physical activity was not as important as the total energy expenditure [7]. It is important to note, however, that while 38% of this

sample 'avoided weight gain of >5% in 5 years', data from the Australian Longitudinal Study on Women's Health (ALSWH) can be used to show that a 4.5% increase in weight for a 20-year-old woman of average weight and height (62.7 kg, 1.66 m) would mean a one unit increase in BMI every 5 years. If this rate of weight gain was to continue, then this woman's BMI would increase from 22.8 (healthy range) to 27.1 (overweight) by the time she was 40 [8].

Researchers from the United States Women's Health Study (WHS) have also recently reported on the amount of physical activity required to prevent weight gain [9]. Average weight gain in this sample of 34,079 mid to older aged women (age 54.2 years at baseline) was 2.6 kg over 13 years, or 200 g/year, which is much lesser than in the younger nurses' cohort described earlier (713 g/year over 8 years) [7], and lesser than that observed in the mid-age cohort of the ALSWH (292 g/year over 14 years from 45–50 to 59–64 years of age) [10]. In the WHS, physical activity was associated with less weight gain *only* in women with initial BMI < 25 kg/m². Women in this BMI category, who maintained their weight and gained <2.3 kg over 13 years, averaged physical activity equating with 21.5 MET-hours/week at six follow-ups over 13 years. This translates to about an hour a day of moderate-intensity activity.

This study is important as it highlights the fact that physical activity was not protective against weight gain in women who were overweight at baseline. Results from the ALSWH have also shown that the rate of weight gain over 10 years is higher in younger adult women (age 18–23 years at baseline) with BMI > 25 than those with healthy BMI [8,11]. Data from that study also show that women who report doing no physical activity gained an average of 7.9 kg in 10 years, while those in the low (40–600 MET-min/week), moderate (600–1200) and high (>1200) physical activity categories gained 7.1, 6.6 and 4.3 kg, respectively. As the women in the highest physical activity category (corresponding to about 50 min of daily moderate-intensity activity) gain (on average) more than 4 kg in 10 years, it is reasonable to assume that more activity is required for prevention of weight gain [8].

3.6.3 Physical fitness and body weight: does being unfit lead to weight gain?

There is evidence of an inverse association between physical fitness and body weight status. The term 'physical fitness' is typically used to describe cardiovascular fitness, which is expressed as maximal oxygen uptake (VO_2max; ml/kg/min). VO_2max is usually estimated using treadmill or cycling tests. In Australia, cardiovascular fitness, estimated using the PWC 75% submaximal cycle test, and BMI and skinfolds were measured in more than 1000 people for the DASET survey in 1992 [12]. The data show a small but significant inverse correlation between fitness and body weight status – that is, the higher an individual's fitness, the lower their BMI. Although the correlation (±95% CI) between VO_2max and BMI was small ($r = -0.17 \pm 0.06$; $n = 1084$, age range 18–78 years), there was a stronger correlation between VO_2max and the sum of four skinfolds ($r = -0.40 \pm 0.05$). There was no significant difference in these relationships by gender.

There is also evidence to suggest a longitudinal relationship between physical fitness and weight gain. Di Pietro and colleagues [13] conducted a cohort study with a sample of 4599 men and 729 women. Physical fitness (estimated using a timed treadmill test) and body weight were measured at least three times over 7.5 years. The results of this study showed inverse relationships between fitness and weight change. Each 1-min improvement in treadmill time was associated with a 14% reduction in the odds of a ≥5 kg weight gain in men (OR = 0.86; 95% CI: 0.83–0.89), and with a 9% reduction in women (OR = 0.91; 95% CI: 0.83–1). There was also a 21% reduction in the odds of a ≥10 kg weight gain in both men (OR = 0.79; CI: 0.75–0.84) and women (OR = 0.79; 95% CI: 0.67–0.93). The results of these cross-sectional and longitudinal studies suggest that individuals who have higher levels of physical fitness are likely to weigh less than their unfit counterparts, but also that improvements in physical fitness over time can attenuate weight gain.

It is also important to note, however, that recent work suggests that individuals who are obese but physically fit have similar morbidity and mortality outcomes as their normal-weight counterparts. This has been termed the 'metabolically healthy but obese' phenotype [14]. Ortega and colleagues analysed data from the Aerobics Center Longitudinal Study, which classified 43,265 US adults (24.3% female) as metabolically healthy or not healthy at baseline (based on standard metabolic syndrome criteria, excluding waist circumference), and tracked health and mortality outcomes over a minimum period of 7 years. The results showed that metabolically healthy but obese individuals were fitter (maximal treadmill test) than their metabolically unhealthy but obese peers ($P < 0.001$). Furthermore, individuals with the metabolically healthy but obese phenotype had a 20–50% lower risk than their metabolically unhealthy but obese peers of all-cause mortality (hazard ratio, HR = 1.44; 95% CI: 1.06–1.96); non-fatal (HR = 1.39; 95% CI: 0.92–2.10) and fatal (HR = 1.48; 95% CI: 0.87–2.52) cardiovascular disease; and cancer mortality (HR = 1.17; 95% CI: 0.73–1.88). Importantly, the metabolically healthy but obese participants had similar morbidity and mortality outcomes as the metabolically unhealthy but normal-weight participants.

3.6.4 Sedentary behaviour and body weight: does being sedentary lead to weight gain?

Sedentary behaviours include activities during waking time that involve sitting or lying down and require low levels of energy expenditure, typically in the range of 1–1.5 METs (metabolic equivalents) [15]. They include many activities at work (e.g. sitting at a desk or machine), during leisure time (e.g. watching TV, reading, socialising) and in transport (e.g. sitting in a car, bus or train). Recently, time spent in sedentary behaviours has been linked to adverse health outcomes, including overweight/obesity and weight gain, with some studies showing that relationships are independent of the time spent in physical activity [16,17]. To date, much of the research in this field has been limited by self-report questionnaires that are restricted to one domain (e.g. watching TV); however, the evidence base is rapidly developing, with more studies using device-based measurement and prospective designs.

Several recent reviews have suggested that there is a positive cross-sectional relationship between time spent in sedentary behaviour and overweight and/or obesity [17–20]. For example, a review of the time spent watching TV vs. health outcomes identified 25 cross-sectional studies that found associations between TV viewing and overweight and/or obesity, using a variety of self-report and objective measures. This finding does not mean that watching TV *causes* overweight and obesity, but could be interpreted to mean that heavier individuals spend more time watching TV than their healthy-weight counterparts. In some studies, these significant relationships only remained in women when analyses were controlled for other factors, such as demographic variables and physical activity [17]. In a cross-sectional study of data from 8233 ALSWH participants, each additional hour of self-reported sitting time was associated with 110 g (95% CI: 40–180) and 260 g (95% CI: 140–380) of additional weight, in overweight and obese women, respectively [18]. As stated, these cross-sectional studies demonstrate associations between sedentary behaviour and overweight and obesity, but cannot determine whether increased amounts of sitting or sedentary behaviour cause weight gain over time.

Prospective studies with a time delay between the measure of sedentary behaviour and the outcome (weight gain) are required to do this, and several recent reviews of such studies have reported mixed findings [16–18,21]. For example, a systematic review of longitudinal studies by Thorp and colleagues identified 10 studies, of which six found that sedentary behaviour significantly predicted adverse changes in BMI, largely independent of baseline BMI and physical activity, while four either showed gender-specific associations, no association or that the time spent sedentary was a determinant of changes in body weight [16]. Using the same data set that demonstrated the cross-sectional association described in the preceding text, the ALSWH researchers found that,

after adjustment for other variables, sitting time was not associated with weight change over a 9-year period [18]. Overall, these results suggest that, while there are cross-sectional relationships between sedentary behaviour and weight, it is not yet clear whether high sedentary behaviour time results in weight gain.

3.6.5 Current physical activity guidelines and their relationship to weight change

Current physical activity guidelines, including those from the UK, USA and Australia, generally recommend a minimum of 150 min of moderate-intensity or 75 min of vigorous-intensity physical activity, or an equivalent combination of both moderate and vigorous activities each week [22–25]. The Australian guidelines are the only ones to provide a *range* of recommended activity levels, with an upper level of 300 min of moderate or 150 min of vigorous activity each week. The high end of the range was added to the Australian guidelines because evidence suggests that 50–60 min/day of moderate-intensity activity, or the equivalent volume of more vigorous activity, is the dose of physical activity required for the prevention of weight gain [26,27]. It is important to note that meeting the minimum physical activity recommendations is likely to result in substantial health benefits (e.g. lower risk of cardiovascular disease, type 2 diabetes, musculoskeletal and mental health problems), but that physical activity at the upper end of the range is required for the prevention of weight gain.

Reflecting on the emerging nature of the evidence, and the current lack of a strong dose–response relationship between sedentary behaviour and weight gain, population-based guidelines for sedentary behaviour for adults are limited to a general message, with no specific recommendations on time limits for the time spent sitting. Guidelines in Australia and the UK recommend minimising the amount of time spent in prolonged sitting [22,23], with Australian guidelines also recommending breaking up long periods of sitting whenever possible.

3.6.6 Summary

Multiple cross-sectional studies have shown relationships between physical activity, fitness, sedentary time and weight. Most seem to indicate that less movement and lower fitness are associated with greater weight, but the direction of these relationships is unclear. A growing body of evidence from prospective cohort studies suggests that more movement is associated with lower weight gain over time, with the equivalent of about 1 hour of moderate-intensity activity each day required to prevent weight gain in adults. Given the growing prevalence of overweight and obesity in most countries, and the difficulty of losing weight once it is gained, there is an urgent need for well-designed studies to inform the development of population-based strategies to prevent weight gain in adulthood. Based on the results of the studies reviewed here, physical activity is likely to be a key component of these strategies.

3.6.7 Summary box

Key points

- An inverse relationship appears evident with increased or higher levels of physical activity resulting in less weight gain over time; however, the exact dose–response relationships are unclear.
- Evidence on the links between activity and body weight are consistently limited by the large variations in study and analytical design; accuracy and reliability of the measures used to capture physical activity; and the inability to control for relevant confounding factors.
- Increasing activity levels may be important in disrupting the typical homeostatic mechanisms that tend to promote energy conservation and, therefore, weight gain over time.
- Metabolically healthy but obese participants had similar morbidity and mortality outcomes as metabolically unhealthy but normal-weight participants – highlighting the benefits of physical activity in reducing the negative metabolic impact of obesity.

- There are cross-sectional relationships between sedentary behaviour and weight, but it is not yet clear whether high sedentary behaviour time results in weight gain.
- Meeting the minimum physical activity recommendations is likely to result in substantial health benefits (e.g. lower risk of cardiovascular disease, type 2 diabetes, and musculoskeletal and mental health problems), but physical activity at the upper end of the range is required for the prevention of weight gain.

References

1. World Health Organization. Obesity and overweight. World Health Organization. 2013. Available from: http://www.who.int/mediacentre/factsheets/fs311/en/, cited 6 August 2013.
2. Hill J, Wyatt H, Peters J. Energy balance and obesity. *Circulation* 2012; **126**(1): 126–132.
3. Di Pietro L. Physical activity, body weight, and adiposity: an epidemiological perspective. *Exercise and Sport Sciences Reviews* 1995; **23**: 275–303.
4. Petersen L, Schnohr P, Sørensen T. Longitudinal study of the long-term relation between physical activity and obesity in adults. *International Journal of Obesity and Related Metabolic Disorders* 2004; **28**(1): 105–112.
5. Wane S, van Uffelen J, Brown W. Determinants of weight gain in young women: a review of the literature. *Journal of Women's Health* 2010; **19**(7): 1327–1340.
6. Schmitz K, Jacobs D, Leon A, Schreiner P, Sternfeld B. Physical activity and body weight: associations over ten years in the CARDIA study. Coronary artery risk development in young adults. *International Journal of Obesity and Related Metabolic Disorders* 2000; **24**(11): 1475–1487.
7. Mekary RA, Feskanich D, Malspeis S, Hu F, Willet W, Alison EF. Physical activity patterns and prevention of weight gain in premenopausal women. *International Journal of Obesity* 2009; **33**(9): 1039–1047.
8. Brown W, Hockey R, Dobson A. Effects of having a baby on weight gain. *American Journal of Preventive Medicine* 2010; **38**(2): 163–170.
9. Lee I, Djoussé L, Sesso H, Wang L, Buring J. Physical activity and weight gain prevention. *JAMA: The Journal of the American Medical Association* 2010; **303**(12): 1173–1179.
10. Gomersall S, Dobson A, Brown W. Weight gain, overweight and obesity: determinants and health outcomes from the Australian Longitudinal Study on Women's Health. *Current Obesity Reports* 2014; **3**: 46–53.
11. Brown W, Hockey R, Dobson A. Physical activity, sitting and weight gain in Australian women. *Journal of Science and Medicine in Sport* 2011; **2011**(14): 7.
12. Department of the Arts, the Environment and Territories. Pilot survey of the fitness of Australians. Canberra, 1992.
13. Di Pietro L, Kohl, HW, Barlow, CE, Blair, SN. Improvements in cardiorespiratory fitness attenuate age-related weight gain

in healthy men and women: The Aerobics Center Longitudinal Study. *International Journal of Obesity and Related Metabolic Disorders* 1998; **22**(1): 55–62.

14. Ortega F, Lee D, Katzmarzyk P, Ruiz J, Sui X, Church T, et al. The intriguing metabolically healthy but obese phenotype: cardiovascular prognosis and role of fitness. *European Heart Journal* 2013; **34**(5): 389–397.

15. Ainsworth BE, Haskell WL, Herrmann SD, Meckes N, Bassett DRJ, Tudor-Locke C, et al. Compendium of physical activities: a second update of codes and MET values. *Medicine and Science in Sports and Exercise* 2011; **43**(8): 1575–1581.

16. Thorp A, Owen N, Neuhaus M, Dunstan D. Sedentary behaviors and subsequent health outcomes in adults: a systematic review of longitudinal studies, 1996–2011. *American Journal of Preventive Medicine* 2011; **41**(2): 207–215.

17. Williams D, Raynor H, Ciccolo J. A review of TV viewing and its association with health outcomes in adults. *American Journal of Lifestyle Medicine* 2008; **2**(3): 250–259.

18. van Uffelen J, Watson M, Dobson A, Brown W. Sitting time is associated with weight, but not with weight gain in mid-aged Australian women. *Obesity* 2010; **18**(9): 1788–1794.

19. Xie Y, Stewart S, Lam T, Viswanath K, Chan S. Television viewing time in Hong Kong adult population: associations with body mass index and obesity. *PLos One* 2014; **9**(1): e85440.

20. Foster J, Gore S, Smith West D. Altering TV viewing habits: an unexplored strategy for adult obesity intervention? *American Journal of Health Behavior* 2006; **30**(1): 3–14.

21. Proper K, Singh A, van Michelen W, Chinapaw MJM. Sedentary behaviors and health outcomes among adults: a systematic review of prospective studies. *American Journal of Preventive Medicine* 2011; **40**(2): 174–182.

22. Australian Government Department of Health. Australia's physical activity and sedentary behaviour guidelines. 2014. Available from: http://www.health.gov.au/internet/main/publishing.nsf/Content/health-pubhlth-strateg-phys-act-guidelines/$File/FS-Adults-18-64-Years.PDF, cited 20 February 2014.

23. United Kingdom Department of Health. Physical activity guidelines for adults (19–64 years). 2011. Available from: https://www.gov.uk/government/uploads/system/uploads/attachment_data/file/213740/dh_128145.pdf, cited 20 February 2014.

24. United States Department of Health and Human Services. Physical activity guidelines for Americans. United States of America. 2008. Available from: http://www.health.gov/paguidelines/, cited 23 June 2012.

25. World Health Organisation. Global recommendations on physical activity for health: 18–64 years old. 2011. Available from: http://www.who.int/dietphysicalactivity/physical-activity-recommendations-18-64years.pdf?ua=1, cited 3 March 2014.

26. Saris W, Blair S, van Baak M, Eaton SB, Davies P, Di Pietro L, et al. How much physical activity is enough to prevent unhealthy weight gain? Outcome of the IASO 1st Stock Conference and consensus statement. *Obesity Reviews* 2003; **4**(2): 101–114.

27. Donnelly A, Blair S, Jakicic JM, Manore M, Rankin J, Smith B, et al. American College of Sports Medicine Position Stand. Appropriate physical activity intervention strategies for weight loss and prevention of weight regain for adults. *Medicine and Science in Sports and Exercise* 2009; **41**(2): 459–471.

Chapter 3.7

Obesogenic environment and obesogenic behaviours

Jeroen Lakerveld[1], Joreintje D Mackenbach[1], Harry Rutter[2] and Johannes Brug[1]

[1] EMGO Institute for Health and Care Research, Amsterdam, Netherlands
[2] London School of Hygiene and Tropical Medicine, London, UK

3.7.1 Introduction

Poor diets, physical inactivity and sedentary behaviour are the major drivers of obesity, with a wide range of chronic diseases directly or indirectly linked to these 'obesogenic' behaviours [1,2]. Lack of physical activity and excessive eating have been described as a normal response, by normal people, to an abnormal environment [3]. To a large extent, these obesogenic behaviours are driven by environmental characteristics that were absent until very recently in human evolution. Environmental characteristics can affect an individual's level of physical activity (e.g. through the availability of opportunities to walk, interconnectivity of streets, proximity of parks [4–6]) and dietary behaviours (e.g. through availability, accessibility and affordability of foods and variety of fast-food outlets) [7]. In turn, certain environments and aspects of the environments may be more 'obesogenic' than others, as they contain elements that are more likely to promote obesogenic behaviours, weight gain and obesity in individuals or populations [8]. The physical, sociocultural, political and economic environments, in powerful interaction with individual factors, are thus likely to be driving the obesity epidemic [9–12]. A large number of potential environmental-level determinants of obesity have been considered in the scientific literature. In this chapter, we aim to provide an overview of the current knowledge about environ-

mental determinants of obesity in adults, with special reference to the physical (built) environment (i.e. the places and spaces created by people, including buildings, parks and transport systems).

3.7.2 Environmental correlates of obesity

How our environment affects our body weight

The relatively new scientific approach of studying a broad range of environmental dimensions can be supported by a comprehensive framework to understand and characterise the 'obesogenic environment' [13]. The obesogenic environment has been described as 'the sum of influences that the surroundings, opportunities, or conditions of life have on promoting obesity in individuals or populations' [8], or simply put, any environmental characteristic that acts as a barrier to the maintenance of a healthy body weight [13]. Building on this, Swinburn et al. have created the ANGELO framework (the ANalysis Grid for Elements Linked to Obesity) for conceptualising the obesogenic environment and prioritising potential areas for intervention. The focus of this framework is to characterise the elements within environments that may have an influence on diet, physical activity and sedentary behaviour [8]. The framework is divided in two axes, one for the level (micro or macro) of the environment and one for the type of environment (physical, sociocultural, economic and political; Figure 3.7.1).

Micro environments are defined as environmental settings where groups of people gather and meet. Such settings are often geographically distinct, and there may be direct mutual influence between individuals and the environment. Examples of micro environments are homes, workplaces, supermarkets, bars and restaurants, and recreational facilities and neighbourhoods. *Macro environments* include the broader infrastructure (sectors) that may support or hinder health behaviours such as the spatial characteristics of urban form, transport infrastructure, the health system, legislation regarding food marketing and distribution, and the media [8] (although specific marketing activities may fall in the micro environment category). Although it is not fully understood how components affect behaviour and weight status [14], the ANGELO framework supports the analysis of all relevant environmental elements while providing a relatively simple scheme for describing a complex system [13].

Not all persons living near a fast-food outlet will regularly buy and consume unhealthy foods, nor will everyone increase their physical activity when there is a sports ground or appealing green space nearby. Individual-level factors such as motivation, attitudes and socio-demographic background play important roles in the relations between the physical environment and behaviour [15–17], and genetic factors strongly underlie the propensity of individuals to be physically active [18] and to become obese [19]. Kremers et al. [20], in their Environmental Research framework for weight Gain prevention (EnRG) framework, conceptualised how environmental factors may have an impact on obesogenic behaviours, and how these environmental influences are also likely to be mediated and moderated by individual-level factors [4]. For example, the presence of a high-quality cycling infrastructure may improve people's motivation to ride bikes and, subsequently, develop actual cycling habits (mediating pathway). This is, however, influenced by individual-level factors: research conducted in the Netherlands shows that adolescents from ethnic minority groups may be less likely to respond to the cycling infrastructure than ethnic Dutch [21–22]. Likewise, people with a genetic or learned stronger taste preference for sweet flavours may be more affected by the high availability and accessibility of sweet foods (moderating pathway). The model has

Size Type	Micro (settings) Neighbourhood, workplace, school, household, institutions, community	Macro (sectors) National, international levels
Physical What is available?	**Food retailers,** e.g. supermarkets **Food service outlets,** e.g. restaurants	**Food importing/production** **Food distribution**
Sociocultural What are the attitudes and beliefs?	**Community's norms and values related to food** Food traditions	**Mass media,** e.g. advertising and marketing for (un)healthy food products **'Common culture'**
Political What are the rules?	**Institutional rules and policies** For example, school food rules, family food rules	**Governmental policies, regulations, and laws,** e.g. on food labelling, advertising
Economic What are the costs?	**Prices of food** **Household income**	Costs of food importing, production, distribution Pricing policies, taxes

Figure 3.7.1 The ANGELO framework with examples of the levels and types of food environments. Adapted from [8].

been adapted and used by others [21] in order to accommodate other potential mediating and moderating characteristics, and links to outcomes such as body composition (Figure 3.7.2).

What environmental factors have been identified thus far?

The association between environmental characteristics, obesogenic behaviours and obesity is in some ways well established. Firstly, the obesity epidemic has developed in parallel with changes in the food and physical activity environments. In extreme environments, for example, in very poor and nutritionally-insecure countries or population groups, the environment – what is available and accessible, rather than individual choices – dictates what people can eat, and obesity is far less likely. For instance, the Cuban situation in the 1980s showed that dramatic

changes to the food and physical activity environments very strongly affected the prevalence of obesity and related diseases [23]. In experimental studies in which micro-environments are manipulated, strong effects on eating behaviour and dietary intake have been observed [24]. For example, research from Wansink and colleagues illustrates that making food only slightly less available or accessible can result in observable changes in food intake [24].

The number of studies that report physical environmental correlates with overweight or obesity has increased significantly in recent years, with a number of review articles published, each of which has taken a slightly different focus [4,5,25–30]. These reviews have shown that the outcomes of individual studies are not consistent. For instance, where some studies have reported significant positive associations between obesity and exposure to fast-food restaurants [31], or the physical activity environment [32], other

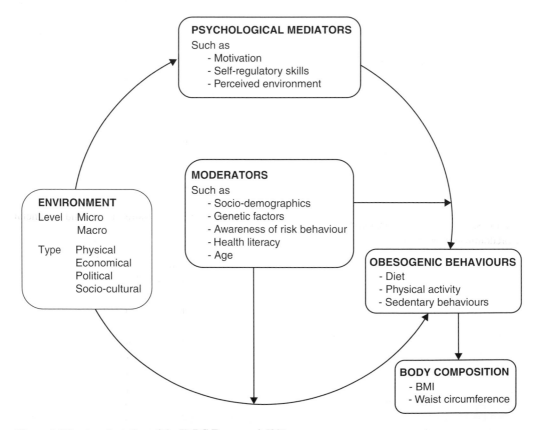

Figure 3.7.2   An adaptation of the EnRG Framework [20].

studies have not [33], or have reported negative associations [34]. This may reflect genuine differences in effect, or it may be a consequence of limitations within the published literature. Overall, among the many studies in which a large range of environmental characteristics have been studied, only two environmental characteristics appear to be consistently associated with weight status: indicators of urban sprawl (often based on population density, and positively associated with obesity) and measures of land use mix (negatively associated with obesity) [29,35]. It is important to note that almost all studies that have examined urban sprawl and land use mix were conducted in North America, where neighbourhood design tends to be very different from that in Europe.

There are numerous potential environmental factors associated with obesity for which there is no robust evidence of an association. Examples include access to recreational areas, proximity to fast-food outlets or the presence of infrastructure to support walking and cycling [36–39]. The micro environmental level (e.g. household, direct neighbourhood, workplace) has been studied relatively more often than the macro environmental level (see also Figure 3.7.1) [40]. This is unsurprising when one considers how much more straightforward it is to study individual-level interventions than it is to assess the impact of upstream, population-level activities.

Evidence for environmental determinants of obesity

Systematic reviews considering which aspects of the environment may influence obesity and obesogenic behaviours, and how they might exert that influence, are predominantly based on cross-sectional, observational studies, and thus cannot provide conclusive evidence of causation. The lack of robust evidence for the impact of environmental correlates of obesity may well reflect the quality and design of studies rather than representing the absence of a true relationship [5,29]. These quality and design issues include:

(1) *A lack of variation.* In Western countries, almost all environments exceed a threshold that would characterise them as obesogenic; hence, studying environmental determinants in one area does not allow for explanation of variation of obesity within that area.

(2) *Mediation and moderation.* Although they are highly influential, environmental factors do not directly cause obesity. Instead, they act by influencing human behaviour, mediated and moderated by a range of factors (see Figure 3.7.2).

(3) *Comprehensiveness.* It is not possible to consider all potential environmental factors in a research project, so studies of environmental influences are unavoidably only able to consider a partial view of the environment.

(4) *Measurement.* Equally, there are no gold standards against which the parts of the environment that we do consider can be judged. There is a lack of consensus as to the most appropriate measures and the definitions of exposure to the environment, while detailed measures may not be feasible in large projects. In addition, the act of measurement may itself have an influence on behaviour, and is subject to biases and measurement errors.

(5) *Research designs and analyses.* Most studies that attempt to identify the environmental characteristics related to obesity use cross-sectional designs. However, individuals are not randomly distributed among areas; healthy and active people may, for example, choose to reside in neighbourhoods that allow them to be physically active. This may be partially offset by longitudinal observational studies and natural experiments, which have the advantage of allowing for temporal associations and disentangling causation and selection, but these designs require more time and financial resources.

3.7.3 Conclusion

Despite a consensus that the physical environment has an important influence on individuals' weight status (in environments where there is no food, one cannot eat; in environments where there are no cars, buses or machines, one cannot avoid being physically active for transport, daily activities or work), a large body of research has failed to identify robust associations between the physical environment and weight status. Thus far, there is no consistent evidence for an association between specific characteristics of the physical environment and overweight or obesity in adults. It remains a challenge to identify the physical environmental factors with a measurable impact on overweight and obesity. However, it may be that even influences with effect sizes that are too small to detect using the research tools we have available could still have an important role to play at the population level [41].

Future researchers should consider the complexity of the relationship between the environment with individual weight status, as simplistic interventions aimed at limited aspects of the physical environment have not been shown to provide the desired changes in obesity-related behaviours, let alone in outcomes such as weight status. It needs to be understood which health-related activities people conduct where, when, for how long, with whom and so on. This will facilitate a thorough appraisal of the different tools that measure perceptions of the environment in terms of validity, reliability and applicability.

3.7.4 Summary box

Key points

- There is increased interest in the impact of our environment on behaviour and weight.
- The existing literature does not provide consistent or robust evidence for associations between environmental characteristics and weight status, other than for urban sprawl and land use mix.
- This inconsistency is, to some extent, a result of the inadequate design and quality of studies, but is also an unavoidable consequence of influences acting together within a complex system.
- Future studies should attempt to take a more comprehensive approach and acknowledge the mediating and moderating factors, measurement issues and designs to identify true obesogenic environmental determinants.
- There is a need to develop new research tools and approaches to consider the ways in which these factors may influence behaviour, and how they might be modified to improve health.

3.7.5 List of useful websites

www.spotlightproject.eu
www.dedipac.eu
www.ipenproject.org

References

1. Fisher E, Fitzgibbon M, Glasgow R, Haire-Joshu D, Hayman L, Kaplan R, et al. Behavior matters. *American Journal of Preventive Medicine* 2011; **40**(5, May): e15–e30.
2. World Health Organization: Obesity. Preventing and managing the global epidemic. Report of a WHO Consultation on Obesity. Geneva, 1998.
3. Egger G, Swinburn B. An 'ecological' approach to the obesity pandemic. *BMJ* 1997; **315**: 477–480.
4. Sallis J, Floyd M, Rodriguez D, Saelens B. Role of built environments in physical activity, obesity, and cardiovascular disease. *Circulation* 2012; **125**(5, Feb 7): 729–737.
5. Mackenbach JD, Rutter H, Compernolle S, Glonti K, Oppert J-M, Charreire H, et al. Obesogenic environments: a systematic review of the association between the physical environment and adult weight status, the SPOTLIGHT project. *BMC Public Health* 2014; **14**(1): 233.
6. Brug J. Determinants of healthy eating: motivation, abilities and environmental opportunities. *Family Practice* 2008; **25**(1, Dec 1): i50–i55.
7. Boone-Heinonen J, Gordon-Larsen P, Kiefe CI, Shikany JM, Lewis CE, Popkin BM. Fast food restaurants and food stores: longitudinal associations with diet in young to middle-aged adults: the CARDIA study. *Archives of Internal Medicine* 2011; **171**(13): 1162–1170.
8. Swinburn B, Egger G, Raza F. Dissecting obesogenic environments: the development and application of a framework for identifying and prioritizing environmental interventions for obesity. *Preventive Medicine* 1999; **29**: 563–570.
9. Robertson A, Lobstein T, Knai C. Obesity and socio-economic groups in Europe: evidence review and implications for action. Available from: http://ec.europa.eu/health/ph_determinants/life_style/nutrition/documents/ev20081028_rep_en.pdf, last accessed 18 August 2016.
10. Brug J, van Lenthe FJ (eds). *Environmental Determinants and Interventions for Physical Activity, Nutrition and Smoking: A Review*. Rotterdam: Zoetermeer, 2005, pp. 204–239.
11. Giskes K, Kamphuis CB, van Lenthe FJ, Kremers S, Droomers M, Brug J. A systematic review of associations between environmental factors, energy and fat intakes among adults: is there evidence for environments that encourage obesogenic dietary intakes? *Public Health Nutrition* 2007; **10**: 1005–1017.
12. Hill JO, Wyatt HR, Reed GW, Peters JC. Obesity and the environment: where do we go from here? *Science* 2003; **299**(5608): 853–855.
13. Kirk SF, Penney TL, McHugh TL. Characterizing the obesogenic environment: the state of the evidence with directions for future research. *Obesity Reviews* 2010; **11**(Feb): 109–117.

14. Lewin K. *Field Theory in Social Science; Selected Theoretical Papers*. New York: Harper and Row, 1951.
15. Van Dyck D, Cerin E, Conway TL, De Bourdeaudhuij I, Owen N, Kerr J, et al. Perceived neighborhood environmental attributes associated with adults' leisure-time physical activity: findings from Belgium, Australia and the USA. *Health & Place* 2012; **19**: 59–68.
16. Giskes K, Avendano M, Brug J, Kunst AE. A systematic review of studies on socioeconomic inequalities in dietary intakes associated with weight gain and overweight/obesity conducted among European adults. *Obesity Reviews* 2009; **11**: 413–429.
17. Kamphuis CB, Giskes K, de Bruijn GJ, Wendel-Vos W, Brug J, van Lenthe FJ. Environmental determinants of fruit and vegetable consumption among adults: a systematic review. *British Journal of Nutrition* 2006; **96**: 620–635.
18. Den Hoed M, Brage S, Zhao JH, Westgate K, Nessa A, Ekelund U, et al. Heritability of objectively assessed daily physical activity and sedentary behavior. *American Journal of Clinical Nutrition* 2013; **98**(5): 1317–1325.
19. Comuzzie AG, Allison DB. The search for human obesity genes. *Science* 1998; **280**: 1374–1377.
20. Kremers SP, de Bruijn GJ, Visscher TL, van MW, de Vries NK, Brug J. Environmental influences on energy balance-related behaviors: a dual-process view. *International Journal of Behavioral Nutrition and Physical Activity* 2006; **3**: 9.
21. De Munter JSL, Agyemang C, van Valkengoed IGM, Bhopal R, Zaninotto P, Nazroo J, et al. Cross national study of leisure-time physical activity in Dutch and English populations with ethnic group comparisons. *European Journal of Public Health* 2013; **23**: 440–446.
22. Lakerveld J, Brug J, Bot S, Teixeira PJ, Rutter H, Woodward E, et al. Sustainable prevention of obesity through integrated strategies: The SPOTLIGHT project's conceptual framework and design. *BMC Public Health* 2012; **12**(1): 793.
23. Franco M, Bilal U, Orduñez P, Benet M, Morejón A, Caballero B, et al. Population-wide weight loss and regain in relation to diabetes burden and cardiovascular mortality in Cuba 1980–2010: repeated cross sectional surveys and ecological comparison of secular trends. *BMJ* 2013; **346**: f1515.
24. Wansink, B. *Mindless eating: Why We Eat More Than We Think*. New York: Bantam Dell, 2006.
25. Booth KM, Pinkston MM, Poston WSC. Obesity and the built environment. *Journal of the American Dietetic Association* 2005; **105**: S110–S117.
26. Papas MA, Alberg AJ, Ewing R, Helzlsouer KJ, Gary TL, Klassen AC. The built environment and obesity. *Epidemiologic Reviews* 2007; **29**: 129–143.
27. O. Ferdinand A, Sen B, Rahurkar S, Engler S, Menachemi N. The relationship between built environments and physical activity: a systematic review. *American Journal of Public Health* 2012; **102**: e7–e13.
28. Feng J, Glass TA, Curriero FC, Stewart WF, Schwartz BS. The built environment and obesity: a systematic review of the epidemiologic evidence. *Health & Place* 2010; **16**: 175–190.
29. Ding D, Gebel K. Built environment, physical activity, and obesity: what have we learned from reviewing the literature? *Health & Place* 2012; **18**: 100–105.
30. Durand CP, Andalib M, Dunton GF, Wolch J, Pentz MA. A systematic review of built environment factors related to physical activity and obesity risk: implications for smart growth urban planning. *Obesity Reviews* 2011; **12**: e173–e182.
31. Burgoine T, Forouhi NG, Griffin SJ, Wareham NJ, Monsivais P. Associations between exposure to takeaway food outlets, takeaway food consumption, and body weight in Cambridgeshire, UK: population based, cross sectional study. *BMJ* 2014; **348**: g1464.
32. Black JL, Macinko J, Dixon LB, Fryer, GE. Neighborhoods and obesity in New York city. *Health & Place* 2010; **16**: 489–499.
33. Richardson AS, Boone-Heinonen J, Popkin BM, Gordon-Larsen P. Neighborhood fast food restaurants and fast food consumption: a national study. *BMC Public Health* 2011; **11**(1): 543.
34. Pearce J, Hiscock R, Blakely T, Witten K. A national study of the association between neighbourhood access to fast-food outlets and the diet and weight of local residents. *Health & Place* 2009; **15**: 193–197.
35. Grasser G, Van Dyck D, Titze S, Stronegger W. Objectively measured walkability and active transport and weight-related outcomes in adults: a systematic review. *International Journal of Public Health* 2013; **58**: 615–625.
36. Humpel N, Owen N, Leslie E. Environmental factors associated with adults' participation in physical activity: a review. *American Journal of Preventive Medicine* 2002; **22**: 188–199.
37. Saelens BE, Handy SL. Built environment correlates of walking: a review. *Medicine and Science in Sports and Exercise* 2008; **40**: S550–S566.
38. Fleischhacker SE, Evenson KR, Rodriguez DA, Ammerman AS. A systematic review of fast food access studies. *Obesity Reviews* 2011; **12**: e460–e471.
39. Holsten JE. Obesity and the community food environment: a systematic review. *Public Health Nutrition* 2009; **12**: 397–405.
40. Brug J, van Lenthe FJ, Kremers SP. Revisiting Kurt Lewin: how to gain insight into environmental correlates of obesogenic behaviors. *American Journal of Preventive Medicine* 2006; **31**: 525–529.
41. Rose G. *The Strategy of Preventive Medicine*. Oxford: Oxford University Press, 1994.

SECTION 4

Weight management in adults

Chapter 4.1

Macronutrient composition for weight loss in obesity

Rebecca Mete[1], Ekavi N Georgousopoulou[1] and Duane D Mellor[2]
[1] University of Canberra, Canberra, Australia
[2] University of Coventry, Coventry, UK

The topic of the best dietary approach for optimising weight loss has long historical roots. There are considerable amounts of theories and literature as to whether there is an optimal macronutrient composition to support weight management and maintenance. The debate particularly challenges the principles of the energy balance theory (energy in vs. energy out) and the first law of thermodynamics. It has been proposed that the thermic effect of feeding is greater for fats and proteins than for carbohydrates [1,2]. The absolute effect of this has also been misreported as having a considerable effect on the total energy expenditure. Although the effects of different nutrients on energy expenditure are variable between individuals, the overall effect of the thermic effect of nutrients is only thought to account for around 4–15% of the total energy expenditure – far less than that of physical activity, which is responsible for >30% of energy expenditure [1,2].

There is a limited body of scientific evidence, along with a considerable volume of non-evidence-based marketing messages, about the properties of different macronutrients with respect to body weight and weight loss. These include differences in the greater thermic effects of fats and proteins on metabolism; impact on host physiology; and potential impacts on satiety and satiation. The challenge in interpreting these types of data can be considerable, as they are dependent on interactions between physiology and self-reported human behaviour. However, to date, there is no evidence that manipulating macronutrients to influence satiety has a

long-term effect on energy intake or energy balance, and therefore no demonstrable indication of its impact on weight [3].

There are, however, a number of potential mechanisms through which manipulating macronutrient intake can support weight loss and weight management. There are several thousand studies, ranging from epidemiological observational research to randomised controlled trials (RCTs), investigating various ratios of macronutrients for weight loss. The rationale and evidence for why these approaches may or may not be more effective (in the short term or chronically) need to be considered.

4.1.1 Carbohydrates and weight loss

The potential of a low-carbohydrate diet was initially developed as palliative treatment for type 1 diabetes prior to the discovery of insulin [4]. The earliest clear definition of a low-carbohydrate diet and its application with respect to weight management was perhaps in 'Letters on Corpulence', published in the mid-nineteenth century by William Banting [5]. In this, Banting described what appears to be predominately a low-energy diet, which is limited with respect to carbohydrate content (around 15–20 g per meal). This is not in complete agreement with some commentators who use 'Banting' as a term for very-low-carbohydrate diets.

Table 4.1.1   Definition of high or low macronutrient intakes as defined in research literature or as per consensus definitions [6,7,23,34,46–49]

	Amount of macronutrients per day (grams)	Energy from macronutrients (%)*
Carbohydrate intake [6,7]		
Very-low-carbohydrate diet	20–50	6–10
Low-carbohydrate diet	<130	<26
Moderate-carbohydrate diet	130–225	26–45
High-carbohydrate diet	>225	>45
Fat intake [23,47]		
Typical fat intake	67–89	30–40
Low-fat diet	67	≤30
Lower limit recommended	44	20
Protein intake [34,48,49]		
Range of high intake (90th–97th centile in Europe)	85–135	17–27
Upper limit proposed	175	35
High-protein diet	125	25

*Based on 2000 kcal/day.

Currently, there is no universal definition of what constitutes a low-carbohydrate diet, and perhaps the most widely used definition is that by Feinman et al. [6], adapted by McCardle et al. [7] to include the percentage of dietary energy (Table 4.1.1). The proposed definitions of low-carbohydrate diets should consider the findings of the safety review on total diet replacements by the European Food Safety Agency (EFSA). This review proposed a minimum carbohydrate content of energy-restricted diets of 30 g/day (for brain, renal medulla and erythrocyte metabolism, which cannot be met by other substrates, e.g. ketone bodies, and based on the assumption that 75 g of proteins is provided), which represents an 80–90% reduction in carbohydrate intake from a typical Western-type diet or that advised in many national guidelines. This review highlighted the challenges of viewing macronutrients in isolation [8].

When considering reviews of the effectiveness of low-carbohydrate diets, there are mixed data, typically varying according to the duration and intensity of the intervention. A number of studies suggest that low-carbohydrate diets can be superior to low-energy or low-fat diets, with up to 2 kg more weight found to be lost in low-carbohydrate diets [9]. However, these findings were not replicated by

Naude et al. [9] in a meta-analysis reviewing studies of 12 weeks or longer in duration, having defined 'low carbohydrate' as being <45% of total energy, and therefore including studies with carbohydrate intakes in the range of 4–40% of total energy. This review analysed data from 19 studies, splitting them into higher-fat and higher-protein variants of low-carbohydrate diets. The conclusion of this meta-analysis was that there was little or no difference in weight loss up to 2 years when diets were isoenergetic but differed in macronutrient content, further supporting the view that the energy deficit is the key, rather than the macronutrient profile.

Very-low-carbohydrate, ketogenic diets

It has been theorised that very-low-carbohydrate diets (less than 25–50 g per day), may have additional benefits over a normal low-carbohydrate diet. As these types of diets are unlikely to meet the requirements of the brain for glucose even with gluconeogenesis (glucose synthesis from amino acids and glycerol), they lead to a metabolic shift linked to starvation to preserve lean tissue through ketogenesis, the synthesis of ketone bodies from fatty acids, which occurs when there is a saturation of Krebs' cycle with acetyl Co-A, resulting in the synthesis of acetone and beta-hydroxy-butyrate. These can then be used as energy substrates in a range of tissues, including muscle and brain, as well as the heart, where it is a preferred substrate. It has been hypothesised that a moderately raised level of ketones may increase the metabolic rate and help supress hunger. Therefore, a dietary pattern that is ketogenic, being higher in fat with a moderate protein content, could be more effective with respect to weight loss than simply low-energy diets or diets less restrictive in carbohydrates [10]. However, this evidence is largely from one short-term (4-month) study, where the actual between-group weight changes in a very-low-calorie ketogenic diet were not significantly different. It remains unproven whether ketosis has any additional benefits over a diet containing more carbohydrate that results in an equivalent energy deficit [11].

Does reducing carbohydrates simply lead to a greater energy deficit?

At first glance, the view that low-carbohydrate diets offer little additional benefits with respect to weight loss appears to conflict with much of the literature, which seems to support the beneficial role of low-carbohydrate diets in weight management. However, when more closely scrutinised, reducing carbohydrate consumption from a habitual intake of 45–55% of energy to 5–10% may simply result in a greater energy deficit than seen when reducing fat intake from 40% to 30% of energy. If this is reflected in an energy intake of 2000 kcal (8400 kJ) per day, a 10% reduction in energy from fat would equate to a 200 kcal (840 kJ) per-day energy deficit, whereas a 40–45% reduction in dietary energy by reducing carbohydrate down to 5–10% of total energy intake would result in a per-day energy deficit of 800–900 kcal (3360–3780 kJ), which is likely to lead to more rapid and greater weight loss. This can be most clearly seen in the study by Bazzano et al. [12]. This study additionally reported the *dietary intake consumed*, which in obese people itself has questionable value, in addition to the *dietary intake advised*. This discrepancy in the degree of carbohydrate restriction and the definition of low-carbohydrate diets (Table 4.1.1) could, in part, explain, along

with variabilities in study duration, why some meta-analyses suggest greater efficacy of low-carbohydrate approaches [13], whereas others do not [9]. Nevertheless, all this detail in terms of dietary prescription really depends on actual dietary compliance (which is difficult to measure), and, although weight change may be considered to be an objective measure of dietary compliance, this to can vary considerably between individuals.

Potential risks of very-low-carbohydrate/ketogenic diets (less than 50 g per day)

A concern raised about low-carbohydrate diets is about safety [14], that is, whether it can be nutritionally adequate. There is no obligate physiological requirement for dietary carbohydrate in adults in the short-to-medium term, with evidence from studies lasting at least 12–24 months in duration, suggesting there are no clear safety concerns [15]. There are some findings from epidemiological studies suggesting positive associations between mortality rates seen in populations consuming low carbohydrates and greater quantities of animal proteins [16]. However, it needs to be acknowledged that individuals in these studies were not actively engaged in weight loss. Additionally, there are at least three reported case studies of ketosis becoming ketoacidosis in individuals following extremely low-carbohydrate diets. The logical inference is that reducing carbohydrates can be effective, but that there is no clear advantage in the very-low-carbohydrate ketogenic diets for weight management, and that there may be risks as seen with the case reports of non-diabetes-related ketoacidosis [8].

4.1.2 Fat intake and weight loss

Being the most energy-dense macronutrient, providing twofold higher energy per gram when compared to proteins and carbohydrates (9 vs. 4 vs. 4 kcal/g, respectively), fat was the first nutrient to be positively associated with obesity [17]. Supporting the fat–obesity hypothesis, in addition to its high energy density, many high-fat foods (fried foods and the majority of confectionary and cakes) are highly palatable and associated with pleasure, and elicit a relatively weak satiety signal. Thus, it has been suggested that increased dietary fat intake could promote passive overconsumption of energy [18]. This, together with the observation that it is difficult to overeat carbohydrates when following a low-fat diet that replaces fat with carbohydrates (fruits, vegetables, legumes, cereals, etc.), was hypothesised to enable *ad libitum* weight control [19]. As a result, approximately 60 years ago, reduction of dietary fat intake was the first public health recommendation made, aiming to reduce the burden of obesity, and was granted great acceptance worldwide [20].

Despite the application of these guidelines, the prevalence of obesity has increased several-fold over the past decades, while its incidence was inversely associated with the proportion of dietary fat intake [21] – suggesting that the key intervention against weight gain might not be in dietary fat reduction alone. This matter still remains controversial, with some commentators suggesting that reducing dietary fat intake is linked to the inevitable overconsumption of carbohydrates (and particularly added sugar and refined carbohydrates), which have been linked to hyperinsulinemia, lower metabolic rate and increased hunger [21]. Moreover, the low-fat era was not linked to healthier dietary habits as initially hoped (more fruits, vegetables and whole-grain cereals), but with a tendency to consume more highly processed products based on refined grains and sugary foods and drinks [22]. Concerning these controversial public health results, nutrition research has focussed in answering whether low-fat diet interventions are actually effective in achieving weight loss.

Low-fat diets and weight loss

One of the very first meta-analyses performed to answer the question of the effectiveness of low-fat diets in weight loss included 32 RCTs with approximately 54,000 participants and data from 25 cohort studies. The effect of eating less fat (defined as ≤30% of total energy being derived from fat, compared with usual dietary fat intake, considered as >30% energy from fat) was a mean weight reduction of 1.5 kg (95% CI = −2 to −1.1 kg), with greater weight loss resulting from greater fat reductions, suggesting a dose-related response. However,

a lower fat intake was associated with smaller increases in weight in middle-aged but not elderly adults in the cohort studies (>65 years of age) [23]. However, it was not possible to quantify this effect, owing to the different methodologies used in these intervention studies; hence, interpretation needs to be treated with caution.

In a recent meta-analysis of RCTs that endured at least 6 months, the effects of low-carbohydrate diets compared to low-fat diets were assessed, and 11 RCTs with 1369 participants met the eligibility criteria. Compared with participants on low-fat diets (<30% energy from fat), participants on low-carbohydrate diets (defined as <20% energy from carbohydrates, or in accordance with the 'Atkins' diet programme) experienced a greater reduction in body weight (weight mean difference = −2.17 kg; 95% CI = 3.36, −0.99), suggesting consistent results regarding the complex and unexpected roles of fat intake in weight loss [13].

Mediterranean diet and 'healthy fats'

Mancini et al. (2016) [24] performed a meta-analysis that studied the healthy high-fat Mediterranean dietary pattern, which is defined in this study as a regional diet rich in vegetables, fruits, monounsaturated fats (mainly from olive oil) and cereals; with moderate consumption of poultry, fish and dairy produce; and little or no consumption of red meat. This was compared with low-fat diet (not formally defined), a low-carbohydrate diet (not formally defined) and the American Diabetes Association diet, for weight loss in overweight or obese individuals in RCTs having at least a 12-month follow-up period. Five RCTs with 998 individuals met the inclusion criteria, and the Mediterranean diet resulted in greater weight loss (range of mean values: −4.1 to −10.1 kg) than the low-fat diet (2.9 to −5 kg) at ≥12 months, but produced similar weight loss as the other comparator diets (range of mean values: −4.7 to −7.7 kg). These results were the first to support the notion that a healthy but higher-fat diet could be more effective in weight loss interventions than low-fat diets, under the context of compliance and satisfaction, as seen through the comparable or greater mean weight loss described [24].

Regarding specific fat types, in a meta-analysis of 13 RCTs with 749 individuals, medium-chain triglyceride (MCT) intake decreased body weight as compared to long-chain triglyceride intake (−0.51 kg; 95% CI = −0.80 to −0.23 kg). This effect is thought to be linked to the increased thermic effect of MCTs, along with their satiating properties. Unfortunately, many trials lacked sufficient information for a complete quality assessment, and commercial bias was detected [25]. Moreover, in an RCT that provided rapeseed oil and olive oil as mono-unsaturated fatty acid sources to assess their potential incremental roles in weight loss programmes, both were proved after 6 months to significantly reduce body weight more effectively than diet alone [26].

All findings of the aforementioned studies are in accordance with recent evidence, suggesting that the role of total dietary fat intake in obesity epidemics may possibly have less importance than first suggested, a rationale linked to potentially limited data and perhaps linked to general poor adherence by the general population [27]. As a result, the 2015 USDA Dietary Guidelines significantly raised the upper limit on the recommended dietary saturated fatty acid intake of <10% of total energy [28]; however, the results remain to be seen in practice. These changes perhaps reflect a change in the view of the diet–heart hypothesis more than diet–weight, with critiques proposing that reducing fat only served to increase refined carbohydrate intake. Perhaps the overall message is to consider the overall dietary pattern, rather than focussing on single nutrients?

4.1.3 Proteins and weight loss

Similar to low-carbohydrate diets, there has been renewed interest in the outcome of high-protein diets in weight management in recent years [29]. Before considering the benefits of increasing proteins directly, it is important to reflect on the diluting effect that increasing proteins may have on the fat and carbohydrate content in the diet, which in turn may reduce dietary energy intake. There is a theoretical basis, with some empirical evidence suggesting that these have produced modest evidence that higher protein intakes may facilitate weight

loss, encourage weight maintenance, and improve body composition and clinical outcomes [29,30]. This potential benefit is thought to be via the influence of increased satiety through the elevated dietary protein intake, which may result in lower energy intake. Increased diet-induced thermogenesis (DIT) has also been proposed, but the net effect of this alone, as previously described, is very modest. However, the combined effects of increased protein intake have been reported to support weight loss and maintenance in a number of studies [29–32]. However, the size of this effect is unlikely to be large enough to result in clinically meaningful weight loss, although it may be statistically significant, causing a maximum variation of around 100 kcal (420 kJ) per day, based on extrapolations from clinical studies.

There are a number of recommendations for protein intake. For example, the Australian dietary protein recommendations for adults suggest an acceptable macronutrient distribution range of 15–25% of total energy intake [33]. While there has been little agreement on the classification of a high-protein diet, a recent meta-analysis suggested that protein intake in high-protein diets range from 1.07 to 1.60 g/kg/day, as compared to 0.55–0.88 g/kg/day in standard-protein diets [29]. However, it is important to consider the effects that this will have on the intake of fats and carbohydrates.

Effects of proteins on body weight

Several studies comparing high- and standard-protein diets have documented that high-protein diets produce greater short-term mean weight loss as compared to standard-protein diets [29–31,34–38]. In a randomised 12-month trial, 50 overweight and obese participants were given a reduced-fat diet (<30% energy from fat), which was either a high-protein (25% of total energy from proteins) or a medium-protein (12% total energy intake) diet, for 6 months [34]. Consistent with other reported findings, participants assigned to the high-protein diet achieved greater weight loss outcomes (9.4 kg vs. 5.9 kg) and improved body composition outcomes, including greater loss of fat mass [34], with 8% dropping out in the high-protein group and 28% in the medium-protein group.

Despite the short-term success of the high-protein diet, after a 12-month follow-up period, no difference in weight loss was found between both groups [34]. The long-term success of high-protein diets has also been reported by other studies to be relatively unclear [34,35,38], with many studies reporting a loss of benefit after 12–24 months [34,35,39]. While modest-quality evidence supports the short-term benefits of high-protein diets in facilitating weight loss and maintenance, the long-term benefits (12–24 months) of high-protein diets are currently under debate due to inconclusive findings [38].

Dietary protein intake and satiety

Strong satiation effects have been commonly cited as the primary mechanism of weight loss associated with high-protein diets [30,35,36]. Affirming that proteins are the most satiating macronutrients as compared to carbohydrates or fats, it is theorised that high-protein diets have the potential to induce a negative energy balance and facilitate weight loss in overweight individuals [30,36,37]. Although not conclusive, it has been suggested that increasing the protein content of meals by 25–81% will result in overall suppressed hunger and enhanced satiety [36,37,40]. However, this represents a wide range of interventions, making it impossible to conclude anything clinically meaningful from these data.

In several studies investigating high-protein diets, with typically 25% of the total energy from protein, it was a common theme that continual elevated protein consumption for 1–5 days produced higher satiety as compared to the standard-protein diets of the control group, with no difference apparent in dietary energy intake [40,41]. While the mechanisms behind protein-induced satiety are still elusive, it is thought to be a multifactorial relationship between an effect on satiety hormones (glucagon-like peptide 1, cholecystokinin, PYY), concentrations of metabolites (amino acids) and gluconeogenesis, all contributing to the protein-induced satiety [40].

Emerging research has suggested that different protein sources influence energy intake differently, with whey proteins found to be more satiating than casein and other proteins (egg-albumin and soy) [40,42,43]. The differences in satiety between protein sources are considered to be due to the

variations in amino acid concentrations and metabolic efficacies of protein oxidation [40]. However, the reason why different protein types contribute differently to protein-induced satiety still remains relatively unclear, and as such should be treated with caution when making recommendations for dietary interventions.

Dietary protein intake and diet-induced thermogenesis

DIT is the metabolic response to food and the associated increase in energy expenditure related to the nutrient processing of food (digestion, absorption and disposal) [37,44]. Consensus within the literature postulates that proteins stimulate DIT (~15–30%) to a greater extent than other macronutrients, including carbohydrates (~5–10%) and fats (~0.3%) [29,35,37,44]. While explanations behind the mechanisms associated with the thermogenic nature of proteins have been made, they largely remain elusive [30]. Little is still known concerning how DIT contributes to metabolic expenditure and weight loss [44]. However, explanations from within the literature, regarding how a high-protein diet may induce thermogenesis to a greater extent than other macronutrients, include the following:

(1) *Owing to the body's inability to store proteins* [32,44]. As a consequence, proteins need to be metabolically processed immediately, a process that demands a high ATP cost. However, to date, the clinical impact in terms of effect on weight and overall energy balance is not clear [32,44,45].
(2) *Due to the potential relationship between DIT and satiety* [44]. While this mechanism is yet to be clearly articulated, a correlation between satiety and DIT has been suggested [44,45].

There is emerging evidence to suggest that, in the short term (less than 12 months), high-protein diets (~25% energy from proteins) can facilitate greater weight loss and encourage weight maintenance, as compared to standard-protein diets (~12% energy from proteins) [30]. However, more research is needed to establish what the ideal high-protein diet intake for weight loss is, along with a classification of what high-protein diets are. Table 4.1.1 collates definitions from consensus groups and clinical trials. This is necessary to assess the effectiveness of high-protein diets within longer time periods (of >12 months) on weight maintenance and outcomes, and to investigate further the roles of satiety and DIT in higher protein intakes.

4.1.4 Summary and conclusion

The focus of the scientific and media communities has moved, over the past century, to the different combinations of macronutrients as the optimal approach to managing weight. However, the best dietary approaches with respect to macronutrient distribution are the ones that are: nutritionally adequate with respect to proteins and micronutrients; that maximise health effects, including minimising lean tissue loss; that are ecologically sustainable; and that can be adhered to for long periods.

The evidence to date does not support the view that any particular macronutrient profile is superior to another. Differences are only observed when manipulations of macronutrient intake result in a greater energy deficit. These differences can be illustrated by a very-low-carbohydrate diet (5–10% of dietary energy) as compared to a low-fat diet (30% of dietary energy). The respective energy deficits based on 2000 kcal (8200 kJ) per day diet of approximately 400 (3360 kJ) or just 200 kcal (840 kJ) per day, respectively. This is further complicated by the fact that the fat-intake recommendations in the national guidelines of many countries are similar, whereas the carbohydrate-intake suggestions are very different. The apparent differences reported in a number of studies can largely be attributed to these differences in energy deficit. Further challenges in interpretation result from the lack of consensus definitions on what the low and high intakes of each of these macronutrients should be. While, in the short term, a range of dietary approaches have been reported as being safe, it should be noted that a meta-analysis of observational studies found that low-carbohydrate diets, although not associated with increased risk of cardiovascular mortality, were associated with a significantly higher risk of all-cause mortality [46].

Additionally, perhaps too much focus has been placed on trials investigating the hypothesised optimal ratios and altering intakes of macronutrients. Based on published evidence, trials are required that investigate customised approaches based on individual preferences towards macronutrient content to induce energy deficits. This is especially the case when long-term adherence is considered.

4.1.5 Summary box

Key points

- Energy restriction and energy balance remain the key elements in achieving weight loss.
- A key concern is that dietary intakes should remain nutritionally adequate, and therefore balanced, with respect to micronutrients.
- Short-term interventions with higher protein and lower carbohydrate intakes appear to be more effective (up to 12 weeks).
- No particular combination of macronutrients or approach to restricting macronutrients leads to greater long-term weight loss or improved maintenance.
- Clinical guidelines for weight loss recommend an individualised energy-deficit approach with macronutrient intakes as advocated for the general adult population.

References

1. Westerterp KR, Wilson SAJ, Rolland V. Diet induced thermogenesis measured over 24h in a respiration chamber: effect of diet composition. *International Journal of Obesity* 1999; **23**: 287–292.
2. Westerterp KR. Diet induced thermogenesis. *Nutrition & Metabolism* 2004; **1**: 5. doi: 10.1186/1743-7075-1-5.
3. Booth DA, Nouwen A. Satiety. No way to slim. *Appetite* 2010; **55**(3): 718–721.
4. Westman EC, Yancy WS Jr, Humphreys M. Dietary treatment of diabetes mellitus in the pre-insulin era (1914–1922). *Perspectives in Biology and Medicine* 2006; **49**(1): 77–83.
5. Banting W. Letters on corpulence, addressed to the public (1863). *Obesity Research* 1993; **1**(2): 153–163. doi: 10.1002/j.1550-8528.1993.tb00605.x.
6. Feinman RD, Pogzelski WK, Astrup A, Bernstein RK, Fine EJ, Westman EC, et al. Dietary carbohydrate restriction as the first approach in diabetes management: critical review and evidence base. *Nutrition* 2015; **31**(1): 1–13.

7. McArdle PD, Mellor D, Rilstone S, Taplin J. The role of carbohydrate in diabetes management. *Practical Diabetes* 2016; **33**(7): 237–242.

8. EFSA NDA Panel (EFSA Panel on Dietetic Products, Nutrition and Allergies). Scientific opinion on the essential composition of total diet replacements for weight control. *EFSA Journal* 2015; **13**(1): 3957, 52. doi:10.2903/j.efsa.2015.3957.

9. Naude CE, Schroonees A, Senekal M, Young T, Garner P, Volmink J. Low carbohydrate versus isoenergetic balanced diets for reducing weight and cardiovascular risk A systematic review and meta-analysis. *PLoS ONE* 2014. Available from: https://doi.org/10.1371/journal.pone.0100652.

10. Goday D, Bellido D, Sajoux I, Crujeira B, Burguera B, Garcia-Luna PP, et al. Short-term safety, tolerability and efficacy of a very low-calorie-ketogenic diet interventional weight loss program versus hypocaloric diet in patients with type 2 diabetes mellitus. *Nutrition & Diabetes* 2016; **6**: e230. doi: 10.1038/nutd.2016.36.

11. Bazzano LA, Hu T, Reynolds K, Yao L, Chen CS, Klag MJ, et al. Effects of low-carbohydrate and low fat diets: a randomized trial. *Annals of Internal Medicine* 2014; **161**(5): 309–318.

12. Crowe TC. Safety of low-carbohydrate diets. *Obesity Reviews* 2005; **6**(3): 235–245.

13. Mansoor N, Vinknes KJ, Veierod MB, Retterstol K. Effects of low-carbohydrate diets v. low-fat diets on body weight and cardiovascular risk factors: a meta-analysis of randomised controlled trials. *British Journal of Nutrition* 2016; **115**(3): 466–479.

14. Shai I, Schwarzfuchs D, Henkin Y, Shahar DR, Witkow S, Greenberg I, et al. Weight loss with a low-carbohydrate, Mediterranean, or low fat diet. *The New England Journal of Medicine* 2008; **359**: 229–241.

15. Fung TT, van Dam RM, Hankinson SE, Stempfer M, Willett WC, Hum FB. Low carbohydrate diets and all cause and cause specific mortality: two cohort studies. *Annals of Internal Medicine* 2010; **153**(5): 289–298.

16. Sackner-Bernstein J, Kanter D, Kaul S. Dietary intervention for overnight and obese adults: comparison of low carbohydrate and low fat diets. A meta-analysis. *PLoS ONE* 2015. Available from: http://dx.doi.org/10.1371/journal.pone.0139817.

17. Brewer WD, Cederquist DC, Williams B, Beegle RM, Dunsing D, Kelley AL, et al. Weight reduction on low-fat and low-carbohydrate diets. *Journal of the American Dietetic Association* 1952; **28**(3): 213–217.

18. Blundell JE, MacDiarmid JI. Fat as a risk factor for overconsumption: satiation, satiety, and patterns of eating. *Journal of the American Dietetic Association* 1997; **97**(7): S63–S69.

19. Stubbs RJ, Mazlan N, Whybrow S. Carbohydrates, appetite and feeding behavior in humans. *Journal of Nutrition* 2001; **131**(10): 2775s–2781s.

20. Department of Health. Dietary Reference Values for Food, Energy and Nutrients for the United Kingdom. Report on Health and Social Subjects. No. 41. HSMO. London, UK, 1991.

21. Ludwig DS. Lowering the bar on the low-fat diet. *JAMA* 2016; **316**: 2087–2088.

22. Mozaffarian D, Hao T, Rimm EB, Willett WC, Hu FB. Changes in diet and lifestyle and long-term weight gain in women and men. *The New England Journal of Medicine* 2011; **364**(25): 2392–2404.

23. Hooper L, Abdelhamid A, Bunn D, Brown T, Summerbell CD, Skeaff CM. Effects of total fat intake on body weight. *The Cochrane Database of Systematic Reviews* 2015; (8): Cd011834.

24. Mancini JG, Filion KB, Atallah R, Eisenberg MJ. Systematic review of the Mediterranean diet for long-term weight loss. *The American Journal of Medicine* 2016; **129**(4): 407–415.e4.

25. Mumme K, Stonehouse W. Effects of medium-chain triglycerides on weight loss and body composition: a meta-analysis of randomized controlled trials. *Journal of the Academy of Nutrition and Dietetics* 2015; **115**(2): 249–263.

26. Baxheinrich A, Stratmann B, Lee-Barkey YH, Tschoepe D, Wahrburg U. Effects of a rapeseed oil-enriched hypoenergetic diet with a high content of α-linolenic acid on body weight and cardiovascular risk profile in patients with the metabolic syndrome. *British Journal of Nutrition* 2012; **108**(4): 682–691.

27. Walker TB, Parker MJ. Lessons from the war on dietary fat. *Journal of the American College of Nutrition* 2014; **33**(4): 347–351.

28. Mozaffarian D, Ludwig DS. The 2015 US dietary guidelines: lifting the ban on total dietary fat. *JAMA* 2015; **313**(24): 2421–2422.

29. Wycherley TP, Moran LJ, Clifton PM, Noakes M, Brinkworth GD. Effects of energy-restricted high-protein, low-fat compared with standard-protein, low-fat diets: a meta-analysis of randomized controlled trials. *American Journal of Clinical Nutrition* 2012; **96**(6): 1281–1298.

30. Paddon-Jones D, Westman E, Mattes RD, Wolfe RR, Astrup A, Westerterp-Plantenga M. Protein, weight management, and satiety. *American Journal of Clinical Nutrition* 2008; **87**(5): 1558S–1561S.

31. Santesso N, Akl EA, Bianchi M, Mente A, Mustafa R, Heels-Ansdell D, et al. Effects of higher- versus lower-protein diets on health outcomes: a systematic review and meta-analysis. *European Journal of Clinical Nutrition* 2012; **66**(7): 780–788.

32. Yang D, Liu Z, Yang H, Jue Y. Acute effects of high-protein versus normal-protein isocaloric meals on satiety and ghrelin. *European Journal of Nutrition* 2014; **53**(2): 493–500.

33. Council ANHaMR. Nutrient reference values for Australia and New Zealand including recommended dietary intakes. In: *Aging DHa*, editor, 2005.

34. Due A, Toubro S, Skov A, Astrup A. Effect of normal-fat diets, either medium or high in protein, on body weight in overweight subjects: a randomised 1-year trial. *International Journal of Obesity* 2004; **28**(10): 1283–1290.

35. Astrup A, Raben A, Geiker N. The role of higher protein diets in weight control and obesity-related comorbidities. *International Journal of Obesity* 2015; **39**(5): 721–726.

36. Dhillon J, Craig BA, Leidy HJ, Amankwaah AF, Anguah KO-B, Jacobs A, et al. The effects of increased protein intake on fullness: a meta-analysis and its limitations. *Journal of the Academy of Nutrition and Dietetics* 2016; **116**(6): 968–983.

37. Pesta DH, Samuel VT. A high-protein diet for reducing body fat: mechanisms and possible caveats. *Nutrition & Metabolism* 2014; **11**(1): 1.

38. Clifton P. Effects of a high protein diet on body weight and comorbidities associated with obesity. *British Journal of Nutrition* 2012; **108**(S2): S122–S129.

39. Clifton PM, Condo D, Keogh JB. Long term weight maintenance after advice to consume low carbohydrate, higher protein diets – a systematic review and meta analysis. *Nutrition Metabolism and Cardiovascular Diseases* 2014; **24**(3): 224–235.

40. Veldhorst M, Smeets A, Soenen S, Hochstenbach-Waelen A, Hursel R, Diepvens K, et al. Protein-induced satiety: effects and mechanisms of different proteins. *Physiology & Behavior* 2008; **94**(2): 300–307.

41. Lejeune MP, Westerterp KR, Adam TC, Luscombe-Marsh ND, Westerterp-Plantenga MS. Ghrelin and glucagon-like peptide 1 concentrations, 24-h satiety, and energy and substrate metabolism during a high-protein diet and measured in a respiration chamber. *American Journal of Clinical Nutrition* 2006; **83**(1): 89–94.

42. Anderson GH, Tecimer SN, Shah D, Zafar TA. Protein source, quantity, and time of consumption determine the effect of proteins on short-term food intake in young men. *Journal of Nutrition* 2004; **134**(11): 3011–3015.

43. Hall WL, Millward DJ, Long SJ, Morgan LM. Casein and whey exert different effects on plasma amino acid profiles, gastrointestinal hormone secretion and appetite. *British Journal of Nutrition* 2007; **89**(2): 239–248.

44. Halton TL, Hu FB. The effects of high protein diets on thermogenesis, satiety and weight loss: a critical review. *Journal of the American College of Nutrition* 2004; **23**(5): 373.

45. Westerterp-Plantenga MS. Protein intake and energy balance. *Regulatory Peptides* 2008; **149**(1–3): 67–69.

46. Noto H, Goto A, Tsujimoto T, Noda M. Low carbohydrate diets and all-cause mortality: a systematic review and meta-analysis of observational studies. *PLoS ONE* 2013; **8**(1): e55030.

47. Panel on Dietetic Products, Nutrition and Allergies. Scientific opinion on dietary reference values for fats, including saturated fatty acids, polyunsaturated fatty acids, monounsaturated fatty acids, trans fatty acids, and cholesterol. *EFSA Journal* 2010; **8**(3): 1461 [107pp.].

48. IoM (Institute of Medicine). *Dietary Reference Intakes for Energy, Carbohydrate, Fiber, Fat, Fatty Acids, Cholesterol, Protein, and Amino Acids.* Washington DC, USA: National Academies Press, 2005, 1357 pp.

49. Panel on Dietetic Products, Nutrition and Allergies. Scientific opinion on dietary reference values for protein. *EFSA Journal* 2012; **10**(2): 2557.

Chapter 4.2

Meal replacements for weight loss in obesity

Joan Khoo and Magdalin Cheong
Changi General Hospital, Singapore

4.2.1 Introduction

Meal replacements are food substitutes containing fixed portions of energy and nutrients and can be instrumental in weight-loss diets as the sole energy source, or in combination with other foods. Meal replacements encompass a wide range of commercially available solid or liquid products that provide 200–400 kcal (840–1680 kJ) of energy, with 25–50% of the total energy as proteins and ≤30 % as fats [1], fortified with vitamins and minerals (Table 4.2.1).

Energy-restricted diet prescriptions, designed to lower energy intake by 500–1000 kcal/day (2100–4200 kJ/day) can incorporate meal replacements into low-calorie diets (LCDs) and very-low-calorie diets (VLCDs). LCDs, which provide 800–1600 kcal/day (3360–6720 kJ/day), may include one or more meals replaced by a meal replacement, or at least one daily meal consisting of regular food in a 'partial-meal-replacement' plan, while VLCDs provide 400–800 kcal/day (1680–3360 kJ/day), using meal replacements as the sole nutrient source [2]. LCDs and VLCDs induce greater weight loss than conventional approaches, with even greater results when combined with regular physical activity and behavioural therapy [3]. Weight loss is similar to that induced with the weight-lowering medications orlistat and sibutramine [4]. This chapter will discuss the use of meal replacements for weight management in obese adults.

4.2.2 Weight loss with meal-replacement plans

Prescription of LCDs

A reduction of 500–1000 kcal/day (2100–4200 kJ/day) from usual intake will provide a weight loss of approximately 0.5–1 kg/week (~1–2 lb/week) [2]. LCDs usually begin at 1000–1200 kcal/day (4200–5040 kJ/day), with diets below 1000 kcal/day (4200 kJ/day) sufficient in older, smaller and inactive individuals. A more accurate and individualised means of prescribing the energy deficit uses calculation of the daily energy requirement, which is resting metabolic rate (RMR) multiplied by activity factor based on the level of physical activity (i.e. 1.2 for sedentary, 1.4 for low–moderate active and 1.6 and above for active lifestyles) [2]. Where measurement of the RMR is not available, the Mifflin–St Jeor equation is the most accurate means for estimating RMR for overweight and obese individuals [5]:

RMR (male) = ([10 × weight in kg] + [6.25 × height in cm] − [5 × age in years] + 5)

RMR (female) = ([10 × weight in kg] + [6.25 × height in cm] − [5 × age in years] − 161)

For example, a 46-year-old woman, 165 cm tall and weighing 90 kg (body mass index [BMI] 33.1 kg/m^2), working a sedentary office job and doing little exercise (activity factor 1.2), requires approximately 1850 kcal/day (7770 kJ/day). A reduction of 750

Table 4.2.1 European Communities (foods intended for use in energy-restricted diets for weight reduction) Regulations 2007

Nutrients & energy content	Specifications
Energy	3360 kJ (800 kcal) to 5040 kJ (1200 kcal) for the total daily ration. 840 kJ (200 kcal) to 1680 kJ (400 kcal) per meal
Protein	25–50% of the total energy; ≤125 g per product
Fat	<30% of the total available energy of the product
Dietary fibre	10–30 g for the daily ration
Vitamins and minerals	Meet 100% of the requirements of vitamins and minerals in the daily diet; 30% of the amounts of vitamins and minerals specified available per meal; 500 mg potassium per meal

kcal/day (3150 kJ/day) would give an energy prescription of ~1100 kcal/day (4620 kJ/day). Achieving this through meal replacements might involve replacing two meals with two sachets of a liquid meal replacement, each containing 160–170 kcal or 672–714 kJ (20 g carbohydrate, 14 g protein, 3–4 g fat, 4–5 g fibre) and the recommended daily allowances of minerals, vitamins and omega-3 and omega-6 essential fatty acids, thus providing 340 kcal/day (1428 kJ/day) as meal replacements. The remaining 760 kcal (3192 kJ) would come from the one other regular meal, with <30% of total energy intake as fats (<10% saturated fats) and at least 20% as proteins.

Benefits of meal-replacement plans compared to conventional diet

Weight loss of at least 10% is known to lower cardiovascular disease risk [2], and has been achieved in 12–16 weeks using meal-replacement plans [3]. In a meta-analysis of six randomised trials (N = 487, duration 3–51 months), weight loss at 12 months in the conventional diet group approximated 3–7% (2.6–4.3 kg), a significant difference of 2.5–3 kg overall from subjects on partial meal replacements, who lost 7–8% body weight (7–7.3 kg) [6]. Improvements in blood glucose, triglyceride, systolic blood pressure, and total and LDL cholesterol levels in this meta-analysis were also highly significant (P < 0.001) in both diet groups, with reduction in insulin being significantly greater in the partial-meal-replacement group [6]. In a subsequent meta-analysis of seven

studies (N = 416, duration 1–5 years), weight reduction was greater at 6 months in subjects on meal-replacement-based LCDs (9.6%) or VLCDs (16%), as compared to losses in those on conventional diets with (8.5%) or without (5%) exercise advice [7]. A recent randomised controlled study found that the Medifast 5 & 1 Plan (a commercially available low-fat meal-replacement plan, manufactured by Medifast Inc, Maryland, USA, consisting of five pre-packaged meal replacements plus a user-selected meal consisting of a lean protein source and three servings of vegetables, thus providing 800–1000 kcal/day) induced significantly greater reductions in weight (−7.5 kg) and waist circumference (−5.7 cm) than an isocaloric food-based diet (−3.8 kg, −3.7 cm), at 26 weeks and 52 weeks (−4.7 vs. −1.9 kg, −5 vs. −3.6 cm), with lower attrition rate at 52 weeks in the meal-replacement group (16.7% vs. 25%) [8]. This plan also induced significantly greater reductions in BMI and fat mass than the food-based diet at 26 weeks, which were maintained at 52 weeks, in association with larger improvements in total and LDL cholesterol levels. Serum glucose, insulin, blood pressure, triglyceride and LDL cholesterol levels decrease in association with weight loss induced with meal-replacement plans [2,3,6,7,9–12], as do visceral adiposity, inflammation and oxidative stress [9,11]. Meal-replacement plans are therefore associated with more rapid improvement in cardiovascular risk factors [3], facilitate exercise and cognitive-behavioural therapy [2,3,7], reduce anxiety and depression and improve quality of life [6]. Moreover, in a meta-analysis, the dropout rate at 1 year of follow-up was significantly lower ($P < 0.001$) in subjects on meal-replacement plans (47%), as compared to that in the conventional diet group (64%) [6]. Portion-controlled meal replacements, therefore, promote significantly greater weight loss, in addition to reduction in cardiometabolic risk and lower attrition rates.

How do meal replacements induce greater weight loss?

During the active weight-reduction phase, the predicted rate of weight loss is proportional to the prescribed energy deficit (intake minus expenditure), as observed in a meta-analysis of 35 studies of diet-induced weight loss published between 1995 and 2009 [13]. By prescribing larger energy deficits, the likelihood of reaching the point where energy expenditure surpasses energy intake is greater and allows a larger margin of noncompliance or error in energy estimation [10,13]. Since dietary adherence is inversely associated with the deficit between intake and expenditure, as observed in a study of overweight and obese women restricted to 800 kcal/day (3360 kJ/day) [14], moderate energy restriction (relative to estimates of energy requirements rather than a fixed intake regardless of activity level) facilitates compliance when prescribing portion-controlled diets. Comparison of weight changes to reported energy intakes using equations to estimate basal metabolic rate [15] is of value as obese adults in population studies tend to underestimate their energy intake by 40–50% [16,17].

Wing and Jeffrey found that food provision in a study that supplied meal replacements for 18 months (pre-packaged meals: five breakfasts and five dinners per week designed to provide 1000 or 1500 kcal, depending on calculated requirement) increased initial weight loss by 31% and structured portion-controlled meal plans by 61% in obese subjects, compared to subjects given standard behavioural therapy (SBT) [18]. The mean weight losses in subjects provided food were significantly greater at 6 (10.9 vs. 7.7 kg), 12 (9.1 vs. 4.5 kg) and 18 (6.4 vs. 4.1 kg) months compared to the SBT group, while attrition rates were 30%

in the SBT and 10% in the food-provision group. Diet adherence was also better in the food provision group, as demonstrated by the higher completion rates of eating and exercise diaries: 87% during weeks 1–20, 61% in weeks 21–52 and 37% during weeks 53–78, compared to 67%, 33% and 23%, respectively, during the same periods in the SBT group. The authors suggested that subjects provided with food had increased compliance and nutritional knowledge, and snacked less, leading to better adherence. In a cross-over study of healthy volunteers who were randomised to a self-selected meal from a buffet or a lunch-only meal replacement, using the meal replacements induced a 250 kcal (1050 kJ) deficit in total daily intake without compensatory intake at the other *ad libitum* meals [19]. Similarly, calculated total energy intake in obese men found approximately 150 kcal/day (630 kJ/day) greater deficit in subjects on partial meal replacements (~1400 kcal/day, or 5880 kJ/day), as compared to those prescribed an isocaloric reduced-fat diet on self-recorded 3-day dietary records and physical activity diaries that were monitored at weeks 4, 8 and 12 of the diet intervention [9], which was associated with a 2 kg difference in weight loss between the groups after 12 weeks. Similarly, adults using different methods for weight loss reported greater reduction in mean daily energy intake using meal replacements (360 kcal vs. 71 kcal with a commercial weight loss programme, and 159 kcal with a self-guided weight management regime) in the STOP Regain trial [20], with correspondingly greater weight loss in this group (24.1% vs. 16.6% with the commercial programme, and 17.1% in the self-guided group). Although the accuracy of self-reported records is lower in obese as compared to lean individuals, the use of meal replacements appears to facilitate diet adherence, as compared to conventional foods.

Overall, partial-meal-replacement plans are associated with higher diet satisfaction and lower dropout rates [6,8,13,21]. The ease of using meal replacements is likely to account for lower energy intake, as seen in overweight and obese Australians on a meal-replacement-based weight-loss diet, who reported greater ease of dining out and compliance, scoring significantly ($P < 0.05$) higher on questionnaires related to understanding and complying with food amounts, as compared to a control group given shopping vouchers and instructions for a low-fat/energy diet [11]. The stress of meal preparation is reduced for people who have difficulty understanding portion sizes and calorie counting, or finding the time or inclination to cook [6], by providing calorie-controlled alternatives to self-selected calorie-dense foods.

4.2.3 Weight maintenance with meal-replacement plans

Beyond 6 months of energy restriction, energy requirements generally decrease with weight loss due to reductions in metabolically active muscles, which decrease resting energy expenditure (REE) and possibly adaptive thermogenesis [22]. *Adaptive thermogenesis* (AT) refers to the underfeeding-associated decrease in non-resting and resting energy expenditure, leading to greater-than-expected reductions in REE after weight loss (measured directly, or calculated using a quantitative model that includes weight and body composition). The discrepancy (~0.5 MJ or 120 kcal) may be up to 25% of the expected reduction in REE [23]. The non-REE components – which include activity-related energy expenditure (exercise and non-exercise activity thermogenesis) and diet-induced (thermic effect of food) and cold-induced thermogenesis (in brown adipose tissue and skeletal muscle) – also decrease after weight loss, in association with reductions in sympathetic nervous system activity, 3,5,3'-tri-iodo-thyronine and leptin [22]. AT reduced the underfeeding-induced loss in energy stores by ~50% [24], which may explain the weight regain after diet-induced weight loss and the accelerated fat gain during refeeding [25].

Changes in concentrations of brain and gut hormones that mediate appetite (ghrelin, cholecystokinin, peptide YY, pancreatic polypeptide and leptin), which persist even at 1 year after diet-induced weight loss, facilitate weight regain by increasing hunger and preoccupation with thoughts of food, while reducing fullness after a standard meal, compared to before weight loss [26]. These changes suggest that the high rate of relapse may have a physiological basis and is not solely owing to the resumption of poor eating habits (such as uninhibited, stress-driven or binge eating) or behavioural fatigue in the presence of a toxic environment – all of which are well-established contributors to weight regain [3].

Extended use of meal replacements improved weight-loss maintenance over 12 months in a recent meta-analysis ($N = 3017$) of 20 randomised controlled trials [27] with similar initial mean weight losses in the VLCD/LCD run-in period (11.1–13.5 kg over median 8–12 weeks). Meal replacements improved weight-loss maintenance by 3.9 kg (95% CI = 2.8, 5.5 kg) as compared to controls, which was greater in comparison to a high-protein diet (1.5 kg; 95% CI = 0.8, 2.1 kg), non-protein macronutrients (1.2 kg; 95% CI = 0.4, 2 kg), anti-obesity drugs (3.5 kg; 95% CI = 1.5, 5.5 kg) and exercise (0.8 kg; 95% CI = −1.2, 2.8 kg). Substantial initial weight loss predicts larger long-term weight loss: weight loss of 17.9 kg (16%) at 6 months using VLCDs was followed by rapid regain, such that net weight loss at 12 months was 10.9 kg (10%) and 5.6 kg (5%) by 36 months [28].

4.2.4 Risks of meal-replacement plans

Complications of energy restriction

Medical and dietetic supervision is indicated with the use of VLCDs due to the increased risks of nutrient inadequacy, dehydration and electrolyte imbalances (such as hypokalaemia from reduced intake and/or gastrointestinal losses), which may lead to hypotension and cardiac arrhythmias. Gallstones develop in 10–25% of people on VLCDs [2]. Rapid weight loss reduces body fat and therefore sex steroid production, which can lead to loss of libido, menstrual irregularity in women and osteoporosis [29]. Dizziness, constipation, loss of muscle mass, hair loss, cold intolerance, poor wound healing, headache, fatigue, depression and irritability may also occur. The risks are dependent on the rate and magnitude of weight reduction.

LCDs and VLCDs are not recommended for pregnant or breastfeeding women; individuals with severe or unstable psychiatric illnesses (particularly eating disorders such as bulimia and anorexia nervosa) or substance abuse tendencies; and patients with illnesses that are adversely affected by energy restriction (e.g. active malignancy, severe renal or liver impairment, unstable angina or recent cardiac events, recent cerebrovascular accidents, recurrent gout, uncontrolled epilepsy, gastrointestinal malabsorption) [2]. These diets should be used with caution and under close medical supervision in children and the elderly, who are more vulnerable to dehydration and nutrient inadequacy and/or have comorbidities that predispose them to complications of extreme energy restriction.

Unsupervised use of meal replacements and challenges with weight maintenance

While meal replacements are effective for short-term weight loss, the expense of initiating and maintaining a meal-replacement plan, with need for medical and dietetic supervision and possibilities of complications, is a major barrier to continued compliance. In the STOP Regain study, an 18-month stand-alone weight maintenance analysis that evaluated obese individuals who had lost at least 10% of their body weight using VLCDs, only 21% of those who had used VLCDs were maintaining their weight loss under 2 kg after 6 months of continued supervision and follow-up by study investigators, compared to 75% in groups using a commercial programme or self-guided approach. The effects of meal replacements may be even more unpredictable in individuals who buy and use meal replacements themselves. The variable costs and lack of regulation of different commercially available plans, especially those sold over the Internet and through advertisements, may lead to 'shopping around', which adversely affects dietary adherence. Meal-replacement plans that are used as a 'quick-fix' solution to achieve short-term weight loss goals, with little or no supervision by

healthcare professionals, increase the risks of complications and are less likely to be effective for weight maintenance in the absence of learning and retention of healthy eating habits [2]. Difficulties with compliance may also be due to lack of dietary variation and unpalatability, or unfamiliarity in relation to local diet and cultural norms, which were cited as reasons for the low adherence and high drop-out rates in one of the centres in the Diet, Obesity and Genes Project, which evaluated the use of VLCDs for weight loss in eight European cities [30].

4.2.5 Use of meal replacements for weight loss in special populations

Diabetes

Meta-analyses indicate that LCDs and VLCDs are safe and effective in reducing insulin resistance and other cardiovascular risk factors in obese adult populations, including significant proportions with type 2 diabetes [2,3,6,7], and they were also associated with better adherence [21]. Similarly, meal-replacement plans incorporated into group lifestyle interventions in obese patients with type 2 diabetes were associated with significantly greater mean weight loss (7.3 kg vs. 2.2 kg) and reduction in glycated haemoglobin, in comparison to a group programme of diabetes self-management education that prescribed similar energy intake (1250–1550 kcal/day, or 5250–6510 kJ/day) and physical activity levels [31]. The increase in the proportion of proteins in relation to carbohydrates in meal-replacement plans, as compared to conventional diets, may also contribute to superior glycaemic control, owing to the lower carbohydrate content [32].

Before bariatric surgery

As preoperative weight loss is associated with decreased liver volume (thereby reducing risks of hepatic injury), 2 weeks of VLCDs has been recommended before bariatric surgery, particularly in patients with uncontrolled diabetes with HbA1c >64 mmol/mol (8%) and hepatomegaly or fatty liver disease [33]. Improvements in glycaemic control and other comorbidities may also decrease risks of anaesthesia, poor wound healing and infection. Hence, meal replacements can help ensure a controlled VLCD preoperatively.

Improving fertility in polycystic ovarian syndrome (PCOS)

Weight loss studies in women with PCOS typically show high drop-out rates: 26–38% over 1–4 months for women with PCOS, as compared to 8–9% over 4 months in women without PCOS [34]. In women with PCOS, the higher prevalence of depression and anxiety can increase stress-driven overconsumption of comfort food. Lifestyle modification is effective in restoring reproductive function in up to 80% of individuals with PCOS who achieve at least 5% weight loss [34]. Women with PCOS who followed an 8-week weight-loss regimen (two meal replacements daily, ~5000 kJ), followed by 6 months of weight maintenance, demonstrated significantly reduced androgen concentrations and improved menstrual cyclicity, which were sustained for the period of weight maintenance [35]. Hence, by enhancing dietary adherence and weight loss, the use of meal replacements can improve fertility.

4.2.6 Conclusion

Meal replacements are portion-controlled low-energy alternatives to self-selected foods, which improve adherence to energy restriction by simplifying diet planning, thereby inducing greater weight loss in comparison to food-based diets when used as LCDs or VLCDs. Individual activity level and local diet norms should be considered in the prescription. Low-energy diets are ideally incorporated into a comprehensive weight-management programme, including exercise and behavioural therapy. Although meal-replacement plans are associated with numerous health benefits, judicious patient selection and supervision by healthcare professionals are necessary to reduce complications and minimise weight regain.

4.2.7 Summary box

Key points

- Meal replacements, with fixed proportions of energy and nutrients, are effective in weight-loss diets as the sole energy source for a meal, or in combination with other foods (partial-meal-replacement diet plan).
- The use of meal replacements results in larger early energy deficits and weight loss, improving diet compliance and completion rates and demonstrating better weight loss maintenance in comparison to conventional diets. This is likely due to their ease of use, leading to enhanced nutritional understanding and greater diet satisfaction.
- Meal-replacement plans are also useful in specific medical conditions, being associated with improved glycaemic control and weight loss in patients with type 2 diabetes, reduced preoperative complications before bariatric surgery and enhanced fertility in women with PCOS.

References

1. Commission Directive 96/8/EC of 26 February 1996 on foods intended for use in energy-restricted diets for weight reduction. OJ L 55, 6.3.1996, p. 22. Amended by 2007/29/EC of 30 May 2007. Internet: http://ec.europa.eu/food/food/labellingnutrition/weight/index_en.htm, accessed 21 April 2014.
2. Gonzalez-Campoy JM, St Jeor ST, Castorino K, Ebrahim A, Hurley D, Jovanovic L, et al. Clinical practice guidelines for healthy eating for the prevention and treatment of metabolic and endocrine diseases in adults: cosponsored by the American Association of Clinical Endocrinologists/the American College of Endocrinology and the Obesity Society. *Endocrine Practice* 2013; **19**: 1–82.
3. Tsai AG, Wadden TA. The evolution of very-low-calorie diets: an update and meta-analysis. *Obesity* (Silver Spring) 2006; **14**: 1283–1293.
4. Rucker D, Padwal R, Li SK, Curioni C, Lau DC. Long term pharmacotherapy for obesity and overweight: updated meta-analysis. *BMJ* 2007; **335**: 1194–1199.
5. Mifflin MD, St Jeor ST, Hill LA, Scott BJ, Daugherty SA, Koh YO. A new predictive equation for resting energy expenditure in healthy individuals. *American Journal of Clinical Nutrition* 1990; **51**: 241–247.
6. Heymsfield SB, van Mierlo CAJ, Knaap van der HCM, Heo M, Frier HI. Weight management using a meal replacement strategy: meta and pooling analysis from six studies. *International Journal of Obesity and Related Metabolic Disorders* 2003; **27**: 537–549.

7. Franz MJ, VanWormer JJ, Crain AL, Boucher JL, Histon T, Caplan W, Bowman JD, et al. Weight-loss outcomes: a systematic review and meta-analysis of weight-loss clinical trials with a minimum 1-year follow-up. *Journal of the American Dietetic Association* 2007; **107**: 1755–1767.

8. Shikany JM, Thomas AS, Beasley TM, Lewis CE, Allison DB. Randomized controlled trial of the Medifast 5 & 1 Plan for weight loss. *International Journal of Obesity* 2013; **37**: 1571–1578.

9. Khoo J, Ling PS, Chen RYT, Ng KK, Tay TL, Tan E, et al. Comparing effects of meal replacements with isocaloric reduced-fat diet on nutrient intake and lower urinary tract symptoms in obese men. *Journal of Human Nutrition and Dietetics*. epub 20 Sep 2013. doi: 10.1111/jhn.12151.

10. Montani JP, Viecelli AK, Prévot A, Dulloo AG. Weight cycling during growth and beyond as a risk factor for later cardiovascular diseases: the 'repeated overshoot' theory. *International Journal of Obesity* 2006; **30**: S58–S66.

11. Noakes M, Foster PR, Keogh JB, Clifton PM. Meal replacements are as effective as structured weight-loss diets for treating obesity in adults with features of metabolic syndrome. *Journal of Nutrition* 2004; **134**: 1894–1899.

12. Davis LM, Coleman C, Kiel J, Rampolla J, Hutchisen T, Ford L, et al. Efficacy of a meal replacement diet plan compared to a food-based diet plan after a period of weight loss and weight maintenance: a randomized controlled trial. *Nutrition Journal* 2010; **9**: 11. doi: 10.1186/1475-2891-9-11.

13. Finkler E, Heymsfield SB, St-Onge MP. Rate of weight loss can be predicted by patient characteristics and intervention strategies. *Journal of the Academy of Nutrition and Dietetics* 2012; **112**: 75–80.

14. Del Corral P, Chandler-Laney PC, Casazza K, Gower BA, Hunter GR. Effect of dietary adherence with or without exercise on weight loss: A mechanistic approach to a global problem. *Journal of Clinical Endocrinology and Metabolism* 2009; **94**: 1602–1607.

15. Thompson FE, Subar AF. Dietary assessment methodology. In: Coulston AM, Boushey CJ (eds) *Nutrition in the Prevention and Treatment of Disease*, 2nd edn. San Diego, CA: Academic Press, 2008.

16. Macdiarmid J, Blundell J. Assessing dietary intake: who, what and why of under-reporting. *Nutrition Research Reviews* 1998; **11**: 231–233.

17. Lichtman SW, Pisarska K, Berman ER, Pestone M, Dowling H, Offenbacher E, et al. Discrepancy between self-reported and actual caloric intake and exercise in obese subjects. *The New England Journal of Medicine* 1992; **327**: 1893–1898.

18. Wing RR, Jeffery RW. Food provision as a strategy to promote weight loss. *Obesity Research* 2001; **9**: 271S–275S.

19. Levitsky DA, Pacanowski C. Losing weight without dieting. Use of commercial foods as meal replacements for lunch produces an extended energy deficit. *Appetite* 2011; **57**: 311–317.

20. Marinilli-Pinto A, Gorin AA, Raynor HA, Tate DF, Fava JL, Wing RR. Successful weight-loss maintenance in relation to method of weight loss. *Obesity* (Silver Spring) 2008; **16**: 2456–2461.

21. Cheskin LJ, Mitchell AM, Jhaveri AD, Mitola AH, Davis LM, Lewis RA, et al. Efficacy of meal replacements versus standard food-based diet for weight loss in type 2 diabetes: a controlled clinical trial. *Diabetes Educator* 2008; **34**: 118–127.

22. Mayor GC, Doucet E, Trayhurn P, Astrup A, Tremblay A. Clinical significance of adaptive thermogenesis. *International Journal of Obesity* 2007; **31**: 204–212.

23. Müller MJ, Bosy-Westphal A. Adaptive thermogenesis with weight loss in humans. *Obesity* (Silver Spring) 2013; **21**: 218–228.

24. Westerterp KR, Donkers JHHL, Fredrix EWHM, Boekhudt P. Energy intake, physical activity and body weight: a simulation model. *British Journal of Nutrition* 1995; **73**: 337–347.

25. Rosenbaum M, Hirsch J, Gallagher D, Leibel RL. Long-term persistence of adaptive thermogenesis in subjects who have maintained a reduced body weight. *American Journal of Clinical Nutrition* 2008; **88**: 906–912.

26. Sumithran P, Prendergast LA, Delbridge E, Purcell K, Shulkes A, Kriketos A, et al. Long-term persistence of hormonal adaptations to weight loss. *The New England Journal of Medicine* 2011; **365**: 1597–1604.

27. Johansson K, Neovius M, Hemmingsson E. Effects of anti-obesity drugs, diet, and exercise on weight-loss maintenance after a very-low-calorie diet or low-calorie diet: a systematic review and meta-analysis of randomized controlled trials. *American Journal of Clinical Nutrition* 2014; **99**: 14–23.

28. Anderson JW, Konz EC, Frederich RC, Wood CL. Long-term weight-loss maintenance: a meta-analysis of US studies. *American Journal of Clinical Nutrition* 2001; **74**: 579–584.

29. Dirks AJ, Leeuwenburgh C. Caloric restriction in humans: potential pitfalls and health concerns. *Mechanisms of Ageing and Development* 2006; **127**: 1–7.

30. Papadaki A, Linardakis M, Plada M, Larsen TM, van Baak MA, Lindroos AK, et al. Diet, Obesity and Genes (DiOGenes) Project. A multicentre weight loss study using a low-calorie diet over 8 weeks: regional differences in efficacy across eight European cities. *Swiss Medical Weekly* 2013; **143**: w13721.

31. Foster GD, Wadden TA, LaGrotte CA, Vander Veur SS, Hesson LA, Homko CJ, et al. A randomized comparison of a commercially available portion-controlled weight-loss intervention with a diabetes self-management education programme. *Nutrition & Diabetes* 2013; **3**: e63. doi: 10.1038/nutd.2013.3.

32. Wing RR, Marcus MD, Salata R, Epstein LH, Miaskiewicz S, Blair EH. Effects of a very-low-calorie diet on long-term glycemic control in obese type 2 diabetic subjects. *Archives of Internal Medicine* 1991; **151**: 1334–1340.

33. Mechanick JI, Youdim A, Jones DB, Garvey WT, Hurley DL, McMahon MM, et al., American Association of Clinical Endocrinologists, Obesity Society, American Society for Metabolic & Bariatric Surgery. Clinical practice guidelines for the perioperative nutritional, metabolic, and nonsurgical support of the bariatric surgery patient – 2013 update: cosponsored by American Association of Clinical Endocrinologists, The Obesity Society, and American Society for Metabolic & Bariatric Surgery. *Obesity* (Silver Spring) 2013; **21**: S1–S27.

34. Moran LJ, Lombard CB, Lim S, Noakes M, Teede HJ. Polycystic ovary syndrome and weight management. *Women's Health* (London, England) 2010; **6**(2, Mar): 271–283.

35. Moran LJ, Noakes M, Clifton PM, Wittert GA, Williams G, Norman RJ. Short-term meal replacements followed by dietary macronutrient restriction enhance weight loss in polycystic ovary syndrome. *American Journal of Clinical Nutrition* 2006; **84**: 77–87.

Chapter 4.3

Formula diets for weight loss in obesity

Anthony R Leeds
University of Surrey, Guildford, UK

4.3.1 Introduction

Very-low-energy diets (VLEDs, or VLCDs – very-low-calorie diets) are diets providing 800 kcal/day or less, composed of three or four portions of formula food products based on skimmed milk powder or other protein sources providing approximately one-third of the micronutrients and essential fatty acids in each portion. They are usually presented in powdered form for reconstitution as soups or shakes to make a fully liquid diet. Devised over 30 years ago to deliver sufficient proteins and micronutrients to facilitate weight loss (usually 1 kg/week or more) while minimising lean body mass loss and nutrient depletion, they have been unpopular with healthcare professionals in some (but not all) countries, owing to largely unfounded anxieties about adverse effects and perceived clinical management issues.

Low-calorie liquid diets (LCLDs) are liquid diets based on the same products, with energy made up using liquid skimmed milk when necessary to deliver 800–1200 kcal/day. Some manufacturers divide an 800 kcal/day intake among five portions in the context of a total diet replacement, providing the full daily nutritional requirement across the five portions. While energy intakes of up to 1500 kcal/day are possible, in practice, 1000 kcal/day is the highest level usually used as a liquid diet. For requirements of above 1000 kcal/day, a small conventional meal is usually given to achieve the higher total dietary energy intake. Part food, part formula diets can incorporate meal replacements providing 200–400 kcal/portion, but products carrying a weight maintenance claim relating to substitution

of two conventional meals within the context of an energy-restricted diet in Europe are legally required to not exceed 250 kcal/portion.

The UK National Institute for Health and Care Excellence partial update guideline [1], which is clearly stated as not being a guideline for use in a commercial context, states that VLCDs should not be used routinely in clinical practice to manage obesity. The guideline states that VLCDs should only be considered 'as part of a multicomponent weight management strategy for people who are obese and who have clinically assessed need to rapidly lose weight (e.g. people who need joint replacement surgery or who are seeking fertility services)'. The guideline development group did not review evidence for the use of LCLDs, thus missing an opportunity to consider all the potential applications of formula diets in the present-day context of the rising prevalence of severe and complex (morbid) obesity, which will increasingly drain the resources of health providers across the globe. The recommendation to consider VLCDs for one increasingly prevalent pre-operative application (weight loss before knee replacement) followed a decision to exclude a review of evidence for the use of VLCDs in the preparation for bariatric surgery, because the guideline development group 'were concerned that clinicians would use VLCDs routinely instead of bariatric surgery, and that the patient's treatment may be delayed as a consequence' [1]. Since obesity can influence many aspects of the process of induction of anaesthesia – such as physical difficulty with intubation, and postoperative recovery and outcomes, including respiratory recovery time, wound

Advanced Nutrition and Dietetics in Obesity, First Edition. Edited by Catherine Hankey.
© 2018 John Wiley & Sons Ltd. Published 2018 by John Wiley & Sons Ltd.

infections and, in the case of knee arthroplasty, long-term outcomes [2–3] – a review of evidence for the preoperative use of formula diets was indeed necessary, but not delivered.

4.3.2 Mechanism of action of formula diets

Formula diets are believed to work via several mechanisms. First, it involves the substitution of conventional food with defined portions, facilitating portion control in those for whom controlling food portion size is a problem. Second, lower energy intakes can be achieved than would be possible with a restricted conventional food intake, while still maintaining micronutrient and protein intake. The energy and carbohydrate restriction (which in most commercial products does not go down to the very low carbohydrate levels used in the ketogenic diets used for treating intractable epilepsy in children) results in physiological ketosis, which has recently been shown to suppress the usual rise of the hunger

hormone, ghrelin [4]. This evidence is consistent with the anecdotal evidence that users of VLCDs tend not to feel hungry, and that they are able to achieve a high degree of compliance with their prescribed diet. The energy and carbohydrate restriction results in a rapid increase of insulin sensitivity with decreased liver glucose output, which can cause improved metabolic variables in people with diabetes [5]. Third, the greater energy deficit that can be achieved (1000–2000 kcal/day) can result in greater rates of weight loss than possible with the 500–600 kcal/day energy deficit in a conventional diet. VLCD use in men with severe and moderate obstructive sleep apnoea can cause an average 19 kg weight loss in 7–9 weeks, and caused five out of six men to show improvement in obstructive sleep apnoea, with nearly 50% no longer using positive airway pressure machines after 1 year of weight maintenance [6–7] (see Figure 4.3.1). The use of VLCDs for 16 weeks in men and women with type 2 diabetes caused an average 23 kg weight loss over 16 weeks, with improved metabolic variables [8]. VLCD use in older people with knee osteoarthritis

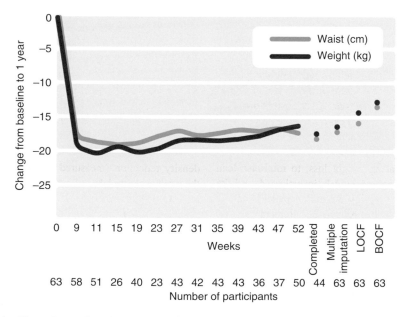

Figure 4.3.1   Mean change from baseline in weight and waist circumference during and after treatment with very-low-calorie diets for men with severe or moderate obstructive sleep apnoea. Results at 52 weeks are given for completers ($n = 44$); with multiple imputation for missing data ($n = 63$); with last observation carried forward (LOCF; $n = 63$); and baseline observation carried forward (BOCF; $n = 63$). Low attendance at 15 and 23 weeks was attributed to summer holidays. Redrawn from reference [6].

over 8 weeks, followed by an 8-week part-food-part-formula diet (1200 kcal/day), gave the same weight loss (around 12–13 kg) as LCLD followed by 8 weeks 1200 kcal/day diet. However, importantly, it reduced pain in more than 60% of the subjects, thus improving mobility and quality of life [9].

4.3.3 Weight regain and lean body mass loss

Healthcare professionals believe that rapid weight loss results in rapid weight regain and will cause excessive lean loss. Purcell has reported a study on over 200 subjects who were prepared with a weight loss of 15 kg by either the use of VLCDs (over 12 weeks) or conventional diets (over 36 weeks) [10]. Weight regain over nearly 3 years, during which subjects met with a dietitian monthly and followed the Australian healthy eating guidelines, was the same in both groups, being about 10 kg regain so the net weight loss from baseline of 5 kg. The Purcell study proved that weight regain was not influenced by the preceding rate of weight loss. The composition of body weight lost after VLCDs can be influenced by exercise, as established by Snel [8], who showed that the addition of a vigorous exercise programme in people with type 2 diabetes reduced lean loss from 29% to 19%. In elderly people with osteoarthritis who started relatively immobile with a probable degree of muscle atrophy, the lean mass losses following VLCDs or LCLDs and a food reintroduction diet (1200 kcal/day) were low at just under 20%, reflecting adequate protein intake and a relative increase in activity [7,11]. The protein requirement during weight loss, to minimise lean loss, has not been adequately investigated, and the European Food Safety Authority panel's current recommendation on protein requirement for formula food products (>70 g/day) is based on guidelines for healthy-weight stable subjects rather than solid experimental evidence [12], and represents a sensible interim compromise [13]. The pattern of protein intake is probably important, and there may be merit in examining whether the delivery of a bolus of 25–30 g proteins after the day's main episode of physical exercise [14] will be proved to facilitate lean retention during weight loss with formula programmes.

Consequences of rapid weight loss with formula diets

Rapid weight loss can have tangible benefits, such as reduced joint pain and shortness of breath, which are highly motivating and encourage compliance. While this is an anecdotal remark based on clinical observation, it is supported by Purcell's finding that drop-out rates were much higher in the slow-weight-loss group than in the rapid-weight-loss group [6–10].

Weight loss with formula diets may cause a range of secondary changes – some beneficial, others not. Cardiovascular risk factors such as blood pressure, blood lipids and calculated insulin sensitivity can improve [11], and there is evidence for improved coronary flow reserve following weight loss in obese women who have severe coronary heart disease or have suffered heart attacks [15,16]. Nutritional status, which can be impaired in the obese [17], can improve following weight loss with formula diets. Nearly 50% of elderly obese people with knee osteoarthritis living in Copenhagen were vitamin D deficient at the commencement of weight loss treatment; this reduced to 22% after the 16-week weight loss programme [11], and to 8% after 1 year of weight maintenance with one formula food portion in place of one conventional meal. The National Institute for Health and Care Excellence (NICE) obesity guideline development group wrote that they 'felt that reduction in bone density may occur because of insufficient calcium in the diet and may result in fragility and fracture' [1], without referring to published evidence showing that those same elderly Danes who lost weight with formula diets showed less bone mineral loss and less bone density reduction (measured by DEXA scanning) than was expected based on their fat mass losses [18]. Constipation can be a problem, but is easily forestalled by asking about the history of constipation, diverticular disease and anal disease, and by providing extra stool-bulking fibre such as a psyllium preparation (3.5 g twice daily). Gout has occurred, but rarely, in some trials, but can be prevented by adequate early detection of raised uric acid followed by treatment. A large survey undertaken in Sweden showed that the rate for clinical gallstone events requiring hospitalisation was low in absolute numbers after weight loss, but three times more likely after weight loss with VLCDs (at 44 cases per 1000 person-years), than after a 1200 kcal/day diet (at 15 cases per 1000 person-years) [19]. Postural hypotension with dizziness and a risk of falling is possible, especially in older people with treated hypertension. Formula diet products contain adequate sodium and potassium, but much less sodium than the usual food-based diet. The typical systolic blood pressure reduction in an older person using a formula diet programme is about 12 mmHg, sufficient to cause dizzy spells. Users of formula diet programmes need to be warned of this possible effect, and some need to have regular blood pressure monitoring and medication adjustment. Use of some other medications (insulin, oral hypoglycaemic agents and warfarin) require careful patient monitoring and dose adjustment during weight loss. Other drug groups such as lipid-lowering agents can be left in place, and their dose can be reassessed after weight loss.

4.3.4 Potential applications

Formula diet weight reduction programmes are eminently suitable for achieving defined amounts of weight loss for specific purposes in a short period of time. Preoperative weight loss for use before bariatric surgery is established in many but not all surgical centres. Food-based 1000 kcal/day diets are still used in some centres. Although formula-based 1000 kcal/day diets have been shown to cause liver shrinkage, some surgeons believe that no preoperative preparation is necessary. A number of studies have shown that liver fat content and liver volume are reduced rapidly, and just 2 weeks of 1000 kcal/s liquid formula diet is effective [20,21]. A randomised controlled trial of weight loss before knee replacement surgery using formula-based 810 kcal/day liquid diets has been completed in Denmark. Effective weight loss has been achieved, and quality of life and function assessment results at 6 and 12 months are awaited [22]. High levels of compliance and predictability of outcome facilitate the process of managing surgical sessions. Weight loss programmes can be delivered during the 8-week period from initial assessment to the surgical knee replacement. Delivery of surgical treatment is not delayed by this planned intervention. Weight loss with

VLCDs can induce changes associated with increased fertility [23], and the predictability of weight loss in compliant patients may help them achieve target weights set by gynaecologists operating fertility programmes.

When bariatric surgery is not medically indicated, where the patient rejects a surgical option or where surgical resources are limited, formula diet programmes may be considered to achieve the 10–20 kg weight loss needed to reverse type 2 diabetes, improve obstructive sleep apnoea, improve psoriasis [24,25], improve cardiovascular function or improve quality of life in those with knee osteoarthritis. Regarding weight maintenance, the evidence derived from randomised controlled trials of interventions after initial weight loss with VLCDs or LCLDs was reviewed in a meta-analysis by Johansson and colleagues [26], who showed that diets with higher-than-usual protein content, drugs (studies on sibutramine and orlistat) and one-a-day formula food replacement were all shown to result in statistically significantly greater weight maintenance at variable lengths of time after weight loss (see Figure 4.3.2).

Setting

VLCDs and LCLDs can be used in primary community and secondary hospital clinical settings, but are also available in commercial settings provided by diet counsellors or consultants who are mostly non-healthcare professionals trained to provide the diet programmes with educational, physical activity and psychological components in a community setting. In the commercial setting, medical management remains with the patient's primary care team, and written protocols are designed to ensure the appropriate use of VLCDs and LCLDs, but the unfortunate trend towards Internet and over-the-counter sales can result in little or no control over the use of formula diets sold in this way.

Research needs

Since considerable weight loss and health benefits have been shown following LCLDs, it is likely that future research on formula diets will focus on those delivering 800–1200 kcal/day. At this energy intake level, it is easier to deliver the needed 70 g/day

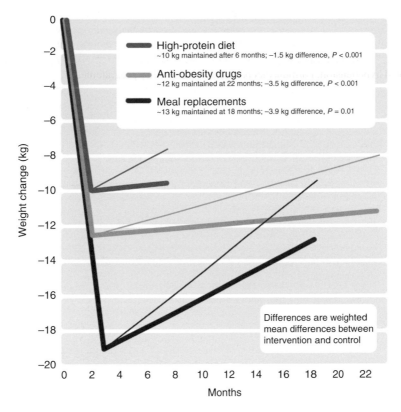

Figure 4.3.2 Body weight change during the VLCD or LCD period followed by the weight loss maintenance period. The thin lines represent the control subjects in each category, while the thick lines represent the active intervention. Redrawn from reference [26].

proteins. Also, when compared directly to VLCDs in elderly people with knee osteoarthritis, there appears to be no disadvantage in using LCLDs. A number of large-scale randomised controlled trials are already underway to investigate diabetes reversal in pre-diabetes [27], early type 2 diabetes [28] and advanced insulin-treated diabetes. The underlying mechanism in the reversal of insulin resistance has been understood for some time [29]. Large multicentre studies are planned to follow-on from the promising findings in women who have severe coronary heart disease or suffered heart attacks [15,16] and in people with psoriasis [24,25]. Translation into practice trials is planned for weight loss in knee osteoarthritis and obstructive sleep apnoea, and need to be undertaken for idiopathic intracranial hypertension [30]. There is a need for studies on mechanisms using which acute weight loss before anaesthesia in obese,

morbidly obese and super-obese individuals leads to improved peri-operative outcomes, including reduced healthcare costs. Trials not yet organised include weight loss in women after pregnancy and after a diagnosis of gestational diabetes; in those with leg or postoperative arm lymphoedema; and in severe–moderate stress incontinence in women.

4.3.5 Conclusion

Weight loss programmes that utilise 800 kcal/day formula diets and above with intense education programmes, regular support and lifestyle guidance have been proven to be effective. Bischoff has reported on a multicentre programme operating in 37 centres in Germany, giving results in over 8000 individuals using a 52-week programme that incorporates 12 weeks of 800 kcal/day diet [31]. At the end of the 1-year intervention, average weight loss was 19.6 kg in women and 26 kg in men (15.2 kg and 10.4 kg, respectively, using intention-to-treat analyses). Incidence of adverse events was low. Taking this in conjunction with the disease-specific studies described earlier, there is clearly a role for nonsurgical weight loss programmes that include short periods of LCLDs (above 800 kcal/day). In Australia, Germany, Sweden and the USA, these programmes are utilised to an increasing degree. A number of European countries discourage the use of VLCDs, and the recent NICE guidance in the UK [1] is somewhat discouraging too. However, in the UK, in the absence of guidelines on the use of LCLDs, dietitians and doctors can utilise the meta-analysis from Sweden as a guideline on weight maintenance after weight loss with VLCDs or LCLDs [26], and use the results of randomised controlled trials in specific conditions – diabetes [8], osteoarthritis [9], obstructive sleep apnoea [6,7] and psoriasis [24,25] – to judge whether and when to use LCLDs for their patients.

4.3.6 Conflict of interest

Anthony R Leeds is a salaried medical director of Cambridge Weight Plan, but holds no shares or share options, nor any shares in any other food or pharmaceutical company.

4.3.7 Summary box

Key points

- Weight loss programmes that utilise formula diets of 800 kcal/day and above along with intense education programmes, regular support and lifestyle guidance have been proven to be effective.
- A 1-year VLCD intervention achieved average weight loss of 19.6 kg in women and 26 kg in men (15.2 kg and 10.4 kg, respectively, using intention-to-treat analyses).
- Use of VLCDs was associated with few adverse events.

- A meta-analysis from Sweden can be used as a guideline on weight maintenance after weight loss with VLCDs or LCLDs.
- A role exists for nonsurgical weight loss programmes that include short periods of LCLDs (above 800 kcal/day) in the treatment of obese and morbidly obese individuals.

References

1. National Institute for Health and Care Excellence. Obesity identification, assessment and management of overweight and obesity in children, young people and adults. CG 189 being a partial update of CG43 Methods, evidence and recommendations, November 2014. Available from: http://www.nice.org.uk/guidance/cg189, accessed 14 December 2014.
2. Liljensøe A, Lauersen JO, Søballe K, et al. Overweight preoperatively impairs clinical outcome after knee arthroplasty: a cohort study of 197 patients 3–5 years after surgery. *Acta Orthopaedica* 2013; **84**(4): 392–397.
3. Kerkhoffs GMM, Servien E, Dunn W, Dahm D, Bramer JAM, Haverkamp D. The influence of obesity on the complication rate and outcome of total knee arthroplasty: a meta-analysis and systematic literature review. *Journal of Bone and Joint Surgery-American Volume* 2012; **94**: 1839–1844.
4. Sumithran P, Prendergast LA, Delbridge E, Purcell K, Shulkes A, Kriketos A, Proietto J. Ketosis and appetite-mediating nutrients and hormones after weight loss. *European Journal of Clinical Nutrition* 2013; **67**: 759–764.
5. Lim EL, Hollingsworth KG, Aribisala BS, et al. Reversal of type 2 diabetes: normalisation of beta cell function in association with decreased pancreas and liver triacylglycerol. *Diabetologia* 2011; **54**: 2506–2514.
6. Johansson K, Hemmingsson E, Harlid R, et al. Longer term effects of very low energy diet on obstructive sleep apnoea in cohort derived from randomised controlled trial: prospective observational follow-up study. *British Medical Journal* 2011; **342**: d3017. doi:10.1136/bmj.d3017.
7. Johansson K, Hemmingsson E, Neovius M. Effects of anti-obesity drugs, diet, and exercise on weight-loss maintenance after a very-low-calorie diet or low-calorie diet: a systematic review and meta-analysis of randomized controlled trials. *American Journal of Clinical Nutrition* 2013. doi: 10.3945/ajcn.113.070052.
8. Snel M, Gastaldelli A, Ouwens DA, Hesselink MKC, Schaart G, Buzzigoli E, et al. Effects of adding exercise to a 16-week very low-calorie diet in obese, insulin-dependent type 2 diabetes mellitus patients. *Journal of Clinical Endocrinology and Metabolism* 2012; **97**(7): 2512–2520.
9. Christensen P, Bliddal H, Riecke BF, et al. Comparison of a low-energy diet and a very low-energy diet in sedentary obese individuals: a pragmatic randomised controlled trial. *Clinical Obesity* 2011; **1**: 31–40.
10. Purcell K, Sumithran P, Prendergast LA, Bouniu CJ, Delbridge E, Proietto J. The effect of rate of weight loss on long-term

weight management: a randomised controlled trial. *The Lancet Diabetes & Endocrinology* 2014 Published online 16 October 2014. Available from: http://dx.doi.org/10.1016/S2213-8587(14)70200-1.

11. Christensen P, Bartels EM, Riecke BF, et al. Improved nutritional status and bone health after diet-induced weight loss in sedentary osteoarthritis patients: a prospective cohort study. *European Journal of Clinical Nutrition* 2011; **66**: 504–509.

12. European Food Safety Authority. Scientific opinion on dietary reference values for protein. *EFSA Journal* 2012; **10**(2): 2557.

13. European Food Safety Authority. Scientific opinion on composition of formula diet for weight loss. *EFSA Journal* 2015; **13**(1): 3957 [1–52 pp].

14. Moore DR, Areta J, Coffey VG, Stellingwerff T, Phillips SM, Burke LM, et al. Daytime pattern of post-exercise protein intake affects whole-body protein turnover in resistance-trained males. *Nutrition & Metabolism* 2012; **9**: 91.

15. Pedersen LR, Olsen RH, Jürs A, Astrup A, Chabanova E, Simonsen L, et al. A randomised trial comparing weight loss with aerobic exercise in overweight individuals with coronary artery disease: the CUT-IT trial. *European Journal of Preventive Cardiology* 2014. Published online 31 July 2014. doi: 10.1177/2047487314545280.

16. Olsen RH, Pedersen LR, Snoer M, Jurs A, Haugaard SB, Prescott E. The effect of a 12-week interval training or weight loss program on coronary flow reserve in overweight patients with coronary artery disease: primary outcome of the randomised controlled CUT-IT trial. *European Journal of Preventive Cardiology* 2014; **21**: S46–S48, 175. doi:10.1177/2047487314534577.

17. Xanthakos SA. Nutritional deficiencies in obesity and after bariatric surgery. *Pediatric clinics of North America* 2009; **56**(5): 1105–1121. doi:10.1016/j.pcl.2009.07.002.

18. Christensen P, Frederiksen R, Bliddal H, et al. Comparison of three different weight maintenance programs on cardiovascular risk, bone, an vitamins in sedentary older adults. *Obesity* 2013; **21**: 1982–1990. doi: 10.1002/oby.20413.

19. Johansson K, Sundström J, Marcus C, et al. Risk of symptomatic gallstones and cholecystectomy after a very-low-calorie diet or low-calorie diet in a commercial weight loss programme: 1-year matched cohort study. *International Journal of Obesity* 2013; **38**: 279–284. doi:10.1038/ijo.2013.83.

20. Colles SL, Dixon JB, Marks P, et al. Preoperative weight loss with a very low-energy diet: quantitation of changes in liver and abdominal fat by serial imaging. *American Journal of Clinical Nutrition* 2006; **84**: 304–311.

21. Bottin J, Balogun B, Thomas E, Fitzpatrick J, Moorthy K, Leeds A, et al. Changes in body composition induced by preoperative liquid low-calorie diet in morbid obese patients undergoing Roux-en-Y gastric bypass. *Obesity Reviews* 2014; **15**(2): 129–176. doi/10.1111/obr.12151/T5:S24.05.

22. Liljensøe A, Laursen J, Bliddal H, Søballe K, Mechlenburg I. Weight loss intervention before total knee replacement. A safety study. *Obesity Reviews* 2014. doi/10.1111/obr.12151/T5:S25.59.

23. van Dam EW, Roelfsema F, Veldhuis JD, Hogendoorn S, Westenberg J, Helmerhorst FM, et al. Retention of estradiol negative feedback relationship to LH predicts ovulation in response to caloric restriction and weight loss in obese patients with polycystic ovary syndrome. *American Journal of Physiology – Endocrinology and Metabolism* 2004; **286**(4): E615–E620. doi: 10.1152/ajpendo.00377.2003.

24. Jensen P, Zachariae C, Christensen R, et al. Effect of weight loss on the severity of psoriasis: a randomized clinical study. *Journal of the American Medical Association Dermatology* 2013; **149**: 795–801. doi:10.1001/jamadermatol.2013.722.

25. Jensen P, Zachariae C, Christensen R, et al. Effect of weight loss on the cardiovascular risk profile of obese patients with psoriasis. *Acta Dermato-Venereologica* 2014; **94**: 691–694. doi: 10.2340/00015555-1824.

26. Johansson K, Hemmingsson E, Neovius M. Effects of anti-obesity drugs, diet, and exercise on weight-loss maintenance after a very-low-calorie diet or low-calorie diet: a systematic review and meta-analysis of randomized controlled trials. *American Journal of Clinical Nutrition* 2013; **99**: 14–23. doi: 10.3945/ajcn.113.070052.

27. PREVIEW. Effect of diet and physical activity on incidence of type 2 diabetes (weight loss with CWP LCD in people with pre-diabetes in 2200 adults in a multicentre study in 6 EU countries and Australia and New Zealand). Available from: http://clinicaltrials.gov/show/NCT01777893, accessed 25 November 2014.

28. DiRECT (Diabetes Remission Clinical Trial). Using CWP LCD to achieve weight loss in people with early type 2 diabetes in a primary care setting. Available from: http://www.diabetes.org.uk/DiRECT, accessed 25 November 2014.

29. Williams K, Bertoldo A, Kinahan P, Cobelli C, Kelley DE. Weight loss-induced plasticity of glucose transport and phosphorylation in the insulin resistance of obesity and type 2 diabetes. *Diabetes* 2003; **52**: 1619–1626.

30. Sinclair AJ, Burdon MA, Nightingale PG, et al. Low energy diet and intracranial pressure in women with idiopathic intracranial hypertension: prospective cohort study. *British Medical Journal* 2010; **340**: c2701. doi:10.1136/bmj.c2701.

31. Bischoff SC, Damms-Machado A, Betz C, Herpertz S, Legenbauer T, Löw T, et al. Multicenter evaluation of an interdisciplinary 52-week weight loss program for obesity with regard to body weight, comorbidities and quality of life: a prospective study. *International Journal of Obesity* 2012; **36**: 614–624.

Chapter 4.4

Group-based interventions for weight loss in obesity

Karen Allan
NHS Education for Scotland, Edinburgh, Scotland, UK

4.4.1 Introduction

Interventions for obesity can be delivered in a variety of ways – using a one-to-one approach, within group settings and online using web-based programmes. Group-based approaches to weight management are popular in commercial weight management organisations (CWMOs) and have gained popularity in healthcare and community settings. Interventions using a group format offer a model of obesity treatment that facilitates social interaction and peer support and can allow health professionals to reach a wider number of people. There are examples of the effectiveness of group interventions in other areas of health improvement such as diabetes education [1] and smoking cessation [2]; however, evaluation of effective weight management group processes has received less attention.

It is often assumed that programmes provided in a one-to-one setting are transferable to group-based settings and vice versa. However, planning, leading and managing groups call for different skills from those employed in one-to-one interventions for weight management. In addition, there are considerations such as the group composition, group setting, treatment length and leadership style. Health professionals currently have very little guidance on how to deliver effective group interventions. This chapter explores the use of group-based interventions across a range of obesity treatments and examines evidence for the effectiveness of group-based approaches for obesity management in adults.

4.4.2 Defining group-based interventions for weight management

'Groups' are a fundamental part of society and feature in social, political, cultural, educational, therapeutic and work contexts. Research literature relating to group processes and group dynamics comes mainly from fields such as behavioural and social psychology and sociology. However, aspects such as defining groups and their characteristics in health-improvement contexts have not been adequately described [3].

Existing literature has explored the use of group interventions for weight management in a variety of contexts and settings. It is common for behavioural programmes for obesity to be delivered in a group format, but few studies describe the group-specific components in terms of outcomes. The National Institutes for Health and Clinical Excellence (NICE) guidelines on behavioural change include groups in the category of community interventions but does not provide any specific guidance on group settings *per se* [4].

In the field of eating disorders, therapies such as cognitive-behavioural therapy and interpersonal behavioural therapy for binge eating disorder have been tested using a group format. These studies do not always outline the factors underlying the decision to provide therapy using a group modality, but it is thought to relate to the broader reach, interpersonal support and cost-effectiveness, as compared to individual one-to-one therapy [5].

Advanced Nutrition and Dietetics in Obesity, First Edition. Edited by Catherine Hankey.
© 2018 John Wiley & Sons Ltd. Published 2018 by John Wiley & Sons Ltd.

In addition to focussing on weight management, groups are often linked by another common factor, particularly in relation to group composition. For example, studies have examined outcomes where members of the group have the same health condition; are of a specific racial composition or sexual orientation; are based in a specific geographical location, such as a rural setting or a worksite setting; or are of common gender, such as men-only groups [6–10].

The literature also suggests significant variation in the structure, underlying theoretical models and the intervention delivered within weight management groups. In some groups, the interaction between members may form part of the intervention, such as in peer support and self-care groups. In other groups, the intervention will be delivered by a recognised group leader who will follow a particular programme based on changing diet and physical activity levels. Some groups will also include 'activities' such as physical activity within the group session itself.

4.4.3 Evidence for obesity interventions delivered in a group setting

Studies support the view that the social and peer support provided by group-based treatments improves outcomes [11]. A systematic review of the impact of social support on weight loss following bariatric surgery showed that attendance at a support group following bariatric surgery was associated with greater postoperative weight loss; however, the studies identified were observational, cohort studies, and not randomised controlled trials [12].

The impact of matching participants to treatments on the basis of their preference for group or individual therapy for obesity was investigated by Renjilian and colleagues [13]. Their study randomised 75 participants to either their preferred or non-preferred treatment modality. The results showed that, overall, group intervention was more effective than one-to-one intervention, and that, even in people who expressed a preference for one-to-one therapy, weight loss was greater if they were allocated to a group.

Paul-Ebhohimhen and Avenell conducted a systematic review of group vs. individual treatments for adult obesity [14]. They identified five trials using a randomised controlled design that compared group-based with individual-based treatment in adults with BMI > 28 kg/m², who were followed-up for at least 1 year and a meta-analysis of weight change conducted. They concluded that group-based interventions were more effective than individual-based interventions, with a significantly greater weight change for group over individual treatment at 12 months ($P = 0.03$). Further sub-analyses showed that better outcomes were achieved with the inclusion of financial incentives and where groups were led by psychologists. The limitations of their review are that only one of the studies included men; there was little information on the socioeconomic status of the participants; and there was no information on the training provided to those running the groups. In addition, the review focussed primarily on weight loss outcomes, and the studies provided little insight into the characteristics and processes that might enhance the effectiveness of group-based interventions. Despite the theory that group-based interventions are potentially less resource intensive than individual-based interventions, limited studies have been reported on the cost-effectiveness of group interventions as compared to individual treatments for obesity.

4.4.4 Evidence for CWMO programmes delivered in a group setting

CWMOs are accessible in communities and online, and are a popular method used by people to support self-management of their weight (Chapter 4.5). More women than men attend such groups, the format of which usually involves payment for weekly attendance, following a branded dietary programme, with support from a recognised group leader and additional support online and through magazines. In the UK, the most popular commercial organisations include Weight Watchers, Rosemary Conley and Slimming World. Tsai and Wadden conducted a review of CWMO programmes in the USA and reflected that there were little or no high-quality controlled trials reporting on the effectiveness on weight loss [15]. They identified only one large ran-domised controlled trial that compared Weight Watchers with a standard self-help programme, with the results showing a mean weight loss of 2.9 kg in the Weight Watchers attendees, as compared to 0.2 kg in the self-help programme, after 2 years [16].

Health service leaders have more formal qualifica-tions but less access to ongoing training specific to developing skills in group facilitation and manage-ment as compared to commercial group leaders. The personality and people skills of the group leader were consistently valued, regardless of the type of group attended. The desirability of the leader having per-sonal experience of weight loss varied, with men in particular being indifferent to this and placing more emphasis on the leader's expert knowledge and credi-bility. The authors highlight that there were no guide-lines for how groups should be operationalised within health service settings, and recommend paying atten-tion to leader training, extending access and targeting populations who are less likely to attend or have the means to attend commercial groups. Further review of CWMOs can be found in Chapter 4.5.

4.4.5 Gender in relation to weight loss groups

The prevalence of overweight and obesity is higher among men than women, yet men are much less likely than women to seek interventions for weight management. Men-only groups have been provided by a number of CWMOs, with Bye et al. evaluating the outcomes for men attending men-only groups at Slimming World [17]. They observed a mean weight reduction of 9.2 % at 12 weeks of attend-ance in 53 men enrolled across seven of their com-mercial weight loss groups. The study was observational in design and did not provide any qualitative data about why men joined and what their experience of the group was. Gray et al. [10] conducted a qualitative and quantitative evaluation of men attending a 12-week, primary-care-based, men-only group in Scotland. Their evaluation concluded that men will engage with group interventions that are specifically tailored to them. The participants in their study appreciated the flexible approach to weight management that the

programme offered. They valued the use of humour, the educational emphasis on nutrition, the rapport they had with the group leader, as well as the peer support gained from other participants. This con-curs with qualitative research from Allan et al., who observed that men valued an educational-style health-service-based group, as compared to com-mercial groups, whom they perceived as being aimed at women and unsuitable for them [18]. In the Football Fans in Training (FFIT) study, Hunt et al. conducted an innovative randomised trial of a 12-week, men-only, group-based weight manage-ment programme with football fans from 13 Scottish Professional Football League clubs [19]. At 12 months, the men participating in the FFIT programme ($n = 374$) had a mean weight loss of 5.56 kg, as compared to 0.58 kg in the men in the minimal intervention comparison group ($n = 373$). This is a higher weight loss than other trials report-ing weight loss outcomes in interventions aimed at men. The authors suggest that this may have been due to the fact that their intervention was a group-based programme that was gender sensitised in content and context (held at football clubs), and that the style of delivery (participative, peer supported with emphasis on learning) was more appealing to the male participants. The intervention was deliv-ered by community coaching staff employed by the football clubs, and they received training for 2 days in preparation for running the groups.

4.4.6 Important components of group-based approaches in obesity management

The quality of reporting on the group-specific elements of weight management interventions is poor. Few studies provide information on elements such as the group setting, group composition, optimum group size, length, style and content of sessions and leader attrib-utes and training. In response to the lack of guidelines for designing, evaluating or reporting health improve-ment interventions in a group setting, Hoddinott et al. proposed a framework to support a more systematic approach to the development and interpretation of group-based interventions [3]. Their article highlights that behaviour change interventions delivered in a group setting are complex processes, with interactions among group participants, the leader and the wider environment occurring, which differ from individual-based approaches. They recommend:

- Taking consideration of how aspects of the setting (e.g. meeting place, surroundings and venue) will impact on all aspects of the group processes, composition and outcomes
- Defining what the intervention is, what quantity will be delivered and how this will be delivered
- Defining who will participate in the group and how they will access the group
- Describing how being part of the group may influence participants
- Defining clearly what happens in the group

Currently, the evidence base is weak with regard to understanding what components of group programmes work in which settings and for whom. Better reporting is required in studies applying a group-based approach, and more research is required to support health professionals with the design, implementation and evaluation of group interventions.

4.4.7 Conclusion

Group-based interventions are an important option in the range of weight management strategies. The advantages of groups are that they can lessen feelings of social isolation and stigmatism that are associated with obesity, but they may not be practicable or appealing to all people wanting to manage their weight. Groups can provide opportunities for health professionals to reach a wider number of people and have the potential to be less resource intensive. However, cost-effectiveness studies are lacking, and randomised controlled trials that directly compare current models of group care with each other and with models of individual treatment are limited. Those that have been conducted show that there is evidence to support the application of group-based approaches, but the poor description and reporting of group-specific elements in many studies mean that the components of group-based approaches that are most effective or show most promise in different settings and contexts are not known.

Facilitating weight management groups has been described as 'giving a performance', and calls for a different skill set as compared to one-to-one interventions [18]. Existing literature is scarce on the practicalities of implementing groups within community and health settings, and training in group facilitation skills is variable and rarely described. The knowledge and skills required to lead groups will, to some extent, be determined by the style and composition of the group, but what makes for an effective group leader in relation to weight management has not been well defined. Gender in relation to groups warrants further investigation, as does the context and group setting.

Given the extent to which groups are utilised, both within commercial settings and in the health service, surprisingly little research has focussed on which group strategies and techniques are most useful and which are not helpful for maximising outcomes. A one-size-fits-all approach is unlikely to be useful in the design and implementation of group-based programmes, but more evidence-based guidelines are required that would support health professionals in setting up, managing and evaluating groups.

4.4.8 Summary box

Key points

- Group-based interventions in weight management strategies can lessen the feelings of social isolation and stigmatism that are associated with obesity.
- Groups can provide opportunities for health professionals to reach a wider number of people and have the potential to be less resource intensive, but are not attractive to all patients.
- Evidence of the cost-effectiveness of current models of group care as compared to each other and to models of individual treatment are limited.
- Poor description and reporting of group-specific elements in many studies mean that the most effective components in different settings and contexts are unknown.
- Facilitating weight management groups calls for a different skill set as compared to one-to-one interventions.

- Existing literature is scarce on the practicalities of implementing group interventions in community and health settings.
- A one-size-fits-all approach is unlikely to be useful in the design and implementation of group-based programmes. Evidence-based guidelines would support health professionals in setting up, managing and evaluating group treatments.

References

1. Deakin T, McShane CE, Cade JE, Williams RD. Group based training for self-management strategies in people with type 2 diabetes. *Cochrane Database of Systematic Reviews* 2005; **2**: CD003417.
2. Stead LF, Lancaster T. Group behaviour therapy programmes for smoking cessation. *Cochrane Database of Systematic Reviews* 2005; **2**: CD001007.
3. Hoddinott P, Allan K, Avenell A, Britten J. Group interventions to improve health outcomes: a framework for their design and delivery. *BMC Public Health* 2010; **10**: 800.
4. National Institute for Health and Clinical Excellence. Behaviour change at population, community and individual levels, 2007. Available from: http://www.nice.org.uk/PH6.
5. Peterson CB, Mitchell JE, Crow SY, Crosby RD, Wonderlich SA. The efficacy of self-help group treatment and therapist led group treatment for binge eating disorder. *American Journal of Psychiatry* 2009; **166**: 1347–1354.
6. Ard JD, Kumanyika S, Stevens VJ, Vollmer WM, Samuel-Hodge C, Kennedy B, et al. Effect of group racial composition on weight loss in African Americans. *Obesity* 2008; **16**(2): 306–310.
7. Fogel S, Young L, McPherson B. The experience of group weight loss efforts among lesbians. *Women & Health* 2009; **49**(6–7): 540–554.
8. Befort CA, Donnelly JE, Sullivan DK, Ellerbeck EF. Group versus individual phone-based obesity treatment for rural women. *Eating Behaviors* 2010; **11**: 11–17.
9. Rigsby A, Gropper DM, Gropper SS. Success of women in a worksite weight loss program: Does being part of a group help? *Eating Behaviors* 2009, **10**: 128–130.
10. Gray C, Anderson A, Clarke A, Dalziel A, Hunt K, Leishman J, et al. Addressing male obesity: an evaluation of a group-based weight management intervention for Scottish men. *JMH* 2009; **6**(1): 70–81.
11. Wing R, Jeffery R. Benefits of recruiting participants with friends and increasing social support for weight loss and maintenance. *Journal of Consulting and Clinical Psychology* 1999; **67**(1): 132.
12. Livhits M, Mercado C, Yermilov I, Parikh J, Dutson E, Mehran A, et al. Is social support associated with greater weight loss after bariatric surgery? A systematic review. *Obesity Reviews* 2011; **12**(2): 142–148.
13. Renjilian D, Perri M, Nezu A, Mckelvey W, Shermer R, Anton S. Individual versus group therapy for obesity: effects of matching participants to their treatment preferences. *Journal of Consulting and Clinical Psychology* 2001; **69**(4): 717.
14. Paul-Ebhohimhen V, Avenell A. A systematic review of the effectiveness of group versus individual treatments for adult obesity. *Obesity Facts* 2009; **2**(1): 17–24.
15. Tsai A, Wadden T. Systematic review: an evaluation of major commercial weight loss programs in the United States. *Annals of Internal Medicine* 2005; **142**(1): 56–66.
16. Heshka S, Anderson J, Atkinson R, Greenway F, Hill J, Phinney S, et al. Weight loss with self-help compared with a structured commercial program: a randomized trial. *JAMA* 2003; **289**(14): 1792–1798.
17. Allan K, Hoddinott P, Avenell A. A qualitative study comparing commercial and health service weight loss groups, classes and clubs. *Journal of Human Nutrition and Dietetics* 2011; **24**(1): 23–31.
18. Bye C, Avery A, Lavin J. Tackling obesity in men--preliminary evaluation of men-only groups within a commercial slimming organization. *Journal of Human Nutrition and Dietetics* 2005; **18**(5): 391–394.
19. Hunt K, Wyke S, Gray C, Anderson A, Brady A, Bunn C, et al. A gender-sensitised weight loss and healthy living programme for overweight and obese men delivered by Scottish Premier League football clubs (FFIT): a pragmatic randomised controlled trial. *Lancet* 2014; **383**(9924): 1211–1221.

Chapter 4.5

Commercial weight management organisations for weight loss in obesity

Amanda Avery
University of Nottingham, Nottingham, UK

Commercial weight management organisations (CWMOs) are well positioned to be able to support the large numbers of people who need weight management guidance.

In the UK, the National Institute for Health and Clinical Excellence (NICE) [1,2] and Scottish Intercollegiate Guidelines Network (2010) [3] recommended that CWMOs, alongside self-help and community weight management programmes, may be endorsed if they meet specific criteria (Box 4.5.1).

This chapter will critically examine the supporting published literature, including data on cost-effectiveness; briefly describe three examples of large commercial providers – Rosemary Conley (RC), Slimming World (SW) and Weight Watchers (WW); and then summarise the strengths, weaknesses, opportunities and threats of CWMOs that conform to the guidance (Box 4.5.2).

4.5.1 Evidence for effectiveness of CWMOs

Tod and Lacey (2004), in their qualitative survey, concluded that limited public resources mean that patients with obesity may not receive the support

---

Box 4.5.1 Essential criteria for CWMO programmes approved by NICE

- Provide a multicomponent programme, including dietary and physical activity support, employing behaviour change techniques.
- Focus on lifelong lifestyle change and the prevention of future weight gain – people need to be equipped with the necessary skills to develop lasting self-determined behaviour change.
- Developed by a multidisciplinary team to include registered dietitians, nutritionists, psychologists, behavioural scientists and experts in physical activity.
- Personnel involved in the delivery of the programme are appropriately trained and supported and receive regular professional development – training content to be based on current evidence and latest thinking in weight management.
- Last at least 3 months, offering at least fortnightly sessions, including a 'weigh-in'.
- Ensure achievable goals for weight loss are agreed on for different stages of the weight loss journey.
- Ensure specific dietary targets are agreed on, tailored to individual needs.
- Provide support on how to reduce sedentary behaviour and how to incorporate physical activities into everyday life.
- Employ a variety of behaviour change methods.
- Tailor programmes to support the needs of different population groups – for example, women, men, younger people, people from different cultural backgrounds and ethnic groups.
- Adopt a respectful, non-judgemental approach to overweight/obese individuals.

Box 4.5.2 A brief overview of the content of common CWMO programmes in the UK (programmes in other countries may vary)

Rosemary Conley (RC) is group-based; participants are able to join at any time. Meetings take place in community venues for 1.5 hours. There is one-to-one support during weighing and to establish an energy allowance. Additional support is available via email and telephone. Goals are staged: either 1–1.5 kg/week with goal of 1 stone loss, or 0.5–1 kg/week with 3.2 kg (7 lb) initial goal. Sessions include a 45-min optional exercise class. Extra exercise sessions may be offered for an additional fee. The theoretical background is based on role modelling and group support, and uses visualisation and reframing to support behaviour change. Predominant behaviour change strategies used include rewards for slimmers who lose or maintain weight; slimmer of the week; and certificates for the 3.2 and 6.35 kg milestones.

Slimming World (SW) is group-based; participants are able to join at any time. Meetings take place in community venues for a duration of 1.5 hours. Also included is access to website, magazines and one-to-one telephone support from the consultant or other members. Members are encouraged to mainly eat low-energy-dense foods to achieve satiety, plus some extras rich in calcium and fibre, with controlled amounts of high-energy-dense foods. Weight-loss goals are set by the individual. Physical activity is encouraged, with a gradual build up to 30 min of moderately intense activity 5 days a week. The theoretical background is based on transactional analysis and motivational interviewing. Predominant behaviour change strategies used included weekly weighing; group support; and group praise for weight loss, new decisions and continued commitment even in absence of weight loss. Awards for 3.2 kg (7 lb) lost and loss of 10% of body weight. Individual support if needed using self-monitoring of food and emotions, for and against evaluations, visualisation techniques and personal eating plans.

Weight Watchers (WW) is group-based; participants are able to join at any time. There is one-to-one support for new members and during weighing. This is followed by a group talk from the leader with discussions. Meetings take place in community venues for 1 hour. Core programme material delivered over 5 weeks included a food points system (based on age, sex, height, weight and activity), beating hunger, taking more physical activity, eating out and keeping motivated. Other sessions delivered to the whole group cover recipes, health and nutrition and keeping active. The plan aims for 500 kcal/day deficit, leading to 0.5–1 kg weight loss per week. Physical activity such as walking is encouraged, with the objective to gradually build up to 10,000 steps daily. Predominant behaviour change strategies used include stages of change, food and activity diaries, goal setting and evaluation of progress. Rewards are given for every 3.2 kg (7 lb) lost, and at 5% and 10% of body weight lost.

---

they require to move through the stages of change, improve their self-esteem and achieve successful weight loss [4]. The authors proposed that partnership working between the National Health Service and a CWMO may help to make more efficient use of public resources to maximise weight loss.

Lavin et al. (2006) first reported the feasibility and benefits of a referral programme from primary care to a CWMO with 107 patients recruited from the UK National Health Service (NHS) [5]. Of these patients, 85% attended a local slimming group, with 58% completing the full 12-week programme. A mean weight loss of 6.4% was reported, and significant improvements in mental well-being were also observed. Of the original population sample, 44% chose to self-fund further attendance at the CWMO

groups, and study follow-up continued until the end of the 12-week self-funding period. Of these patients, 72% completed the second 12-week self-funding period, achieving a mean weight loss of 11.3%.

A more recent evaluation of 34,271 adults referred into a CWMO primary care partnership scheme (SW) (Stubbs et al., 2011) [6] reported a mean BMI change of -1.5 kg/m^2, a mean percentage weight change of -4%, a rate of weight change of -0.3 kg/week and a mean attendance of 8.9 weekly sessions out of the 12 offered. For the 19,907 patients who attended at least 10 of the 12 sessions, the results were even better, with a mean BMI change of -2 kg/m^2, mean percentage weight change of -5.5% and rate of weight change of -0.4 kg/week. In addition, 35.8% of all patients enrolled and

54.7% of patients attending 10 or more sessions achieved >5% weight loss at 12 weeks. Weight gain was prevented in 92.1% of all patients. Weight loss was significantly greater ($P < 0.001$) in the 3651 men compared to the larger number of women (30,620).

Results from further work investigating referral over a 6-month period in a study population of 4754 suggest that, if patients are offered a second 12-week referral and continue to attend after the initial 12-week referral period, these weight losses persist [7]. Extending the evaluation period to 24 weeks resulted in a mean weight loss of 8.6% and a mean BMI change of −3.3 kg/m^2. In total, 74.5% of all patients offered the programme achieved at least a 5% weight loss, and weight gain was prevented in 96.3%.

A similar observational study of WW including 29,326 patients showed similar results [8]. Median weight change for all commenced referrals was −2.8 kg, equating to a 3.1% weight loss from baseline after the 12-week initial period. Median weight loss increased as the number of meetings attended increased. For the 11,851 participants who attended all 12 sessions, a median weight loss of 5.4 kg, representing a 5.6% median loss, was reported. Overall, 57% lost greater than 5% of their starting weight, and 12% lost greater than 10% of their starting weight.

A randomised control trial showed that, in all analyses, participants in the CWMO programme (WW) lost twice as much weight as those in the standard care group [9]. All of the study participants were referred through primary care practices in Germany, Australia or the UK ($n = 772$ overweight and obese). Participants randomised to the standard care group received healthcare advice from a primary care professional at their local general practitioner practice. Professionals delivering the standard care were encouraged to use the relevant national clinical guidelines for treatment and were directed to the available resources. Mean weight change at 12 months was −5.06 kg for those in the commercial programme, as compared to −2.25 kg for those receiving standard care. When outcomes were analysed conservatively, with a 'last observation carried forward' analysis the values were, −2.99 to −1.58 kg, respectively. Participants assigned to the

commercial programme had increased odds of losing >5% (OR = 3; CI = 2–4.4) and >10% (OR = 3.2; CI = 2–5.3) of initial body weight at 12 months than those assigned to standardised care. The greater weight loss in participants attending the commercial programme also resulted in larger reductions in both waist circumference and fat mass in all the analyses, and significant improvements in circulating insulin and total HDL cholesterol levels. Participants randomised to the commercial programme may have been advantaged, in that they were also able to access online support in addition to the weekly group meetings and attended a mean of three meetings per month (UK), as compared to one appointment per month with the healthcare provider. As with many other clinical obesity trials, the dropout rate was high, but more participants completed the commercial programme (61%) as compared to those completing the standard care programme (54%). The numbers of men recruited to the study were low – 12% referred to the commercial programme and 14% to standard care, but these figures are very consistent with similar referral data reported [5,6].

Lighten Up is a randomised control trial conducted in the UK that involved the comparison of a range of commercial and NHS weight reduction programmes with a control group, where patients were provided with 12 vouchers enabling free access to a local leisure centre [10]. All programmes resulted in a significant weight loss at 12 weeks, with the commercial options resulting in a significantly greater weight loss than the primary-care-led options (mean difference 2.3 kg). The NHS dietetic-led programme and the commercial options all led to significant weight loss at 1 year, but not the general practice and pharmacy provision when compared to the control group. The authors suggest that, because the primary care programmes were the more costly to provide, commercially provided weight management services are more cost-effective. A further non-inferiority analysis has been reported by the Lighten Up study group with a larger population sample, but just comparing weight loss outcomes at 12 months for those people referred to either the NHS group-based programme, RC or SW, and comparing outcomes with those achieved by people selecting to go to WW [11]. Follow-up rates at 3 months were 74.5% for NHS, 69.9% for RC, 81.4% for SW and 77.6% for WW, and, at 12 months, 80.2%, 60.7%, 71.8% and 63.1%, respectively. As in the earlier Lighten Up study, the NHS group programme was inferior to WW in terms of weight loss at 12 months. At the 12-month follow-up, the weight losses for both SW and RC were similar to those achieved by people attending WW, with the losses being slightly greater for the SW programme (4.5 vs. 3.7 kg).

The Diet Trials study, a randomised, controlled trial comparing WW, RC, as well as Atkins and Slimfast, concluded that clinically useful weight and fat loss can be achieved in adults who are motivated to follow CWMO for 6 months [12]. Loss of body fat and weight was significantly greater in all groups, compared with the control group. Furthermore, the follow-up data at 12 months suggested that participants had made considerable changes to their dieting and activity behaviours, but more participants in the unsupported programmes had withdrawn compared to those in the WW and RC group programmes ($P = 0.04$). The weight rebound after the 6-month intervention period was also higher in the unsupported programmes, although all diets resulted in a clinically useful (~10%) weight loss at 12 months for those participants who had continued with the weight management programme allocated. More participants from the control group who decided to make changes to their diet and lifestyle after the 6-month test period went on to choose group-based support, achieving a mean weight loss of 6.4 kg in 12 months [12].

For all programmes achieving successful weight loss over a short time period, there are concerns that the weight lost is easily regained [13]. However, most of the data on weight regain was from research conducted within either university or hospital environments, and hence the study populations are not representative of a typical overweight/obese population using CWMO [14]. From a sample of 1002 target members at 5 years after achieving their target weight, 19.4% were still within 5 lb of this weight, 18.8% maintained a loss of >10%, 42.6% maintained a loss of >5% and 70.3% were still below their initial weight.

Heshka et al. (2003) reported greater weight loss in a population who received support through

CWMO groups than a clinically matched group who received two 20-min counselling sessions with a dietitian plus supporting self-help materials [15]. The 423 overweight/obese people were randomly assigned to one of the two interventions, and weight loss compared over a 2-year period. While the self-help group lost a mean of 1.4 kg in 1 year, there was a return to baseline weight observed at 2 years. In contrast, the CWMO group lost 5 kg in 1 year, and the mean weight loss was still 2.8 kg lower than baseline at 2 years. Those participants who attended 78% or more (70% overall completion rate vs. 75% for the self-help group) of the CWMO weekly sessions maintained a mean weight loss of 5 kg at the end of the 2-year study period. Waist circumference was also reduced in the commercial group by 4.5 cm at 1 year and 2.5 cm at 2 years.

Weight loss maintenance is particularly important in any obesity strategy. Many CWMOs have strategies in place, including free membership, to incentivise weight loss maintenance for those members achieving their personal target weights.

To evaluate the benefits of setting up men-only CMWO groups, Bye et al. (2005) analysed data collected from seven men-only SW groups ($n = 67$) [16]. Mean weight loss at 12 weeks was 9.2% (range 0.2–21.1%). At least 5% weight loss had been achieved by 90% of the sample since joining. In those who had been members for 24 weeks, the mean weight loss was 11.4% (range 5–17.9%), and 69% achieved a 10% weight loss. The remaining 31% had all achieved at least a 5% weight loss. At the point of data collection, mean BMI had decreased from 35.9 to 32.5 kg/m^2. Barraj et al. (2014) presented men's data from a pooled analysis of weight loss and the related physiological parameter data from two randomised clinical trials [17]. After 12 months, analysis of covariance tests showed that men in the CWMO group ($n = 85$) lost significantly more weight ($P < 0.01$) than men in the control group ($n = 84$); similar significant differences were observed for body mass index and waist circumference. These results suggest that participation in a commercial weight loss programme may be an effective means for men to lose weight and maintain weight loss, but there needs to be greater insight into the barriers to men attending CWMO group sessions and how engagement can be improved.

Women can find it difficult to lose excess weight gained during pregnancy [18]. With repeated pregnancies, maternal weight can often increase progressively. A survey of members attending SW up to 2 years postnatally was hosted on the members' website for 2 weeks. Of the respondents, 42.5% (*n* = 590) said that they had reached their pre-pregnancy weight, and 41.5% said that they were lighter than before becoming pregnant. Of the respondents who were members for >6 months (*n* = 152), 56.5% had reached their pre-pregnancy weight and 55.3% were lighter than before becoming pregnant [19].

It is also suggested that CWMOs may have a positive influence on the diet and physical activity behaviours of both members and their families. Of the SW group members who were responsible for providing food for a family (*n* = 709), 63% said that they had changed their eating habits and were eating more healthily [20]. Among the study population who had become more active (*n* = 718), 33% included their partners and 28% included their children in their physical activity sessions. It is difficult to cost these wider benefits.

A qualitative study comparing commercial and health service weight loss groups suggests that health service leaders had less opportunity for supervision, peer support or specific training in how to run a group when compared to group facilitators from the commercial sector [21].

Self-esteem and mental well-being are important outcome measures of any weight management programme. To sustain behaviour change, such as adopting healthier eating habits and increasing physical activity levels, self-esteem needs to be enhanced. Mental well-being was reported in the referral feasibility study [5]. Compared to a representative sample, obese patients had a lower level of 'well-being' before enrolment (assessed using a validated questionnaire). Improvements in all aspects measured (feeling calm and peaceful, having a lot of energy, feeling downhearted and low) were seen in those attending a CWMO at both 12 weeks (*P* = 0.001, 0.001, 0.015, respectively) and 24 weeks (*P* = 0.02, 0.001, 0.001). The emphasis of the training received by the lay people facilitating CWMO groups is very much on developing behaviour change techniques and using a compassionate approach to promote self-worth.

A qualitative study comparing CWMO and health service weight loss groups suggests that health service leaders had less opportunity for supervision, peer support, or specific training in how to run a group when compared to group facilitators from the commercial sector [21].

Commercial programmes use many of the techniques that are used in more intensive behavioural treatments, delivered by healthcare professionals, such as self-monitoring, goal setting, problem-solving, stimulus control and relapse prevention [9]. In a survey examining self-reported behaviour changes associated with weight loss and maintenance in a group of 292 longer-term SW members, primary factors reported by participants as important in achieving their weight loss included not going hungry by satisfying appetite with low-energy-density food eaten *ad libitum*, following a flexible diet, peer-group support and having tools to cope with small lapses. A range of eating and activity behaviours was associated with weight loss maintenance, and the paper concluded that it was important to offer consumers flexible solutions that they can adapt to their individual lifestyle needs to support long-term weight control [22].

In the modern healthcare system, and given the scale of the obesity epidemic, finding cost-effective solutions to obesity is of paramount importance. Trueman and Flack used an economic model to determine the cost-effectiveness of WW groups in the prevention and management of obesity [23]. In the base case analysis, the incremental cost per quality-adjusted life year (QALY) gained compared to no treatment was £1022. This compares favourably with other interventions – for example, the incremental cost of other non-pharmacological interventions was reported to range from £174 to £9971 per QALY, with anti-obesity medication costing £3200–£24,431 per QALY and surgery costing £6289–£8527 per QALY [1].

More recently, the cost-effectiveness of primary care referral to SW has been reported [24]. At 12 months, the incremental cost-effectiveness ratio was £6906, indicating that referral was cost-effective. Over a lifetime, referral to the CWMO was dominant, as it led to a cost saving of £924 and an incremental benefit of 0.22 QALY over usual care, defined as information provision but with no active component.

Box 4.5.3 Strengths, weaknesses, opportunities and threats of CWMOs in the management of weight loss and obesity

Strengths of CWMOs
- Well-established infrastructures focussing solely on weight management.
- Input from advisory panels that consist of a range of experts, including psychologists and physical activity advisers, to support company dietitians and nutritionists.
- Comprehensive electronic databases allow the monitoring and reporting of attendance and weight change data.
- Already large capacity, but with the scope to expand further.
- Weekly group support, with in-between support offered in different forms, such as through mobile applications, appealing recipe ideas, cookbooks, online access and magazines, as required, and usually at no additional cost.
- Use of local community venues with a range of meeting times made available to ensure equal access opportunities.
- The groups are often run by locally recruited people who themselves had been overweight and have lost weight through group support.
- A range of motivational and behavioural modification tools are available to support members to make lifestyle changes, including an increase in physical activity.
- Able to support people with a range of starting BMIs.
- Members of the group are able to access on-going support for as long as they feel the need, rather than the support being made available for a set number of weeks.
- Well-established subsidised referral partnership schemes available to help reduce health inequalities
- Cost-effectiveness has been demonstrated.

Weaknesses of CWMOs
- Limited knowledge of how they support people from different ethnic minority groups.
- Predominantly attended by females – at least 90% of the self-referred membership will be female.
- The weekly group fee may be expensive for people with low incomes
- A group approach may not be the first choice of support for everyone.
- Not all members will be able to stay for the whole group session, and they will thus not benefit from the behavioural group support.
- There may be some variability in the group facilitation skills of the person leading the group, although quality checks are in place.

Opportunities for CWMOs
- To take a family approach to weight management to help support more men and adolescents.
- To work with local authorities to offer the opportunity for people from local ethnic minority groups to become trained and be able to lead the groups.
- To continue to forge partnerships with healthcare professionals to ensure that all members with associated chronic conditions are appropriately supported – for example, overweight members with diabetes.
- To continue to forge partnerships with physical activity specialists, and thus encourage more overweight and obese people to become more physically active.
- To further increase capacity by looking at geographical locations where there is limited access.
- To ensure an even greater involvement from local communities by using a whole-systems approach to weight management.
- To provide support in the workplace setting, including working with catering teams.
- To continue to develop appropriate behavioural therapy techniques that are best suited for motivating overweight or obese people.
- To continue to publish scientific literature that explores efficacy – particularly long-term data. Also, to include outcome measures other than just weight change.

Threats to CWMOs
- The very fact that CWMOs need to be financially viable means there may be cynicism from some health professionals that they make money out of overweight people.
- Some healthcare professionals may view CWMOs as a direct threat to services that they would wish to deliver.
- Evidence produced by CWMOs may never be perceived as being as robust as that presented by academic institutes, irrespective of the rigor involved in the data analysis.
- In the past, 'fad diets' have been inappropriately associated with CWMOs, giving them an unfounded poor reputation.

Threshold analyses suggested that a weight loss of 1.25 kg was sufficient to make 12 weeks of the commercial programme cost-effective at 12 months. Subgroup analyses showed that the programme is even more cost-effective for men [24].

In many areas, be they public-, private- or voluntary-sector weight management providers may be commissioned to provide individual or group lifestyle weight management services. People can also self-refer to voluntary or commercial lifestyle weight management programmes. Local policies vary, but funded referrals to a lifestyle weight management programme (in tier 2 services/usually in the community) generally lasts for around 12 weeks or 12 sessions.

In 2013, approximately 69,000 adults in the UK were referred to WW and SW under NHS referral schemes. According to evaluation data, 71% of adults who attended a weight management programme opted for a CWMO or not-for-profit programme [10]. Inflating the figure of 69,000 to account for the 29% of people who attended other types of weight management programmes gives a total of approximately 97,000 adults in the UK. This is equivalent to around 0.3% of overweight or obese adults, or 170 adults per 100,000 population. Going forward, NICE, in their costing model, have assumed that the proportion of overweight or obese adults attending lifestyle weight management programmes each year will increase by 1% [25]. This would represent a quadrupling of existing levels of uptake for these programmes. The 1% increase equates to approximately 680 overweight or obese adults per 100,000 population. The potential cost impact for this proposed model, recognising the role of CWMOs as a commissioned service, is illustrated in the recent work by NICE [25], examining the potential costs over time, per 100,000 population, for referral to commissioned lifestyle weight management programmes [25].

The strengths, weaknesses, opportunities and threats of CWMOs in the management of weight loss and obesity are summarised in Box 4.5.3.

4.5.2 Conclusion

Over the recent years, there has been an increase in published scientific literature supporting the role of CWMOs in tackling overweight and obesity.

Clearly, this needs to continue – particularly with an emphasis on the reporting of long-term weight changes, and also the extended role of CWMOs in a whole-systems approach as a community provider of services. The experience and wealth of knowledge of these organisations should not be overlooked.

4.5.3 Summary box

Key points

- CWMOs have well-established infrastructures, focussing solely on weight management, with large capacities to support the overweight and obese population.
- CWMOs which meet current NICE criteria for community weight management programmes can be endorsed. This allows commissioning to provide local tier 2 weight management through subsidised referral packages.
- The efficacy of CWMOs has been considered through a number of different study designs, with 12-month outcome data reported for large sample sizes.
- The published RCTs suggest that the weight loss outcomes achieved through CWMO support is approximately twice that of the control arm, with lower attrition rates generally observed.
- More research is required that considers how CWMOs support different population groups – for example, people of different ethnic origins, people with learning disabilities, people with diabetes and those with other chronic diseases.

References

1. National Institute for Health and Care Excellence (NICE). CG43, Obesity: guidance on the prevention, identification, assessment and management of overweight and obesity in adults and children, 2006, London.
2. National Institute for Health and Care Excellence (NICE). PH53 Obesity: managing overweight and obesity in adults – lifestyle weight management services, 2014a, London.
3. Scottish Intercollegiate Guidelines Network (SIGN). Guideline 115: management of obesity, 2010, Edinburgh.
4. Tod AM, Lacey A. Overweight and obesity: helping clients to take action. *British Journal of Community Nursing* 2004; **9**: 59–66.
5. Lavin JH, Avery A, Whitehead SM, Rees E, Parsons J, Bagnall T, et al. Feasibility and benefits of implementing a slimming on referral service in primary care using a commercial weight management partner. *Public Health* 2006; **120**: 872–881.

6. Stubbs RJ, Pallister C, Whybrow S, Avery A, Lavin JH. Weight outcomes audit for 34,271 adults referred to a primary care/commercial weight management partnership scheme. *Obesity Facts* 2011; **4**: 113–120.

7. Stubbs RJ, Brogelli DJ, Pallister CJ, Whybrow S, Avery AJ, Lavin JH. Attendance and weight outcomes in 4,754 adults referred over 6 months to a primary care/commercial weight management partnership scheme. *Clinical Obesity* 2012; **2**: 6–14.

8. Ahern A, Olson A, Aston L, Jebb S. Weight Watchers on prescription: an observational study of weight change among adults referred to Weight Watchers by the NHS. *BMC Public Health* 2011; **11**: 434.

9. Jebb SA, Ahern AL, Olson AD, Aston LM, Holzapfel C, Stoll J, et al. Primary care referral to a commercial provider for weight loss treatment versus standard care: a randomised controlled trial. *Lancet* 2001; **378**: 1485–1492.

10. Jolly K, Lewis A, Beach J, Denley J, Adab P, Deeks JJ, et al. Comparison of a range of commercial or primary care led weight reduction programmes with minimal intervention control for weight loss in obesity: lighten up randomised controlled trial. *BMJ* 2011; **343**: d6500.

11. Madigan C, Daley A, Lewis A, Jolly K, Aveyard P. Which weight-loss programmes are as effective as Weight Watchers? Non-inferiority analysis. *British Journal of General Practice* 2014; **64**: e128–e136.

12. Truby H, Baic S, Delooy A, Fox KR, Livingstone MBE, Logan CM, et al. Randomised controlled trial of four commercial weight loss programmes in the UK: initial findings from the BBC 'diet trials'. *BMJ* 2006; **332**: 1309–1314.

13. Wing RR, Phelan S. Long-term weight loss maintenance. *American Journal of Clinical Nutrition* 2005; **82**: 222–225S.

14. Lowe MR, Miller-Kovach K, Phelan S. Weight-loss maintenance in overweight individuals one to five years following successful completion of a commercial weight loss program. *International Journal of Obesity and Related Metabolic Disorders* 2001; **25**: 325–331.

15. Heshka S, Anderson JW, Atkinson RL, Greenway FL, Hill JO, Phinney SD, et al. Weight loss with self-help compared with a structured commercial program: a randomized trial. *JAMA* 2003; **289**: 1792–1798.

16. Bye C, Avery A, Lavin JH. Tackling obesity in men: a preliminary evaluation of men only groups within a commercial slimming organisation. *Journal of Human Nutrition and Dietetics* 2005; **18**: 391–394.

17. Barraj LM, Murphy MM, Heshka S, Katz DL. Greater weight loss among men participating in a commercial weight loss program: a pooled analysis of 2 randomised controlled trials. *Nutrition Research* 2014; **34**: 174–177.

18. Linné Y, Dye L, Barkeling B, Rössner S. Long-term weight development in women: a 15-year follow-up of the effects of pregnancy. *Obesity Research* 2004; **12**: 1166–1178.

19. Avery A, Allan J, Lavin JH, Pallister C. Supporting post-natal women to lose weight. *Journal of Human Nutrition and Dietetics* 2010; **23**: 439.

20. Pallister C, Avery A, Stubbs RJ, Lavin JH. Influence of Slimming World's lifestyle programme on diet, activity behaviour and health of participants and their families. *Journal of Human Nutrition and Dietetics* 2009; **24**: 351–358.

21. Allan K, Hoddinott P, Avenell A. A qualitative study comparing commercial and health service weight loss groups, classes and clubs. *Journal of Human Nutrition and Dietetics* 2011; **24**: 23–31.

22. Stubbs RJ, Brogelli D, Pallister C, Avery A, McConnon A, Lavin JH. Behavioural and motivational factors associated with weight loss and maintenance in a commercial weight management programme. *The Open Obesity Journal* 2012; **4**: 35–43.

23. Trueman P, Flack S. Economic evaluation of Weight Watchers in the prevention and management of obesity. Poster presentation at the Conference of the National Institute of Health and Clinical Excellence, December 2006.

24. Meads DM, Hulme CT, Hall P, Hill AJ. The cost-effectiveness of primary care referral to a UK commercial weight loss programme. *Clinical Obesity* 2014; **4**: 324–332.

25. National Institute for Health and Care Excellence (NICE). Costing report: managing overweight and obesity in adult's lifestyle weight management services; Implementing the NICE guidance on overweight and obese adults: lifestyle weight management (PH53) costing report, 2014b, London. Available from: https://www.nice.org.uk/guidance/ph53/resources/costing-report-69241357, accessed November 2016, figure 1, page 5.

Chapter 4.6

Fad diets and fasting for weight loss in obesity

Katherine Hart
University of Surrey, Guildford, UK

4.6.1 Introduction

A 'fad' is defined as 'something that is embraced very enthusiastically for a short time, especially by many people'. While there is no definitive meaning of the term 'fad diet' this, for health professionals at least, may have negative connotations of crazes and celebrity-endorsed regimes lacking in a sound evidence base. Labelling a particular diet as a 'fad' may be socially, culturally and time dependent, and, even for a given individual at a given time, the term 'fad diet' may still encompass a very heterogeneous group of practices.

Therefore, for the purposes of this chapter, the term 'fad diet' will be taken to mean any dietary regime promoted for weight loss that does not form part of standard dietetic-led weight management advice, and is not covered elsewhere in this section concerning approaches for weight management in adults. Fad approaches will be cited but, given the diversity and ever-changing nature of this classification, the focus will be primarily on general, rather than regime-specific, issues.

Fasting could be classified as the oldest 'fad diet'; however, while fasting shares many common issues, fasts, specifically alternate-day fasts (ADF) and intermittent fasting (IF), will be discussed separately in recognition of the greater historical body of evidence relating to fasting, starvation and semi-starvation practices.

While it is easy to dismiss fads, it is essential that health professionals understand the regimes that their patients may be exposed and attracted to, and

appreciate their motivation for following them, to effectively communicate risk and benefit.

4.6.2 Popularity of fad diets

Regardless of their evidence base, or lack of it, fad diets remain extremely prevalent and popular in the field of weight management. Over 1500 diet books are published each year, and data suggests that consumers are willing to pay for the 'rapid weight loss with minimal effort' promoted by many fads – an industry worth US$35 billion per year in the USA alone [1]. In Australia, 78% of obese adults searched online for information about obesity and weight loss, exposing them to the wealth of fads available [2], while 14–15% of Americans report having used short-term fasting or supplements to facilitate weight loss [3,4]. Many fad diets also avoid the face-to-face contact that overweight or obese people may find intimidating, yet provide extensive support and encouragement via online forums, further encouraging their uptake.

4.6.3 Classification of fad diets

While a definitive list of fad diets is not possible or particularly useful, given the ever-changing market, Table 4.6.1 lists some of the common categories of fad diets promoted as tools for weight loss.

Advanced Nutrition and Dietetics in Obesity, First Edition. Edited by Catherine Hankey.
© 2018 John Wiley & Sons Ltd. Published 2018 by John Wiley & Sons Ltd.

Table 4.6.1 Types of 'fad' regimes or supplements promoted for weight loss

Classification	Example
Herbal or other supplements	Synephrine (bitter orange)
Physical/physiological testing	Hair mineral analysis
	Kinesiology
	Face/tongue reading
	Blood group analysis
Very-low calorie diets	Cabbage soup diet
	Baby food diet
Fasting	Alternate-day fasting (ADF)
	Alternate-day modified fasting (ADMF)
	Intermittent fasting (IF) (e.g. 5:2 diet)
	Time-restricted feeding (TRF)

Table 4.6.2 'Red flags' to identify unhealthy weight loss regimes

- Promise of rapid weight loss (>0.5–1 kg/week, 1–2 lb/week)
- Restricts large number of foods and/or whole food groups
- Recommends consumption of large amounts of one food or food type
- Suggests foods should be eaten in a specific order or specific combinations
- Suggests that certain foods or ingredients 'burn' fat
- Is nutritionally imbalanced
- Does not include or encourage exercise
- Based on anecdotal evidence and/or testimonials rather than robust clinical trials and/or simplistic conclusions drawn from complex studies
- Makes dramatic claims not supported by evidence or seem 'too good to be true'
- Requires purchase of specific products, supplements or resources
- Provides no health warning to those with pre-existing medical conditions
- Focus on appearance-related outcomes rather than health benefits

Adapted from [5], [14] and [21].

There are many different forms of fasting diets. ADF involves alternate feed and fast days, whereas ADMF involves alternate feed followed by partial fast days (usually 25–50% energy requirements); IF involves as little as one fast day per week (e.g. the 5:2 diet), whereas TRF allows *ad libitum* dietary intake within a controlled time frame each day (e.g. 3–12-hour range).

While not all fad diets are inherently detrimental to health, there are certain 'red flags' that can help in identifying those regimes and practices that are less likely to promote successful or sustainable weight loss, or are unlikely to support overall health (Table 4.6.2).

4.6.4 Mechanism of action

Short-term weight loss is certainly achievable with many fad diets, but, contrary to the claims often associated with these regimes, this is unlikely to be due to any specific ingredient or component [5]. Despite the various 'phenotypes' of these diets (Table 4.6.1), the vast majority facilitate weight loss via a simple reduction in food and therefore energy intake, often due to decreased total or refined carbohydrate intake.

Fasting is an extreme but simple example of reduced intake whereby all food, and therefore all nutrients, are severely restricted. This usually results in rapid weight loss, but this is characterised by large losses of water, glycogen and muscle, and as such may be associated with greater side-effects and greater regain once a normal diet is resumed than when predominantly fat is lost.

There is, however, evidence that fasting may have longer-term benefits independent of weight loss *per se*. Energy restriction has been shown to exert a nutrigenomic effect via the activation of a 'skinny gene',

SirT1, whose potential effects include increasing insulin sensitivity and the efficiency of fat oxidation while inhibiting fat storage and inflammation [6,7].

The ability of energy restriction, via various fasting protocols, to facilitate acute negative energy balance and/or to activate adaptive stress response pathways have been proposed as the potential mechanisms underlying the metabolic improvements seen [8].

4.6.5 Advantages of fad diets

Fad diets may have a number of perceived advantages over traditional approaches to weight management. These include the novelty value of a 'new' diet, which may counter 'diet fatigue' and promote greater compliance. Fad diets can offer a choice of weight loss strategies in recognition that 'one size does not fit all' [9], and are frequently accompanied by an active and supportive online community.

In addition, fasting has numerous perceived advantages above those of general fad diets. For example, fasting may be perceived to offer a 'quick fix' to achieve substantial weight loss in a short duration (up to 5% in 6 days or 8% in 8–12 weeks) [8,10,4]. Intermittent fasting may promote greater adherence with an 'on–off' approach to eating, which is potentially more preferable and achievable [11] than standard dietary regimes that require daily dietary restrictions [12]. Fasting may also preserve a greater proportion of lean body mass during weight loss (10% FFM:90% FM) in comparison to continuous energy restriction (25% FFM:75% FM) [13]. There may also be additional benefits for chronic disease risk, similar to those associated with long-term energy restriction (Figure 4.6.1), although these effects may be partially or fully explained by the weight loss achieved, rather than being independent effects of the regime itself. Finally, they may equip users with a successful long-term weight management strategy via repeated ADF episodes, leading to greater maintenance of weight loss (compared to a low-calorie or very-low-calorie diet) at 3 months and 1 year [4].

4.6.6 Disadvantages of fad diets

Despite these advantages, there are considerable disadvantages to the use of fad diets. Fad diets encourage the notion of a 'diet' as a short-term behaviour rather than a sustainable lifelong change. Regular dieting itself is associated with weight gain [14], possibly due to the adoption of negative behaviours such as binge eating, skipping breakfast and not exercising [15]. Persistent dieting attempts may be associated with weight cycling, itself associated with a number of physiological effects, including the suppression of natural killer cells necessary for immune response [16] and potential increased risk of hypertension, hypercholesterolaemia and gall bladder disease [17]. Fad diets fail to re-educate consumers about healthy eating and portion control as they often focus on 'unlimited' eating and/or very restrictive eating. They fail to address the causes of poor eating behaviour and, therefore, are unlikely to help change underlying behaviours.

Fad diets rarely focus attention on energy expenditure (e.g. by promoting increased activity). They can be expensive and time consuming, and therefore may be inaccessible to a large proportion of the population who would benefit most from weight loss. Some fad diets can be difficult to sustain due to boredom, monotony, cost and unsociable eating practices, and consumers may blame themselves if they are unable to conform to the unrealistic expectations of the fad diet, with a subsequent reduction in self-esteem and body image [2]. Many fad diets are nutritionally imbalanced, with lower diet quality scores, particularly where the focus is on macronutrient composition rather than micronutrient intakes [18,19].

Low-carbohydrate regimes (see Chapter 4.1) may result in fatigue, irritability and impaired athletic performance due to depletion of glycogen reserves. The resulting ketosis may manifest itself as bad breath, and there may also be significant fluid losses, and therefore dehydration, itself a risk factor for impaired oral health (e.g. xerostomia).

Those who follow fad diets that include supplement use should be cautioned. Supplements are largely unregulated, and, while some ingredients such as ephedra are now banned, their chemical alternatives are easily available online. No independent health check is required to purchase weight loss supplements online, despite a number of potential vascular, hepatic and cardiac-related contraindications.

In terms of fasting regimes, these require drastic changes to eating patterns to reduce energy intake sufficiently, and support may therefore be essential for success in the free-living environment (as compared to clinical trials). Many fasting regimes result

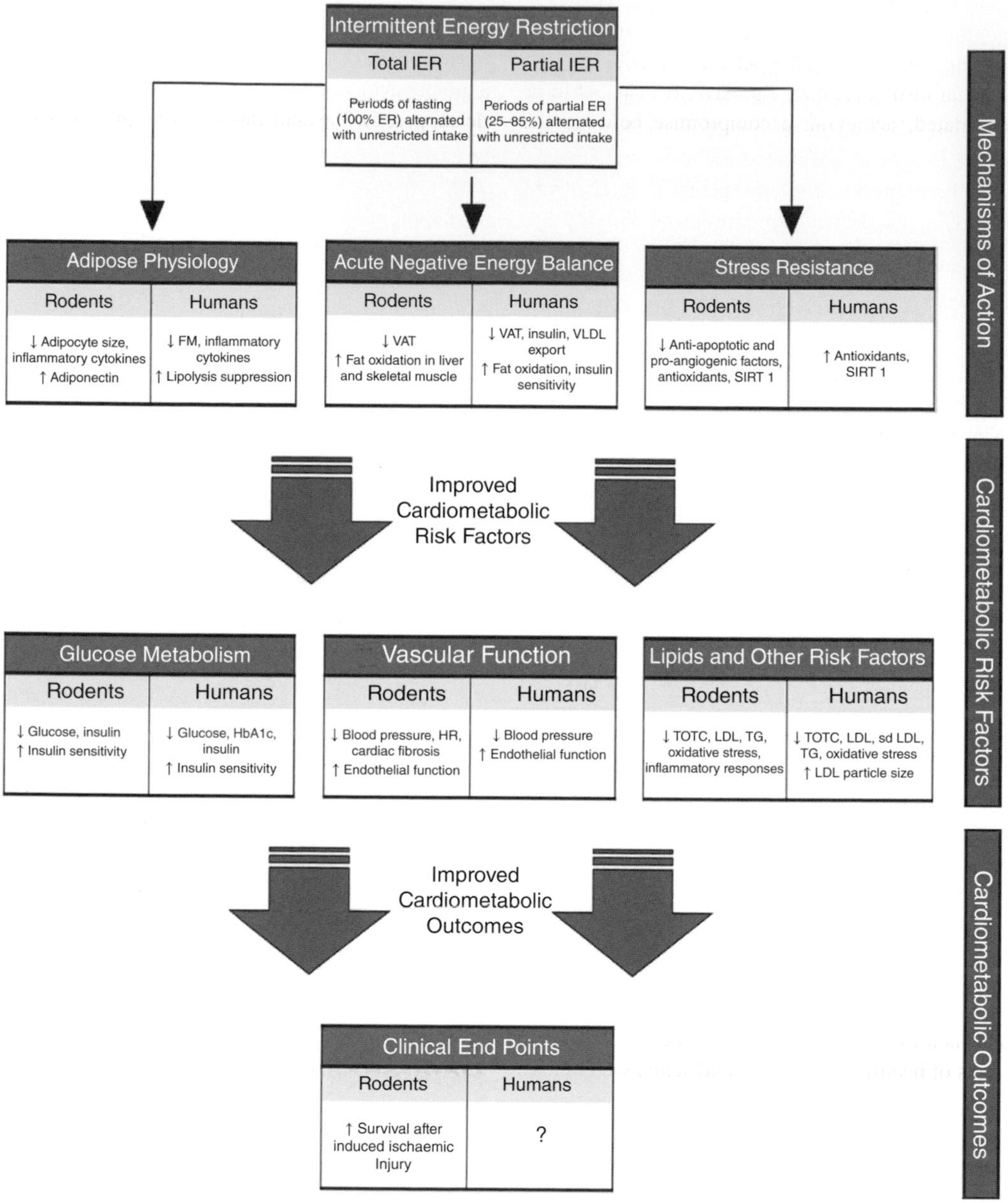

Figure 4.6.1 Intermittent energy restriction: mechanisms of its action, effects upon cardiometabolic risk factors and clinical endpoints reported by animal and human IER studies to date. Taken from [8].

in hyperphagia on 'feed' days and/or elevated hunger or motivation to eat, although the evidence is inconclusive. Low fullness ratings during ADF may compromise long-term adherence [12].

Fasting cannot be used as a widespread public health strategy due to the potential medical issues, and because it is as yet unclear which strategies and/or characteristics are required to convert short-term weight loss success into long-term weight loss and maintenance. This is complicated as outcomes are variable between individuals. The optimal fasting regime (e.g. ADF, IF) has yet to be elucidated, achieving a compromise between the advantages for adherence of allowing some intake on fast days and the disadvantages in terms of slower weight and fat loss. For this, more well-controlled human trials are required [8]. Adherence may be correlated with fatigue – that is, the stricter/longer the fast and more rapid the weight loss, the greater the reported fatigue and, subsequently, the lower the energy expenditure [4].

Fasting will inevitably affect intakes of vital nutrients if not managed very carefully, and will likely require micronutrient supplementation to compensate. Fibre intakes may be inadequate, particularly where energy restriction is achieved via the use of liquid diets. Finally, there is a lack of longer-term studies (>8 weeks) to investigate changes in the eating practices of fasters over time. Anecdotal evidence suggests that the level of restriction on fast days may diminish over time, but may be counteracted by a simultaneous reduction in intake on feed days. Excessive limitation in the variety of foods consumed on 'fast' days [20], in addition to their quantity, may be linked to lower sustainability [8].

4.6.7 Conclusion

The term 'fad diets' encompasses an extremely heterogeneous group of weight loss practices varying considerably in their approach and evidence base, and therefore also in their subsequent outcomes in terms of health risk, benefits and actual weight loss. At best, these regimes may offer a novel and engaging means of energy reduction, often accompanied by an active and supportive online community. However, at worst, they may be nutritionally imbalanced, medically unsuitable, unsustainable and unable to effectively re-educate consumers about behaviour change, portion control, healthy eating and physical activity.

It is essential that health professionals in the field of weight management maintain a working knowledge of current trends and fads in order to have effective discussions with their clients and equip them to

make informed choices. Although the detail of their dietary regimes may be equally susceptible to trends, fasting is one of the longer-standing 'fads' for which a greater evidence base does exist. While there is little support for the application of true fasts or starvation practices, alternate or intermittent fasting has become increasingly popular, and may confer psychological and physiological benefits compared to the more conventional chronic energy restriction. However, the evidence base is by no means complete, focussing heavily on animal models. Also, fasting should not be portrayed as an 'easy option'.

In conclusion, contrary to the claims associated with most fad diets and fasting regimes, it is clear that, unfortunately, a 'no effort, quick fix' does not exist for those in pursuit of sustainable healthy weight loss and management.

4.6.8 Summary box

Key points

- There is no single definition for 'fad diets', making these a very varied group of approaches with subsequently varied outcomes, advantages and disadvantages.
- In general, 'fads' may lack a 'whole diet' and 'whole lifestyle' approach to weight loss.
- Fasting regimes that incorporate varying periods and levels of energy restriction have the potential to confer physiological, metabolic and psychological benefits for weight loss and maintenance.

References

1. Cleland RL, Gross WC, Koss LD, Daynard M, Muoio KM. Weight-loss advertising: an analysis of current trends, Washington, D.C. Federal Trade Commission, 2002. Available from: https://www.ftc.gov/reports/weight-loss-advertisingan-analysis-current-trends, accessed 16 August 2016.
2. Lewis S, Thomas SL, Blood RW, Castle D, Hyde J, Komesaroff PA. 'I'm searching for solutions': why are obese individuals turning to the Internet for help and support with 'being fat'? *Health Expectations* 2011; **14**(4): 339–350.
3. Blanck HM, Serdula MK, Gillespie C, Galuska DA, Sharpe PA, Conway JM, et al. Use of nonprescription dietary supplements for weight loss is common among Americans. *Journal of the American Dietetic Association* 2007; **107**(3): 441–447.

4. Johnstone AM. Fasting: the ultimate diet? *Obesity Reviews* 2006; **8**: 211–212.
5. Daniels J. Fad diets: slim on good nutrition. *Nursing* 2004; **34**(12): 22–23.
6. Gillum MP, Erion DM, Shulman GI. Sirtuin-1 regulation of mammalian metabolism. *Trends in Molecular Medicine* 2011; **17**(1): 8–13.
7. Fulco M, Sartorelli V. Comparing and contrasting the roles of AMPK and SIRT1 in metabolic tissues. *Cell Cycle* 2008; **7**(23): 3669–3679.
8. Antoni R, Johnston KL, Collins A, Robertson MD. The effects of intermittent energy restriction on indices of cardiometabolic health. *Research in Endocrinology* 2014. doi: 10.5171/2014.459119.
9. Herriot AM, Thomas DE, Hart KH, Warren J, Truby H. A qualitative investigation of individuals' experiences and expectations before and after completing a trial of commercial weight loss programmes. *Journal of Human Nutrition and Dietetics* 2008; **21**: 72–80.
10. Johnson JB, Summer W, Cutler RG, Martin B, Hyun DH, Dixit VD, et al. Alternate day calorie restriction improves clinical findings and reduces markers of oxidative stress and inflammation in overweight adults with moderate asthma. *Free Radical Biology & Medicine* 2007; **42**(5): 665–674.
11. Collier R. Intermittent fasting: the next big weight loss fad. *CMAJ* 2013; **185**(8): E321–E322.
12. Klempel MC, Bhutani S, Fitzgibbon M, Freels S, Varady KA. Dietary and physical activity adaptations to alternate day modified fasting: implications for optimal weight loss. *Nutrition Journal* 2010; **9**: 35.
13. Varady KA. Intermittent versus daily calorie restriction: which diet regimen is more effective for weight loss? *Obesity Reviews* 2011; **12**: e593–e601.
14. British Dietetic Association. Fad diets, 2006. Available online at: https://www.bda.uk.com/foodfacts/faddiets.pdf, accessed 16 August 2016.
15. Neumark-Sztainer D, Wall M, Haines J, Story M, Eisenberg ME. Why does dieting predict weight gain in adolescents? Findings from project EAT-II: a 5-year longitudinal study. *Journal of the American Dietetic Association* 2007; **107**: 448–455.
16. Shade ED, Ulrich CM, Wener MH, Wood B, Yasui Y, Lacroix KA, et al. Frequent intentional weight loss is associated with lower natural killer cell cytotoxicity in postmenopausal women: possible long-term immune effects. *Journal of the American Dietetic Association* 2004; **104**: 903–912.
17. Goldfarb DS, Coe FL. Prevention of recurrent nephrolithiasis. *American Family Physician* 1999; **60**: 2269–2276.
18. Gardner CD, Kim S, Bersamin A, Dopler-Nelson M, Otten J, Oelrich B, Micronutrient, et al. Quality of weight-loss diets that focus on macronutrients: results from the A TO Z study. *American Journal of Clinical Nutrition* 2010; **92**: 304–312.
19. Yunsheng MA, Pagoto SL, Griffith JA, Merriam PA, Ockene IS, Hafner AR, et al. A dietary quality comparison of popular weight-loss plans. *Journal of the American Dietetic Association* 2007; **107**(10): 1786–1791.
20. Harvie MN, Pegington M, Mattson MP, Frystyk J, Dillon B, et al. The effects of intermittent or continuous energy restriction on weight loss and metabolic disease risk markers: a randomised trial in young overweight women. *International Journal of Obesity* 2011; **35**: 714–727.
21. Stegeman C, Kunselman B, McClure E, Pacak D. Fad diets: implications for oral health care treatment. *Access* 2006; **20**(3): 30–35.

Chapter 4.7

Pharmacological management of weight loss in obesity

Aileen Muir
NHS Greater Glasgow and Clyde, Glasgow, UK

Drug treatment of obesity has had a chequered past, with amphetamines proving popular for much of the twentieth century, until their cardiovascular adverse effects resulted in them being withdrawn from the market in the late 1970s. Medicines are required to be tested for efficacy and safety, and their benefits and risks assessed, before they are given a license for use. In Europe, this is done by the European Medicines Agency (EMA), and, in the USA, by the US Food and Drug Administration (FDA). While products are required to go through rigorous testing and clinical trials, some rarer adverse effects are only recognised once many people have taken the medicine. There seemed to be a resurgence in developing drugs to treat obesity in the early twenty-first century. Orlistat, rimonibant and sibutramine, all were licensed for long-term use in the UK, until the withdrawal of rimonabant in 2008, when the European Medicines Agency (EMA) concluded that the risks outweighed the benefits, and the subsequent withdrawal of sibutramine in 2010, owing to cardiovascular risks.

In the UK, orlistat remains the only drug specifically licensed for the long-term treatment of obesity. This is in contrast to the USA, where lorcaserin and the phentermine/topiramate combination are both licensed by the FDA but have been rejected by the EMA. However, as is clear from previous experience, this is an area of constant change, and there may be differences in indications in different areas.

Use of other drugs is being investigated, with an application for liraglutide and a fixed combination of naltrexone/bupropion having been approved by the FDA. The naltrexone/bupropion combination has received a positive opinion from the EMA, and is now approved for use. Exenatide, a glucagon-like peptide 1 receptor agonist, is in late-phase clinical trials.

Drugs used for obesity management are licensed in conjunction with diet and exercise, and show overall modest benefits in some patients, with weight loss in the region of 3–5% of initial weight, as compared to placebo. Studies, regardless of the medicine, have shown that there is a 30–50% attrition rate in those patients randomised for treatment [1]. A patient's response in the first 12 weeks of treatment provides a good indication of his or her long-term response, and results in the discontinuation of obesity medication if the patient does not lose at least 5% of initial weight after 12 weeks of therapy (after assessment for adherence and, where appropriate, an increase in dosage). Reviews of the effectiveness of these products should also be part of the treatment plan, as the benefit–risk ratio of using long-term medication for weight management requires to be assessed.

4.7.1 Orlistat

Orlistat inhibits gastrointestinal and pancreatic lipases, which results in the inability to hydrolyse dietary fat, in the form of triglycerides, into absorbable free fatty acids. It is available as a prescription product at a dose of 120 mg three times daily, and also as an over-the-counter preparation at a dose of 60 mg three times a day.

Advanced Nutrition and Dietetics in Obesity, First Edition. Edited by Catherine Hankey.
© 2018 John Wiley & Sons Ltd. Published 2018 by John Wiley & Sons Ltd.

A recent systematic review found that orlistat at 120 mg three times a day caused weight loss of average 3.4 kg (3.1% of initial weight) more than placebo-treated patients at 12 months. Patients were also participating in a behavioural weight control programme and had a lower-fat diet that contained around 30% of energy from fat. The review also found two trials of orlistat 60 mg three times a day that resulted in a pooled estimate of 2.5 kg greater weight loss at 52 weeks than placebo [1].

It has also been shown in a 4-year study to significantly reduce the risk of developing type 2 diabetes. The cumulative incidence rate of type 2 diabetes at 4 years was 2.9% with orlistat, as compared to 4.2% for placebo-treated patents [2].

As orlistat acts by decreasing the fat that is absorbed, this can result in considerable gastrointestinal side effects, which may lead to discontinuation. The possibility of these effects being experienced increases if the patient continues with a high-fat diet or if orlistat is taken with a meal that is very high in fat [3].

Within the licensed indication, orlistat should not be continued beyond 12 weeks if at least a 5% decrease from the initial body weight has not been achieved.

4.7.2 Lorcaserin

Lorcaserin is licensed for use by the FDA, but not by the EMA in Europe. It is a selective serotonin 2C (5HT2c) receptor agonist, and is administered as a 10 mg tablet twice a day. In the pivotal trials in non-diabetic patients, lorcaserin decreased body weight by about 3.2 kg more than placebo, and significantly more patients lost >5% body weight (47% vs. 20% in BLOOM and 47 vs. 25% in BLOSSOM, respectively) [4,5]. Blood pressure, total cholesterol, LDL cholesterol and triglycerides were also improved.

However, there have been concerns about the adverse effects associated with lorcaserin, including about the risk of tumours and also the potential risk of psychiatric disorders and valvulopathy (problems with heart valves). Indeed, problems with heart valves led to the withdrawal of a previous product, fenfluramine (5HT2B agonist), in the 1990s [6]. These concerns led to the EMA being of the opinion that the benefits did not outweigh the risks of this medicine, and the application for a marketing authorisation was subsequently withdrawn [7]. The FDA granted approval on condition that a post-marketing study to evaluate long-term cardiovascular safety was carried out [8].

4.7.3 Phentermine/topiramate extended release

The combination of phentermine and topiramate is another product that has been granted approval for treatment of obesity by the FDA, but not by the EMA. Phentermine is an appetite suppressant/stimulant, and topiramate is marketed as an anti-epileptic, but has been found to have weight loss side effects. There are four fixed-dose combinations that allow upward dosage titration. The main pivotal studies showed clinically relevant weight loss, but adverse effects have once again proven to be a concern [1]. The cardiovascular effects of phentermine on long-term use, in addition to concerns about the long-term psychiatric effects and cognitive effects related to topiramate, resulted in the EMA concluding that the benefits did not outweigh the risks, and refusing marketing authorisation [9]. An additional concern is the teratogenic effects from the topiramate component. The majority of potential users of the product are women of childbearing age, and therefore a risk-evaluation and -mitigation strategy was developed to minimise this risk in the USA [10].

4.7.4 Glucagon-like peptide-1 (GLP-1) receptor agonists

Liraglutide and exenatide are two drugs currently licensed for the treatment of type 2 diabetes that are undergoing clinical trials for the treatment of obesity. Applications have been made to both the FDA and the EMA for liraglutide, seeking a license for the treatment of obesity, and liraglutide is now licensed for use by the FDA and in the EU. It is licensed as a treatment option for chronic weight management, along with a low-energy diet and physical activity.

Liraglutide is a glucagon-like peptide-1 (GLP-1) receptor agonist, and is administered via a once-daily subcutaneous injection using a pre-filled multi-dose pen [11]. GLP-1 reduces appetite in normal and obese individuals, and liraglutide mimics this effect on the receptors [13].

There were three clinical trials presented for licensing that includes obese and overweight patients with and without significant weight-related conditions [11,12,13]. All patients received counselling regarding lifestyle modifications that consisted of a low-energy diet and regular physical activity.

The main pivotal trial, which was a 56-week clinical trial that enrolled 3731 patients without diabetes, showed a significant difference when compared to placebo, with patients having an average weight loss of 4.5% from baseline. In this trial, 62% of patients treated with liraglutide lost at least 5% of their body weight, as compared to 34% of patients treated with placebo [11]. Liraglutide was studied in patients who had previously achieved weight loss by adopting a low-calorie diet [13]. Maintenance of ≥5% weight loss was achieved by 81.4% of those taking liraglutide, as compared to 48.9% of those on placebo, and 50.5% lost ≥5% of randomisation weight, as compared to 221.8% of those on placebo. The most common side effects observed in patients treated with liraglutide were nausea, diarrhoea, constipation, vomiting and hypoglycaemia. The FDA requires post-marketing trials investigating medullary thyroid tumours, breast cancer and cardiovascular safety.

Exenatide is from the same group of drugs as liraglutide, and is currently being studied for its effectiveness on weight loss in non-diabetic obese patients. This study is due for completion in 2016 [14].

4.7.5 Naltrexone/bupropion

Naltrexone/bupropion use in combination in the treatment of addiction is sold under the brand names Contrave (in the USA) and Mysimba (in European markets). Naltrexone is an opioid antagonist, and bupropion is a dopamine and norepinephrine re-uptake inhibitor used in some countries as an antidepressant, although it is used as an adjunct for smoking cessation in the UK.

Four 56-week, multicentre, double-blind, placebo-controlled obesity trials (CONTRAVE Obesity Research, or COR-I, COR-II, COR-BMOD and COR-Diabetes) were conducted to evaluate the effect of naltrexone/bupropion in conjunction with lifestyle modification in 4536 patients, randomised to combination drug or placebo. Baseline mean weight across the trials was in the region of 100 kg [15,16,17,18].

In the 56-week COR-I trial, the mean change in body weight was −5.4% among patients assigned to naltrexone/bupropion (32 mg/360 mg), as compared to −1.3% among patients assigned to placebo, and at least 5% reduction in body weight was achieved by 44% of those receiving naltrexone/bupropion, as compared to 17% receiving placebo.

There was a large proportion of withdrawals from both arms across the studies, with the majority doing so within the first 12 weeks. In those randomised to naltrexone/bupropion, 46% withdrew (24% due to adverse reactions), as compared to 45% in the placebo group (12% due to adverse reactions). Indeed, adverse reactions may be a limiting factor to the success of this combination drug. Risks of developing suicidal ideation and neuropsychiatric disorders are well-recognised concerns in relation to bupropion use. The most common adverse effects in studies for weight loss, however, were nausea, constipation, headache and dizziness [15].

4.7.6 Cost-effectiveness of pharmacological interventions in obesity

A systematic review assessed the cost-effectiveness of orlistat by analysing the combined results of 54 studies [19]. The authors found that the average estimated cost of the drug was £1665 per quality-adjusted life year (QALY), which is well below accepted thresholds for cost-effectiveness.

The QALY is a widely used economic indicator, or tool, that allows a consistent approach to comparing the value of different interventions. A QALY takes into account how a treatment affects a patient's quantity of life (how long he or she lives) and quality of life (the quality of his or her remaining years of life). It combines both these factors into a single measure that puts a figure on the health benefits for any treatment, including medicines. QALY provides a benchmark that can be used to measure and compare the benefits that an intervention is likely to offer.

There has yet to be a cost-effectiveness analysis of the more recently licensed medicines for obesity. However, in the USA, the cost of liraglutide is almost 25 times that of orlistat, so there are affordability implications for the healthcare system. However, in view of the large costs associated with the health impact of obesity, these newer medicines may still be found to be cost-effective.

4.7.7 Conclusion

Pharmaceutical interventions for weight loss and maintenance produce modest benefits, and should be combined with lifestyle modifications. Experience in the development of medicines for the treatment of obesity has shown that some of the more serious adverse effects may not be seen until a large number of patients have received the product post-marketing, and this strategy should be considered when using all newly licensed medicines. The recent license submissions and approvals will no doubt increase interest in the pharmaceutical solutions for weight management. It remains to be seen whether the most recent approvals for drugs licensed for treatment of overweight and obese patients will have a major impact on the care of these patients. However, it seems likely that they will remain as adjuncts to treatment.

4.7.8 Summary box

Key points

- Pharmacological therapy for obesity should only be used in combination with lifestyle interventions.
- Pharmacological therapy has shown modest weight loss of 3–5% of body weight, as compared to placebo.
- Response should be assessed after 12 weeks and treatment discontinued if the patient has not lost 5% of his or her body weight.
- Pharmacological treatment is a rapidly changing marketplace with continued interest in developing new medicines.
- Many rarer adverse effects from medicines do not become apparent until many patients have taken it over a period of time.

References

1. Yanovski SJ, Yanovski JA. Long-term drug treatment for obesity: a systematic and clinical review. *JAMA* 2014; **311**(1): 74–86.
2. Torgerson JS, Hauptman J, Boldrin MN, Sjostrom L. XENical in the prevention of diabetes in obese subjects (XENDOS) study. *Diabetes Care* 2004; **27**(1): 155–161.
3. Electronic Medicines Compendium. Summary of product characteristics Xenical (orlistat 120 mg hard capsules). Internet: https://www.medicines.org.uk/emc/medicine/33323, accessed 28 July 2017.
4. Smith SR, Weissman NJ, Anderson CM, et al. Multicenter, placebo-controlled trial of lorcaserin for weight management. *The New England Journal of Medicine* 2010; **363**(3): 245–256.
5. Smith SR, Weissman NJ, Anderson CM, Sanchez M, Chuang E, Stubbe S, et al. A one-year randomized trial of lorcaserin for weight loss in obese and overweight adults: the BLOSSOM trial. *Journal of Clinical Endocrinology and Metabolism* 2011; **96**(10): 3067–3077.
6. FDA announces withdrawal of fenfluramine and dexfenfluramine, 15 September 1997. Internet: http://www.fda.gov/Drugs/DrugSafety/PostmarketDrugSafetyInformationforPatientsandProviders/ucm179871.htm, accessed 17 January 2016.
7. European Medicines Agency Assessment Report. Belviq. 17 January 2013.
8. New Drug Application Approval Letter. Belviq (lorcaserin). Food and drug agency 27/06/12.
9. European Medicines Agency. Refusal of marketing authorisation for Qsiva (phentermine/topiramate). Questions and answers, 21 February 2013. Internet: http://www.ema.europa.eu/docs/en_GB/document_library/Summary_of_opinion_-_Initial_authorisation/human/002350/WC500139215.pdf, accessed 17 January 2016.
10. New Drug Approval Letter. Qsymia (phentermine/topiramate) Food and drug agency, 17/07/12. Internet: http://www.accessdata.fda.gov/drugsatfda_docs/appletter/2012/022580Origs000ltr.pdf, accessed 17 January 2016.
11. Saxenda. Prescribing information. Internet: http://novo-pi.nnittest.com/saxenda.pdf, accessed 17 January 2016.
12. Astrup A, Carraro R, Finer N, Harper A, Kunesova M, Lean ME, Niskanen L, Rasmussen MF, Rissanen A, Rössner S, Savolainen MJ, Van Gaal L. Safety, tolerability and sustained weight loss over 2 years with the once-daily human GLP-1 analog, liraglutide. *International Journal of Obesity* 2012; **36**(6): 843–854.
13. Wadden TA, Hollander P, Klein S, Niswender K, Woo V, Hale PM, Aronne L. Weight maintenance and additional weight loss with liraglutide after low-calorie-diet-induced weight loss: the SCALE Maintenance randomized study. *International Journal of Obesity* 2013; **37**(11): 1443–1451.
14. The effects of exenatide (Byetta) on energy expenditure and weight loss in nondiabetic obese subjects. Internet: https://clinicaltrials.gov/ct2/show/NCT00856609, accessed 17 January 2016.
15. Contrave. Prescribing information. Internet: http://general.takedapharm.com/content/file.aspx?filetypecode=CONTRAVEPI&CountryCode=US&LanguageCode=EN&cacheRandomizer=c9e7f7fc-5f99-4556-8b6c-e675c13d1e02, accessed 17 January 2016.

16. Greenway FL, Fujioka K, Plodkowski RA, Mudaliar S, Guttadauria M, Erickson J, et al. Effect of naltrexone plus bupropion on weight loss in overweight and obese adults (COR-I): a multicentre, randomised, double-blind, placebo-controlled, phase 3 trial. *Lancet* 2010; **376**(9741): 595–605.

17. Apovian CM, Aronne L, Rubino D, Still C, Wyatt H, Burns C, et al. A randomized, phase 3 trial of naltrexone SR/bupropion SR on weight and obesity-related risk factors (COR-II). *Obesity* 2013; **21**: 935–943.

18. Wadden TA, Foreyt JP, Foster GD, Hill JO, Klein S, O'Neil PM, et al. Weight loss with naltrexone SR/bupropion SR combination therapy as an adjunct to behavior modification: the COR-BMOD trial. *Obesity* 2011; **19**: 110–120.

19. Ara R, Blake L, Gray L, Hernandez M, Crowther M, Dunkley A, Warren F, Jackson R, Rees A, Stevenson M, Abrams K, Cooper N, Davies M, Khunti K, Sutton A. What is the clinical effectiveness and cost-effectiveness of using drugs in treating obese patients in primary care? A systematic review. *Health Technology Assessment* 2012; **16**(1): 1–195.

Chapter 4.8

Diet to support pharmacological management of weight loss

Ghalia Abdeen

King Saud University, Riyadh, Saudi Arabia

Treating obesity with medication does not represent a cure, but rather the management of a chronic condition. Lifestyle and behavioural modifications, including diet and exercise as recommended by the American College of Physicians (ACP) and the Scottish Intercollegiate Guideline, are part of the long-term management of the obese [1–5]. People with a BMI of ≥30 kg/m², or those with a BMI of ≥27 kg/m² with comorbidities such as type 2 diabetes, cardiovascular disease and sleep apnoea, are good candidates for pharmacological therapy [1]. A combination of medication with lifestyle measures are better than either medication or lifestyle modifications alone [6]. Obesity should thus be treated within the healthcare system, just like any other complex and chronic disease.

Physicians and other healthcare specialists find it challenging to assist obese patients to lose weight and to maintain weight loss. The combination of regular physical activity, cognitive-behavioural modification of lifestyle and effective anti-obesity drugs (Chapter 4.7) is more likely to achieve weight loss maintenance. Treatment for obesity should be personalised to address age, sex, severity of obesity, comorbidities, psychological–behavioural characteristics and history of previous weight loss efforts.

4.8.1 Anti-obesity drugs

Orlistat

Orlistat is a reversible gastrointestinal lipase inhibitor that reduces fat absorption by attenuating hydrolysation of dietary fat in the gut [7]. The effects of orlistat when taken in combination with a high-fat diet are unpleasant, and include diarrhoea, steatorrhoea, flatulence, bloating, dyspepsia and abdominal pain [8]. Prior to patients starting the drug, these effects are not always clearly linked to the overconsumption of fat. During the consultation between healthcare professionals and patients, this aspect of treatment should be emphasised. The lack of this crucial information can lead patients to experience these predictable effects and subsequently reduce compliance with medication and diet. If explained appropriately to patients, the drug results in a change from 'mindless eating' to 'mindful eating', with patients changing their diet and consuming less energy from fat to avoid steatorrhoea. A deficiency of the fat-soluble vitamins (vitamins A, D, E and K) is rare, and, although no signal exists for either positive or negative effects, definitive data on long-term cardiovascular outcomes are still awaited [9].

The X-PERT study showed good weight loss and reductions of the components of the metabolic syndrome when lifestyle changes were combined with diverse dietary interventions and orlistat [10]. Patients received 120 mg orlistat three times/day. They were randomly divided into two groups (500 or 1000 kcal/day deficit) and followed for a year, with assessments at 3 and 6 months, in addition to the primary outcome measure the change in weight after 12 months as compared to the baseline. It showed that both groups had similar improvements in blood pressure, lipid levels, waist circumference and weight loss (−11.4 kg vs. −11.8 kg, respectively;

$P = 0.78$). In addition, owing to treatment with orlistat, 84% and 85% of patients in the 500 and 1000 kcal/day deficit groups, respectively, achieved ≥5% weight loss; and 50% and 53% of patients, respectively, achieved ≥10% weight loss [11]. The results of a systematic review and meta-analysis of 10 studies to assess the effects of orlistat on cardiometabolic risk factors [12] were similar to the findings of a multicentre, randomised, double-blind, placebo-controlled study (RCT). This trial also compared orlistat to placebo. All groups had a nutritionally balanced diet with a 600-kcal energy deficit. The orlistat groups lost significantly more weight and maintained the weight loss over 2 years [13]. The role of the diet is thus crucial for the medication to be optimally effective. The diets with the best potential effects will enhance satiety – for example, by increasing the protein content and reducing the glycaemic index of carbohydrates – but it is critical that the diet also be low in fat. The latter component is required to prevent the predictable side effects of orlistat when taken with a high-fat diet. The advice to improve long-term compliance should thus be focussed on enhancing satiety and reducing the risk of side effects of the medication.

Contrave

Contrave, a combination of naltrexone sustained-release (SR) and bupropion (SR), is a norepinephrine/dopamine reuptake inhibitor and opioid receptor antagonist. All these patients underwent simultaneous intensive behaviour modification, portion size control, calorie counting and were advised to undertake increased physical activity, in addition to keeping detailed daily records of their food intake. Patients were instructed to consume a balanced low-energy diet, with 15–20% of energy from protein, 30% or less energy from fat and 50% from carbohydrate. They had group sessions with dietitians, behavioural psychologists and exercise specialists weekly during the first 4 months of the study, followed by monthly sessions thereafter. The group sessions used multimodal therapies to improve the patients' compliance with the medication and lifestyle approaches. Information was given on how to sustain the interventions in the long term, but these sessions also allowed the patients to 'belong to the club' and to feel that they were not in this on their own (see Chapter 4.7). A combination of Contrave with intensive behavioural modification produced significantly greater weight loss than behavioural modification alone [14].

Qsymia

Qsymia (Qnexa) is a combination of low-dose phentermine and the antiepileptic agent topiramate [15]. The combination can maintain approximately 10% body weight loss over 1 year. The drug is meant to complement lifestyle modifications, low-fat diet, exercise, behavioural changes and surgical approaches [16,17]. In the trial setting, the drug was combined with techniques from *The LEARN Program for Weight Management* [18], which represented a balanced 500 kcal/day deficit with increased water intake and physical exercise. *The LEARN Program for Weight Management* advocates working on changes in *L*ifestyle, *E*xercise, *A*ttitudes, *R*elationships, and *N*utrition. It uses diets low in fat and high in low-glycaemic-index carbohydrate, and was founded on national guidelines that aimed to achieve precise goals for energy restriction. The LEARN books propose multiple strategies, such as relapse preparation, planning strategies and goal setting. In general, the LEARN manual emphasises behaviour alteration strategies [19]. Patients in the trials were also offered a monthly nutritional and lifestyle modification counselling [16,18,20–24]. For example, *The LEARN Program for Weight Management* provides 16 step-by-step lessons for modifying eating, activities and thinking habits. The dietary recommendations are based on the 'Food Guide Pyramid', introduced in 1992 by the United States Department of Agriculture. Keeping a daily record of their food intake, including the amount of energy consumed, is encouraged. An increase in physical activity (by walking up to 30 min/day) and practicing other weight control behaviours (e.g. stimulus control, cognitive restructuring, slowing eating) are encouraged [18].

Liraglutide

In the SCALE Obesity and Prediabetes study as well as the SCALE Diabetes study, patients were randomised to either liraglutide (3 mg) or placebo.

All patients also received a 500 kcal/day deficit that reflected the usual practice of the centre where they were treated [25]. There was no statistically significant difference in weight loss, depending on the macronutrient contribution of the 500-kcal deficit diet that patients received. The SCALE Maintenance study used a low-energy diet approach to achieve at least 5% weight loss prior to patients being randomised to a 500 kcal/day deficit with or without liraglutide. This combination approach resulted in almost 15% total weight loss on average in the liraglutide group, and weight maintenance in the placebo group [26]. The diet approaches can vary with liraglutide, but the principles of combining a diet approach that enhances satiety together with the satiety-enhancing effects of the medication appears to work best.

4.8.2 Diet to support anti-obesity drugs

Pharmacotherapy can be useful for managing obesity as part of a comprehensive approach, which includes lifestyle modifications [27,28], diet, exercise and behavioural therapy [10]. The most successful strategy initially to use with pharmacotherapy are low-calorie-diets (LCDs) of 800–1500 kcal/day and a balanced deficit diet typically of around 1500 kcal/day, which results in approximately 8% body weight loss over 6 months. The National Institute of Diabetes and Digestive and Kidney Diseases and the National Heart, Lung, and Blood Institute convened the first Expert Panel on the Identification, Evaluation, and Treatment of Overweight and Obesity in Adults, which suggested a 500–1000-kcal/day deficit for obese people aimed at 0.5–1 kg/week weight loss. However, it remains challenging to determine patients' daily energy requirements, and thus energy-intake guidelines are often based largely on a patient's original body weight and gender [29].

Regular adjustment of the energy content of any prescribed diet is needed in response to a patient's weight loss response and treatment goals. Low-fat diets are the typical approach, defined as diets deriving 30% of energy from fat [30], but an increase in proteins and low-glycaemic-index carbohydrates may be equally helpful [31]. Obese people undertaking

long-term weight maintenance ought to consume only 25% of their energy intake from fat [32].

A low-carbohydrate ketogenic diet (LCKD) has been shown to lead to improvements comparable to orlistat plus a low-fat diet (O+LFD) [33,34]. The LCKD restricts carbohydrate intake initially to less than 20 g/day [33,34]. Patients in the LCKD group were allowed to eat *ad libitum* amounts of meat, eggs, hard cheese, low-carbohydrate vegetables (e.g. leafy greens) and moderate-carbohydrate vegetables (e.g. broccoli, asparagus) daily, with no restrictions on energy intake. All types of fats and oils, even butter, were allowed. Patients did not avoid the fat that came with meat, poultry, fish and eggs. Olive oil and peanut oil, which are particularly healthy oils, were encouraged in cooking. Margarine and other hydrogenated oils that contain trans unsaturated fats were avoided. Approximately 5 g/day from other carbohydrates were added to the patients' intake each week as they approached their goal weight, or if cravings threatened their compliance. The second group took orlistat therapy (120 mg orally three times before meals per day) plus a low-fat diet which constituted <30% of daily energy, saturated fat <10% of daily energy and cholesterol <300 mg per day. The study showed that both the very-high-fat and the very-low-fat diets had similar health benefits. Brinkworth et al. [35] also confirmed that compliance with low-carbohydrate diets could be maintained for 1 year, by testing the mean carbohydrate intake in the LCKD group (62 g/day, 15% of energy intake), although the impact of carbohydrate intake in the longer term (>1 year) is unclear. The combination of orlistat with LCKDs has not been tested.

Weight loss is considerably greater in the obese who regularly attend group sessions. Attending 80% or more of the group counselling sessions resulted in more weight loss – −14.9% and −13.9% among the LCKD and low-fat groups, respectively – regardless of whether the patients were taking medications or not. This inclusion led to the selected population probably representing the motivated patients. Incorporating intensive weight loss programmes into medical practice and identifying the motivated patients require extra efforts from healthcare providers, which may not always be possible [36].

Reduction in energy intake is the cornerstone of reducing weight, while appropriate nutrition counselling, behaviour modification therapy and lifestyle changes could aid weight loss maintenance. The addition of medications to reduce long-term energy intake or absorption can have added benefits [37], such as improving the risks of type 2 diabetes, cardiovascular problems, hyperlipidaemia and sleep apnoea, but only in partnership with dietary and lifestyle management.

4.8.3 Conclusion

Despite initial promise, most anti-obesity drugs have either not been approved or had to be withdrawn from the market. Orlistat is the anti-obesity drug that has been internationally available for the longest period [38]. The development of new and safe anti-obesity drugs is urgently needed, and the recent progress of liraglutide, tesofensine, Qsymia (Qnexa), Contrave and Empatic is exciting [39], although the dietary strategies to optimise the outcomes of these drugs remain to be defined. The majority of the clinical trials of anti-obesity drugs have been in combination with low-energy diets, which may have included behaviour change advice. Given that compliance is frequently better in clinical trials than in clinical practice, weight loss expectations may have to be adjusted [9]. The diet types that need to be used in conjunction with specific obesity drugs were often left up to the research centres that participated in the studies. In some instances, these diets were poorly defined, and only the energy deficit was specified. This heterogeneity represents an important aspect that requires further study, as it will be helpful to understand how to use specific diets or specific macronutrient composition of diets to further enhance the effects of medication.

4.8.4 Summary box

Key points

• Reduction in energy intake: establishing a negative energy balance is the cornerstone for reducing weight, while appropriate nutrition counselling, behaviour modification therapy and lifestyle changes could aid weight loss maintenance.

• Pharmacotherapy can be useful for treating obesity as part of a comprehensive approach that addresses issues with dietary and lifestyle behaviours.
• A combined therapy for weight management is better for weight loss and diabetes prevention as compared to a single therapy.
• Obesity should be treated in a multidisciplinary healthcare system.

References

1. Snow V, Barry P, Fitterman N, Qaseem A, Weiss K. Pharmacologic and surgical management of obesity in primary care: a clinical practice guideline from the American College of Physicians. *Annals of Internal Medicine* 2005; **142**(7): 525–531.
2. Bravata DM, Sanders L, Huang J, Krumholz HM, Olkin I, Gardner CD, et al. Efficacy and safety of low-carbohydrate diets: a systematic review. *JAMA* 2003; **289**(14): 1837–1850.
3. Samaha FF, Iqbal N, Seshadri P, Chicano KL, Daily DA, McGrory J, et al. A low-carbohydrate as compared with a low-fat diet in severe obesity. *The New England Journal of Medicine* 2003; **348**(21): 2074–2081.
4. Yancy WS, Olsen MK, Guyton JR, Bakst RP, Westman EC. A low-carbohydrate, ketogenic diet versus a low-fat diet to treat obesity and hyperlipidemia: a randomized, controlled trial. *Annals of Internal Medicine* 2004; **140**(10): 769–777.
5. Network SIG. *Management of Obesity: A National Clinical Guideline*. Edinburgh: Scottish Intercollegiate Guidelines Network, 2010.
6. Wadden TA, Berkowitz RI, Womble LG, Sarwer DB, Phelan S, Cato RK, et al. Randomized trial of lifestyle modification and pharmacotherapy for obesity. *The New England Journal of Medicine* 2005; **353**(20): 2111–2120.
7. Guerciolini R. Mode of action of orlistat. *International Journal of Obesity* 1997; **21**: S12–S23.
8. Maahs D, Serna DGd, Kolotkin RL, Ralston S, Sandate J, Qualls C, et al. Randomized, double-blind, placebo-controlled trial of orlistat for weight loss in adolescents. *Endocrine Practice* 2006; **12**(1): 18–28.
9. Li MF, Cheung BM. Rise and fall of anti-obesity drugs. *World Journal of Diabetes* 2011; **2**(2): 19–23.
10. Hainer VÜ, Toplak H, Mitrakou A. Treatment modalities of obesity: what fits whom? *Diabetes Care* 2008; **31**(2): S269–S277.
11. Toplak H, Ziegler O, Keller U, Hamann A, Godin C, Wittert G, et al. X-PERT: weight reduction with orlistat in obese subjects receiving a mildly or moderately reduced-energy diet. Early response to treatment predicts weight maintenance. *Diabetes Obesity & Metabolism* 2005; **7**(6): 699–708.
12. Zhou YH, Ma XQ, Wu C, Lu J, Zhang SS, Guo J, et al. Effect of anti-obesity drug on cardiovascular risk factors: a systematic review and meta-analysis of randomized controlled trials. *PloS ONE* 2012; **7**(6): e39062.

13. Rossner S, Sjostrom L, Noack R, Meinders AE, Noseda G, on behalf of the European Orlistat Obesity Study. Weight loss, weight maintenance, and improved cardiovascular risk factors after 2 years treatment with orlistat for obesity. *Obesity Research* 2000; **8**(1): 49–61.
14. Wadden TA, Foreyt JP, Foster GD, Hill JO, Klein S, O'Neil PM, et al. Weight loss with naltrexone SR/bupropion SR combination therapy as an adjunct to behavior modification: the COR-BMOD trial. *Obesity* 2011; **19**(1): 110–120.
15. Rodgers RJ, Tschop MH, Wilding JP. Anti-obesity drugs: past, present and future. *Disease Models Mechanisms* 2012; **5**(5): 621–626.
16. Allison DB, Gadde KM, Garvey WT, Peterson CA, Schwiers ML, Najarian T, et al. Controlled-release phentermine/topiramate in severely obese adults: a randomized controlled trial (EQUIP). *Obesity* 2012; **20**(2): 330–342.
17. Garvey WT. Phentermine and topiramate extended-release: a new treatment for obesity and its role in a complications-centric approach to obesity medical management. *Expert Opinion on Drug Safety* 2013; **12**(5): 741–756.
18. Brownell KD. *The LEARN Program for Weight Management*, 10th edn. Dallas, TX: American Health Publishing Company, 2004.
19. Gardner CD, Kiazand A, Alhassan S, Kim S, Stafford RS, Balise RR, et al. Comparison of the Atkins, Zone, Ornish, and LEARN diets for change in weight and related risk factors among overweight premenopausal women: the A to Z weight loss study: a randomized trial. *JAMA* 2007; **297**(9): 969–977.
20. Allison DB, Gadde KM, Garvey WT, Peterson CA, Schwiers ML, Najarian T, et al. Controlled-release phentermine/topiramate in severely obese adults: a randomized controlled trial (EQUIP). *Obesity* 2012; **20**(2): 330–342.
21. Gadde KM, Allison DB, Ryan DH, Peterson CA, Troupin B, Schwiers ML, et al. Effects of low-dose, controlled-release, phentermine plus topiramate combination on weight and associated comorbidities in overweight and obese adults (CONQUER): a randomised, placebo-controlled, phase 3 trial. *Lancet* 2011; **377**(9774): 1341–1352.
22. Garvey WT, Ryan DH, Look M, Gadde KM, Allison DB, Peterson CA, et al. Two-year sustained weight loss and metabolic benefits with controlled-release phentermine/topiramate in obese and overweight adults (SEQUEL): a randomized, placebo-controlled, phase 3 extension study. *American Journal of Clinical Nutrition* 2012; **95**(2): 297–308.
23. Cameron F, Whiteside G, McKeage K. Phentermine and topiramate extended release. *Drugs* 2012; **72**(15): 2033–2042.
24. Fala L. Qsymia: combination oral therapy a new weight-loss option for obese or overweight patients. *American Health & Drug Benefits* 2013; **6**: 1389.
25. Pi-Sunyer X, Astrup A, Fujioka K, Greenway F, Halpern A, Krempf M, et al. A randomized, controlled trial of 3.0 mg of liraglutide in weight management. *The New England Journal of Medicine* 2015; **373**(1): 11–22.
26. Wadden TA, Hollander P, Klein S, Niswender K, Woo V, Hale PM, et al. Weight maintenance and additional weight loss with liraglutide after low-calorie-diet-induced weight loss: the SCALE maintenance randomized study. *International Journal of Obesity* 2013; **37**(11): 1443–1451.
27. Alpert MA, Terry BE, Kelly DL. Effect of weight loss on cardiac chamber size, wall thickness and left ventricular function in morbid obesity. *American Journal of Cardiology* 1985; **55**(6): 783–786.
28. Salans LB, Cushman SW, Weismann RE. Studies of human adipose tissue adipose cell size and number in nonobese and obese patients. *Journal of Clinical Investigation* 1973; **52**(4): 929.
29. Klein S, Wadden T, Sugerman HJ. AGA technical review on obesity. *Gastroenterology* 2002; **123**(3): 882–832.
30. Panel NOEIE. Clinical guidelines on the identification, evaluation, and treatment of overweight and obesity in adults, 1998.
31. Astrup A, Grunwald GK, Melanson EL, Saris WH, Hill JO. The role of low-fat diets in body weight control: a meta-analysis of ad libitum dietary intervention studies. *International Journal of Obesity and Related Metabolic Disorders* 2000; **24**(12): 1545–1552.
32. Klem ML, Wing RR, McGuire MT, Seagle HM, Hill JO. A descriptive study of individuals successful at long-term maintenance of substantial weight loss. *American Journal of Clinical Nutrition* 1997; **66**(2): 239–246.
33. Borushek A. The Doctor's Pocket Calorie, Fat & Carbohydrate Counter 2004: Plus 170 Fast-Food Chains & Restaurants. Family Health Pub, 2003.
34. Atkins. *The Atkins Trial Kit Handbook: A Simple Guide to Doing Atkins*. Ronkonkoma, NY: Atkins Nutritionals Inc, 2001.
35. Brinkworth GD, Noakes M, Buckley JD, Keogh JB, Clifton PM. Long-term effects of a very-low-carbohydrate weight loss diet compared with an isocaloric low-fat diet after 12 mo. *American Journal of Clinical Nutrition* 2009; **90**(1): 23–32.
36. Yancy WS, Westman EC, McDuffie JR, Grambow SC, Jeffreys AS, Bolton J, et al. A randomized trial of a low-carbohydrate diet vs. orlistat plus a low-fat diet for weight loss. *Archives of Internal Medicine* 2010; **170**(2): 136–145.
37. Klein S, Burke LE, Bray GA, Blair S, Allison DB, Pi-Sunyer X, et al. Clinical implications of obesity with specific focus on cardiovascular disease: a statement for professionals from the American Heart Association Council on Nutrition, Physical Activity, and Metabolism: endorsed by the American College of Cardiology Foundation. *Circulation* 2004; **110**(18): 2952–2967.
38. Kang JG, Park CY, Kang JH, Park YW, Park SW. Randomized controlled trial to investigate the effects of a newly developed formulation of phentermine diffuse-controlled release for obesity. *Diabetes Obesity & Metabolism* 2010; **12**(10): 876–882.
39. Kang JG, Park CY. Anti-obesity drugs: a review about their effects and safety. *Diabetes & Metabolism* 2012; **36**(1): 13–25.

Chapter 4.9

Surgical management of weight loss in obesity

Natasha P Ross[1] and Duff Bruce[2]
[1] NHS Grampian, Aberdeen, UK
[2] Robert Gordon University, Aberdeen, UK

4.9.1 Introduction

Conventional strategies for weight loss and maintenance have modest long-term outcomes in severe obesity [1]. A variety of surgical weight loss procedures and operations have been developed that offer effective and persistent weight loss that may contribute to improvements of comorbidities with associated survival benefits [2]. These were typically termed 'bariatric' or 'metabolic' procedures, in recognition of the beneficial impact they may have on conditions such as type 2 diabetes, cardiac disease and stroke [2–4], in addition to weight-related musculoskeletal and degenerative conditions [5], hypertension, hyperlipidaemia reflux disease, sleep apnoea [6], asthma [7], cancer risk [8] and infertility [9]. This chapter will explore the indications, benefits and risks of weight loss surgery; types of procedures available and their controversies; future developments in bariatric surgery; and translational work in the field.

Bariatric surgery is effective, evidence based, cost-effective and safe, associated with a 0.5% mortality rate, although this is dependent on procedure and patient comorbidity [10,11]. Initially, it developed following recognition that gastric surgery, for peptic ulceration and cancer, resulted in significant weight loss and improvement or resolution of established type 2 diabetes in some. The onset of the obesity epidemic has prompted clinicians to explore this management option for obesity and related comorbidity.

There is now acceptance that conventional weight control strategies are unable to replicate the magnitude and durability of weight loss afforded by surgical options for the severely obese [2]. Several factors contributed to early controversy around the use of surgical options. These included the paucity of an evidence base regarding optimal patient selection, preparation and support. Furthermore, information on the technical safety of procedures, the choice of optimal approaches and the lack of any useful audit data were also shortcomings.

4.9.2 Patient selection, assessment and preparation

Early patient selection focussed on preoperative weight or BMI, and the associated risk of mortality. A National Institutes of Health consensus meeting held in North America in 1991 defined a BMI of >40 kg/m^2, or a BMI of >35 kg/m^2 in association with obesity-related comorbidity, as appropriate indications for bariatric surgery. These remain core to most healthcare systems, although requiring adjustment for high-risk demographic groups – such as South Asian populations (increased type 2 diabetes risk at lower BMI); 'lighter' patients with established or impending type 2 diabetes; and adolescents [10]. Hence, the selection criteria used often include a BMI of >30 kg/m^2 with impaired glucose tolerance or type 2 diabetes, and South Asian or ethnic high-risk groups with a BMI of >27 kg/m^2 [12].

Selection, assessment and preparation of patients to ensure best outcomes with least adverse effects

Advanced Nutrition and Dietetics in Obesity, First Edition. Edited by Catherine Hankey.

require a team of healthcare professionals, including dietitians, psychologists, specialist nurses, pharmacists, physical activity specialists, physicians, anaesthetists, patient mentors and surgeons. Patients should have an opportunity to engage with structured healthy eating and lifestyle programmes through specialised weight management services. These ought to be compulsory prior to the consideration of invasive options. Engagement, often congruent with a good outcome, can be gauged during these structured programmes through attendance and weight change. Such programmes inform patients of the potential benefits, limitations and adverse effects of bariatric procedures [13].

Within the UK, the National Bariatric Surgery Registry reported over 17,000 bariatric surgical procedures between 2011 and 2013. These were predominately gastric bypass, with gastric band and sleeve gastrectomy taking second and third place, respectively. Over 1300 of these were revisional procedures. Obesity surgery in adolescents is rare, with few studies in the literature and in the UK register. Over 3 years, only 62 patients who were ≤18 years underwent bariatric surgery.

Key contraindications to surgical interventions include active mental health issues, eating disorders (especially binge eating), substance dependence and high anaesthetic and surgical risks, although definitive evidence around these is scant and often seen as relative contraindications if these conditions are managed appropriately. Learning difficulties may impact on safe or effective engagement with changes in eating behaviour and lifestyle following bariatric surgery [14]. All active comorbidities and other illnesses should be optimised prior to surgery, and smoking should be ceased, due to the increased risk of respiratory complications, surgical site infections and anastomotic breakdowns [15].

Controversy still surrounds the assumed benefits of preoperative weight loss. Modest preoperative weight loss may decrease peri-operative risk and provide a surrogate marker of patients whose higher levels of engagement in preparation for surgery has been associated with greater weight loss and overall outcomes. It has been suggested that it is therefore appropriate to prioritise 'engaged' individuals, given the scarcity of publicly funded access to bariatric surgery. However, such prioritization remains subjective, and cannot be considered as evidence-based practice [16].

A number of screening tools have been described for sleep apnoea, including the Epworth and STOP-BANG scores. While there is a high prevalence of this condition in the obese, evidence of the benefits of formal diagnosis and prolonged treatment prior to weight loss surgery has not been comparatively studied [10].

Many overweight patients are prescribed medications as treatment for comorbidities. Early involvement of a pharmacist is advised, since cessation or modification of medications may be required prior to or after surgery (insulin, anticoagulants), where the consumption and absorption changes can necessitate change, or negate requirements [17].

4.9.3 Surgical and endoscopic procedures

Endoscopic weight loss procedures

Bariatric procedures now fall into two categories: temporary endoscopic procedures and permanent surgical procedures. Temporary procedures include intragastric balloon, endo-duodenal sleeve placement and mucosal-based stapling to parts of the stomach. Short-term studies are increasingly demonstrating weight loss and comorbidity improvement with some procedures, but long-term evidence is as yet unavailable. Most are likely associated with weight regain when removed. Patients should be informed of the limits of current evidence and the likelihood of long-term weight regain.

Operative weight loss procedures

There are a number of established surgical procedures that aim to provide long-term benefits. Worldwide, three laparoscopic procedures account for the majority of surgeries: gastric bypass with Roux-en-Y reconstruction, adjustable gastric band and sleeve gastrectomy.

The gastric bypass, first performed in 1965, involves forming a small pouch from the proximal stomach, immediately below the oesophagus, using surgical staples, anastamosed to a divided portion of small bowel. The stomach and duodenum are left in place to act as a channel for digestive juice from the liver, pancreas and gastric remnant and are joined to the small bowel approximately 100 cm below its attachment to the pouch. Key effects significantly suppress appetite (due to the small gastric pouch), decrease the volume of food eaten, and cause a degree of malabsorption. The procedure results in rapid weight loss, to around 30–35%, in 2 years [18].

An early and popular weight loss procedure was the vertical banded gastroplasty (VBG). This formed a small pouch of proximal stomach using staples and a fixed band of special reinforcing mesh. The gastric band developed later with the advantage of adjustability. These are positioned like a collar around the top part of the stomach. A thin tube attaches to a subcutaneous port, which may be accessed to fill or empty the band, causing a variable mixture of appetite suppression and volume restriction, which decreases intake. Patients are encouraged to avoid filling the band in excess of a level that causes appetite suppression, as this can result in conversion to a high-calorie liquid intake, regurgitation and poor oesophageal function. On average, a gastric band patient will lose 20% of his or her overall weight in 2 years, and this change may persist.

Sleeve gastrectomy is a recent popular procedure in which stapled removal of the left portion of the stomach leaves a thin gastric conduit of 1–1.3 cm. The resected stomach is completely removed, making this procedure irreversible. This results in 25–27% weight loss [18] by reducing the volume of food eaten and through appetite suppression. Although the resulting hormonal disturbance has been hypothesised, there is no clear evidence that this contributes to weight loss postoperatively.

A small number of procedures are primarily malabsorptive: duodenal switch, bilio-pancreatic diversion and distal gastric bypass. These appear to result in greater, prolonged weight loss and improved diabetic control, particularly in heavier patients, but are associated with more nutritional deficiency, which limits their use to well-engaged patients with follow-up provided in expert units [18] (Table 4.9.3).

4.9.4 Risks and benefits of surgical procedures

As bariatric surgeries increase in number, the associated risks and adverse outcomes are being better scrutinised. Many of the risks of surgery are generic to abdominal surgery in the severely obese, including venous thromboembolism (VTE) [19], respiratory complications, wound herniation and surgical site infection [6]. In procedures that involve the division of gastrointestinal tissue, the possible complications include bleeding [20], leaks and internal hernias [21] (Figure 4.9.1).

Postoperative mortality must be considered in the context of untreated obesity. In those eligible for surgery, the annual mortality risk is 0.5%, which is higher than the mortality risk from surgery, estimated to be around 0.07–0.3% [10]. Furthermore, bariatric surgery is associated with a long-term reduction in overall mortality (hazard ratio 0.71) [2]. The obesity surgery mortality risk score has been validated to predict risk based on five factors: (1) male sex, (2) age >45 years, (3) BMI >50 kg/m^2, (4) hypertension and (5) risk of venous VTE

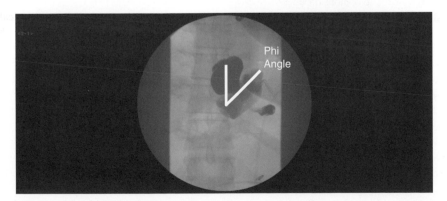

Figure 4.9.1 Gastric band: Contrast study demonstrating gastric band in position. Normally, the Phi angle (between spine and longitudinal axis of the gastric band) is 4–58°.

(includes sleep apnoea). However, recent data challenges this [10].

Some of the risks are particular to specific bariatric procedures. Gastric bypass is associated with stromal ulcer [21] and dumping syndrome, where hormonal responses to excess sugar intake result in hypoglycaemia [22]. Orientation of the small bowel mesentery results in two potential internal hernia spaces – between mesenteric loops, and in Petersen's space (behind the Roux-en-Y loop) – and such defects can result in internal hernia and catastrophic strangulation of the small bowel [21].

Some gastric bands will be removed over time due to intolerance; ineffective oesophageal motility; gastric pouch dilatation [23] and slippage [21] (Figures 4.9.2 and 4.9.3); stomach band erosion [21] and technical failure [21]. Rates of removal are described up to 40%, and port site infections are relatively common [18].

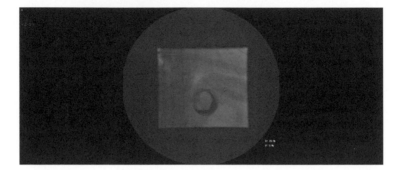

Figure 4.9.2 Gastric band slippage. A typical 'O' sign of a slipped gastric band.

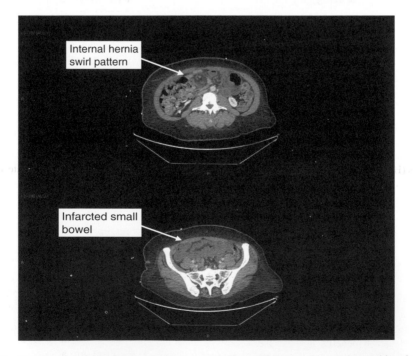

Figure 4.9.3 Complication following Roux-en-Y gastric bypass. CT images show an internal hernia (swirl pattern) through Peterson's space and mesenteric–jejunal defects resulting in small bowel infarction demonstrated with poor enhancement.

Table 4.9.1 Frequent complications of common bariatric surgical procedures

Complication	Risk (%)
Mortality	0.05–0.3
VTE	0.4–2.4
Surgical site infection	0.4–3.7
Bleeding	3
Gastric bypass	
Dumping symptoms	40
Internal hernia	0.75–1.1
Small bowel obstruction	3.9
Leak	0.5
Stromal ulcer	0.75
Gastric sleeve	
Dehydration	19
Leak	0.1–0.3
Narrow conduit/stricture	0.59
Gastric band	
Port site complications	2.6
Pouch dilatation	12
Band slippage	9.09
Band erosion	1.19
Failure to lose weight	1.58

Table 4.9.2 Advantages of bariatric surgery and procedures

Benefits of bariatric surgery
Reduced mortality
• Long-term, all-cause
• Cardiovascular, stroke and cancer associated
Improved quality of life
Improved comorbidities, including:
• Diabetes (HbAic)
• Cholesterol
• Hypertension
• Obstructive sleep apnoea
• Reflux

Sleeve gastrectomy can be complicated by an overly narrow conduit, bleeding and leaks that can be particularly troublesome and may require further surgery [20] (Table 4.9.1).

All the risks of bariatric surgery come with remarkable potential benefits in all-cause, cardiovascular, stroke and cancer-related mortality [24], in addition to improvements in quality of life and comorbidities [6] (Table 4.9.2).

4.9.5 Selection of weight loss procedure

Much attention has been given to the choice of an optimal surgical procedure for any individual, and a number of studies have compared these, focussing on outcomes of either weight loss or the control of type 2 diabetes. However, the range of outcomes for any individual includes many other factors, such as complications and psychological impact. We currently do not have sufficient information to definitively allocate patients to an optimal procedure. Health professionals should ensure that patients understand current evidence-based information regarding the benefits and limitations of different procedures to aid informed patient choice as several procedures may provide acceptable degrees of weight loss and equal reduction in comorbidity for an individual patient [18]. Recent work has suggested that simple genetic factors may impact procedure outcomes, and, once matured, this may impact procedure choice [25,26].

4.9.6 Novel procedures

Several novel procedures have been described and are performed in limited numbers. The mini-gastric bypass is formed by leaving a long, gastric-sleeve-like pouch, anastomosed to a jejunum loop approximately 200 cm from the duodenum. This is technically straightforward, and early results show satisfactory weight loss of 80% of excess body weight in 1 year. Although patients may suffer bile reflux, and similar reconstructions for ulcer surgery were historically associated with a late increase in cancer development, changes in drainage of the pouch may alter this [27]. Gastroplication involves sewing the left side of the stomach in on itself. Early outcomes are reasonable, with loss of 31–74% of excess weight in ≤2 years and lowered glucose levels, but long-term outcomes are awaited [28]. A common modification of the sleeve gastrectomy and gastric bypass is to place a small non-distensible band around the upper part of the pouch, termed the 'banded sleeve/bypass' [29]. This correlates with increased, persistent weight loss, and studies are underway to compare any adverse effects, such as band slippage and infection. These procedures exemplify the large amount of experimental work being undertaken in this field, although long-term data is required before these may be recommended beyond research study.

4.9.7 Long-term management

Revisional surgery

Procedure complications or failure to lose weight can necessitate revision or conversion to another procedure. Typical revision procedures include endoscopic or laparoscopic removal or revision of gastric bands; conversion of gastric bands to sleeve gastrectomy or gastric bypass; and conversion of sleeve gastrectomy to gastric bypass or duodenal switches. These are typically more complex procedures than primary ones, and have higher risk of major morbidities such as leak rates [30].

Long-term follow-up

The goal of surgery is to have a lifelong impact on eating behaviour and nutrition, and traditional lifelong follow-up has therefore been indicated. Early follow-up should ensure good surgical outcome and monitor for complications. Follow-up should provide an opportunity for advice and support around dietary change, nutritional supplementation and psychological challenges. It offers a crucial opportunity to screen and identify common nutritional deficiencies [13,20,31–35] (Table 4.9.3).

Body contouring surgery

Patients successful in weight loss – often estimated as around 50% of excess body weight loss with bariatric surgery – may be left with large amounts of loose skin at the lower abdominal apron, breasts, upper arms and thighs. Approximately 15–40% of patients seek body contour surgery (BCS), most commonly for cosmetic reasons, psychological distress or difficulties with movement and skin ulceration. Access to treatment is often limited due to clinical risk or limited access, and less than 20% achieve the local requirements for contour surgery. For clinical reasons, many surgeons will only perform the surgery at a BMI of <30 kg/m^2, a

cut-off that is difficult for most people undergoing surgery to achieve. Access in some healthcare systems is limited to those with a BMI of <28 kg/m^2 with associated comorbidities such as skin ulceration or infection. As there is a limit to weight loss from bariatric procedures, a majority of patients are unable to satisfy these criteria [36,37].

4.9.8 Challenges and future developments

Differences in philosophy, geography and resources present various challenges throughout the world in the management of severe obesity. However, certain key themes emerge, such as patient selection (who will benefit) and decisions around which procedure will best serve an individual. There is no doubt that the healthcare community strives to improve the options available for the management of obesity. This requires innovative techniques – both improved surgical procedures and translation of surgically induced benefits to conservative interventions. Such improvements will require structured research and comparable audit of interventions and their outcomes.

Patient selection

Patient selection has primarily been defined by absolute weight or BMI, or, in the past, 'ideal weight' as modified by associations with comorbidities. The Edmonton classification describes categories of comorbidities and levels of impact on function with reversibility. It attributes a score of 0–4 based on metabolic, psychological and physical parameters to determine optimal obesity management. Classifications such as this have been validated and demonstrate more accurate outcome prediction than current patient selection based on BMI and diabetes.

Procedure selection

Numerous comparisons have examined differences between bariatric procedures. While differences in weight loss outcomes are easily measured, integrating

Table 4.9.3 Common nutritional deficiencies and the supplements that should be considered, based on British Obesity and Metabolic Surgery Society Guidelines 2015 [41]

Potential nutritional deficiency	Associated procedure	Cause	Complications	Patients deficient (%)	Supplement
Urea and electrolytes	All	Early postoperative poor fluid intake	Dehydration	19	Fluids
Albumin	Duodenal switch	Poor nutritional compliance	Malnutrition	–	–
Iron	Bypass Duodenal switch	Poor intake Limited absorption Loss (menstruation, pathology)	Iron deficiency anaemia	49	Complete multivitamin and mineral supplements
Vitamin B_{12}, folate deficiency	Bypass Duodenal switch Sleeve	Deficient diet Loss of intrinsic factor Poor absorption/intake	Macrocytic anaemia Neuropathy	3.6–64	B_{12} injections (every 3 months)
Protein	Duodenal switch	Poor intake Malnutrition	Muscle wasting Oedema Fatigue	–	Dietary advice
Vitamin D and calcium (monitor 25-hydroxy vitamin D)	Duodenal switch Gastric bypass sleeve	Preoperatively common Malabsorption	Secondary hyperparathyroidism Osteomalacia	7	Calcium and vitamin D
Fat-soluble vitamins (vitamins A, K and E)	Duodenal switch Gastric bypass	Fat malabsorption	Visual disturbance Anaemia Neuropathy Coagulopathy Osteoporosis	11–23	Supplements
Thiamine	All	Excessive weight loss Reduced appetite Vomiting High alcohol intake	Oedema Neuropathy Wernikes encephalopathy	18	Consider additional thiamine
Trace mineral deficiency (zinc, copper, selenium, magnesium)	Bypass Duodenal switch	Poor absorption Chronic diarrhoea	Chronic diarrhoea Cardiomyopathy Bones Fatigue Neuropathy	30 (zinc) Most rare	Dietary supplementation

differences in comorbidity and nutritional and lifestyle outcomes has made recommendations largely subjective. Some prospective randomised (ByBrand) and observational (ScOTS) studies are attempting to answer this [18]. There are early indications that some genetic or demographic factors may impact on clinical outcomes, such as gender, hormonal status (oestrogen) and age. In the future, matrices of measurable factors may guide selection [25].

Innovative procedures

Many surgical research groups attempt to improve outcomes by further developing existing surgical procedures or inventing new surgical concepts. These include minimally invasive approaches, such as altering stimulation of the foregut and endoscopic manipulation of the gastrointestinal tract. Autonomic innervation in relation to gut hormones is a focus of research, as is the study of gut microbiome. Anatomical manipulation with transposition of the ileum has been suggested as a future area of study, and appears to alter gut function and delay onset, or improve severity, of metabolic syndrome in rat models [38].

Audit

With the plethora of surgical innovations being used to combat obesity, it is increasingly important that we understand the cumulative outcomes of individual practitioners, institutions and organisations, and the breadth of procedures offered. Many organisations are developing extensive data collection tools. The National Bariatric Surgery Registry in the UK has already given reassurance about individual surgeons and national outcomes data, and the International Federation of Surgical Obesity is developing international databases, collecting similar information for comparison. Similarly, the American Society of Metabolic and Bariatric Surgery has developed the Bariatric Outcomes Longitudinal Database. Aligning and examining this information in centres of excellence worldwide will enable improved recommendations for future patients.

Much work is going on to examine the pathophysiological mechanisms that underlie the benefits of weight loss surgery. This includes work examining potential gut hormones and gut microbiome changes from surgery [39,40].

4.9.9 Summary box

> **Key points**
>
> - Weight loss surgical procedures have revolutionised the current management of severe and complicated obesity.
> - Laparoscopic gastric bypass with Roux-en-Y reconstruction, adjustable gastric band and sleeve gastrectomy are the most popular procedures worldwide.
> - Improved understanding of the mechanisms of action, patient selection and advances in techniques are making these interventions safer and more effective.
> - Further advances may improve outcomes and reveal new, less invasive options for patient management.

References

1. Ryan DH, Johnson WD, Myers VH, Prather TL, McGlone MM, Rood J, et al. Nonsurgical weight loss for extreme obesity in primary care settings: results of the Louisiana Obese Subjects Study. *Archives of Internal Medicine* 2010; **170**(2): 146–154.
2. Sjostrom L. Review of the key results from the Swedish Obese Subjects (SOS) trial a prospective controlled intervention study of bariatric surgery. *Journal of Internal Medicine* 2013; **273**(3): 219–234.
3. Dixon JB, O'Brien PE, Playfair J, Chapman L, Schachter LM, Skinner S, et al. Adjustable gastric banding and conventional therapy for type 2 diabetes: a randomized controlled trial. *JAMA* 2008; **299**(3): 316–323.
4. Schauer PR, Bhatt DL, Kirwan JP, Wolski K, Brethauer SA, Navaneethan SD, et al. Bariatric surgery versus intensive medical therapy for diabetes – 3-year outcomes. *The New England Journal of Medicine* 2014; **370**(21): 2002–2013.
5. Iossi MF, Konstantakos EK, Teel DD 2nd, Sherwood RJ, Laughlin RT, Coffey MJ, et al. Musculoskeletal function following bariatric surgery. *Obesity* 2013; **21**(6): 1104–1110.
6. Burton P, Brown W, Chen R, Shaw K, Packiyanathan A, Bringmann I, et al. Outcomes of high-volume bariatric surgery in the public system. *ANZ Journal of Surgery* 2016; **86**(7–8): 572–577.
7. van Huisstede A, Rudolphus A, Castro Cabezas M, Biter LU, van de Geijn GJ, Taube C, et al. Effect of bariatric surgery on

asthma control, lung function and bronchial and systemic inflammation in morbidly obese subjects with asthma. *Thorax* 2015; **70**(7): 659–667.

8. Casagrande DS, Rosa DD, Umpierre D, Sarmento RA, Rodrigues CG, Schaan BD. Incidence of cancer following bariatric surgery: systematic review and meta-analysis. *Obesity Surgery* 2014; **24**(9): 1499–1509.

9. Musella M, Milone M, Bellini M, Sosa Fernandez LM, Leongito M, Milone F. Effect of bariatric surgery on obesity-related infertility. *Surgery for Obesity and Related Diseases* 2012; **8**(4): 445–449.

10. Inge TH, Zeller MH, Jenkins TM, Helmrath M, Brandt ML, Michalsky MP, et al. Perioperative outcomes of adolescents undergoing bariatric surgery: the Teen-Longitudinal Assessment of Bariatric Surgery (Teen-LABS) study. *JAMA Pediatrics* 2014; **168**(1): 47–53.

11. Ackroyd R, Mouiel J, Chevallier JM, Daoud F. Cost-effectiveness and budget impact of obesity surgery in patients with type-2 diabetes in three European countries. *Obesity Surgery* 2006; **16**(11): 1488–1503.

12. Lakdawala M, Bhasker A, Asian Consensus Meeting on Metabolic Surgery (ACMOMS). Report: Asian Consensus Meeting on Metabolic Surgery. Recommendations for the use of bariatric and gastrointestinal metabolic surgery for treatment of obesity and type II diabetes mellitus in the Asian population: August 9th and 10th, 2008, Trivandrum, India. *Obesity Surgery* 2010; **20**(7): 929–936.

13. Mechanick JI, Youdim A, Jones DB, Timothy Garvey W, Hurley DL, Molly McMahon M, et al. Clinical practice guidelines for the perioperative nutritional, metabolic, and nonsurgical support of the bariatric surgery patient – 2013 update: cosponsored by American Association of Clinical Endocrinologists, the Obesity Society, and American Society for Metabolic & Bariatric Surgery. *Surgery for Obesity and Related Diseases* 2013; **9**(2): 159–191.

14. Pull CB. Current psychological assessment practices in obesity surgery programs: what to assess and why. *Current Opinion in Psychiatry* 2010; **23**(1): 30–36.

15. Haskins IN, Amdur R, Vaziri K. The effect of smoking on bariatric surgical outcomes. *Surgical Endoscopy* 2014; **28**(11): 3074–3080.

16. Brethauer S. ASMBS position statement on preoperative supervised weight loss requirements. *Surgery for Obesity and Related Diseases* 2011; **7**(3): 257–260.

17. Elliott JP, Gray EL, Yu J, Kalarchian MA. Medication use among patients prior to bariatric surgery. *Bariatric Surgical Practice and Patient Care* 2015; **10**(3): 105–109.

18. Colquitt JL, Pickett K, Loveman E, Frampton GK. Surgery for weight loss in adults. *Cochrane Database of Systematic Reviews* 2014; **8**: CD003641.

19. Winegar DA, Sherif B, Pate V, DeMaria EJ. Venous thromboembolism after bariatric surgery performed by Bariatric Surgery Center of Excellence Participants: analysis of the Bariatric Outcomes Longitudinal Database. *Surgery for Obesity and Related Diseases* 2011; **7**(2): 181–188.

20. Alvarenga ES, Lo Menzo E, Szomstein S, Rosenthal RJ. Safety and efficacy of 1020 consecutive laparoscopic sleeve gastrectomies performed as a primary treatment modality for morbid obesity. A single-center experience from the metabolic and bariatric surgical accreditation quality and improvement programme. *Surgical Endoscopy* 2016; **30**(7): 2673–2678.

21. Fridman A, Moon R, Cozacov Y, Ampudia C, Lo Menzo E, Szomstein S, et al. Procedure-related morbidity in bariatric surgery: a retrospective short- and mid-term follow-up of a single institution of the American College of Surgeons Bariatric Surgery Centers of Excellence. *Journal of the American College of Surgeons* 2013; **217**(4): 614–620.

22. Tack J, Deloose E. Complications of bariatric surgery: Dumping syndrome, reflux and vitamin deficiencies. *Best Practice & Research Clinical Gastroenterology* 2014; **28**(4): 741–749.

23. Moser F, Gorodner MV, Galvani CA, Baptista M, Chretien C, Horgan S. Pouch enlargement and band slippage: two different entities. *Surgical Endoscopy* 2006; **20**(7): 1021–1029.

24. Adams TD, Mehta TS, Davidson LE, Hunt SC. All-cause and cause-specific mortality associated with bariatric surgery: a review. *Current Atherosclerosis Reports* 2015; **17**(12): 74-015-0551-4.

25. Manning S, Carter NC, Pucci A, Jones A, Elkalaawy M, Cheung WH, et al. Age- and sex-specific effects on weight loss outcomes in a comparison of sleeve gastrectomy and Roux-en-Y gastric bypass: a retrospective cohort study. *BMC Obesity* 2014; **1**: 12-9538-1-12.

26. Sevilla S, Hubal MJ. Genetic modifiers of obesity and bariatric surgery outcomes. *Seminars in Pediatric Surgery* 2014; **23**(1): 43–48.

27. Rutledge R, Walsh TR. Continued excellent results with the mini-gastric bypass: six-year study in 2,410 patients. *Obesity Surgery* 2005; **15**(9): 1304–1308.

28. Ji Y, Wang Y, Zhu J, Shen D. A systematic review of gastric plication for the treatment of obesity. *Surgery for Obesity and Related Diseases* 2014; **10**(6): 1226–1232.

29. Fobi MA, Lee H, Felahy B, Che-Senge K, Fields CB, Sanguinette MC. Fifty consecutive patients with the GaBP ring system used in the banded gastric bypass operation for obesity with follow up of at least 1 year. *Surgery for Obesity and Related Diseases* 2005; **1**(6): 569–572.

30. Shimizu H, Annaberdyev S, Motamarry I, Kroh M, Schauer PR, Brethauer SA. Revisional bariatric surgery for unsuccessful weight loss and complications. *Obesity Surgery* 2013; **23**(11): 1766–1773.

31. O'Kane M, Pinkney J, Aasheim E, Barth J, Batterham R, Welbourn R. British Obesity and Metabolic Surgery Society – guidelines on perioperative and postoperative monitoring and micronutrient replacement for patients undergoing bariatric surgery, 2014. Available at: http://www.bomss.org.uk/wp-content/uploads/2014/09/BOMSS-guidelines-Final-version1Oct14.pdf, accessed 19 August 2016.

32. Halverson JD. Micronutrient deficiencies after gastric bypass for morbid obesity. *American Surgeon* 1986; **52**(11): 594–598.

33. Clements RH, Katasani VG, Palepu R, Leeth RR, Leath TD, Roy BP, et al. Incidence of vitamin deficiency after laparoscopic Roux-en-Y gastric bypass in a university hospital setting. *American Surgeon* 2006; **72**(12): 1196–202; discussion 1203–1204.

34. Boylan LM, Sugerman HJ, Driskell JA. Vitamin E, vitamin B-6, vitamin B-12, and folate status of gastric bypass surgery patients. *Journal of the American Dietetic Association* 1988; **88**(5): 579–585.

35. Xanthakos SA. Nutritional deficiencies in obesity and after bariatric surgery. Pediatric Clinics of North America 2009; **56**(5): 1105–1121.

36. Breiting LB, Lock-Andersen J, Matzen SH. Increased morbidity in patients undergoing abdominoplasty after laparoscopic gastric bypass. *Danish Medical Bulletin* 2011; **58**(4): A4251.

37. British Association of Plastic Reconstructive and Aesthetic Surgeons. Commissioning guide: massive weight loss body contouring, 2014. Available at: http://www.bapras.org.uk/docs/default-source/commissioning-and-policy/body-contouring-surgery-commissioning-guide-published.pdf?sfvrsn=0, accessed 18 August 2016.

38. Tam CS, Berthoud HR, Bueter M, Chakravarthy MV, Geliebter A, Hajnal A, et al. Could the mechanisms of bariatric surgery hold the key for novel therapies? Report from a Pennington Scientific Symposium. *Obesity Reviews* 2011; **12**(11): 984–994.

39. Cole AJ, Teigen LM, Jahansouz C, Earthman CP, Sibley SD. The influence of bariatric surgery on serum bile acids in humans and potential metabolic and hormonal implications: a systematic review. *Current Obesity Reports* 2015; **4**(4): 441–450.

40. Peat CM, Kleiman SC, Bulik CM, Carroll IM. The intestinal microbiome in bariatric surgery patients. *European Eating Disorders Review* 2015; **23**(6): 496–503.

41. Members of the Working Party, Nightingale CE, Margarson MP, Shearer E, Redman JW, Lucas DN, Cousins JM. Peri-operative management of the obese surgical patient 2015: Association of Anaesthetists of Great Britain and Ireland Society for Obesity and Bariatric Anaesthesia. *Anaesthesia* 2015; **70**(7): 859–876.

Chapter 4.10

Diet to support surgical management of weight loss

Mary O'Kane
Leeds Teaching Hospitals NHS Trust, Leeds, UK

4.10.1 Introduction

Lifestyle interventions including changes in eating behaviour, energy intake and physical activity are key components in weight management for the morbidly obese adult patient. Bariatric surgery too is a treatment option, provided certain criteria are met (Box 4.10.1) [1].

There are a number of considerations when determining whether bariatric surgery is an appropriate treatment option for the individual. These include the degree of obesity, comorbidities and psychological and social factors, alongside the benefits and risks of surgery. Nutrition is affected by surgery, and it is essential that patients have a comprehensive nutritional assessment. Positive changes in lifestyle are still required to obtain optimum results following bariatric surgery.

The current bariatric procedures include the adjustable gastric band (AGB), Roux-en-Y gastric bypass (RYGB), sleeve gastrectomy (SG) and duodenal switch (DS). Within the UK and Ireland, the most common surgical procedure reported by the National Bariatric Surgery Registry [2] is RYGB (52.3% of all operations in 2011–2013), followed by AGB (22.4%) and SG (20.9%).

4.10.2 Preoperative assessment and preparation for surgery

A comprehensive assessment by the bariatric multidisciplinary team (MDT) is essential, and the dietitian, as a core member, plays a lead role in this. All surgical procedures affect the volume of food consumed and, therefore, the diet and nutritional content. The absorption of micronutrients and/or macronutrients may be affected, increasing the risk of nutritional deficiencies [3,4,5]. Surgery may lead to deterioration in eating patterns and nutritional status [6,7].

Box 4.10.1   Criteria for bariatric surgery, NICE CG 189: obesity [1]

Bariatric surgery is recommended as a treatment option for people with obesity if all the following criteria are fulfilled:

- They have a BMI of 40 kg/m² or more; or a BMI of 35–40 kg/m² along with other significant diseases (e.g. type 2 diabetes or high blood pressure) that could be improved if they lost weight.
- All appropriate nonsurgical measures have been tried, but the person has not achieved or maintained adequate, clinically beneficial weight loss.
- The person has been receiving or will receive intensive management in a tier 3 service.
- The person is generally fit for anaesthesia and surgery.
- The person commits to the need for long-term follow-up.

Advanced Nutrition and Dietetics in Obesity, First Edition. Edited by Catherine Hankey.
© 2018 John Wiley & Sons Ltd. Published 2018 by John Wiley & Sons Ltd.

Weight and dieting history

To be eligible for surgery, patients must have exhausted all nonsurgical methods to lose weight [1]. Most patients report many dieting attempts but failure to maintain the lower weight [8]. Those who have never attempted to lose weight may be ill-prepared for the dietary and lifestyle modifications required following surgery [9]. They may need further support to make dietary and lifestyle changes before going forward.

Dietary and nutritional assessment

The specialist dietitian will explore eating behaviour and the patient's ability to manage the postoperative dietary changes. Many obese patients feel ashamed of their failed weight loss attempts [9] and are more likely to under-report food intake and over-report energy expenditure than lean people [10]. The dietitian will assess patients' eating patterns, regularity of meals, grazing, favourite foods, food cravings, emotional cues and triggers for eating. The impact of surgery on eating behaviour will be discussed alongside the postoperative diet. Current alcohol misuse is seen as a contraindication for surgery [11].

The nutritional assessment may reveal pre-existing nutritional deficiencies that will be further exacerbated by the bariatric surgery [4,12,13,14]. Nutritional deficiencies must be corrected prior to surgery [12]. The risk of nutritional problems following surgery and the need to comply with postoperative dietary advice and follow-up should be emphasised.

Eating disorders

Screening for eating disorders such as binge eating disorder, night eating syndrome and bulimia nervosa is important. For patients with binge eating disorder or night eating syndrome, consideration should be given as to whether they need specialist support, as it may affect the ability to comply with the postoperative diet [11]. Bariatric surgery in patients with active bulimia nervosa is contraindicated because of the high risk of vomiting [9], and specialist help is recommended.

Social and psychological factors

The patient's social environment should also be considered as part of the overall assessment. Unfortunately, some patients have limited cooking skills, or state that they have little time to prepare or cook meals. Patients need to consider how they will manage the postoperative diet and potential barriers.

Preoperative courses that discuss the various surgical procedures, the impact on food and eating behaviours and the psychological implications have been found to be of value [15]. Many find it helpful to attend bariatric surgery patient support groups.

Knowledge of bariatric surgery and expectations

The patient's expectations and level of understanding of bariatric surgery need to be explored. Those who have attended preoperative weight management programmes are more likely to be prepared, in contrast to those who have little knowledge or who have gained information via media sources. The dietetic interview is an opportunity to discuss the surgical procedures, impacts on diet and lifestyle and the need for regular follow-up. Expectations about the weight loss achieved by surgery should also be discussed, as the purpose is to reduce excess weight and improve comorbidities rather than achieve a BMI of 25 kg/m^2. Weight regain is possible after all procedures. Written information and contact details should be provided, along with opportunities to ask further questions.

Preoperative diet/'liver shrinking' diet

Many bariatric surgery centres require patients to follow a strict preoperative low-energy diet to decrease the liver volume and intra-abdominal fat [16]. There is no consensus as to the type of diet or the length of time needed prior to surgery [17]. However, this period can be used as a time for the patient, along with the family, to prepare for the bariatric surgery.

4.10.3 Postoperative dietary intervention

Postoperative dietary intervention depends on the nature of the bariatric surgery performed (Box 4.10.2).

All surgical procedures require a phased introduction to foods and textures. Initially, a liquid diet will be recommended, followed by a pureed diet, soft foods and then progressing to normal food textures. The rate of progression will depend on the surgical procedure and the recommendations of the bariatric centres.

Liquid diet

Following surgery, patients initially commence on clear fluids for 1–2 days before progressing to nourishing fluids such as milk, yoghurt, liquid meal replacement and fortified soup. Liquids should be sipped slowly over the day. This may be for a couple of days only, although many centres do recommend longer times. For SG, a minimum of 2 weeks is usually advised because of the greater risk of anastomotic leaks. There may be a small risk of secondary lactose intolerance, and patients would need to be advised accordingly. Carbonated drinks should be avoided.

Pureed/blended diet

Patients are advised to progress to pureed/blended foods, keeping portions small (1–2 tablespoons per meal). Small, frequent meals and nourishing fluids are encouraged. Drinks and meals must be taken separately, and a gap of 30–45 min is recommended. Care should be taken to ensure that there is adequate protein intake. This phase may continue for 2–3 weeks.

Soft diet

During the soft phase, patients should be encouraged to further expand the range of food and textures. Meat and poultry should be moist and tender – for example, slow-cooked casseroles and stews. Fish may need to be served with a sauce. Cheese, eggs, beans, pulses, quorn and tofu are suitable soft protein sources. Many starch sources such as pasta, rice and bread may be difficult for patients to tolerate initially.

Patients need to be reminded to keep the portions small, and to eat slowly.

Gradually, over a few weeks, portions will start to slowly increase. Melba toast, crisp breads, crackers and, eventually, toasted bread can be introduced. The expansion in food groups enables the patient to return to a balanced diet and develop a regular meal

---

Box 4.10.2 Bariatric surgical approaches

Adjustable gastric band
This involves the placement of a band around the upper part of the stomach (Figure 4.10.1a). The band is inflated or deflated by injecting or withdrawing fluid via a port. The first band adjustment will take place 4–8 weeks after surgery. Care must be taken to not overinflate the band, else dysphagia will result.

Roux-en-Y gastric bypass
A small gastric pouch is created and a section of the small intestine attached to the pouch bypassing the stomach, duodenum and part of the jejunum (Figure 4.10.1b). This procedure impacts on the absorption of iron, calcium, vitamin D and vitamin B_{12} [3–4,12].

Sleeve gastrectomy
A sleeve is created by stapling along the lesser curvature of the stomach and removing the outer section of stomach (Figure 4.10.1c). Absorption is less likely to be affected compared with the gastric bypass.

Duodenal switch
This may be done as a one stage or two stage procedure. A sleeve gastrectomy is performed and then a large section of the small intestine bypassed leaving 50–100 cm common channel for absorption (Figure 4.10.1d). There is malabsorption of protein, fat, calcium, fat soluble vitamins and zinc [5].

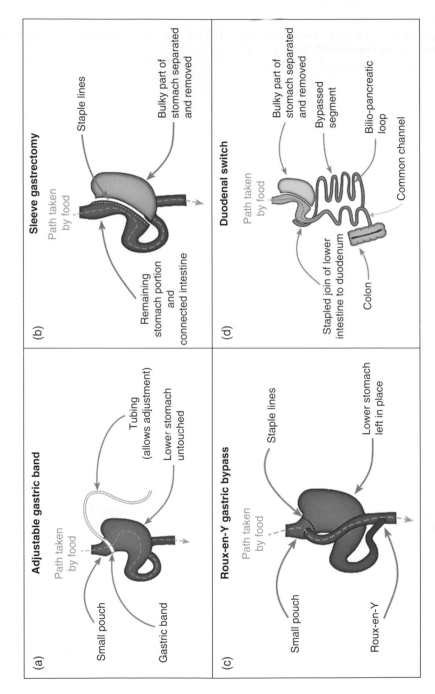

Figure 4.10.1 Bariatric surgical approaches. Diagrams reproduced with permission from Dendrite and NBSR Committee.

pattern. Support may be needed to help with menu planning, especially when the patient returns to work or is away from home.

The importance of chewing food and eating slowly cannot be overemphasised. Some patients struggle with the phased approach, choosing food textures that are inappropriate for that stage. This may result in the food becoming lodged in the gastric pouch, causing discomfort, followed by regurgitation or vomiting. Patients may then become reluctant to try new foods and choose soft foods or liquids of poor nutritional content [18]. This is likely to result in nutritional deficiencies and/or poor weight loss results. Patients who self-reported that they had adhered to the postoperative dietary advice as directed by the dietitian experienced a greater weight loss than those who said they had not [19].

4.10.4 Impact of bariatric surgery on nutrition

All bariatric surgical procedures impact on nutrition. This may be by altering the volume and type of food eaten, or by affecting absorption [3–7,12], and thus increasing the risk of nutritional deficiencies. A survey of current practice of members of the British Obesity and Metabolic Surgery Society (BOMSS) found variation in preoperative nutritional screening, postoperative nutritional monitoring and recommendations regarding vitamin and mineral supplements [20], following which the BOMSS guidelines on preoperative and postoperative biochemical monitoring and micronutrient replacement for patients undergoing bariatric surgery were developed [21]. These guidelines give practical guidance around long-term nutritional monitoring and vitamin and mineral supplementation. Table 4.10.1 summarises the main recommendations for nutritional monitoring and micronutrient supplementation. The SurgiCal Obesity Treatment Study (SCOTS) includes the monitoring of nutritional parameters over 10 years, and will provide valuable information [22].

Protein

Adequate protein intake can be difficult to achieve postoperatively [12,19,23]. DS results in additional protein requirements because of malabsorption. A protein intake of 60 g/day should be the target following gastric bypass, and 90 g/day following DS [12,23]. The risk of protein energy malnutrition is greatest following DS. An emphasis on proteins may also help prevent weight regain in the longer term, but the diet should still include complex carbohydrates to prevent loss of muscle mass [24].

Calcium and vitamin D

RYGB and DS increase the risk of calcium and vitamin D deficiency [4,5,12,23,25,26]. This may result in secondary hyperparathyroidism and, eventually, metabolic bone disease [26]. Low vitamin D and increased parathyroid hormone (PTH) levels have been reported in SG patients [27]. Vitamin D deficiency should be corrected prior to surgery and monitored postoperatively. The National Osteoporosis Society's guidelines document, titled 'Vitamin D and bone health: A practical clinical guideline for patient management', contains practical recommendations for vitamin D replacement in primary care [28]. There is ongoing debate about the levels of calcium and vitamin D supplementation required following surgery, but it is acknowledged that the monitoring of calcium, vitamin D and PTH levels following RYGB, SG and DS is essential [5,12,23,26].

Iron, folate and vitamin B_{12}

Patients may struggle to tolerate red meat, thereby reducing iron intake. As iron is mainly absorbed in the duodenum and proximal jejunum, absorption is reduced following RYGB, SG and DS, and the risk of iron deficiency anaemia increases [3,5,12,20,23,27,29]. Additional iron supplementation is needed, especially in women of menstruating age.

Poor folate status has been reported following AGB, SG and RYGB [30–32]. This may indicate a low-folate diet or noncompliance with vitamin and mineral supplements.

Vitamin B_{12} absorption requires the intrinsic factor, secreted by the gastric parietal cells, and so vitamin B_{12} levels are decreased following RYGB [12,23,29,31]. There are variable reports of vitamin B_{12} deficiency in SG [27,32]. Vitamin B_{12} deficiency

Table 4.10.1 Nutritional monitoring and vitamin and mineral supplements following bariatric surgery

Surgical procedure and monitoring/supplements	Biochemical monitoring	AGB	SG, RYGB, DS
Vitamin and mineral supplements (complete, containing water- and fat-soluble vitamins, iron, zinc, copper and selenium)		One daily	One to two daily
Iron and folate	Monitor ferritin and folate levels	Within vitamin and mineral supplements	Additional iron recommended, providing 45–60 mg iron. 100 mg iron recommended for menstruating women
Vitamin B$_{12}$	Monitor vitamin B$_{12}$ levels in SG, RYGB, DS	Should not need additional vitamin B$_{12}$	Three monthly intramuscular vitamin B$_{12}$ injections
Calcium and vitamin D	Monitor calcium, vitamin D and PTH levels	Continue with maintenance doses of calcium and vitamin D as identified preoperatively	Continue with maintenance doses of calcium and vitamin D as identified preoperatively. Treat and adjust vitamin D supplementation to maintain serum vitamin D levels in line with National Osteoporosis Society guidelines. Patients are likely to be on at least 800 mg calcium and 20 µg vitamin D. Additional vitamin D supplementation is likely to be required for DS
Vitamin A	Monitor vitamin A in DS and RYGB patients in case of severe malabsorption	Contained within vitamin and mineral supplements	Contained within vitamin and mineral supplements. Consider additional fat-soluble vitamin supplementation for DS
Zinc, copper and selenium	Monitor zinc and copper in RYGB, SG and DS. Monitor selenium in unexplained anaemia, metabolic bone disease or cardiomyopathy	Contained within vitamin and mineral supplements	Contained within vitamin and mineral supplements. If additional zinc required, ensure ratio of 8–15 mg of zinc per mg of copper
Thiamine		Sufficiently contained in multivitamins and minerals; however, if patient experiences prolonged vomiting, always prescribe additional thiamine (200–300 mg daily, vitamin B compound strong, one or two tablets, three times a day), and urgent referral to a bariatric centre.	Sufficiently contained in multivitamins and minerals; however, if patient experiences prolonged vomiting, always prescribe additional thiamine (200–300 mg daily, vitamin B compound strong, one or two tablets, three times a day), and urgent referral to a bariatric centre

Adapted from reference [21].

results in megaloblastic anaemia and peripheral neuropathy. Oral supplementation with vitamin B_{12} following RYGB may not be sufficient to prevent vitamin B_{12} deficiency, and intramuscular vitamin B_{12} injections are recommended [33]. Vitamin B_{12} concentrations should be monitored, and patients should receive supplementation as appropriate. However, postoperative nutritional monitoring may not be as robust as it should be, so vitamin B_{12} supplementation is recommended following SG and DS [31]. Vitamin B_{12} deficiency should be excluded as a cause of megaloblastic anaemia before giving additional folate supplements.

Vitamins A, E and K

The risk of vitamin A deficiency in patients following DS is increased as a result of fat malabsorption [5,25]. Although the risk of vitamin A deficiency is small following RYGB, poor vitamin A status has been reported [34]. Poor vitamin K status has been reported in patients following DS [35]. Routine screening for vitamin A deficiency is recommended following DS [23], with higher doses of fat-soluble vitamins provided in a water-soluble form to aid absorption [12]. For other procedures, multivitamin and mineral supplements should be sufficient.

Thiamine

Thiamine deficiency leading to Wernicke's encephalopathy has been reported following bariatric surgery [36]. Causes included poor dietary intake, prolonged vomiting and noncompliance with vitamin and mineral supplements. Healthcare professionals need to be aware of the risk of thiamine deficiency and should treat with additional thiamine.

Zinc, copper and selenium

Routine screening for zinc deficiency is recommended following RYGB and DS, especially if there are symptoms of zinc deficiency [23]. Zinc supplementation is routinely recommended following DS, but not RYGB. As zinc and copper share a common absorption pathway, over-supplementation with zinc will affect copper and *vice versa* [37], so the supplements must contain the appropriate copper–zinc ratio

[23]. There is insufficient evidence to support routine screening for selenium status, but deficiency should be considered if there are specific conditions such as persistent diarrhoea or unexplained anaemia [23].

Managing weight regain

Although many patients achieve significant weight loss following bariatric surgery, a small minority will have inadequate weight loss or even weight regain [38]. In the Swedish Obesity Surgery (SOS) study, in which patients had a gastric band, vertical banded gastroplasty or gastric bypass, the average weight loss at 12 months was 25.3% [38]. After 10 years, the average weight loss was 16%. There was variability in the weight loss results, ranging from around 12% who lost more than 30% of their initial body weight, to 9% who had gained weight. The SOS is not a randomised control trial, so it is not possible to decide which surgical procedure may result in optimum weight loss and weight maintenance. For this reason, a multicentre trial that randomises patients to gastric band, gastric bypass or sleeve gastrectomy is being undertaken [39].

Weight regain is disheartening for patients, whether they have had surgery or not. In surgical patients, factors include dietary noncompliance and maladaptive eating [18–19]. Patients who self-reported that they had complied with the dietary advice had greater weight loss and less regain [19]. Those patients who had a higher baseline level of cognitive restraint had better outcomes, suggesting that the ability to restrict food before surgery may be a predictor of the ability to follow the postoperative diet. Good postoperative dietetic intervention was found to help patients make positive changes in eating behaviours [40]. In the National Control Weight Registry, Bond et al. compared the weight loss between nonsurgical and surgical methods [41]. Both groups had managed to lose around 56 kg and experienced the same amount of weight regain; however, those who had surgery reported a higher-fat diet and were less physically active. Kalarchian et al. randomised patients who were more than 3 years post-surgery, and had less than 50% excess weight loss, to a behavioural intervention or a wait-list control group [42]. This pilot study suggested that ongoing support with weight management following surgery was of benefit. Patients need continued support and behavioural interventions following surgery to aid weight maintenance.

4.10.5 Conclusion

The dietitian has a key role is assessing patients preoperatively, in preparing them for surgery and in supporting them to make the appropriate lifestyle modifications postoperatively. There is a risk of maladaptive eating and nutritional deficiencies, and patients need continued dietetic support and nutritional monitoring following surgery. When accompanied with positive changes in behavioural and lifestyle changes, bariatric surgery is an effective treatment option.

4.10.6 Summary box

Key points

- A comprehensive assessment by the bariatric multidisciplinary team is essential, and the dietitian, as a core member, plays a lead role in this.
- Bariatric surgery impacts on dietary and nutritional intake. The dietitian plays a key role in educating and supporting the patient to ensure a good nutritional intake and avoidance of maladaptive eating.
- The gastric bypass, sleeve gastrectomy and duodenal switch adversely affect the absorption of micronutrients. The duodenal switch also impacts on the absorption of proteins and fats.
- Patients require lifelong nutritional supplements and nutritional monitoring postoperatively.
- Patients need support with behavioural changes and weight maintenance after bariatric surgery.

References

1. National Institute for Health and Clinical Excellence. NICE CG189 Obesity: identification, assessment and management, 2014. Internet: https://www.nice.org.uk/guidance/cg189.
2. Welbourn R, Sarela A, Small P, Somers S, Finlay A, Mahawar K. National Bariatric Surgery Registry of The British Obesity and Metabolic Surgery Society Second Registry Report, 2014. Henley on Thames: Dendrite Clinical Systems Limited. Internet: http://nbsr.co.uk/2014-report/.
3. Malone M, Alger-Mayer S, Lindstrom J, Bailie JR. Management of iron deficiency and anaemia after Roux-en-Y gastric bypass surgery: an observational study. Surgery for Obesity and Related Diseases 2013; 9: 969–974.
4. Carlin AM, Rao S, Meslemani AM, Genaw JA, Parikhb NJ, Levy S, et al. Prevalence of Vitamin D depletion amongst morbidly obese patients seeking gastric bypass surgery. Surgery for Obesity and Related Diseases 2006; 2(2): 98–103.
5. Dolan K, Hatzifotis M, Newbury L, Lowe N, Fielding G. A clinical and nutritional comparison of biliopancreatic diversion with and without duodenal switch. Annals of Surgery 2004; 240: 51–56.
6. Lindroos AK, Lissner L, Sjostrom L. Weight change in relation to intake of sugar and sweet foods before and after weight reducing gastric surgery. International Journal of Obesity and Related Metabolic Disorders 1996; 20: 634–643.
7. Näslund I, Järnmark I, Andersson H. Dietary intake before and after gastric bypass and gastroplasty for morbid obesity in women. International Journal of Obesity 1988; 12: 503–513.
8. Gibbons LM, Sarwer DB, Crerand CE, Fabricatore AN, Kuehnel RH, Lipschutz PE, et al. Previous weight loss experiences of bariatric surgery candidates: how much have patients dieted prior to surgery? Obesity 2006; 14 (3):70S–75S.
9. Wadden TA, Sarwer DB. Behavioural assessment of candidates for bariatric surgery: a patient-oriented approach. Obesity 2006; 14: 53S–62S.
10. Prentice AM, Black AE, Coward WA, Davies HL, Goldberg GR, Murgatroyd PR, et al. High levels of energy expenditure in obese women. BMJ 1986; 292: 983–987.
11. Stevens T, Spavin S, Scholtz S, McClelland L. Your patient and weight loss surgery. Advances in Psychiatric Treatment 2012; 18: 418–425.
12. Aills L, Blankenship J, Buffington C, Furtado M, Parrott J. ASMBS allied health nutritional guidelines for the surgical weight loss patient. Surgery for Obesity and Related Diseases 2008; 4(5): S73–S108.
13. Bates B, Lennox A, Prentice A, Bates CSG. National Diet and Nutrition Survey, London. Headline results from years 1, 2 and 3 (combined) of the rolling programme (2008/2009–2010/11) 2013: Department of Health and the Food Standards Agency. Internet: https://www.gov.uk/government/statistics/national-diet-and-nutrition-survey-headline-results-from-years-1-2-and-3-combined-of-the-rolling-programme-200809-201011, accessed 12 January 2016.
14. Hypponen E, Power C. Vitamin D status and glucose homeostasis in the 1958 British Birth Cohort. Diabetes Care 2006; 29: 2244–2246.
15. Giusti V, De Lucia A, Di Vetta V, Calmes JM, Héraïef E, Gaillard RC, Burckhardt P, Suter M. Impact of preoperative teaching on surgical option of patients qualifying for bariatric surgery. Obesity Surgery 2004; 14: 1241–1246.
16. Fris RJ. Preoperative low energy diet diminishes liver size. Obesity Surgery 2004; 14: 1165–1170.
17. Baldry EL, Leeder PC, Idris IR. Pre-operative dietary restriction for patients undergoing bariatric surgery in the UK: observational study of current practice and dietary effects. Obesity Surgery 2014; 24(3): 416–421.

18. Sarwer DB, Dilks RJ, West-Smith L. Dietary intake and eating behaviour after bariatric surgery: threats to weight loss maintenance and strategies for success. *Surgery for Obesity and Related Diseases* 2011; **7**(5): 644–651.

19. Sarwer DB, Wadden TA, Moore RH, Baker AW, Gibbons LM, Raper SE, et al. Preoperative eating behaviour, postoperative dietary adherence, and weight loss after gastric bypass surgery. *Surgery for Obesity and Related Diseases* 2008; **4**(5): 640–646.

20. O'Kane M. Bariatric surgery, vitamins, minerals and nutritional monitoring: a survey of current practice within BOMSS [M.Sc. dissertation]. Leeds: Leeds Metropolitan University, 2013.

21. O'Kane M, Pinkney J, Aasheim E, Barth J, Batterham R, Welbourn R. BOMSS guidelines on perioperative and postoperative biochemical monitoring and micronutrient replacement for patients undergoing bariatric surgery 2014. Internet: http://www.bomss.org.uk/bomss-nutritional-guidance/, accessed 12 January 2016.

22. Logue J. Surgical obesity treatment study. Available from: http://www.nets.nihr.ac.uk/projects/hta/104202.

23. Mechanick JI, Youdim A, Jones DB, Garvey WT, Hurley DL, McMahon MM, et al. Clinical practice guidelines for the perioperative nutritional, metabolic, and nonsurgical support of the bariatric surgery patient – 2013 update: cosponsored by the American Association of Clinical Endocrinologist, The Obesity Society, and American Society for Metabolic and Bariatric Surgery. *Surgery for Obesity and Related Diseases* 2013; **9**(2): 159–191.

24. Faria SL, Faria OP, Buffington C, Cardeal MdeA, Ito MK. Dietary protein intake and bariatric surgery patients: a review. *Obesity Surgery* 2011; **21**: 1798–1805.

25. Søvik TT, Aasheim ET, Taha O, Engstrom M, Fagerland MW, Bjorkman S, et al. Weight loss, cardiovascular risk factors, and quality of life after gastric bypass and duodenal switch. *Annals of Internal Medicine* 2011; **155**: 281–291.

26. Heber D, Greenway FI, Kaplan LM, Livingston E, Salvador J, Still C. Endocrine and nutritional management of the post-bariatric surgery patient: an endocrine society clinical practice guideline. *Journal of Clinical Endocrinology and Metabolism* 2010; **95**(11): 4823–4843.

27. Aarts EO, Janssen IMC, Berends FJ. The gastric sleeve: losing weight as fast as micronutrients? *Obesity Surgery* 2011; **21**: 207–211.

28. Francis R, Aspray T, Fraser W, Gittoes N, Javaid K, MacDonald H, et al. Vitamin D and bone health: a practical clinical guideline for patient management. National Osteoporosis Society [Internet], 2013. Available from: http://www.nos.org.uk/document.doc?id=1352, accessed 12 January 2016.

29. Cable CT, Colbert CY, Showalter T, Ahluwalia R, Song J, Whitfield P, et al. Prevalence of anaemia after Roux-en-Y gastric bypass surgery: what is the right number? *Surgery for Obesity and Related Diseases* 2011; **7**(2): 134–139.

30. Gasteyger C, Suter M, Calmes JM, Gaillard RC, Giustiet V. Changes in body composition, metabolic profile and nutritional status 24 months after gastric banding. *Obesity Surgery* 2006; **16**(3): 243–250.

31. Gudzune KA, Huizinga MM, Chang H-Y, Asamoah V, Gadgil M, Clarke JM. Screening and diagnosis of micronutrient deficiencies before and after bariatric surgery. *Obesity Surgery* 2013; **23**(10): 1581–1589.

32. Saif T, Strain GW, Dakin G, Gagner M, Costa R, Pomp A. Evaluation of nutrient status after laparoscopic sleeve gastrectomy 1, 3, and 5 years after surgery. *Surgery for Obesity and Related Diseases* 2012; **8**(5): 542–547.

33. Majumder S, Soriano J, Cruz AL, Dasanu CA. Vitamin B$_{12}$ deficiency in patients undergoing bariatric surgery: Preventive strategies and key recommendations. *Surgery for Obesity and Related Diseases* 2013; **9**: 1013–1019.

34. Eckert MJ, Perry JT, Sohn VY, Boden J, Martin M, Rush RM, et al. Incidence of low vitamin A levels and ocular symptoms after Roux-en-Y gastric bypass. *Surgery for Obesity and Related Diseases* 2010; **6**(6): 653–657.

35. Slater GH, Ren CJ, Siegel N, Williams T, Barr D, Wolfe B, et al. Serum fat-soluble vitamin deficiency and abnormal calcium metabolism after malabsorptive bariatric surgery. *Journal of Gastrointestinal Surgery* 2004; **8**(1): 48–55.

36. Aasheim ET. Wernicke encephalopathy after bariatric surgery. *Annals of Surgery* 2008; **248**: 714–720.

37. Rowin R, Lewis SL. Copper deficiency myeloneuropathy and pancytopenia secondary to overuse of zinc supplementation. *Journal of Neurology, Neurosurgery, and Psychiatry* 2005; **76**: 750–751.

38. Karlsson J, Taft C, Rydén A, Sjostrom L, Sullivan M. Ten-year trends in health-related quality of life after surgical and conventional treatment for severe obesity: the SOS intervention study. *International Journal of Obesity* 2007; **31**: 1248–1261.

39. Rogers CA, Welbourn R, Byrne J, Donovan JL, Reeves BC, Wordsworth S, et al. The by-band study: gastric bypass or adjustable gastric band surgery to treat morbid obesity: study protocol for a multi-centre randomised controlled trial with an internal pilot phase. *Trials* 2014; **15**: 53.

40. Sarwer DB, Moore RH, Spitzer JC, Wadden TA, Raper SE, Williams NN. A pilot study investigating the efficacy of postoperative dietary counselling to improve outcomes after bariatric surgery. *Surgery for Obesity and Related Diseases* 2012; **8**: 561–568.

41. Bond DS, Phelan S, Leahey TM, Hill JO, Wing RR. Weight-loss maintenance in successful weight losers: surgical vs. non-surgical methods. *International Journal of Obesity* 2009; **33**: 173–180.

42. Kalarchian MA, Marcus M, Courcoulas AP, Cheng y, Levine MD, Josbeno D. Optimizing long-term weight control after bariatric surgery: a pilot study. *Surgery for Obesity and Related Diseases* 2012; **8**: 710–716.

Chapter 4.11

Physical activity for weight loss in obesity

Mark Hopkins[1], Catherine Gibbons[2] and Neil A King[3]
[1] Leeds Beckett University, Leeds, UK
[2] University of Leeds, Leeds, UK
[3] Queensland University of Technology, Brisbane, Australia

4.11.1 Introduction

Physical activity (PA) is a commonly prescribed means of promoting weight loss in overweight and obese individuals. Increased levels of daily PA can create a negative energy imbalance, which, if maintained over a prolonged period, will result in weight loss. However, the efficacy of PA to promote meaningful and sustained weight loss has been questioned, potentially undermining the important role that PA can (and should) play in obesity management [1]. However, effective obesity management should not simply focus on body weight. This misconception in part stems from a failure to disassociate the independent health benefits of regular PA from changes in body weight, with weight loss often mistakenly perceived as the only reason for promoting PA. Recent guidelines by the American College of Sports Medicine (ACSM; Table 4.11.1) indicate that differing levels of PA are needed to prevent initial weight gain, elicit weight loss and prevent weight regain, and these differences must be recognised when prescribing PA for weight management [2]. These issues are further complicated by recent findings demonstrating that exercise-induced weight loss is characterised by a high degree of inter-individual variability, and compensatory changes in the energy balance system can attenuate exercise-induced increases in total daily energy expenditure (TDEE). As such, this chapter will provide a current overview of the positive role that PA can play in obesity management. Particular attention will be given to the individual variability in exercise-induced weight loss, as well as the compensatory adjustments in energy balance that mediate the propensity for weight loss, as this is vital for a more complete understanding of the relationship between PA and body weight.

4.11.2 Physical activity and weight gain

In many countries, governments and health agencies are strongly promoting PA as a means to prevent the accumulation of fatness that leads to weight gain and obesity. However, there is often a resistance to respond to health promotion initiatives. For example, in the UK, the Chief Medical Officer has recently reported that 71% of women and 61% of men fail to carry out even the minimal amount of PA recommended in the government's guidelines. However, whether the current rates of obesity are primarily driven by decreased PA or increased energy intake (EI) has been debated [3–5]. Recently, it has been argued that increased EI is the key driver [6,7], as PA has remained unchanged since the 1980s [8,6]. It has been suggested that an 'energy gap' of approximately 50 kcal/day (the imbalance between total daily energy intake and expenditure) can explain the average 1 kg/year increase in body weight seen in adult Americans over the last decade [9]. However, inaccuracies inherent to the measurement of PA and EI at the population level mean that this energy gap is likely much larger, with the gap between normal weight and obese individuals likely

Advanced Nutrition and Dietetics in Obesity, First Edition. Edited by Catherine Hankey.
© 2018 John Wiley & Sons Ltd. Published 2018 by John Wiley & Sons Ltd.

Table 4.11.1 ACSM physical activity recommendations for weight management and the level of evidence (NHLBI) for each statement. Adapted from reference [2]

Aim	Recommended level of PA	NHLBI evidence category	Evidence statement
PA to prevent weight gain	150–250 min/week (1200–2000 kcal/week).	A	PA level will prevent excessive weight gain (>3%) in most adults.
PA for weight loss	<150 min/week promotes minimal weight loss. 150–250 min/week results in modest weight loss of approximately 2–3 kg. >225–420 min/week results in approximately 5–7.5 kg weight loss.	B	A clear dose–response relationship exists for weight loss.
PA for weight maintenance after weight loss	Approximately 200–300 min/week during weight maintenance to reduce weight regain after weight loss.	B	While a dose–response relationship appears to exist, there is a lack of appropriate studies to provide evidence for the amount of PA to prevent weight regain.
Resistance training (RT) for weight loss	Evidence does not support RT as effective for weight loss with or without diet restriction.	B	Limited evidence that RT promotes gain or maintenance of lean mass and loss of body fat during energy restriction. Some evidence that RT improves chronic disease risk factors (HDL-C, LDL-C, insulin, blood pressure).

PA, physical activity; ACSM, American College of Sports Medicine; NHLBI, National Heart, Lung, and Blood Institute; RT, resistance training; HDL-C, high-density lipoprotein cholesterol; LDL-C, low-density lipoprotein cholesterol.

to be in the range of 300–1500 kcal/day [10]. Notwithstanding this, the promotion of PA at the individual and population level would seem a viable approach to obesity management, as PA is a readily modifiable component of energy balance that accounts for approximately 30% of TDEE in sedentary individuals [11]. Unfortunately, the complexities in both human behaviour and the biological regulation of body weight can confound this approach. While the psychological benefits and barriers to PA have been discussed elsewhere [12], it is important that the interplay between PA and the physiological regulation of energy balance be discussed if the role of PA in obesity management is to be fully understood.

4.11.3 The impact of physical activity on energy balance

The basic assumption made when prescribing increased PA for weight loss is that the associated increase in energy expenditure will create a negative energy imbalance and lead to weight loss. However, this assumes a static energy balance system in which the individual components of energy balance are rigid. In fact, the regulation of energy balance is a dynamic and integrated process, where components interact in a coordinated fashion and can compensate for perturbations elsewhere in the system [13]. For example, an increase in energy expenditure via PA could produce compensatory changes in EI or non-exercise PA, while changes in EI may influence TDEE through changes in daily PA levels. The need for such flexibility becomes apparent when the variability in day-to-day EI, which can vary by as much as 100%, is considered [14]. Indeed, on a daily or short-term basis, the energy state of the body is constantly fluctuating between periods of positive and negative energy imbalance; yet, body weight remains relatively stable in most individuals over time [15]. Therefore, when an acute exercise-induced increase in energy expenditure is considered in the context of this changeable internal environment, it should not be assumed that TDEE will simply increase in a linear fashion relative to the exercise-induced energy expenditure (ExEE).

The integrated nature of this dynamic regulatory system must be considered when examining the evidence relating to PA and obesity management. The efficacy of exercise for weight loss has been extensively reviewed, with a weight loss of approximately 1.5–3 kg typically reported [16]. Importantly, the observed weight loss is often below that theoretically expected, based on objective measures of ExEE. In such cases, expected weight loss is predicted using objectively measured ExEE, body composition and the energy equivalents of tissue composition. As such, adherence (or the lack of it) cannot explain any differences between actual and predicted weight loss. Indeed, Borer (2008) suggests that, when performed

without dietary restriction, a daily ExEE of 400 kcal produces body fat losses equivalent to approximately one-third of that predicted [17]. This indicates partial compensation in one or more components of the energy balance system that limits perturbations to stored energy and body weight.

4.11.4 Individual variability: biological and behavioural compensatory responses

Until recently, compensation to exercise was not explored, with poor adherence commonly cited as a causal factor for the lower-than-expected weight loss. Findings have revealed marked inter-individual variability in the body weight response to acute [18,19] and medium-term exercise interventions, which cannot be explained by differences in adherence or ExEE [20–23]. For example, Barwell et al. (2009) reported that, following 7 weeks of aerobic exercise in sedentary women, changes in fat mass ranged from −5.3 to +2.1 kg [21]. Differences in ExEE accounted for 36% of this variance, but large variability still existed in the residual changes in fat mass when ExEE was accounted for (Figure 4.11.1). While it is intuitive that individuals will not respond in the same way to exercise (even under conditions of high compliance), this notion has not been reflected

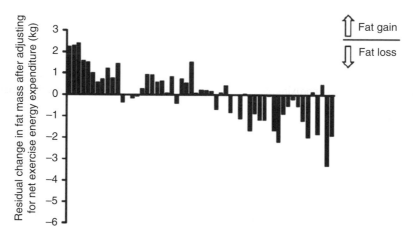

Figure 4.11.1   Individual changes in fat mass following seven weeks of aerobic exercise training in lean women. Data are presented as residual changes in fat mass after net ExEE has been accounted for. Previously published in [21] (permission granted).

in the standard scientific approach to the study of PA and obesity management. Acknowledgement of this variability is of great importance if effective weight management programmes are to be designed. This need is clearly illustrated by the fact that, despite large and verified increases in ExEE, a small number of individuals actually gain weight during supervised exercise interventions [20,21].

Attempts to characterise this variability has revealed that that some individuals are more susceptible to exercise-induced weight loss than others. This susceptibility is likely to be conveyed through one or more compensatory pathways that act as auto-regulatory responses to energy deficit, minimising perturbations to energy homeostasis and body weight [24]. Attempts have been made to identify the key biological and behavioural compensatory mechanisms, but a greater understanding of these, and how they interact to shape body weight during long-term energy deficit, is still needed. While two potential compensatory pathways are briefly summarised in the following text, more detailed reviews concerning energy balance and compensation [25], and the effects of exercise on appetite control [26–28] and spontaneous PA, can be found elsewhere [29,30].

4.11.5 The effect of physical activity on energy intake

While acute exercise does not lead to an automatic increase in EI [31–33], it is becoming clear that eating behaviour in response to acute exercise is highly variable [18,19,34]. When exercise is performed over consecutive days, EI begins to track TDEE, with partial compensation in EI equal to approximately 30% of the ExEE observed following 7–14 days of intense exercise [35–37]. These findings are consistent with longer-term interventions, which demonstrate that exercise-induced compensatory eating is a powerful mediator of weight loss in susceptible individuals [20,23,38]. In some, the same ExEE can result in substantial weight loss and no *concomitant* increase in EI, but minimal weight loss and compensatory increases in hunger in others [23]. However, even in those who experience an increased orexigenic drive, evidence suggests that regular exercise still has a positive effect on appetite control. A 'duel process' has been

observed in which increases in fasting hunger are partially offset by an improved post-meal satiety response following chronic exercise [23,38]. This is consistent with the improved sensitivity in appetite control noted in regular exercisers [39] and those who undertake exercise training [40]. It has been proposed that the primary rationale for promoting PA in obesity management may not relate to its impact on energy expenditure, but to the positive effect it has on appetite regulation [41,42]. Recent evidence indicates a weak coupling between EI and TDEE in sedentary individuals or those displaying low levels of PA, but a stronger coupling between EI and TDEE at high levels of PA [43–45]. A weak coupling at low levels of PA would promote the overconsumption of food, whereas a stronger coupling between EI and TDEE would promote the maintenance of energy balance (albeit at higher absolute levels of intake and expenditure).

4.11.6 Physical activity and non-exercise activity thermogenesis

It has also been suggested that compensatory reductions in non-exercise activity thermogenesis (NEAT) – that is, the energy expenditure of all physical activities other than volitional exercise – may occur in response to increased voluntary exercise [46]. However, some [47,48], but not all, have reported a reduction in NEAT with increased levels of voluntary exercise [49–52]. Such inconsistencies may relate to the duration or mode of the exercise intervention and the variations in the measurement techniques used, with TDEE commonly measured using indirect calorimetry, doubly labelled water, accelerometers, heart rate or activities diaries (or a combination of these). Age and/or exercise intensity may also mediate such compensation, with reductions in non-exercise activity reported in older (55–68 years) but not younger (28–41 years) individuals [53,54], while a delayed increase in NEAT has been reported 3 days after a high-intensity exercise bout, but not a moderate bout [55]. Notwithstanding these methodological inconsistencies, a recent systematic review [30] concluded that there was little evidence to support a compensatory reduction in non-exercise PA during exercise training in healthy adults.

4.11.7 Beyond weight loss: alternative health benefits of physical activity

While body weight is typically (and inappropriately) used as the primary marker of success in exercise-based weight management, it is clear that regular PA can produce clinically meaningful improvements in health that are independent of body weight. Studies have demonstrated that regular exercise can improve insulin sensitivity, reduce the progression of type 2 diabetes and ameliorate hepatic steatosis and blood lipid profiles without changes in body weight [56–58]. Indeed, it has been argued that cardiovascular fitness is a better predictor of all-cause mortality than body weight. This is supported by evidence that adults demonstrating high cardiovascular fitness are at lower risk of all-cause mortality than those with poor cardiovascular fitness [59–62]. Such findings have led to the 'fat but fit' concept, where it has been shown that, for all-cause and cardiovascular mortality, those with a high BMI and good cardiovascular fitness are at lower risk than those with a normal BMI but poor cardiovascular fitness [63]. However, it should be noted that the evidence demonstrating a protective effect of high aerobic fitness for type 2 diabetes and cardiovascular disease is stronger than that for high PA levels [64], and that a high BMI is still a risk factor in type 2 diabetes and cardiovascular disease [65]. As such, body weight and cardiovascular fitness should be considered alongside each other when trying to improve long-term health [66]. While it is clear that the ideal is to be of normal weight and to be physically active, the importance of PA and aerobic fitness should be promoted to the general public as clinically meaningful health improvements can be achieved irrespective of changes in body weight [67].

4.11.8 The optimal dose of physical activity for weight loss and maintenance

A dose–response relationship appears to exist between PA, health and body weight [68]. As shown in Table 4.11.1, the required PA dose will vary depending on the desired outcome. It has been suggested that the relationship between PA and health is curvilinear (see Figure 4.11.2), with the greatest benefits seen in physically inactive individuals who can achieve marked improvements in health with relatively minor increases in PA [68]. However, while 150 min/week of moderate PA appears sufficient to reduce the risk of multiple chronic diseases and all-cause mortality [69], higher levels of PA may be needed for weight loss. The ACSM currently suggests that 150–250 min/week of moderate PA is required for modest weight loss (2–3 kg), while 225–420 min/week is required for more substantial weight loss (5–7.5 kg) [2]. It is worth noting that little attention has been given to how exercise dose affects compensatory responses to exercise. Church et al. (2009) compared actual to predicted weight loss across three doses of ExEE (4, 8 and 12 kcal.kg/week) during 6 months of supervised exercise [22]. Actual weight loss closely mirrored that predicted in the 4 and 8 kcal.kg/week groups, but, in the 12 kcal.kg/week group, the actual weight loss was significantly lower than that predicted (−1.5 vs. −2.7 kg, respectively). Consequently, weight loss was higher in the 8 kcal.kg/week group than the 12 kcal.kg/week group, despite a lower total ExEE [22]. While this suggests that a higher exercise dose may elicit greater compensation, the mechanisms behind such compensation were not examined. Indeed, even within the 4 and 8 kcal.kg/week groups, compensation was still observed in approximately 50% of individuals. It is also important to note that evidence indicates that sedentary behaviour/time is an independent risk factor (distinct to PA levels and other known risk factors) in several chronic and all-cause mortality [70]. Importantly, high levels of PA appear to attenuate, but not completely eliminate, the risks associated with high levels of sedentary behaviour [70].

While research has primarily focussed on the efficacy of specific weight loss strategies, less attention has been given to the prevention of weight regain, despite a high level of recidivism seen in body weight following initial weight loss. Unfortunately, approximately one-third of the initial weight lost is regained within 1 year [71], while much of the weight is typically regained after 5 years [56]. Although identifying predictors of successful weight maintenance is

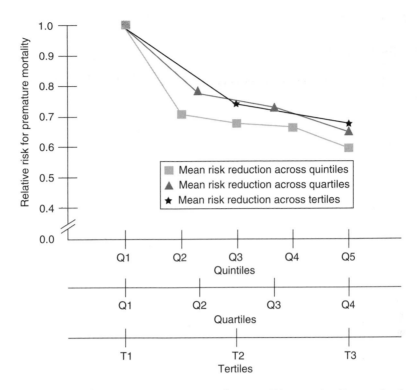

Figure 4.11.2 Relative risk for premature all-cause mortality across PA categories. Data previously published in [78] (permission granted via Rightslink).

problematic [72], PA has been shown to play a key role in preventing or attenuating weight regain [73]. While some have suggested that PA is a stronger determinant of weight maintenance than diet [74,75], other behaviours such as eating a low-calorie and low-fat diet, regular breakfast consumption, self-monitoring of body weight and a consistent pattern of eating across weekdays and weekends have also been shown to predict successful long-term weight maintenance [76]. Again, a dose–response relationship appears to exist between the volume of PA performed and weight regain, with those achieving better weight maintenance regularly engaging in high levels of PA [77]. However, despite the apparent importance of PA in weight maintenance, the optimal dose and type of PA has not been well defined. While noting that there is a lack of quality studies addressing this issue, the ACSM has recommended that 200–300 min/week of moderate-to-vigorous PA is required to prevent weight regain in weight-reduced individuals [2]. As such, it is apparent that the volume of PA

required to prevent weight regain is substantially greater than that initially required to prevent weight gain in the first place. The high volume of PA required to prevent weight regain may in part contribute to the high level of recidivism seen following weight loss.

4.11.9 Conclusions

When considering the importance of PA in obesity management, the independent health benefits derived from regular PA must be considered (and promoted) alongside any changes in body weight. These benefits convey clinically meaningful improvements in health and are not undermined by minimal changes in body weight. When PA is used to promote a negative energy imbalance and weight loss, the interplay between the components of energy balance must be considered. An increase in energy expenditure through PA has the potential to produce compensation in other areas of the energy balance system, with evidence suggesting that changes in hunger and EI may attenuate the increase in energy expenditure in susceptible individuals following acute and chronic exercise. While evidence is equivocal with regard to compensatory changes in NEAT, behavioural and/or biological compensation can partly explain why exercise-induced weight loss is highly variable (even under conditions of high compliance), and often less than that theoretically expected based on objective measures of ExEE. Evidence suggests that a dose–response relationship exists between PA and health, with marked improvements in health seen in physically inactive individuals with relatively modest increases in PA. A similar relationship exists between PA and weight loss, albeit that a greater volume of PA is needed to achieve substantial weight loss when dietary intake is not controlled. Despite the high level of recidivism seen in body weight following weight loss, further work is needed to characterise the factors that contribute to successful weight maintenance. However, it appears that PA plays a key role in the prevention of weight regain.

4.11.10 Summary box

Key points

- Regular PA can improve health, independent of changes in body weight, and these health benefits should be promoted alongside reductions in body weight as a rationale for the use of PA in obesity management.
- Exercise-induced weight loss will vary markedly between individuals performing the same volume of exercise, with behavioural and/or biological compensation partly shaping the response in body weight. However, clinically meaningful improvements in health still occur in those who experience lower-than-expected weight loss.
- A dose–response relationship exists between PA, health and body weight. While marked improvements in health are seen in inactive individuals with modest increases in PA, a greater volume of PA is need for weight loss. The volume of PA performed during weight maintenance appears to be a key factor in preventing or attenuating weight regain.

References

1. Thorogood A, Mottillo S, Shimony A, Filion KB, Joseph L, Genest J, et al. Isolated aerobic exercise and weight loss: a systematic review and meta-analysis of randomized controlled trials. *The American Journal of Medicine* 2011; **124**: 747–755.
2. Donnelly J, Blair S, Jakicic J, Manore M, Rankin J, Smith B. American College of Sports Medicine Position Stand. Appropriate physical activity intervention strategies for weight loss and prevention of weight regain for adults. *Medicine & Science in Sports & Exercise* 2009; **41**: 459–471.
3. Cutler D, Glaeser E, Shapiro J. Why have Americans become more obese? *Journal of Economic Perspectives* 2003; **17**: 93–118.
4. Prentice A, Jebb S. Obesity in Britain: gluttony or sloth? *BMJ* 1995; **311**: 437.
5. Philipson T. The world-wide growth in obesity: an economic research agenda. *Health Economics* 2001; **10**: 1–7.
6. Swinburn B, Sacks G, Lo S, Westerterp K, Rush E, Rosenbaum M, et al. Estimating the changes in energy flux that characterize the rise in obesity prevalence. *American Journal of Clinical Nutrition* 2009a; **89**: 1723.
7. Swinburn B, Sacks G, Ravussin E. Increased food energy supply is more than sufficient to explain the US epidemic of obesity. *American Journal of Clinical Nutrition* 2009b; **90**: 1453–1456.
8. Westerterp K, Speakman J. Physical activity energy expenditure has not declined since the 1980s and matches energy expenditures of wild mammals. *International Journal of Obesity* 2008; **32**: 1256–1263.
9. Hill J, Wyatt H, Reed G, Peters J. Obesity and the environment: where do we go from here? *Science* 2003; **299**: 853–855.
10. Bouchard C. The magnitude of the energy imbalance in obesity is generally underestimated. *International Journal of Obesity* 2008; **32**: 879–880.
11. Ravussin E, Lillioja S, Anderson TE, Christin L, Bogardus C. Determinants of 24-hour energy expenditure in man. Methods and results using a respiratory chamber. *Journal of Clinical Investigation* 1986; **78**: 1568–1578.
12. Biddle S, Mutrie N. *Psychology of Physical Activity: Determinants, Well-being, and Interventions*. Routledge: Psychology Press, 2008.
13. Schoeller D. The energy balance equation: looking back and looking forward are two very different views. *Nutrition Reviews* 2009; **67**: 249–254.
14. Bray G, Flatt J, Volaufova J, Delany J, Champagne C. Corrective responses in human food intake identified from an analysis of 7-d food-intake records. *American Journal of Clinical Nutrition* 2008; **88**: 1504.
15. Bessesen DH. Regulation of body weight: what is the regulated parameter? *Physiology & Behavior* 2011; **104**: 599–607.
16. Shaw K, Gennat H, O'rourke P, Del Mar C. Exercise for overweight or obesity. *Cochrane Database of Systematic Reviews* 2006; **4**: 112–117.
17. Borer K. How effective is exercise in producing fat loss? *Kinesiology* 2008; **2**: 126–137.
18. Finlayson G, Bryant E, Blundell J, King N. Acute compensatory eating following exercise is associated with implicit hedonic wanting for food. *Physiology & Behavior* 2009; **97**: 62–67.

19. Unick J, Otto A, Goodpaster B, Helsel D, Pellegrini C, Jakicic J. Acute effect of walking on energy intake in overweight/obese women. *Appetite* 2010; **55**: 413–419.

20. King N, Hopkins M, Caudwell P, Stubbs R, Blundell J. Individual variability following 12 weeks of supervised exercise: identification and characterization of compensation for exercise-induced weight loss. *International Journal of Obesity* 2008; **32**: 177–184.

21. Barwell N, Malkova D, Leggate M, Gill J. Individual responsiveness to exercise-induced fat loss is associated with change in resting substrate utilization. *Metabolism* 2001; **58**: 1320–1328.

22. Church T, Martin C, Thompson A, Earnest C, Mikus C, Blair S. Changes in weight, waist circumference and compensatory responses with different doses of exercise among sedentary, overweight postmenopausal women. *PLoS ONE* 2009; **4**: 4515.

23. King N, Caudwell P, Hopkins M, Stubbs J, Naslund E, Blundell J. Dual-process action of exercise on appetite control: increase in orexigenic drive but improvement in meal-induced satiety. *American Journal of Clinical Nutrition* 2009; **90**: 921–927.

24. Dulloo A. Suppressed thermogenesis as a cause for resistance to slimming and obesity rebound: adaptation or illusion? *International Journal of Obesity* 2007; **31**: 201–203.

25. King N, Caudwell P, Hopkins M, Byrne N, Colley R, Hills A, et al. Metabolic and behavioral compensatory responses to exercise interventions: barriers to weight loss. *Obesity* 2007; **15**: 1373–1383.

26. Martins C, Morgan L, Truby H. A review of the effects of exercise on appetite regulation: an obesity perspective. *International Journal of Obesity* 2008; **32**: 1337–1347.

27. Hopkins M, King NA, Blundell JE. Acute and long-term effects of exercise on appetite control: is there any benefit for weight control? *Current Opinion in Clinical Nutrition and Metabolic Care* 2010; **13**: 635–640.

28. Donnelly JE, Herrman SD, Lambourne K, Szabo AN, Honas JJ, Washburn RA. Does increased exercise or physical activity alter ad-libitum daily energy intake or macronutrient composition in health adults? A systematic review. *PLoS ONE* 2014; **9**: e83498.

29. Garland T, Schutz H, Chappell MA, Keeney BK, Meek TH, Copes LE, et al. The biological control of voluntary exercise, spontaneous physical activity and daily energy expenditure in relation to obesity: human and rodent perspectives. *Journal of Experimental Biology* 2011; **214**: 206–229.

30. Washburn R, Lambourne K, Szabo A, Herrmann S, Honas J, Donnelly J. Does increased prescribed exercise alter non-exercise physical activity/energy expenditure in health adults? *Clinical Obesity* 2014; **4**: 1–20.

31. King N, Blundell J. High-fat foods overcome the energy expenditure induced by high-intensity cycling or running. *European Journal of Clinical Nutrition* 1995; **49**: 114–123.

32. King N, Snell L, Smith R, Blundell J. Effects of short-term exercise on appetite responses in unrestrained females. *European Journal of Clinical Nutrition* 1996; **50**: 663–667.

33. King N, Lluch A, Stubbs R, Blundell J. High dose exercise does not increase hunger or energy intake in free living males. *European Journal of Clinical Nutrition* 1997; **51**: 478–483.

34. Hopkins M, Blundell JE, King NA. Individual variability in compensatory eating following acute exercise in overweight and obese women. *British Journal of Sports Medicine* 2013; **48**: 1472–1476.

35. Stubbs R, Sepp A, Hughes D, Johnstone A, King N, Horgan G, et al. The effect of graded levels of exercise on energy intake and balance in free-living women. *International Journal of Obesity and Related Metabolic Disorders* 2002; **26**: 866–869.

36. Stubbs R, Sepp A, Hughes D, Johnstone A, Horgan G, King N, et al. The effect of graded levels of exercise on energy intake and balance in free-living men, consuming their normal diet. *European Journal of Clinical Nutrition* 2002; **56**: 129–140.

37. Whybrow S, Hughes D, Ritz P, Johnstone A, Horgan G, King N, et al. The effect of an incremental increase in exercise on appetite, eating behaviour and energy balance in lean men and women feeding ad libitum. *British Journal of Nutrition* 2008; **10**: 1109–1115.

38. Martins C, Kulseng B, King N, Holst J, Blundell J. The effects of exercise-induced weight loss on appetite-related peptides and motivation to eat. *Journal of Clinical Endocrinology and Metabolism* 2010; **95**: 1609–1616.

39. Long S, Hart K, Morgan L. The ability of habitual exercise to influence appetite and food intake in response to high-and low-energy preloads in man. *British Journal of Nutrition* 2002; **87**: 517–523.

40. Martins C, Truby H, Morgan L. Short-term appetite control in response to a 6-week exercise programme in sedentary volunteers. *British Journal of Nutrition* 2007; **98**: 834–842.

41. Blundell J. Physical activity and appetite control: can we close the energy gap? *Nutrition Bulletin* 2011; **36**: 356–366.

42. Chaput JP, Sharma AM. Is physical activity in weight management more about 'calories in' than 'calories out'? *British Journal of Nutrition* 2011; **1**: 1–2.

43. Shook RP, Hand GA, Drenowatz C, Hebert JR, Paluch AE, Blundell JE, et al. Low levels of physical activity are associated with dysregulation of energy intake and fat mass gain over 1 year. *American Journal of Clinical Nutrition* 2015; **102**: 1332–1338.

44. Beaulieu K, Hopkins M, Blundell J, Finlayson G. Does habitual physical activity increase the sensitivity of the appetite control system: a systematic review. *Sports Medicine* 2016; **46**: 1897–1919.

45. Myers A, Finlayson G, Gibbons C, Blundell J. Associations amongst sedentary and active behaviours, body fat and appetite dysregulation: investigating the myth of physical inactivity and obesity. *British Journal of Sports Medicine* 2016; published online.

46. Levine J. Nonexercise activity thermogenesis (NEAT): environment and biology. *American Journal of Physiology, Endocrinology and Metabolism* 2004; **286**: E675–E685.

47. Colley R, Hills A, King N, Byrne N. Exercise-induced energy expenditure: Implications for exercise prescription and obesity. *Patient Education and Counseling* 2010; **79**: 327–332.

48. Manthou E, Gill J, Wright A, Malkova D. Behavioural compensatory adjustments to exercise training in overweight women. *Medicine & Science in Sports & Exercise* 2010; **42**: 1121–1128.

49. Mclaughlin R, Malkova D, Nimmo M. Spontaneous activity responses to exercise in males and females. *European Journal of Clinical Nutrition* 2006; **60**: 1055–1061.

50. Hollowell RP, Willis LH, Slentz CA, Topping JD, Bhakpar M, Kraus WE. Effects of exercise training amount on physical activity energy expenditure. *Medicine and Science in Sports and Exercise* 2009; **41**: 1640–1645.

51. Turner JE, Markovitch D, Betts JA, Thompson D. Nonprescribed physical activity energy expenditure is maintained with structured exercise and implicates a compensatory increase in energy intake. *American Journal of Clinical Nutrition* 2010; **92**: 1009–1016.

52. Rangan VV, Willis LH, Slentz CA, Bateman LA, Shields AT, Houmard JA, et al. Effects of an eight-month exercise training program on off-exercise physical activity. *Medicine and Science in Sports and Exercise* 2011; **43**: 1744–1751.

53. Meijer GAL, Janssen GME, Westerterp K, Verhoeven F, Saris WHM, Ten Hoor F. The effect of a 5-month endurance-training programme on physical activity: evidence for a sex-difference in the metabolic response to exercise. *European Journal of Applied Physiology and Occupational Physiology* 1991; **62**: 11–17.

54. Meijer EP, Westerterp KR, Verstappen FTJ. Effect of exercise training on total daily physical activity in elderly humans. *European Journal of Applied Physiology and Occupational Physiology* 1999; **80**: 16–21.

55. Alahmadi MA, Hills AP, King NA, Byrne NM. Exercise intensity influences nonexercise activity thermogenesis in overweight and obese adults. *Medicine and Science in Sports and Exercise* 2011; **43**: 624–631.

56. Knowler WC, Barrett-Connor E, Fowler SE, Hamman RF, Lachin JM, Walker EA, et al. Reduction in the incidence of type 2 diabetes with lifestyle intervention or metformin. *The New England Journal of Medicine* 2002; **346**: 393–403.

57. Lindstrom J, Louheranta A, Mannelin M, Rastas M, Salminen V, Eriksson J, et al. The Finnish Diabetes Prevention Study (DPS): Lifestyle intervention and 3-year results on diet and physical activity. *Diabetes Care* 2003; **26**: 3230–3236.

58. Johnson NA, George J. Fitness versus fatness: moving beyond weight loss in nonalcoholic fatty liver disease. *Hepatology* 2010; **52**: 370–381.

59. Blair SN, Kohl HW, Barlow CE, Paffenbarger RS, Gibbons LW, Macera CA. Changes in physical fitness and all-cause mortality. *JAMA* 1995; **73**: 1093–1098.

60. Wei M, Kampert JB, Barlow CE, Nichaman MZ, Gibbons LW, Paffenbarger RS, et al. Relationship between low cardiorespiratory fitness and mortality in normal-weight, overweight, and obese men. *JAMA* 1999; **282**: 1547–1553.

61. Kodama S, Saito K, Tanaka S, Maki M, Yachi Y, Asumi M, et al. Cardiorespiratory fitness as a quantitative predictor of all-cause mortality and cardiovascular events in health men and women: a meta-analysis. *JAMA* 2009; **301**: 2024–2035.

62. McAuley PA, Blaha MJ, Keteyian SJ, Brawner CA, Al Rifai M, Dardari ZA, et al. Fitness, fatness and mortality: the FIT (Henry Ford Exercise Testing) Project. *The American Journal of Medicine* 2016; **129**: 960–965.

63. Fogelholm M. Physical activity, fitness and fatness: relations to mortality, morbidity and disease risk factors. A systematic review. *Obesity Reviews* 2009; **11**: 202–221.

64. Blair SN, Cheng Y, Scott Holder J. Is physical activity or physical fitness more important in defining health benefits? *Medicine & Science in Sports & Exercise* 2001; **33**: S379–S399.

65. Lewis CE, Mctigue KM, Burke LE, Poirier P, Eckel RH, Howard BV, et al. Mortality, health outcomes, and body mass index in the overweight range: a science advisory from the American Heart Association. *Circulation* 2009; **119**: 3263–3271.

66. Blair SN, Church TS. The fitness, obesity, and health equation. *JAMA* 2004; **292**: 1232–1234.

67. King N, Hopkins M, Caudwell P, Stubbs J, Blundell J. Beneficial effects of exercise: shifting the focus from body weight to other markers of health. *British Journal of Sports Medicine* 2010; **43**: 924–927.

68. Warburton DER, Charlesworth S, Ivey A, Nettlefold L, Bredin SSD. A systematic review of the evidence for Canada's Physical Activity Guidelines for Adults. *International Journal of Behavioral Nutrition and Physical Activity* 2010; **7**: 1–220.

69. Tremblay MS, Warburton DE, Janssen I, Paterson DH, Latimer AE, Rhodes RE, et al. New Canadian physical activity guidelines. *Applied Physiology Nutrition and Metabolism* 2011; **36**: 36–46.

70. Ekelund U, Steene-Johannessen J, Brown WJ, Fagerland MW, Owen N, Powell K, et al. Physical activity attenuates the detrimental association of sitting time with mortality: a harmonised meta-analysis of data from more than one million men and women. *Lancet* 2016; **24**: 1302–1310.

71. Anderson J, Konz E, Frederich R, Wood C. Long-term weight-loss maintenance: a meta-analysis of US studies. *American Journal of Clinical Nutrition* 2001; **74**: 579–584.

72. Stubbs J, Whybrow S, Teixeira P, Blundell J, Lawton C, Westenhoefer J, et al. Problems in identifying predictors and correlates of weight loss and maintenance: implications for weight control therapies based on behaviour change. *Obesity Reviews* 2011; **12**: 688–708.

73. Mekary RA, Feskanich D, Hu FB, Willett WC, Field AE. Physical activity in relation to long-term weight maintenance after intentional weight loss in premenopausal women. *Obesity* 2010; **18**: 167–174.

74. Wier L, Ayers G, Jackson A, Rossum A, Poston W, Foreyt J. Determining the amount of physical activity needed for long-term weight control. *International Journal of Obesity* 2001; **25**: 613–621.

75. Jeffery RW, Wing RR, Sherwood NE, Tate DF. Physical activity and weight loss: does prescribing higher physical activity goals improve outcome? *American Journal of Clinical Nutrition* 2003; **78**: 684–689.

76. Wing RR, Phelan S. Long-term weight loss maintenance. *American Journal of Clinical Nutrition* 2005; **82**: 222S–225S.

77. Jakicic JM, Marcus BH, Lang W, Janney C. Effect of exercise on 24-month weight loss maintenance in overweight women. *Archives of Internal Medicine* 2008; **168**: 1550–1559.

78. Warburton DE, Bredin SS. Reflections on physical activity and health: what should we recommend? *Canadian Journal of Cardiology* 2016; **32**: 495–504.

Chapter 4.12

Psychological interventions for weight loss in obesity

Bethan R Mead and Emma J Boyland
University of Liverpool, Liverpool, UK

4.12.1 Introduction

Worldwide obesity rates have rapidly increased over several decades [1], and there is a more pressing need for efficacious obesity treatments than ever before. While traditional treatment of obesity has focussed on the provision of dietary counselling and increasing physical activity, health organisations are increasingly recommending the use of psychological interventions as a means of managing and reducing excess weight in adults. For example, a recent report commissioned by the British Psychological Society explicitly identifies the value of adopting a psychological approach to obesity treatment [2]. This is consistent with recommendations by multiple government health bodies [3,4] that identify psychological treatments or referral to a psychologist alongside diet and exercise-based treatments as useful in the management of overweight and obesity.

In recent years, several key reviews have been published to evaluate the effectiveness of current psychological interventions in obesity [5,6]. These have identified behavioural therapy (BT) and cognitive therapy/cognitive-behavioural therapy (CBT) as the commonly used types of psychological interventions for the treatment of obesity in adults. Mindfulness-based therapies have more recently also been suggested as a potentially useful avenue for emerging weight loss interventions [7]. This chapter will consider and evaluate the most common psychological interventions currently employed in the treatment of obesity.

Behavioural therapy for obesity

BT for obesity is based on the behavioural principles of learned behaviour; that is, behaviours have a learned component that can be increased or decreased, depending on their desirability. If a behaviour is adaptive or likely to contribute to the achievement of a goal, its frequency can be increased using behaviour modification techniques. In terms of application to obesity treatment, BT aims to modify behaviours that contribute to the development and maintenance of excess weight. BT programmes tend to focus on developing techniques that enable the individual to adapt their behaviours to promote successful weight loss [8]. They typically hold at their core the three stages of behavioural change identified by Brownell and colleagues [9]: (1) realisation of motivation for change; (2) application of learned weight loss strategies; and (3) cultivating plans for maintaining change.

Whereas early reports of the effectiveness of BT for obesity describe programmes lasting approximately 10 weeks, more recent programmes can be up to 40 weeks in length [10]. This reflects the inclusion of developments in the research areas relevant to therapies that have occurred since their inception several decades previously. Participants will often attend weekly meetings as part of a weight loss programme that may also include a focus on diet and physical activity. The BT aspect of these programmes includes at least the following key components: goal setting, stimulus control and self-monitoring. Detailed descriptions of these components have been

Advanced Nutrition and Dietetics in Obesity, First Edition. Edited by Catherine Hankey.
© 2018 John Wiley & Sons Ltd. Published 2018 by John Wiley & Sons Ltd.

Box 4.12.1 Brief description of the three key components of behavioural therapy for the management of weight loss in obesity

Goal setting: Participants are encouraged to set moderate, achievable goals throughout the course of a programme. The eventual achievement of the 10% reduction in body weight that is recommended by these programmes is broken down into weekly goals of 0.5–1 kg [12]. Breaking down the larger, long-term goal of overall weight reduction into smaller, more immediate goals makes the ultimate aim more manageable and achievable [13].

Stimulus control: The basis of the stimulus control component of BT is that cues related to food intake become associated with eating behaviour [14]. By limiting the presence of, or modifying the associations attached to, internal or external cues, behaviours relevant to weight management can be modified based on their desirability. Stimulus control may take the form of changing the visibility of unhealthy food items in the home to reduce their consumption.

Self-monitoring: Encouraging participants to monitor their own behaviours, energy intake and physical activity has been described as a crucial component of BT for obesity [12]. Participants are encouraged to monitor and record their food intake, physical activity and behaviours during their progression through a BT programme. Effective self-monitoring has been associated with more successful weight loss when incorporated into BT [15].

---

published elsewhere [11], but a brief description is provided in Box 4.12.1.

BT for weight loss is the most commonly studied psychological intervention in obesity management in adults [6]. Reviews and meta-analyses of multiple randomised controlled trials evaluating the effectiveness of behavioural therapies, compared to control or other established therapies, suggest that establishing behavioural modification techniques is a valuable tool in weight loss for the obese [5,12,14]. Indeed, behavioural weight loss therapies can produce a significant weight loss of 8–10% of initial body weight in obese adults [10]. This is a similar reduction to that seen in some pharmacological weight loss options [4], and is highly promising, considering reports that a 5–10% reduction of body weight has been associated with reductions is obesity-related health risks [16]. Furthermore, a review [5] of 18 studies that examined behavioural weight loss therapy showed that greater weight loss was achieved by behavioural weight loss therapy in comparison to no-therapy control groups. BT was also shown to be effective when combined with dietary counselling and physical activity, and when the intervention was more intense than less intense.

Evaluations of the effectiveness of BT clearly show that it is a valuable psychological intervention for obesity when received alone or in addition to a diet and exercise intervention. This is recognised in the inclusion of BT in treatment guidelines and in the recommendations for obesity published by health advisory and regulatory bodies such as the National Institute for Health and Care Excellence (NICE [17]), the National Obesity Observatory (NOO [18]) and the National Heart, Lung, and Blood Institute (NHLBI [3]). BT can be delivered by health practitioners, rather than by specialised psychological therapists, and is often less costly than other forms of interventions (e.g. cognitive therapy/CBT). Despite this, evidence of its efficacy in the *long term* is mixed. The range of follow-up times reported in the preceding reviews and studies is often far less than the recommended 5 years [3]. Wing [10] reports that participants in behavioural weight loss therapies lose most of the weight by 6 months of treatment, and that regain often begins after this point. In fact, some data [19] suggest that, although behavioural weight loss therapy appeared superior to CBT immediately post-treatment, this difference had reversed by the 12-month follow-up point. Weight maintenance following weight loss and the prevention of weight regain are significant issues in any form of weight loss intervention.

Cognitive therapy/CBT for obesity

Cooper and Fairburn [20,21] describe an initial adaptation of CBT as a psychological intervention for obesity. The structured programme they present has been adopted for use in multiple healthcare settings and, as such, is identified as a candidate treatment for obesity in the European Clinical Practice Guidelines for the Management of Obesity in Adults [16].

Cognitive therapies and CBTs have roots in Beck's [22] work, which assumes that defective cognitions are crucial to the development and maintenance of maladaptive behavioural and emotional responses. Current incarnations of CBTs have a combined focus on cognitive, behavioural and emotional components, and have been adapted as treatments for multiple disorders [23]. Applied to the treatment of obesity, these therapies aim to change cognitions and equip participants with strategies and responses that are used to identify and revaluate behavioural and emotional responses, processes and thought patterns likely to help or hinder progress towards an eventual weight loss goal [20,21]. CBT is distinct from traditional BT, as described in the preceding text. While similarities between the two types of interventions are undeniable due to their aims to produce new behavioural patterns and their requirement of active contributions from participants, cognitive therapies also emphasise the importance and role of cognitive processes in successful weight management and maintenance of weight loss [21]. A core

facet of CBT that is absent from behavioural therapies is the aim of creating cognitive change in addition to behavioural change. Behavioural experiments (explicit tests of the predicted outcome of behaviour, aimed at challenging predictions) and working to modify cognitive patterns are key to this [21].

The established programme of CBT for obesity is described in detail by Cooper and Fairburn [20,21], and an overview is presented here. The CBT programme for obesity is divided into two phases, which are further subdivided into a series of nine modules. Phase One focusses on weight loss; Phase Two focusses on weight maintenance. It is worth noting that this focus on weight maintenance is another defining feature of CBT for obesity, not always seen in other types of interventions. The programme was initially designed for one-to-one delivery [20], although examples of group-based delivery are not uncommon [24,25]. Participants work through modules systematically, although not without flexibility, with the guidance of a trained cognitive-behavioural therapist. The intervention produced by Cooper and Fairburn [20,21] is designed to last 11 months, and is depicted in Box 4.12.2.

Box 4.12.2 An 11-month CBT intervention for the management of obesity produced by Cooper and Fairburn [20,21]

Phase One comprises the following modules:
- *Module 1: 'Starting Treatment'* – involves assessment of the participant and introduction to the programme, key requirements and activities.
- *Module 2: 'Establishing and Maintaining Weight Loss'* – introduces the practicalities and considerations of an energy-restrictive diet.
- *Module 3: 'Addressing Barriers to Weight Loss'* – examines the issues that may arise and compromise successful weight loss.
- *Module 4: 'Eating Well'* – nutrition-centred.
- *Module 5: 'Increasing Activity'* – examines the relevance of creating an active lifestyle, and how this is done.
- *Module 6: 'Body Image'* – utilises CBT to address concerns relating to self-acceptance of shape.
- *Module 7: 'Weight Goals'* – focusses participants on the acceptance of their weight goals and explores participants' historical weight management issues.
- *Module 8: 'Primary Goals'* – explicitly explores goals participants may have that are directly related to their weight loss. The importance of planning goal-attainment methods, potential obstacles to this and how to overcome them is also stressed in this module.

Phase Two primarily concerns the longevity of the changes made:
- *Module 9: 'Weight Maintenance'* – provides participants with strategies and techniques that should be adopted in order to maintain weight loss.

CBT appears to be effective in aiding weight reduction, particularly when combined with diet and exercise interventions [5]. Empirical support for its efficacy is provided by a host of studies, as discussed in Shaw et al. [5], although some evidence is mixed, and the long-term effects of treatment are unclear [25]. Some studies indicate that cognitive therapy produced weight reductions of 8.3 kg (compared with no weight change in the wait-list control group) [24] and 8.6 kg (1.4 kg weight gain in the behavioural programme control group) [26]. The beneficial effects of the cognitive therapy groups were maintained until the 18-month follow-up in both studies. Complementary results are also reported by Werrij et al. [27], where significant weight loss was seen when cognitive therapy was added to dietetic treatment and in a control dietetic plus physical exercise intervention, although only the group receiving cognitive treatment maintained this weight loss at the 12-month follow-up. The authors conclude that superior relapse prevention can be achieved by the combination of cognitive therapy and dietetic treatment than is possible through a dietary and exercise intervention.

While evidence suggests that these programmes can produce weight loss of approximately 10% of initial body weight, others have highlighted that this is not always maintained over time [28]. For example, Muggia et al. [25] report no difference in the numbers of participants achieving a 10% weight reduction, regardless of whether they received brief, group-based CBT or standard care. Others report significant, but not differing weight loss in participants of CBT and BT groups, as compared to guided self-help (weight reductions of 10%, 11.3% and 6.7%, respectively) [29]. Follow-up data 3 years post-treatment showed substantial weight regains for BT and CBT participants. These results indicate that, despite its focus on relapse prevention, CBT was no more effective at preventing weight regain than BT. Conversely, evidence from Sbrocco et al. [19] suggests that participation in a BT intervention (vs. a cognitive-therapy-based intervention) led to better initial weight loss, but this pattern was reversed at the 12-month follow-up.

It is clear that more research with longer follow-up periods is desperately needed in order to fully understand the effectiveness of CBT for obesity. While, on one hand, it appears to be an effective treatment and is recognised as such in clinical practice recommendations (see [16]), the disparity between results, such as those discussed here, challenges previous statements of CBT's effectiveness as a psychological intervention for weight management. Furthermore, the practicalities of delivering interventions such as these may impact the types of investigations of efficacy that can be conducted, and also limit the feasibility of delivery of CBT in a healthcare setting. Initial descriptions of CBT are of an 11-month programme delivered by a specialist therapist in a one-to-one setting [20,21]. This relatively time- and labour-intensive structure may be off-putting to some health providers or researchers. CBT typically requires delivery by a graduate-level-qualified cognitive-behavioural therapist, whereas behavioural therapies do not, thus arguably making behavioural therapies more easily deliverable. Furthermore, the delivery of shortened or group-based variations of the treatment has produced disappointing results (e.g. see [25]). Considerations such as these may deter finance- and time-pressured researchers from embarking on the much-needed in-depth and long-term evaluations of CBT for weight loss.

Mindfulness-based interventions for obesity

Mindfulness-based interventions have been suggested as a potential avenue for investigation in the development of new psychological interventions for obesity [7]. Mindfulness has been described as a way of paying attention to the present moment in a purposeful and non-judgemental way [30]. A recent review indicates that a host of mindfulness-based therapies show beneficial effects on weight loss in obese adults [7]. These therapies are hypothesised to act by promoting self-regulation and attention to cues that may trigger unhelpful eating behaviours.

Mindfulness-based therapies include, but are not limited to, Mindfulness-Based Eating Awareness Training (MB-EAT [31]), Mindful Eating Training [32] and Acceptance-Based Treatments (ABTs [33]). Although originally developed for the treatment of obese individuals with binge eating disorder, a 10-session MB-EAT intervention can produce a weight loss of approximately 3.2 kg and shows promise for translation into a non-pathological intervention setting [34]. Comparable weight loss has also been shown in Mindful Eating Interventions [32]. When compared to standard behavioural treatment, ABT for weight loss (which aims to cultivate tolerance of experiences that may provoke unhelpful eating behaviours) yielded superior weight loss achievements in a large sample of overweight and obese adults ('Mind Your Health Project'; [33]). Participants in this study took part in a 40-week intervention and, although both ABT and standard behavioural treatment groups achieved a 10% weight loss by follow-up, the ABT group performed better overall when lead by more experienced therapists and for participants with higher levels of cue reactivity. Additional variations of these therapies have been developed, but a thorough examination of these is beyond the scope of this chapter.

Interventions that incorporate or are centred on mindfulness-based theories and techniques appear to be a promising means of supporting successful weight loss in non-clinical populations of obese adults. Although current evidence does indeed support this, more research is needed to examine the longevity of the effects described in the preceding text [7]. As is often seen in research evaluating the effects of other psychological interventions for obesity, studies of mindfulness-based treatments are limited by their short (or lack of extended) follow-up times. Furthermore, some evidence suggests that these treatments may only achieve their maximum effects when delivered by highly specialised and experienced therapists [33]. This is in contrast to the therapy provision options of behavioural treatments. This specificity and probably increased financial cost is likely to hinder the palatability of mindfulness-based treatments when health bodies consider them alongside existing psychological interventions for obesity. In these respects, in comparison to the long-established bank of literature on behavioural and cognitive therapies, these types of psychological interventions for obesity are in their infancy.

4.12.2 Final considerations

Psychological interventions for obesity in adults are included in many treatment and clinical practice guidelines [3,4]. However, empirical findings supporting their immediate and long-term efficacy are mixed. Evidence suggests that, although BT, CBT and mindfulness-based interventions each have some value as stand-alone interventions for obesity, they are also effective when combined with interventions that include dietary counselling and physical activity [5]. This is reflected in the call for the use of multicomponent weight management interventions seen in clinical practice guidelines and in recommendations published by NICE [17], NOO [18] and the National Health and Medical Research Council [4]. Combined with emerging mindfulness-based interventions, it does appear that psychological interventions for obesity are a valuable treatment option for weight management in obese adults. Importantly, however, more longitudinal research is needed to meet the 5-year follow-up criteria recommended by the National Heart, Lung, and Blood Institute [3].

Extensive reviews of psychological interventions for obesity [5,6] consider results from large numbers of participants across multiple studies (Shaw [5]; 3495 participants). While these provide excellent overviews of the state of the literature on this topic, examination of the studies included by these authors, and also the other studies included in this chapter, indicate common themes that should be addressed by future research. There appears to be an over-reliance on university settings, female participants and prescriptive treatment structures in the existing literature. While it is understandable that these limitations stem from the nature of academic research and research conducted in collaboration with health providers, future evaluations of intervention effectiveness should consider community-based settings, wider participant groups and, perhaps, increasingly participant-directed interventions. In an increasingly Internet-reliant society, Internet-based interventions may become useful tools to maximise intervention audience, accessibility, engagement and personalisation of future psychological interventions for obesity. Online CBT programmes for bulimia nervosa (iCBT) have already been shown to be efficacious for symptom improvement and treatment accessibility in some individuals [35]. Translating these methods for non-clinical purposes may prove to be an effective and modern psychological intervention for obesity.

4.12.3 Summary box

Key points

- Psychological interventions for obesity in adults are included in many treatment and clinical practice guidelines, although empirical findings supporting their immediate and long-term efficacy are mixed.
- Several theory-based interventions have some value as stand-alone interventions for obesity, but are most effective alongside dietary counselling and physical activity.
- Combined with emerging mindfulness-based interventions, it does appear that psychological interventions for obesity are a valuable treatment option for weight management in obese adults. Importantly, however, more longitudinal research is needed to meet the 5-year follow-up criteria.
- Extensive reviews of psychological interventions for obesity reveal an over-reliance on university settings, female participants and prescriptive treatment structures in the existing literature.
- Internet-based interventions may become useful tools to maximise intervention audience, accessibility, engagement and personalisation of future psychological interventions for obesity.

References

1. WHO. Obesity and overweight [Factsheet]. 2013 [17/03/2014]. Available from: http://www.who.int/mediacentre/factsheets/fs311/en/, accessed 17 January 2016.
2. Obesity Working Group. *Obesity in the UK: A Psychological Perspective*. British Psychological Society, 2011. 978-1-85433-714-6.
3. Clinical guidelines on the identification, evaluation, and treatment of overweight and obesity in adults: the evidence report. National Heart, Lung, and Blood Institute, 1998. Available from: https://www.nhlbi.nih.gov/health-pro/guidelines/archive/clinical-guidelines-obesity-adults-evidence-report, accessed 31 July 2017.
4. Clinical practice guidelines for the management of overweight and obesity in adults, adolescents and children in Australia. National Health and Medical Research Council, 2013. Available from: https://www.nhmrc.gov.au/guidelines-publications/n57, accessed 31 July 2017.
5. Shaw K, O'Rourke P, Del Mar C, Kenardy J. Psychological interventions for overweight or obesity – art. no. CD003818. pub2. *Cochrane Database of Systematic Reviews* 2005; (2): 64.
6. Lo Presti R, Lai J, Hildebrandt T, Loeb KL. Psychological treatments for obesity in youth and adults. *Mount Sinai Journal of Medicine: A Journal of Translational and Personalized Medicine* 2010; 77(5): 472–487.

7. O'Reilly GA, Cook L, Spruijt-Metz D, Black DS. Mindfulness-based interventions for obesity-related eating behaviours: a literature review. *Obesity Reviews* 2014; 15(6): 453–461.
8. Van Dorsten B, Lindley EM. Cognitive and behavioral approaches in the treatment of obesity. *Medical Clinics of North America* 2011; 95(5): 971–988.
9. Brownell KD, Marlatt GA, Lichtenstein E, Wilson GT. Understanding and preventing relapse. *American Psychologist* 1986; 41(7): 765–782.
10. Wing RR. Behavioral weight control. In: Wadden TA, Stunkard AJ (eds) *Handbook of Obesity Treatment*. New York, NY: Guilford Press, 2002, pp. 301–316.
11. Brownell KD. *The LEARN Program for Weight Management*. Dallas, TX: American Health, 2000.
12. Butryn ML, Webb V, Wadden TA. Behavioral Treatment of Obesity. *Psychiatric Clinics of North America* 2011; 34(4): 841–859.
13. Bandura A, Simon KM. The role of proximal intentions in self-regulation of refractory behavior. *Cognitive Therapy and Research* 1977; 1(3): 177–193.
14. Foster GD, Makris AP, Bailer BA. Behavioral treatment of obesity. *American Journal of Clinical Nutrition* 2005; 82(1): 230S–235S.
15. Butryn ML, Phelan S, Hill JO, Wing RR. Consistent self-monitoring of weight: a key component of successful weight loss maintenance. *Obesity* 2007; 15(12): 3091–3096.
16. Tsigos C, Hainer V, Basdevant A, Finer N, Fried M, Mathus-Vliegen E, et al. Management of obesity in adults: European clinical practice guidelines. *Obesity Facts* 2008; 1(2): 106–116.
17. NICE. Obesity guidance on the prevention, identification, assessment and management of overweight and obesity in adults and children. *National Institute for Health and Care Excellence*, 2006. Available from: https://www.nice.org.uk/guidance/cg189/evidence/obesity-update-appendix-m-pdf-6960327447, accessed 31 July 2017.
18. NOO. Treating adult obesity through lifestyle change interventions. *National Obesity Observatory*, 2010. Available from: http://studylib.net/doc/8085782/treating-adult-obesity-through-lifestyle-change-intervent.
19. Sbrocco T, Nedegaard RC, Stone JM, Lewis EL. Behavioral choice treatment promotes continuing weight loss: preliminary results of a cognitive-behavioral decision-based treatment for obesity. *Journal of Consulting and Clinical Psychology* 1999; 67(2): 260–266.
20. Cooper Z, Fairburn CG. A new cognitive behavioural approach to the treatment of obesity. *Behaviour Research and Therapy* 2001; 39(5): 499–511.
21. Cooper Z, Fairburn CG. Cognitive-behavioral treatment of obesity. In: Wadden TA, Stunkard AJ (eds) *Handbook of Obesity Treatment*. New York, NY: Guilford Press, 2002, pp. 465–479.
22. Beck AT. Cognitive therapy: nature and relation to behavior therapy. *Behavior Therapy* 1970; 1(2): 184–200.
23. Hofmann SG, Asnaani A, Vonk IJJ, Sawyer AT, Fang A. The efficacy of cognitive behavioral therapy: a review of meta-analyses. *Cognitive Therapy and Research* 2012; 36(5): 427–440.
24. Stahre L, Hällström T. A short-term cognitive group treatment program gives substantial weight reduction up to 18 months

from the end of treatment. A randomized controlled trial. *Eating and Weight Disorders* 2005; **10**(1): 51–58.

25. Muggia C, Falchi AG, Michelini I, Montagna E, De Silvestri A, Grecchi I, et al. Brief group cognitive behavioral treatment in addition to prescriptive diet versus standard care in obese and overweight patients. A randomized controlled trial. *e-SPEN Journal* 2014; **9**(1): e26–e33.

26. Stahre L, Tärnell B, Håkanson CE, Hällström T. A randomized controlled trial of two weight-reducing short-term group treatment programs for obesity with an 18-month follow-up. *International Journal of Behavioral Medicine* 2007; **14**(1): 48–55.

27. Werrij MQ, Jansen A, Mulkens S, Elgersma HJ, Ament AJHA, Hospers HJ. Adding cognitive therapy to dietetic treatment is associated with less relapse in obesity. *Journal of Psychosomatic Research* 2009; **67**(4): 315–324.

28. Maguire T, Haslam D. *The Obesity Epidemic and its Management*. London, UK: Pharmaceutical Press, 2010.

29. Cooper Z, Doll HA, Hawker DM, Byrne S, Bonner G, Eeley E, et al. Testing a new cognitive behavioural treatment for obesity: a randomized controlled trial with three-year follow-up. *Behaviour Research and Therapy* 2010; **48**(8): 706–713.

30. Kabat-Zinn J. *Full Catastrophe Living*. New York, NY: Dell Publishing, 1990.

31. Kristeller JL, Hallett CB. An exploratory study of a meditation-based intervention for binge eating disorder. *Journal of Health Psychology* 1999; **4**(3): 357–363.

32. Dalen J, Smith BW, Shelley BM, Sloan AL, Leahigh L, Begay D. Pilot study: Mindful Eating and Living (MEAL): weight, eating behavior, and psychological outcomes associated with a mindfulness-based intervention for people with obesity. *Complementary Therapies in Medicine* 2010; **18**(6): 260–264.

33. Forman EM, Butryn ML, Juarascio AS, Bradley LE, Lowe MR, Herbert JD, et al. The mind your health project: a randomized controlled trial of an innovative behavioral treatment for obesity. *Obesity* 2013; **21**(6): 1119–1126.

34. Kristeller JL. Mindfulness-based eating awareness training (MB-EAT): theory, research, and practice. *Eating Disorders: The Journal of Treatment & Prevention* 2010; **19**(1): 49–61.

35. Sánchez-Ortiz VC, Munro C, Stahl D, House J, Startup H, Treasure J, et al. A randomized controlled trial of internet-based cognitive-behavioural therapy for bulimia nervosa or related disorders in a student population. *Psychological Medicine* 2011; **41**(2): 407–417.

Chapter 4.13

Weight loss interventions in specific groups: overweight and obese men

Alison Avenell[1], Clare Robertson[1] and Daryll Archibald[2]

[1] University of Aberdeen, Aberdeen, UK
[2] University of Edinburgh, Edinburgh, UK

4.13.1 Epidemiology of obesity in men

Data from the USA from 2007 to 2010 demonstrated that 34.4% of men and 36.1% of women were obese [1]. In the UK, in 2011, 24% of men and 26% of women were obese [2], but the UK Foresight Report [3] predicted that more men (47%) than women (36%) will be obese by 2025. However, morbid obesity (BMI ≥ 40 kg/m^2) is less prevalent in men [1,2].

Men are under-represented in weight loss programmes. In the US National Weight Control Registry [4], only 20% of participants are men. In the UK Counterweight weight loss programme in 65 general practices, only 23% of participants were men [5]. Men comprise only around 10% of participants in commercial weight loss programmes [6,7].

Obesity in men is a risk factor for a very wide range of diseases impacting on health and quality of life [8]. Men with BMI ≥ 30 kg/m^2 and waist circumference ≥ 102 cm have an increased risk of at least one symptom of impaired physical, psychological or sexual function, and these symptoms are also more likely in men with raised waist circumference but lower BMI [9].

4.13.2 Men's attitudes to lifestyle behaviour change

Men's attitudes

Men may be more reluctant to change their lifestyle than women, and may be cynical about government health messages [10]. Media and other cultural influences encourage men to maintain a larger, muscular, masculine body size [11]. Men appear less interested in gaining an ideal body weight, according to medical definitions, and are more interested in physical activity, fitness and body shape [12]. There are also differences in the way that men and women view physical activity as a means of becoming stronger, fitter and healthier [13].

Weight loss programmes and facilities, including commercial weight loss organisations, can be seen as feminised spaces [12,13], while men prefer masculine spaces, such as their workplaces, for such programmes [14,15]. Fear and embarrassment may particularly hinder men from taking part in weight loss programmes [15].

Social, cultural and environmental influences on obesity in men

Men's reluctance to seek help is often explained through theories of masculinity, resting on the concept of 'hegemonic' or dominant masculinity [16]. In debates on health-related help-seeking, hegemonic masculinity is thought to create patterns of behaviour resisting contact with formal services to emphasise self-sufficiency and robustness. However, viewing hegemonic masculinity as the dominant force in health-related decision-making has been criticised. It is argued that masculinity interconnects with other factors such as social class, age and ethnicity [17,18]. Hence, it is impossible to pull men out of the social structures in which they live.

Advanced Nutrition and Dietetics in Obesity, First Edition. Edited by Catherine Hankey.
© 2018 John Wiley & Sons Ltd. Published 2018 by John Wiley & Sons Ltd.

4.13.3 Identifying obesity in men

The desire for muscularity may make it harder for men than women to identify that they are overweight or obese. BMI tends to be used more than waist circumference in clinical practice, but waist circumference might be an easier measurement to raise awareness among men, and less susceptible to conflicts over muscularity. BMI does not distinguish between differences in body composition affected by sex, physique or ethnicity. Thus, men will have lower percentage of fat than women of equivalent BMI [19]. Unlike BMI, waist circumference cut-offs for risks of disease are sex-specific. If waist circumference alone is used to define risks from obesity, then women are more at risk (47% of women and 34% of men) in the UK in 2011 [2]. The National Institute for Health and Care Excellence (NICE) has advised that both BMI and waist circumference should be used to assess the risk of health problems such as type 2 diabetes in people with BMI <35 kg/m^2 [20] (see Table 4.13.1).

4.13.4 Clinical management

We have systematically reviewed the long-term randomised trial and qualitative research evidence on weight loss interventions for men [21]. Some of our findings are similar to those of an earlier systematic review by Young and colleagues on interventions for men [22], which included shorter studies, but excluded studies of men who were all recruited on the basis of comorbidities. Our review shows that long-term weight loss programmes help reduce comorbidities in obese men. Programmes with low-fat, low energy diets, and/or physical activity, with or without behaviour change training, improved erectile function (where there was approximately 10% weight loss after 1 year) [23–25] and prevented diabetes in the Finnish Diabetes Prevention Study (hazard ratio for diabetes incidence 0.43; 95% CI = 0.22–0.81) [26]. However, in type 2 diabetes, successful weight loss might increase the risk of osteoporosis (change in total hip bone density for men after 1 year is −1.48% vs. 0.02% in controls; for women, −1.44% vs. −0.61% in controls; reported $P = 0.04$ for interaction) [27]. Health benefits could help motivate men to try to lose weight. Other benefits for men include taking fewer medications, increased mobility and physical fitness, and outcomes not traditionally associated with obesity, such as fewer headaches [21]. We found no evidence that men are less successful at losing weight than women. Typical weight losses for men are around 5 kg after 1 year [28,29]. In the intensive Look AHEAD trial, diabetic men in the intervention group lost around 8% of body weight by the end of the first year, and half of this weight loss was sustained 8 years later [30,31].

4.13.5 Weight loss in men

Engaging and motivating men with weight loss

By examining randomised trials for men and women, we found that men were significantly less likely to drop out of weight loss programmes than women [21]. Combining long-term data from eight

Table 4.13.1 NICE table for assessing increased risk of obesity-related disease [21]

		Waist circumference		
		Low	High	Very high
	Men	<94 cm	94–102 cm	>102 cm
BMI	Women	<80 cm	80–88 cm	>88 cm
Normal (<25 kg/m^2)		No increased risk	No increased risk	Increased risk
Overweight (25–<30 kg/m^2)		No increased risk	Increased risk	High risk
Obese (30–<35 kg/m^2)		Increased risk	High risk	Very high risk

trials with 3813 participants (31% men), we found that men were 11% (95% CI = 8–14%) less likely to drop out [21]. Men may be harder to engage in current weight loss programmes than women, emphasising the need to improve engagement without diminishing commitment.

The qualitative literature shows that middle-aged men are more likely to attempt to lose weight once they perceive that they have a health problem from a health professional (particularly a health scare or hospitalisation); are told by a health professional that they are 'obese' as opposed to other terms; and/ or are shown their weight position on a chart [21]. Doctors' referral to commercial organisations probably doubles the proportion of men taking part, compared to self-referral [21]. This suggests that, for some men, health professionals' advice acts as a motivator to engage in a programme. Contacts with primary care can provide 'teachable moments' [32], opportunities to motivate people to change unhealthy behaviours and for referral or signposting to available services. Offers of health screening (e.g. cholesterol, blood pressure), particularly checks provided outside health service premises, may be a way of engaging with obese men. 'Jolts' from a partner and word-of-mouth recommendation can help provide motivation to lose weight and engage with programmes.

Improving personal appearance is an important motivator, but men are wary of looking too thin [33]. In contrast to women, social norms mean that men may express the desire to gain weight as a means of living up to bodily ideals for strength and size.

Placing interventions in the community, for example, in sports clubs and workplaces, may be preferable to healthcare settings. The enjoyment associated with attending a football or rugby match in a stadium contrasts with the anxiety that can be experienced while visiting a health setting. Associating such healthcare-related visits with their long-standing loyalty and pleasure from collectively supporting a sporting team (still predominantly a male activity), while challenging men to change behaviour, could also increase the likelihood of 'contagious motivation' among fans. Privileges, such as access to team coaches and gifts of clothing, reinforce the connection between being a supporter

and losing weight. These factors are exemplified by the successful long-term weight loss of men participating in the Football Fans in Training (FFIT) programme, a randomised trial with football clubs in Scotland [28,34]. Men in the FFIT programme attended 12 weekly sessions at their club training ground and received personalised dietary and behaviour change advice, followed by structured exercise classes delivered by the club community coaches. Men were encouraged to increase their walking through the use of pedometers and were taught behaviour change techniques (e.g. goal setting and self-monitoring). The 12-week active phase was followed by email prompts and group reunions at 6 and 12 months. The FFIT trial attracted men at high risk of future ill health, very few of whom had ever attended a weight loss programme with the NHS or in the commercial sector [35].

However, sporting venues are not the most promising points of contact for all obese men. Workplaces offer another opportunity, and programmes could influence productivity and absenteeism. Other venues that are associated with male identities outside health services need to be considered to deliver programmes that could reach and engage disadvantaged groups, such as barbers and pubs. Careful use of humour may attract men in promotional materials, but care should be taken not to trivialise issues.

Diet and alcohol

There is clear evidence from our review of randomised trials that low energy diets, particularly low-fat, low energy diets, are effective for men, and are the most important component of any weight loss intervention [21]. We have been unable to establish that the macronutrient (such as providing more protein) or energy content of low energy diets (provided there is a prescribed calorie deficit) influence the amount of long-term weight loss in men. It is clear that men do not want strict or extreme diets. It may be that terms describing 'healthier eating' are best used to promote reducing diets to men, rather than 'dieting' terms. Allowing some alcohol and food treats is also valued, although high alcohol intake may be an issue for some men. Heavy alcohol intake ($\geq$30 g/day) is strongly associated with weight gain and obesity [36]. Men have reported being particularly interested in the scientific appeal of the energy intake and energy expenditure equation, and the ability to monitor their energy intake [21].

Physical activity

Men do well if physical activity is part of a weight loss programme, and may be more likely to respond to this than women [21]. However, weight loss in men is greater with low energy diets than with a physical activity programme alone, and better if both are provided. Pain and comorbidities may be barriers to increasing physical activity for some men.

Interventions in sport clubs, with their focus on physical activity sessions, are particularly able to provide this important aspect of men's weight loss programmes. Men responded enthusiastically to the use of pedometers, but walking as a means of exercise may not always be liked, and some men may prefer to use the gym [37].

Behaviour change

Our review evidence suggests that behaviour change strategies and techniques should be similar in men and women [21]. NICE recommends that interventions at an individual level contain easy steps over time, coping strategies, goal setting and sharing these goals, and planning for social situations that might undermine changes [38]. In another systematic review of systematic reviews and meta-analyses (including meta-regression), Greaves and colleagues [39] found that engaging social support, increased contact frequency and using a cluster of self-regulatory behaviour change techniques (e.g. goal setting, prompting self-monitoring, providing feedback, review of goals) increased the effectiveness of programmes, mainly based on weight loss outcomes. Phone and email support may be helpful, particularly for long-term follow-up. Feedback on diaries is valued, but men are less likely than women to use web-based discussion groups for weight loss support [21].

Social support

In a systematic review of male inclusion in randomised trials, Pagoto and colleagues [40] found a trend of lower representation of men in groups

(24%) compared to individuals (29%) or mail/email/Internet programmes (34%), but the sex distribution of these groups was not described. To enhance the appeal of group-based programmes, some provision of individual tailoring of fact-based, simple-to-understand advice or counselling is also desirable [21]. A systematic review by Young and colleagues [22] found that group-based face-to-face sessions and increased frequency of contact were associated with greater weight loss in men.

Based on qualitative research, some men clearly wish to attend men-only groups [33,41], but not all men will have a preference [41,42]. Although some men will be reluctant to take part in group programmes, being able to identify with other participants can help, including meeting people with similar health problems. Men who are a minority in a mixed-sex group may be 'cheered on' by the female slimmers [42].

For men, groups provide camaraderie, and the presence of spontaneous humour and banter, which has been shown to be very important, as demonstrated by the FFIT trial [35]. However, although groups may require fewer resources to run, group-based programmes can be logistically difficult to arrange. For group-based programmes, it is important to arrange longer-term follow-up and support after the initial weight loss phase.

Family and friends can play a pivotal role in successful weight loss, providing support for choosing against the expected social norm. If they are not supportive, they can also be very detrimental to men's efforts to lose weight [21].

The 'Healthy Dads, Healthy Kids' randomised trial from Australia evaluated the effect of primary school children attending some group weight loss sessions intended for their fathers. After 6 months, men in the intervention group had lost 7.6 kg more than men in the control group, with significant improvements in physical activity and dietary intake in their children too [43].

Commercial weight loss programmes

Commercial weight loss organisations are effective in producing weight loss in men, especially when delivered in mixed-sex settings, but men are much less likely to enrol in such commercial programmes than women. Some organisations have started to offer men-only groups/sections in their websites. However, it is unclear how much single-sex group sessions are tailored for men. Although referrals by doctors to commercial providers can improve the low take-up, health service programmes appear to be favoured over commercial weight loss organisations, despite the fact that health service settings appear to provoke fear and anxiety among men.

Drug treatment

One randomised trial has examined the effects of orlistat 120 mg three times daily as compared to placebo added to lifestyle counselling for weight maintenance in type 2 diabetes. In the weight maintenance phase, after an 8-week very-low-calorie diet, men were significantly less likely to benefit from orlistat than women after 1 year (calculated difference in weight loss between orlistat and placebo 3.1% for women and 0.8% for men) [44].

Other factors to consider

We found evidence that some men found technology and innovations appealing in their weight loss programmes – for example, using sandbags to demonstrate weight that had been lost, or body scans to show changes in body composition [21].

There is no clear evidence that the sex or profession of the person delivering the intervention affects men's outcomes. In the UK, men appear to be more likely to raise weight problems with primary care nurses than with their family doctor [21].

4.13.6 Conclusions

Policies and services to prevent and treat obesity should take account of sex and gender-related differences, and consult users in the development and evaluation of services. Some points to consider when designing services for men are listed in the summary box. Additional helpful resources are available in the literature [45,46].

4.13.7 Summary box

Key points

- The main features of effective weight loss programmes are the same for men and women.
- Weight reduction for men is best achieved and maintained with a combination of reduced diet, physical activity advice, opportunities to exercise and behaviour change techniques (e.g. self-monitoring, goal setting, providing feedback, review of goals).
- Men prefer more fact-based information on how to lose weight and place more emphasis on physical activity programmes than women.
- For some men, but not all, the opportunity to attend men-only groups may enhance effectiveness. Some individual tailoring and accepting feedback may also be features of more effective services.
- To help recruit men, it may be better to provide weight loss programmes in social settings, such as sports clubs and workplaces, than in health service settings.
- Innovative means of delivering services are needed for hard-to-reach groups, such as younger men, unemployed men and those men who do not see their weight status as a problem.
- Health service staff should be encouraged to recognise 'teachable moments' to initiate discussion and provide opportunities to access weight loss services.

References

1. Centers for Disease Control and Prevention. Healthy weight, overweight, and obesity among adults aged 20 and over, by selected characteristics: United States, selected years 1960–1962 through 2007–2010. Atlanta, USA: CDC, 2010. Internet: http://www.cdc.gov/nchs/data/hus/2012/068.pdf, accessed 31 January 2014.
2. Health Survey for England – 2011. Health, social care and lifestyles [document on the Internet]. Leeds: The Health and Social Care Information Centre, 2012. Internet: http://www.ic.nhs.uk/searchcatalogue?productid=10149&returnid=1685, accessed 31 January 2014.
3. Butland B, Jebb S, Kopelman P, McPherson K, Thomas S, Mardell J, et al. Foresight. Tackling obesities: future choices – project report, 2nd edn [document on the Internet]. London: Government Office for Science, 2007. Internet: http://www.bis.gov.uk/assets/foresight/docs/obesity/17.pdf, accessed 31 January 2014.

4. US National Weight Control Registry. NWCR facts. Internet: http://www.nwcr.ws/Research/default.htm, accessed 31 January 2014.

5. Ross HM, Laws R, Reckless J, Lean M, McQuigg M, Noble P, et al. Evaluation of the counterweight programme for obesity management in primary care: a starting point for continuous improvement. *British Journal of General Practice* 2008; **58**: 548–554.

6. Stubbs RJ, Pallister C, Whybrow S, Avery A, Lavin J. Weight outcomes audit for 34,271 adults referred to a primary care/commercial weight management partnership scheme. *Obesity Facts* 2011; **4**: 113–120.

7. Ahern AL, Olson AD, Aston LM, Jebb SA. Weight Watchers on prescription: an observational study of weight change among adults referred to Weight Watchers by the NHS. *BMC Public Health* 2011; **11**: 434.

8. Prospective Studies Collaboration. Body-mass index and cause-specific mortality in 900,000 adults: collaborative analyses of 57 prospective studies. *Lancet* 2009; **373**: 1083–1096.

9. Han TS, Tajar S, O'Neill TW, Jiang M, Bartfai G, Boonen S, et al. Impaired quality of life and sexual function in overweight and obese men: the European Male Ageing Study. *European Journal of Endocrinology* 2011; **164**: 1003–1011.

10. Gough B, Conner MT. Barriers to healthy eating amongst men: a qualitative analysis. *Social Science & Medicine* 2006; **62**: 387–395.

11. McCabe MP, McGreevy SJ. Role of media and peers on body change strategies among adult men: is body size important? *European Eating Disorders Review* 2011; **19**: 438–446.

12. Hunt K, McCann C, Gray CM, Mutrie N, Wyke S. 'You've got to walk before you run': positive evaluations of a walking program as part of a gender-sensitized, weight-management program delivered to men through professional football clubs. *Health Psychology* 2013; **32**: 57–65.

13. Wolfe BL, Smith JE. Different strokes for different folks: why overweight men do not seek weight loss treatment. *Eating Disorders* 2002; **10**: 115–124.

14. Sabinsky MS, Toft U, Raben A, Holm L. Overweight men's motivations and perceived barriers towards weight loss. *European Journal of Clinical Nutrition* 2007; **61**: 526–531.

15. White A, Conrad D, Branney P. Targeting men's weight in the workplace. *Journal of Men's Health* 2008; **5**: 133–140.

16. Connell R. *Gender and Power: Society, the Person and Sexual Politics*. Cambridge: Polity, 1987.

17. Galdas PM, Cheater F, Marshall P. Men and health help-seeking behaviour: literature review. *Journal of Advanced Nursing* 2005; **49**: 616–623.

18. Galdas PM. Men, masculinity and help seeking behaviour. In: Broom A, Tovey P, (eds) *Men's Health: Body, Identity and Social Context*. Chichester: Wiley-Blackwell, 2009.

19. Ross R, Shaw KD, Rissanen J, Martel Y, De Guise J, Avruch L. Sex differences in lean and adipose tissue distribution by magnetic resonance imaging: anthropometric relationships. *American Journal of Clinical Nutrition* 1994; **59**: 1277–1285.

20. CG43: Obesity: Guidance on the prevention, identification, assessment and management of overweight and obesity in adults and children. London: National Institute for Health and Care Excellence, 2014. Internet: http://www.nice.org.uk/guidance/cg43/resources/guidance-obesity-pdf, accessed 12 August 2014.

21. Robertson C, Archibald D, Avenell A, Douglas F, Hoddinott P, van Teijlingen E, et al. Systematic reviews and integrated report on the quantitative, qualitative and economic evidence base for the management of obesity in men. *Health Technology Assessment* 2014; **35**: v–vi, xxiii–xxis, 1–424.

22. Young MD, Morgan PJ, Plotnikoff RC, Callister R, Collins CE. Effectiveness of male-only weight loss and weight maintenance interventions: a systematic review and meta-analysis. *Obesity Reviews* 2012; **13**: 393–408.

23. Esposito K, Giugliano F, Di Palo C, Giugliano G, Marfella R, D'Andrea F, et al. Effect of lifestyle changes on erectile dysfunction in obese men. *JAMA* 2004; **291**: 2978–2984.

24. Wadden TA, Neiberg RH, Wing RR, Clark JM, Delahanty LM, Hill JO, et al. Four-year weight losses in the Look AHEAD Study: factors associated with long-term success. *Obesity* 2011; **19**: 1987–1998.

25. Wing RR, Rosen RC, Fava JL, Bahnson J, Brancati F, Gendrano I, et al. Effects of weight loss intervention on erectile function in older men with type 2 diabetes in the Look AHEAD trial. *The Journal of Sexual Medicine* 2010; **7**: 156–165.

26. Lindstrom J, Peltonen M, Eriksson JG, Aunola S, Hamalainen H, Ilanne PP, et al. Determinants for the effectiveness of lifestyle intervention in the Finnish Diabetes Prevention Study. *Diabetes Care* 2008; **31**: 857–862.

27. Schwartz AV, Johnson KC, Kahn SE, Shepherd JA, Nevitt MC, Peters AL, et al. Effect of 1 year of an intentional weight loss intervention on bone mineral density in type 2 diabetes: results from the Look AHEAD randomized trial. *Journal of Bone and Mineral Research* 2012; **27**: 619–627.

28. Hunt K, Wyke S, Gray CM, Anderson AS, Brady A, Bunn C, et al. A gender-sensitised weight loss and healthy living programme for overweight and obese men delivered by Scottish Premier League football clubs (FFIT): a pragmatic randomised controlled trial. *Lancet* 2014; **383**: 1211–1221.

29. Jolly K, Lewis A, Beach J, Denley J, Adab P, Deeks JJ, et al. Comparison of range of commercial or primary care led weight reduction programmes with minimal intervention control for weight loss in obesity: lighten up randomised controlled trial. *BMJ* 2011; **343**: 1035.

30. Wadden TA, Neiberg RH, Wing RR, Clark JM, Delahanty LM, Hill JO, et al. Four-year weight losses in the Look AHEAD Study: factors associated with long-term success. *Obesity* 2011; **19**: 1987–1998.

31. The Look AHEAD Research Group. Eight-year weight losses with an intensive lifestyle intervention: The Look AHEAD Study. *Obesity* 2014; **22**: 5–13.

32. Cohen DJ, Clark EC, Lawson PJ, Casucci BA, Flocke SA. Identifying teachable moments for health behavior counseling in primary care. *Patient Education and Counseling* 2011; **85**: e8–e15.

33. Gray CM, Anderson AS, Clarke AM, Dalziel A, Hunt K, Leishman J, et al. Addressing male obesity: an evaluation of a group-based weight management intervention for Scottish men. *Journal of Men's Health* 2009; **6**: 70–81.

34. Gray CM, Hunt K, Mutrie N, Anderson AS, Leishman J, Dalgarno L, et al. Football Fans in Training: the development

and optimization of an intervention delivered through professional sports clubs to help men lose weight, become more active and adopt healthier eating habits. *BMC Public Health* 2013; **13**: 322.

35. Hunt K, Gray CM, Maclean A, Smillie S, Bunn C, Wyke S. Do weight management programmes delivered at professional football clubs attract and engage high risk men? A mixed-methods study. *BMC Public Health* 2014; **14**: 50.

36. Wannamethee SG, Shaper AG. Alcohol, body weight, and weight gain in middle-aged men. *American Journal of Clinical Nutrition* 2003; **77**: 1312–1317.

37. Hunt K, McCann C, Gray CM, Mutrie N, Wyke S. 'You've got to walk before you run': positive evaluations of a walking program as part of a gender-sensitized, weight-management program delivered to men through professional football clubs. *Health Psychology* 2013; **32**: 57–65.

38. PH6: Behaviour change at population, community and individual levels [document on the Internet]. London: National Institute for Health and Clinical Excellence, 2007. Internet: http://guidance.nice.org.uk/PH6/Guidance/pdf/English, accessed 31 January 2014.

39. Greaves CJ, Sheppard KE, Abraham C, Hardeman W, Roden M, Evans PH, et al. Systematic review of reviews of intervention components associated with increased effectiveness in dietary and physical activity interventions. *BMC Public Health* 2011; **11**: 119.

40. Pagoto SL, Schneider KL, Oleski JL, Luciani JM, Bodenlos JS, Whited MC. Male inclusion in randomized controlled trials of lifestyle weight loss interventions. *Obesity* 2012; **20**: 1234–1239.

41. Morgan PJ, et al. Engaging men in weight loss: experiences of men who participated in the male only SHED-IT pilot study. *Obesity Research & Clinical Practice* 2011; **5**: e239–e248.

42. De Souza P, Ciclitira KE. Men and dieting: a qualitative analysis. *Journal of Health Psychology* 2005; **10**: 793–804.

43. Morgan PJ, Lubans DR, Callister R, Okely AD, Burrows TL, Fletcher R, et al. The 'Healthy Dads, Healthy Kids' randomized controlled trial: efficacy of a healthy lifestyle program for overweight fathers and their children. *International Journal of Obesity* 2011; **35**: 436–447.

44. Richelsen B, Tonstad S, Rossner S, Toubro S, Niskanen L, Madsbad S, et al. Effect of orlistat on weight regain and cardiovascular risk factors following a very-low-energy diet in abdominally obese patients: a 3-year randomized, placebo-controlled study. *Diabetes Care* 2007; **30**: 27–32.

45. Banks I. The HGV man manual. Yeovil: JH Haynes & Co Ltd, 2005.

46. McCarthy M, Richardson N. Report on best practice approaches to tailoring lifestyle interventions for obese men in the primary care setting. Centre for Men's health, Department of Health and Science, Institute of Technology, Carlow, Republic of Ireland, 2011. Internet: http://www.hse.ie/eng/health/child/healthyeating/tacklingmaleobesityinprimarycare.pdf, accessed 31 January 2014.

Chapter 4.14

Weight loss interventions in specific groups: Adults with intellectual disabilities and obesity

Dimitrios Spanos[1] and Craig A Melville[2]
[1] Cleveland Clinic Abu Dhabi, Abu Dhabi, UAE
[2] University of Glasgow, Glasgow, UK

To understand the needs of individuals with intellectual disabilities (IDs), this chapter will start with a definition of ID, a summary of the prevalence studies of obesity and an outline of the determinants of obesity in this population group. National clinical guidelines [1–2] recommend the use of multicomponent weight loss interventions for the management of obesity. Therefore, the issues around multicomponent weight loss interventions for adults with ID and obesity are discussed in the final part of the chapter.

4.14.1 Definition of intellectual disability

The American Association on Intellectual and Developmental Disabilities (AAIDD) [3] defines ID as:

> … a disability characterized by significant limitations both in intellectual functioning and in adaptive behaviour, which covers many everyday social and practical skills. This disability originates before the age of 18.

Individuals with IDs have more complex unmet health needs than the general population, and experience significant health inequalities, including increased mortality rates, higher physical and mental health needs and inequitable access to evidence-based healthcare [4].

4.14.2 Obesity in people with intellectual disabilities

Obesity is an important health issue for children and adults with IDs, and comparisons with data from national health surveys consistently report that the prevalence of obesity is higher in this population group than in the general population [5–7].

In children and adolescents, the prevalence of obesity ranges from 7 to 36% [7]. In adults, studies report a range of estimates of obesity from 2 to 50.5% [8]. A review of 12 articles published between 1985 and 2006 showed that the national and international prevalence of obesity in adults with IDs has increased in the last 20 years [9]. However, a recent study showed that the prevalence of obesity in adults with IDs in 20 states in the USA has reached similar levels as that of people without IDs (33.6 vs. 33.8%, respectively) [10].

Caution should be exercised in interpreting the review findings on the prevalence, because of the heterogeneity identified across the study samples. Recruitment of samples from different geographical areas (e.g. urban and suburban areas, individuals

Advanced Nutrition and Dietetics in Obesity, First Edition. Edited by Catherine Hankey.
© 2018 John Wiley & Sons Ltd. Published 2018 by John Wiley & Sons Ltd.

living in the community or living in institutions), as well as the inclusion of people with varying levels of IDs and people who have full time and part time support from carers, all contribute to the heterogeneity of the sample. However, the overall evidence indicates that the rates of obesity are higher for individuals with IDs.

4.14.3 Determinants of obesity in intellectual disability

The identification of the determinants of obesity in adults with IDs is relevant to the prevention of obesity and for the development of weight management interventions [9]. Some of the most commonly recognised risk factors for obesity in IDs are discussed in the following subsections.

Gender

Similar to the general population [11], 11 studies in adults with IDs show higher rates of obesity in women than in men [5]. Bhaumik et al. [7] reported that women with IDs were around three times more likely to be obese than men with IDs (OR 0.36; 95% CI = 0.25–0.53). This finding is supported by a population-based study which found that women were more likely to have obesity (OR 1.68; 95% CI = 1.28–2.21) [5].

Dietary habits

Similar to the general population, people with IDs are susceptible to unhealthy dietary habits, and have the same needs for healthy and balanced diets [12]. Recorded unhealthy dietary habits among people with IDs include high fat intake and very low consumption of fruit and vegetables [13–14]. However, alcohol consumption has not been identified as a big health issue among adults with IDs [13–14].

Very few studies have examined the association between unhealthy dietary habits and the risk of developing obesity in adults with IDs. Druheim et al. [15] assessed the dietary habits of 145 participants with mild IDs living in the community and found that participants with lower dietary fat intakes

($\leq35\%$ of total intake) were at lower risk of developing abdominal obesity. However, Cunningham et al. [16] and Braunschweig et al. [17] reported no significant associations between dietary intakes and BMI or waist circumference.

It is difficult to review the evidence and make an overall estimation of the dietary habits of people with IDs, owing to the methodological differences among the studies. For example, Draheim et al. [15] assessed the nutritional status of the participants by using the "Block Screening Questionnaire for Fat Intake', but Cunningham et al. [16] used semi-weighing techniques over 4 consecutive days. In addition, data was based on reports made by the participants with assistance from the carers who supported them, or via entirely second-hand reporting by the carers. This method can affect the reliability of assessing the health behaviours of people with IDs [13].

Physical activity

Adults with IDs have consistently been shown to lead inactive and sedentary lifestyles. A review of data from national health surveys show that men and women with IDs are less likely to meet public health recommendations for physical activity than the general population [18].

Current guidelines for health improvement in the general population recommend at least 30 min of accumulated moderate-intensity physical activity for 5 days per week or more [1] A review of studies assessing the physical activity levels of adults with IDs reported that the proportion of study participants who follow current clinical guidelines ranges from 17.5 to 33% [19]. Older age, lack of daytime opportunities, immobility, faecal incontinence and epilepsy have been identified as barriers to physical activity in adults with IDs [20].

Finlayson et al. [21] compared the actual levels and patterns of physical activity in adults with IDs against the recommended 10,000 steps per day. The study found that only 27% of the participants, who were mainly public transport users, were achieving the recommended number of steps. The participants (73%) who were not achieving the 10,000 steps were mainly overweight ($P < 0.05$).

There is no consistency in the methodologies used in these studies. There is a variety of physical activity assessment techniques used, such as accelerometers, pedometers and diaries. There is also a variety of definitions used to classify healthy physical activity levels – for example, 10,000 steps, 30 min of moderate physical activity, etc. Measured outcomes included the percentage of inactivity and the hours spent exercising or walking. Regardless of the differences in methodology, research consistently reports low levels of physical activity in adults with IDs.

Environment – living arrangements

Evidence from studies that explore the environmental factors linked to obesity in adults with IDs show a strong association between living in less restrictive environments and obesity.

Bryan et al. [22] assessed the nutritional vulnerability of people with IDs living in the community by measuring weight changes 1 year after discharge from institutions. The study showed that the prevalence of overweight for males and females increased within 1 year by 6% and 5%, respectively. Moran et al. [23] defined more restrictive environments including community training homes, intermediate care facilities and family homes, private boarding homes, supervised apartment living or living in a private home as least restrictive environments. Prevalence of obesity was found to be higher in adults with IDs living in less restrictive environments than in those living in more restrictive environments ($P < 0.05$). This finding is supported by Bhaumik et al. [7], who showed that individuals who live independently, or with family members, were at higher risk of becoming obese than individuals living in residential care.

Proposed pathways for this environmental influence on the development of obesity is the impact of living in a restrictive institution but living in the community where there is greater availability of food choices and access to it. Consequentially, it has been suggested that people with IDs who live independently in the community may not be prepared for the implications of the lifestyle patterns they adopt or follow. This highlights the need to provide accessible information and appropriate support for individuals with IDs.

Level of intellectual disability

Studies that have used bivariate and multivariate analysis to examine the association between levels of IDs and the prevalence of obesity consistently report that obesity is more common in individuals with milder IDs [7,24]. Melville et al. [5] reported that men and women with profound IDs had a 52% and 71% lower risk of obesity, respectively, than men and women with mild IDs. Profound IDs can often be accompanied by neurological problems that affect food intake, and is therefore often associated with the risk of becoming underweight.

Obesogenic medication

A review of 43 studies showed that the medication used for chronic conditions can lead to a weight gain of 10 kg in 52 weeks [25]. Medications known for their obesogenic effect include antipsychotics, antidepressants, lithium, beta blockers and insulin. The side effects of these medications, especially the psychotropic ones, include increased appetite and abnormalities in the metabolic rate, leading to weight gain. These types of medications are more commonly used by adults with IDs [26], and could potentially contribute to the increased rate of obesity.

Genetic syndromes

In a small proportion of individuals with IDs, the genes responsible for the IDs could also contribute to the development of obesity at an early age. It is believed that these genes could act directly in the brain, or in the periphery, to affect food intake and energy metabolism [27]. Research has identified about 30 genetic disorders that have obesity as a clinical feature and are also associated with IDs, dysmorphic features and organ developmental abnormalities [28]. More common genetic syndromes that are associated with obesity include Prader–Willi, Bardet–Biedl, Cohen and Down syndromes.

4.14.4 Weight management interventions for adults with intellectual disabilities

Several reviews that examined the effectiveness of weight loss interventions for adults with IDs have commented on the limited evidence-base and methodological weaknesses of published studies [29]. The limitations of the studies reviewed include small sample sizes, heterogeneous samples, non-randomised designs and generalisability of the results. There is a need for research in adults with IDs and obesity to examine the effectiveness of multicomponent weight loss interventions. These studies are essential to assess the sustainability of the weight loss interventions and their cost-effectiveness. In keeping with the treatments of choice recommended in clinical guidelines [1,2], the focus of investigation in the following section is multicomponent weight loss interventions for adults with a variety of IDs.

Multicomponent weight loss interventions

The studies discussed in this section are multicomponent interventions that focussed on three lifestyle areas: diet, physical activity and behaviour [1,2]. These interventions used behaviour change strategies to improve unhealthy dietary patterns and to increase the physical activity levels of individuals with IDs and obesity.

Of eight studies for adults with IDs identified as multicomponent weight loss interventions, six were mainly delivered in group sessions, and two offered individual interventions [30,31]. The components of the different interventions in these studies are summarised in the following text.

Diet

Only two studies included energy-deficit diets as part of the intervention. Melville et al. [30] recommended dietary change based on a personalised dietary prescription that was calculated to achieve an energy deficit of 600 kcal/day and a weight loss of 0.5–1 kg/week. Saunders et al. [31] recommended

a low-energy diet of 1200–1300 kcal/day, focussing on the consumption of foods that provide the sensation of fullness and offering meal-replacement shakes that provide 110 kcal per serving. This study also developed a 'Stoplight Guide', classifying food into three coloured categories based on their energy content: green for <60 kcal, yellow for 60–100 kcal and red for >100 kcal.

Other studies that involved a dietary change component offered home visits to the participants to develop individualised dietary plans [32,33]. One study provided dietary information based on the diabetic exchange diet [34]. The rest of the studies provided limited information about the nutritional advice that was offered to the participants. These studies mainly took the form of health education programmes providing general information on healthy dietary habits and patterns – for example, healthy meal planning [35–37]. Cooking classes, meal planning and grocery store visits were common activities relevant to diets offered among the interventions [31,33,35,37].

Physical activity

Compared to the multicomponent interventions for adults without IDs, the physical activity component in interventions for adults with IDs recommended less intensive physical activity. Only one study followed current clinical guidelines and recommended that participants work towards 30 min of moderate-intensity physical activity, on at least 5 days per week [30]. Five of the studies incorporated physical activity (sometimes optional) as part of the intervention sessions – offering dancing, aerobic exercises and walking [31,33–35,37]. Ewing et al. [32] and Mann et al. [33] offered home visits to develop an individualised physical activity programme for the participants. Jackson and Thorbecke provided advice on simple changes – for example, taking the stairs instead of the lift [36].

Behaviour

The behavioural techniques that were used as part of the multicomponent interventions included goal setting, strategies to improve motivation, problem-solving, stimulus control and relapse-prevention strategies [30,32–34]. Geller and Crowley [37] mainly focussed on empowering the participants by enhancing their ability to make choices, and by creating feelings of community and success. Self-monitoring was facilitated with weight and food diaries [30,31,36], and reward systems were used to motivate behavioural changes [31,35,36]. None of the multicomponent interventions for adults with IDs that focussed on behaviour modification reported using a specific theory – for example, trans-theoretical therapy or social cognitive theory.

Overview of the outcomes of multicomponent weight loss interventions

The majority of the studies for adults with IDs and obesity have not followed the national guideline recommendations on obesity management, and have not focussed on changing the dietary, physical activity and behavioural aspects of an individual's lifestyle, at the same time [1,2]. Energy-deficit diets were not usually offered as part of the dietary intervention. Physical activity interventions were of low intensity, and did not follow the total recommended minutes and levels of physical activity. However, most of the studies used similar behavioural approach techniques, although none of them reported using a specific behaviour change theory.

Only a few multicomponent studies for adults with IDs helped participants achieve a clinically significant weight loss of 5–10%. All the multicomponent interventions reported decreases in weight (or BMI), but it appears that the biggest instances of weight loss were reported by the two interventions that recommended energy-deficit diets [30,31]. At 6 months follow-up, Saunders et al. [31] reported a 6.3% weight loss from baseline, and Melville et al. [30] reported a mean weight loss of 4.3%. Melville et al. [30] reported that 36% of the participants reached a 5% weight loss. No power calculations or randomisations were used by any of these studies. An intervention that intensively involved the parents of the participants reported a 6% weight loss at

week 17, and a further weight loss of 10.4% from baseline in 12 months [36].

There are several important methodological weaknesses in the evidence base. The majority of the studies of multicomponent weight loss interventions recruited small sample sizes, ranging from 12 to 192, and included obese and overweight participants based on BMI scores. Only one study limited inclusion criteria to participants with obesity [30].

Only two studies reported weight changes at follow-up at least 12 months from baseline [34,36]. All the multicomponent studies reported attrition or dropout rates, with the highest attrition rate up to 35% [35]. The study by Bazzano et al. [35], which had the highest attrition rate, reported that the barriers to attendance included lack of motivation to exercise, transportation issues, childcare problems, conflicting work schedules and language translation needs. Ewing et al. [32] showed that, when home visits were added to the analysis of attendance in more than four classes of the intervention, attendance was higher among the group with home visits (87%) as compared to those without home visits (79%).

The majority of the multicomponent studies for adults with IDs and obesity did not aim for the recommended clinically significant weight loss [1,2]. Studies that incorporated energy-deficit diets as part of their intervention reported bigger weight loss than the studies offering healthy eating advice. Weaknesses in the methodology are similar to those identified by the other reviews, including small sample sizes, heterogeneity in the characteristics of the samples, no randomised designs and no long follow-ups [29].

4.14.5 The role of carers

The supporting role of carers has been recognised as an important factor in meeting the needs of individuals with IDs. Carers can exert a strong influence on the dietary patterns of people with IDs by making food choices on their behalf, based on their own knowledge or preferences [38]. However, carers may have poor knowledge about healthy eating and healthy physical activity patterns [39]. Since carers often have pivotal relationships with the persons they support, and can help in tackling the barriers or difficulties that individuals with IDs experience, it is essential to involve carers in intervention research for adults with IDs.

A limitation of the weight loss intervention literature for adults with IDs is that the role of the carers is not always described in detail. Carers have been invited to be present during interventions to simply support the participants, assist in the consultation where appropriate, encourage the participants during the weight loss process [30] or be involved with the design of activity programmes [31]. In other studies, the carers had more active roles, such as assisting with food intake recording, reinforcing intervention messages and being involved with reward systems [29].

The involvement of carers in the obesity management of adults with IDs can have a positive impact on weight loss. However, to date, there has been only very limited description of the views and experiences of carers supporting individuals with IDs participating in a weight loss intervention.

4.14.6 Conclusion

There is a high prevalence of obesity in adults with IDs, and the determinants are multifactorial and different from the general population. Overall, the studies that examine weight loss interventions in adults with IDs are characterised by significant methodological limitations. Therefore, there is insufficient evidence to support the effectiveness of multicomponent weight loss interventions in adults with IDs and obesity.

Future research should aim to use controlled designs, follow-up participants for at least 12 months and specifically examine weight loss maintenance in adults with IDs. There is also a need to specifically assess the role of carers in supporting the participants in weight loss interventions, and to explore factors that could contribute to clinically effective weight loss (≥5% weight loss from initial body weight).

4.14.7 Summary box

Key points

- There is a high prevalence of obesity in adults with IDs, and the determinants are multifactorial and different from the general population.
- Studies that examine weight loss interventions in adults with IDs are characterised by significant methodological limitations.
- To date, there is insufficient evidence to support the effectiveness of multicomponent weight loss interventions in adults with IDs and obesity.
- Future research should aim to use controlled designs, follow-up participants for at least 12 months and examine weight loss maintenance in adults with IDs.
- The role of carers in supporting the participants in weight loss interventions is important.

References

1. National Institute for Health and Clinical Excellence (NICE). Obesity: the prevention, identification, assessment and management of overweight and obesity in adults and children, 2006. NICE, London.
2. Scottish Intercollegiate Guideline Network (SIGN). Management of obesity: a national clinical guideline, 2010. SIGN, Edinburgh.
3. American Association on Intellectual and Developmental Disabilities. Definition of intellectual disability [accessed 30.11.2011], 2010. Available from: http://aaidd.org/intellectual-disability/definition, last accessed October 2016.
4. Scheepers M, Kerr M, O'Hara D, Bainbridge D, Cooper S, Davis R, et al. Reducing health disparity in people with intellectual disabilities: a report from Health Issues Special Interest Research Group of the International Association for the Scientific Study of Intellectual Disabilities *Journal of Policy and Practice in Intellectual Disabilities* 2005; **2**: 249–255.
5. Melville CA, Cooper SA, Morrison J, Allan L, Smiley E, Williamson A. The prevalence and determinants of obesity in adults with intellectual disabilities. *Journal of Applied Research in Intellectual Disabilities* 2008; **21**: 425–437.
6. Bhaumik S, Watson J, Thorp C, Tyrer F, McGrother C. Body mass index in adults with intellectual disability: distribution, associations and service implications: a population-based prevalence study. *Journal of Intellectual Disabilities* 2008; **52**: 287–298.
7. Maiano C. Prevalence and risk factors of overweight and obesity among children and adolescents with intellectual disabilities. *Obesity Reviews* 2011; **12**: 189–197.
8. Haveman M, Heller T, Lee L, Maaskant M, Shooshtari S, Strydom A. Major health risks in aging persons with intellectual disabilities: An overview of recent studies. *Journal of Policy and Practice in Intellectual Disabilities* 2010; **7**: 59–69.

9. Melville CA, Hamilton S, Hankey CR, Miller S, Boyle S. The prevalence and determinants of obesity in adults with intellectual disabilities. *Obesity Reviews* 2007; **8**: 223–230.

10. Stancliffe RJ, Lakin KC, Larson S, Engler J, Bershadsky J, Taub S, et al. Overweight and obesity among adults with intellectual disabilities who use intellectual disability/developmental disability services in 20 U.S. States. *American Journal on Intellectual and Developmental Disabilities* 2011; **116**: 401–418.

11. Rennie KL, Jebb SA. Prevalence of obesity in Great Britain. *Obesity Reviews* 2005; **6**: 11–12.

12. Rimmer JH. Health promotion for people with disabilities: the emerging paradigm shift from disability prevention to prevention of secondary conditions. *Physical Therapy* 1999; **79**: 495–502.

13. McGuire BE, Daly P, Smyth F. Lifestyle and health behaviours of adults with an intellectual disability. *Journal of Intellectual Disability Research* 2007; **51**: 497–510.

14. Bertoli S, Battezzati A, Merati G, Margonato V, Maggioni M, Testolin G, et al. Nutritional status and dietary patterns in disabled people. *Nutrition Metabolism and Cardiovascular Diseases* 2006; **16**: 100–112.

15. Draheim CC, Williams DP, McCubbin JA. Physical activity, dietary intake, and the insulin resistance syndrome in nondiabetic adults with mental retardation. *American Journal of Mental Retardation* 2002; **5**: 361–375.

16. Cunningham K, Gibney MJ, Kelly A, Kevany J, Mulcahy M. Nutrient intakes in long-stay mentally handicapped persons. *European Journal of Clinical Nutrition* 1990; **64**: 3–11.

17. Braunschweig CL, Gomez S, Sheean P, Tomey KM, Rimmer J, Heller T. Nutritional status and risk factors for chronic disease in urban-dwelling adults with Down syndrome. *American Journal of Mental Retardation* 2004; **109**: 186–193.

18. Bartlo P, Klein PJ. Physical activity benefits and needs in adults with intellectual disabilities: systematic review of the literature. *American Journal on Intellectual and Developmental Disabilities* 2011; **116**: 220–232.

19. Stanish HI, Temple VA, Frey GC. Health-promoting physical activity of adults with mental retardation. *Mental Retardation and Developmental Disabilities Research Reviews* 2006; **12**: 13–21.

20. Finlayson J, et al. Understanding predictors of low physical activity in adults with intellectual disabilities. *Journal of Applied Research in Intellectual Disabilities* 2009; **22**: 236–247.

21. Finlayson J, Turner A, Granat MH. Measuring the actual levels and patterns of physical activity/inactivity of adults with intellectual disabilities. *Journal of Applied Research in Intellectual Disabilities* 2011; **24**: 508–517.

22. Bryan F, Allan T, Russell L. The move from a long-stay learning disabilities hospital to community homes: a comparison of clients' nutritional status. *Journal of Human Nutrition and Dietetics* 2000; **13**: 265–270.

23. Moran R, Drane W, McDermott S, Dasari S, Scurry JB, Platt T. Obesity among people with and without mental retardation across adulthood. *Obesity Research* 2005; **13**: 342–349.

24. Emerson E. Underweight, obesity and exercise among adults with intellectual disabilities in supported accommodation in Northern England. *Journal of Intellectual Disability Research* 2005; **49**: 134–143.

25. Leslie WS, Hankey CR, Lean ME. Weight gain as an adverse effect of some commonly prescribed drugs: a systematic review. *The Quarterly Journal of Medicine* 2007; **100**: 395–404.

26. Robertson J, Emerson E, Gregory N, Hatton C, Kessissoglou S, Hallam A. Receipt of psychotropic medication by people with intellectual disability in residential settings. *Journal of Intellectual Disability Research* 2000; **44**: 666–676.

27. Delrue MA, Michaud JL. Fat chance: genetic syndromes with obesity. *Clinical Genetics* 2004; **66**: 83–93.

28. Farooqi IS, O'Rahilly S. New advances in the genetics of early onset obesity. *International Journal of Obesity* 2005; **29**: 1149–1152.

29. Spanos D, Melville C, Hankey C. Weight management interventions in adults with intellectual disabilities and obesity: a systematic review of the evidence. *Nutrition Journal* 2013; **12**: 132.

30. Melville CA, Boyle S, Miller S, Macmillan S, Penpraze V, Pert C, et al. An open study of the effectiveness of a multi-component weight loss intervention for adults with intellectual disabilities and obesity. *British Journal of Nutrition* 2011; **10**: 1553–1562.

31. Saunders RR, Saunders MD, Donnelly JE, Smith BK, Sullivan DK, Guilford B, et al. Evaluation of an approach to weight loss in adults with intellectual or developmental disabilities. *Intellectual and Developmental Disabilities* 2011; **49**: 103–112.

32. Ewing G, McDermott S, Thomas-Koger M, Whitner W, Pierce K. Evaluation of a cardiovascular health program for participants with mental retardation and normal learners. *Health Education & Behavior* 2004; **31**: 77–87.

33. Mann J, Zhou H, McDermot S, Poston MB. Healthy behaviour change of adults with mental retardation: attendance in a health promotion programme. *American Journal of Mental Retardation* 2006; **111**: 62–73.

34. Harris M, Steven R. A pilot investigation of a behavioural weight control program with mentally retarded adolescents and adults: effects on weight, fitness and knowledge of nutritional and behavioural principles. *Rehabilitation Psychology* 1984; **29**: 177–182.

35. Bazzano AT, Zeldin AS, Diab IR, Garro NM, Allevato NA, Lehrer D. The healthy lifestyle change program: a pilot of a community-based health promotion intervention for adults with developmental disabilities. *American Journal of Preventive Medicine* 2009; **37**: 201–208.

36. Jackson HJ, Thorbecke PJ. Treating obesity of mentally retarded adolescents and adults: an exploratory program. *American Journal of Mental Deficiency* 1982; **87**: 302–308.

37. Geller J, Crowley M. An empowerment group visit model as treatment for obesity in developmentally delayed adults. *Journal of Developmental and Physical Disabilities* 2009; **5**: 345–353.

38. Rodgers J. 'Whatever's on her plate': food in the lives of people with learning disabilities. *British Journal of Learning Disabilities* 1998; **26**: 13–16.

39. Melville CA, Hamilton S, Miller S, Boyle S, Robinson N, Pert C, Hankey CR. Carer knowledge and perceptions of healthy lifestyles for adults with intellectual disabilities. *Journal of Applied Research in Intellectual Disabilities* 2009; **22**: 298–306.

Chapter 4.15

Weight maintenance following weight loss in obesity

Nathalie Jones
University of Glasgow, Glasgow, UK

4.15.1 Introduction

Given that obesity is a chronic condition that brings with it long-term health complications, maintenance of weight loss is essential. Although methods of weight loss are explored in the literature and a focus for many patients, the importance of maintaining the lost weight after the weight loss phase is over is often overlooked. Furthermore, we know that weight loss interventions can achieve varying levels of success, but there is now a growing knowledge base regarding approaches to weight maintenance following weight loss.

This chapter aims to investigate the evidence base for weight maintenance and synthesise the aspects of the individual, the supporting health professional and the weight maintenance intervention that contribute to the successful maintenance of weight loss.

Although there is currently no consensus on the definition of weight maintenance in adults, a meta-analysis of weight maintenance definitions recommended that long-term weight maintenance in adults be defined as a weight change of <3% of body weight [1].

However, studies differ in their definitions of weight maintenance – in terms of the units used (weight loss in kilograms or percentage), timescale (number of years examined following the weight loss phase), numeric cut-offs and from when the measurement was taken (i.e. weight prior to or following the weight loss phase) (Table 4.15.1).

4.15.2 Importance of weight maintenance

The health benefits of a 5–10% weight loss have been well documented. SIGN (2010) [12] lists the health benefits associated with sustained modest weight loss, and includes improved lipid profiles, reduced osteoarthritis-related disability, reduced blood pressure [13], improved glycaemic control and insulin sensitivity [14].

If this modest weight loss is not sustained, these health improvements will be short lived. It is common for people to lose and then regain weight. This 'weight cycling' has been defined by SIGN 115 (2010) [12] as 4.5 kg lost and regained over 3–6 years, and has been linked to a greater weight gain as compared to non-weight cyclers, a risk factor for all-cause mortality, hypertension in obese women and symptomatic gallstones in men.

The financial cost of treating obesity is substantial. The chronic nature of obesity requires long-term treatment for weight loss and weight loss maintenance to limit future weight gain episodes, needing repeated costly weight loss attempts. However, it is also important to consider the cost implications of the weight maintenance programmes themselves, and this will be discussed in more detail.

Table 4.15.1 Definitions of weight maintenance in studies examining weight maintenance following weight loss (taken from reference [1])

First author (year)	Study cohort[a]	Weight loss definition (time interval)	Weight maintenance definition (time interval)	Reference point for weight maintenance	Justification for definition
Crawford (2000) [2]	Community-based study	≥5% BMI change (1 year)	Maintain 'new weight' or less (2 years)	After weight loss	Not stated
Field (2001) [3]	Nurses' Health Study II	Small: 5–9.9% (3 years) Large: ≥10%	Two definitions: 1. Gain no more than 5 lb from 'new weight' (4 years) 2. Gain no more than 5%	After weight loss	Not stated
Lowe (2001) [4]	Participants in a commercial weight loss programme (Weight Watchers)	At least 5 lb less than joining weight Encouraged to be in the BMI range of 20–25 kg/m²	Three definitions: 1. Maintain weight loss of at least 5% 2. Maintain weight loss of at least 10% 3. Remained within 5 lb of goal weight	Initial weight After weight loss	Not stated
McQuire (1999) [5]	Random digit dialling survey	≥10% of maximum lifetime weight	Two definitions: 1. Currently ≥10% below maximum weight 2. Maintained ≥10% weight loss for 1 year or more	Initial weight	Not stated
McGuire (1999) [6]	National weight loss registry	At least 10% of body weight (30 lb)	First phase: maintain at least a 10% weight loss for 1 year or more Second phase: ±5 lb	After weight loss and 1 year of weight maintenance	Also used 5% and 10% – similar results
Moore (2000) [7]	Framingham study	>1 lb/year (8 years)	±1 lb/year (8 years) interval	After weight loss	Not stated
Mogul (2003) [8]	Retrospective analysis of syndrome W patients	≥10% or BMI normalisation	Weight regain ≤3 kg (2 years)	After weight loss	NHLBI guidelines (1998)
Sarlio-Lahteenkorva (2000) [9]	Finnish twin cohort	At least 5% between 1975 and 1984	Remain at least 5% below their original weight in 1990	Initial weight	WHO (1998)
Wadden (1999) [10]	25 obese women who lost weight and maintained the weight loss for 1 year	5–10% or >10%	Two definitions: 1. Maintained 5–10% reduction (100 weeks) 2. Maintained >10% reduction (100 weeks)	Initial weight	IOM guidelines (1995)
Wing (2001) [11]	National Weight Control Registry	At least 10% of body weight (30 lb)	Maintain at least 10% weight loss for 1 year or more	Initial weight	IOM guidelines[7] and NHLBI guidelines[2]

[a] All are cohort studies, except Crawford (2000), which was a weight gain prevention intervention.

4.15.3 Evidence base for weight maintenance after weight loss

There have been many publications of varying durations, study designs and sizes on the subject of weight maintenance. Two large bodies of evidence are: (1) the National Weight Control Registry (NWCR) by Wing et al., who have published their findings since the 1990s; [15] and [12] and (2) the Weight Loss Maintenance Randomised Controlled Trial (WLMRCT) by Svetkey et al. [16]. NWCR is the largest study, covering nearly 3000 individuals successful at long-term weight loss maintenance over 10 years. However, it is a self-selected group, chosen based on self-reported and qualitative data. WLMRCT is an intervention study comparing three different approaches to maintenance over 30 months, following a 6-month weight loss programme of the DASH diet and behavioural techniques.

These will be summarised alongside other studies, including the STOP Regain study by Wing et al. [17] (a randomised controlled trial comparing three different methods of weight maintenance for 314 people over 18 months); a systematic review of 11 studies [18] investigating the importance of extended care; and, finally, a study comparing free-living energy expenditure of 61 women who were successful and unsuccessful in maintaining a normal BMI over a year [19].

This chapter will then explore the evidence surrounding weight maintenance by examining varying methods of weight loss, and will look at the Glasgow and Clyde Weight Management Service as an example of an NHS service offering a weight maintenance programme as part of their weight management service.

National Weight Control Registry

The most recently published data from NWCR showed weight loss trajectories of successful weight losers over 10 years [20]. The 2886 participants included in NWCR at entry had lost at least 13 kg and kept it off for at least a year. Mean weight loss compared to the start of the weight loss phase was 31.6 kg at baseline, 23.5 kg at 5 years and 23.1 kg at 10 years. Over 87% of people were still maintaining a 10% weight loss at years 5 and 10. This study over 10 years shows that long-term weight maintenance after weight loss is possible, but requires sustained behaviour change, as summarised in Table 4.15.2.

Extended care

The 'Study to Prevent Regain' (STOP Regain) identified a need for maintenance programmes that teach skills specific to maintaining weight loss [17]. The randomised controlled trial tested the efficacy of a

Table 4.15.2 Characteristics of participants in NWCR who maintained weight loss

Study	Characteristics of successful weight loss maintainers
Klem et al. (1997) [21]	Limited intake of certain foods (92% of participants), quantities (49.2%), percentage energy from fat (38.1%) and counted calories (35.5%) Were physically active, expending an average of 11830 kJ ± 11682 kJ per week (404 kcal ± 399 kcal/day) Self-monitoring of weight, at least weekly (75%) Used more intensive methods of weight loss than in previous weight loss attempts
Shick et al. (1998) [22]	Low-energy and low-fat diet (women consuming an average of 1306 kcal/day with 23% energy from fat; men consuming 1685 kcal/day with 23.5% energy from fat)
Wing et al. (2001) [11]	Low-fat diet (24% of dietary energy) High-carbohydrate diet (56% of dietary energy from carbohydrate) Frequent self-monitoring of body weight and food intake (44% weighed themselves daily and 31% weighed themselves at least once a week) High levels of physical activity (women expending an average of 2545 kcal/week and men 3293 kcal/week, comparable to 1 hour of moderate physical activity daily)

face-to-face programme, an Internet programme and a newsletter control group in preventing weight regain over 18 months. Participants had to have lost at least 10% body weight before starting the maintenance programme. At 6 months, there was a significant difference between the percentage of participants regaining 2.3 kg in the face-to-face group (27%) and the control group (47%). At 18 months, the control group differed significantly from the face-to-face group and the Internet group (72.4% of participants in the control group regained 2.3 kg, as compared to 45.7% of participants in the face-to-face group and 54.8% of participants in the Internet group). These are clinically important findings that seem to show that more care, for longer duration, results in less weight regain.

Middleton et al. [18] extended the data from the STOP Regain study and emphasised the effect of extended care through a systematic review and meta-analysis of 11 studies. Extended care was defined as 'at least two sessions, in person or by phone, by trained interventionists focussing on continued support of the behaviours associated with weight maintenance'. These included a reduced energy intake, increased physical activity, goal setting, problem-solving and relapse prevention. They found that extended care led to the maintenance of an additional 3.2 kg weight loss over 17.6 months post-intervention, as compared to controls. The 11 papers differed in the duration of extended care (1.5–30 months), the type of contact (in person or by phone) and the frequency of contact (weekly, biweekly or monthly). As only 11 studies were identified, the authors were unable to answer questions about the impact of the type or frequency of contact. The authors acknowledge the cost implications of extended care maintenance programmes, but state that, without continued support, weight regain is likely.

The patients' acceptance of extended care should also be considered. For example, Lantz et al. [23] concluded that successful weight loss maintenance depended upon completion of a 4-year comprehensive programme of a hypocaloric diet and behavioural support, but only 48% of people who started, completed the programme.

However, it may well be the case that, over time, the likelihood of continued weight maintenance will increase. Klem et al. suggested that the risk of relapse reduces after a year [24]. They found that people who had maintained their weights for longer used fewer weight maintenance strategies and reported that less effort was required to maintain their weights. This was supported by Wing and Hill, who found that the chances of longer-term success greatly increased once successful maintainers have maintained a weight loss for 2.5 years [11].

Self-monitoring weight in the National Weight Control Registry

Wing suggests that, by adopting particular behavioural strategies, including self-monitoring, 20% of overweight or obese people can achieve weight loss maintenance in the long term [11]. Frequent monitoring of body weight was associated with lower BMI and higher cognitive restraint. Weight regain at 1 year was significantly greater for participants whose self-weighing frequency decreased between baseline and 1 year (4 ± 6.3 kg), as compared to those whose frequency increased (1.1 ± 6.5 kg) or stayed the same (1.8 ± 5.3 kg). Furthermore, those who decreased their frequency of weighing reported increases in fat intake and reduced cognitive restraint [25]. They reported that consistent self-weighing of varying durations may help individuals maintain weight by allowing them to be aware of weight gains promptly and to make changes to prevent additional weight gain.

The STOP Regain study also examined those who had regained at least 2.3 kg of their lost weight, and compared those who had weighed themselves daily with those weighing themselves less often at 18 months [17]. Figure 4.15.1 shows that the numbers of people with weight regain of at least 2.3 kg was significantly lower in those who weighed themselves daily in a face-to-face and Internet group, but not in a newsletter control group where there was no support. It suggests that some external support, whether face to face or via technology, is needed in addition to self-monitoring weight.

Weight Loss Maintenance Randomised Controlled Trial

WLMRCT compared three different approaches of maintenance over 30 months following a 6-month weight loss programme of the DASH diet and

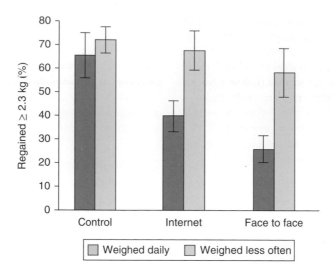

Figure 4.15.1 Proportion of participants who regained 2.3 kg or more among those who reported weighing themselves daily vs. weighing less often at 18 months (taken from reference [17] – reproduced with permission).

behavioural techniques [6]. Participants included in the study were overweight or obese with hypertension and/or dyslipidaemia, and had lost at least 4 kg during the weight loss programme The three approaches were monthly personal contact, unlimited access to an interactive-technology-based intervention or a self-directed control. A total of 71% of people who completed the weight loss programme maintained their weight below the initial level. In this study, where the mean weight loss had been 8.5 kg, the least weight was regained in the 'monthly personal contact' group (4 kg), followed by the interactive technology group (5.2 kg), and then the self-directed group (5.5 kg) [16].

These results mirrored those of Wing et al. and added to the data that personal contact during maintenance results in less weight regain than technology support or no support [17]. In a secondary analysis of the 'interactive technology' arm of the study, it was determined that those who had regained the least weight had used the technology (1) more frequently; (2) for longer each time; and that they had (3) registered their weight and exercise more frequently; and (4) used other website features after weight entry [26]. It seems, therefore, that if people use information technology for weight maintenance, they should use it as much as possible.

Similar to those participants in NWCR, subjects that maintained their weight loss in WLMRCT continued to adhere to their dietary and lifestyle changes. They were physically active for 225 min/ week (measured by a calibrated accelerometer), self-monitored and were skilled in problem-solving and relapse prevention. It has been suggested in the SIGN 2010 obesity guideline that 225 min of weekly physical activity equates to an expenditure of 1800–2500 kcal/week [12]. This is potentially achievable through five sessions of 45–60 min of moderate-intensity activity per week, or lesser amounts of vigorous physical activity.

Weight maintenance programmes in practice

The Glasgow and Clyde Weight Management Service (GCWMS) is a specialist, multidisciplinary NHS weight management programme providing a structured educational lifestyle programme, including a 600 kcal/day deficit diet, cognitive-behavioural therapy and physical activity advice over 16 weeks [27]. Criteria for referral to the service is a BMI of >35 kg/m^2 or >30 kg/m^2 with comorbidities (e.g. hypertension, diabetes or poor mobility). After a 5%

weight loss has been achieved, people are encouraged to follow a 12-month weight maintenance programme. This consists of monthly sessions based around the four key factors shown by NWCR to predict weight maintenance success (follow a low-fat, high-carbohydrate diet; regular meals including breakfast; monitor weight and food intake; and 1 hour of moderate-intensity exercise daily).

Over a 16-week weight loss intervention, 26% of people lost ≥5 kg (21% lost ≥5% of body weight). At around 7 months, 30% of individuals on the maintenance programme lost ≥5 kg (25% lost ≥5% of body weight); and, after 12 months of the maintenance programme, 28% had maintained a loss of ≥5 kg (24% lost ≥5% of body weight) [27].

GCWMS aims to maintain a 5-kg weight loss target for 12 months after the weight loss. Of all successful weight loss patients (defined as losing ≥5 kg), 48% maintained ≥5 kg weight loss at 18 months, and 77% weighed less than the initial weight at follow-up [28]. Weight loss maintenance was associated with a low-fat, low-energy diet, weight monitoring, portion control, 225–300 min of physical activity a week and attending 10 months of the maintenance phase of the programme.

4.15.4 The role of physical activity in weight maintenance

Successful weight maintainers in NWCR and WLMRCT were physically active for around an hour a day.

Weinsier et al. compared the total free-living energy expenditure in 61 women with a BMI of <25 kg/m^2 who were successful and unsuccessful in maintaining a normal body weight over a year [19]. Over the year, the 'maintainers' (those who had gained ≤3%) lost an average of 0.5 kg. The 'gainers' (who had a weight gain of >10%) gained an average of 9.5 kg. The 'maintainers' had a significantly higher physical activity level and muscle strength than the 'gainers'. The lower activity energy expenditure of the 'gainers' explained 77% of their greater weight gain. The authors concluded that the 'gainers' would have to add around 1 hour and 17 min of moderate-intensity physical activity

to their daily routine to achieve the same weight maintenance status as the 'maintainers'. These findings, as well as the information gained from NWCR and WLMRCT, suggest that the current guidelines, recommending a minimum of 30 min of moderate-intensity physical activity a day, may be insufficient for weight maintenance [19].

4.15.5 Method of initial weight loss and subsequent weight maintenance success

Pharmacological intervention (orlistat), very-low-calorie diets (VLCDs), liquid diets and bariatric surgery are recognised weight loss approaches – either in addition to, or instead of, making lifestyle and behavioural changes.

Maintenance after pharmacological intervention

After 6 months of orlistat treatment for weight loss, a 6-month lifestyle modification programme in 55 people of 18–50 years, with and without diabetes and a BMI of ≥25 kg/m^2, was found to be effective in maintaining weight loss [29]. Initially, 60 people were recruited to the weight loss intervention of orlistat plus general advice (not including a low-energy diet or specific lifestyle advice) from a dietitian. At the end of the weight loss period, five participants declined to participate, and the remaining 55 were randomised to a weight maintenance phase to receive either a lifestyle intervention (27 people, 15 with diabetes) or none (28 people, 15 with diabetes) for 6 months.

The lifestyle programme was held monthly in groups of five participants with a nutrition educator. It consisted of dietary advice (balanced diet; food labels; eating out and healthy cooking methods; a eucaloric menu plan calculated from the weight at the end of the orlistat treatment; and a daily food diary), physical activity (30 min aerobic exercise two–three times a week; walking at least 10,000 steps daily; using a pedometer; and completing a daily activity log), peer group support, self-monitoring, stimulus control and cognitive restructuring.

After 6 months, those who had received the intervention gained significantly less weight (−0.2 kg) than the non-intervention group (3.3 kg) (*P* < 0.001). In addition to maintaining weight loss, those in the intervention group also maintained beneficial anthropometric, metabolic, dietary intake, physical activity and quality-of-life profiles. These benefits were not seen in the 'no lifestyle intervention' group. The authors acknowledge that the number of subjects was small and the duration of the intervention programme was short. It is unknown, therefore, whether subjects would be willing or able to continue with the programme in the long term.

Maintenance after VLCDs

VLCDs are sometimes the weight loss method of choice, particularly for those who have high BMI and comorbidities, or those who have not succeeded with low-energy diets. Following an initial 6-week VLCD of 500 kcal/day, one study investigated weight regain during a 2-year weight maintenance period [30]. A total of 133 individuals started the 6-week VLCD programme, and, after the first 3 months of the weight maintenance programme, 13 people withdrew. The remaining 120 subjects completed the first year of the programme, and 103 completed the whole programme of 6 weeks of weight loss and 2 years of weight maintenance. Average weight loss over the 6-week weight loss phase was 7.2 kg, and average weight regain was 69%. Those who regained the least weight (<10% body weight regain) increased and maintained their dietary restraint more over the whole programme, and they also lost the most body fat during the weight loss phase. However, these "successful' individuals only made up 9.7% of the total numbers involved in the study.

A systematic review of 20 studies investigated the effects of anti-obesity drugs, diet and exercise on weight loss maintenance after VLCDs [31]. They showed that, after either VLCDs or low-energy diet interventions followed for 3–16 weeks, improved weight loss maintenance was associated with anti-obesity drugs (3.5 kg), meal replacements (3.9 kg) and high-protein diets (1.5 kg), as compared to controls. However, they found no

significant improvements for dietary supplements and exercise, possibly due to the difficulties in achieving the 60–90 min of exercise necessary for weight control. Similarly, after VLCDs, both orlistat and meal replacements have been shown to be effective in maintaining the lost weight over a year, and did not differ significantly in the levels of weight regain [32].

Maintenance after liquid diet

McGuire et al. investigated the different ways in which individuals on NWCR had lost weight and how they maintained their weight loss [33]. They compared those who had lost weight through lifestyle changes on their own, those who attended an organised programme and those who followed a liquid formula diet (which are often, but not exclusively, VLCDs and LCDs in the region of 800 kcal/day). There was a significant interaction between the method of weight loss and the reported difficulty in maintaining the weight loss. Those who followed a liquid diet found that maintaining their weight loss harder than losing it. The liquid diet group reported a greater use of dietary strategies during maintenance, such as calorie counting and following a low-fat diet. Those who had lost weight on their own found maintenance easier than the initial weight loss phase, suggesting that perhaps they had already developed the skills for maintenance while losing weight. Although the groups differed in their initial weight loss strategies and in their perceptions of the effort required for maintenance (the 'on my own' group reported less difficulty in maintaining weight than the organised programme group and the liquid formula users), all three groups achieved similar weight maintenance.

Maintenance after surgical intervention

Bond et al. investigated 315 individuals from NWCR, of whom 105 had undergone bariatric surgery (58% Roux-en-Y gastric bypass, 18% gastric banding and 24% non-specified surgery) [34]. The surgical and nonsurgical individuals were matched for gender, entry weight, maximum weight loss and weight maintenance duration. Questionnaires were used to gather self-reported information on weight; energy and macronutrient intake (via the Block Food Frequency Questionnaire); physical activity levels (via the Paffenbarger Physical Activity Questionnaire); psychological factors (via the Eating Inventory); and the depression and stress levels (via the Centers for Epidemiologic Studies Depression Scale and the Perceived Stress Scale, respectively). Both groups gained similar, small amounts of weight (the surgical group gained 1.8 kg, and the nonsurgical group gained 1.7 kg). However, the surgical group reported less dietary restraint, less physical activity, more fast food, higher depression and stress levels and higher fat consumption while achieving similar weight regain as those in the nonsurgical group. Therefore, it could be interpreted that, although the surgical and nonsurgical groups regained the same weight over the first year of maintenance, the surgical group seemed to find it easier. The nonsurgical group needs more behavioural efforts to achieve the same results as the surgical group.

4.15.6 Unsuccessful weight maintenance

There will always be some people who do not maintain their weight loss. Wing et al. suggest that there may be a set point for weight, and that reducing weight below this level leads to physiological compensation [17]. A reduced metabolic rate lower than what would be suggested for the person's new weight, reduced fat oxidation, and low leptin and insulin resistance have all been suggested as possible metabolic reasons, but these require further investigation [17]. Alternatively, it may be too difficult for some to maintain the necessary behaviours permanently. Factors that predicted failure to maintain lost weight in NWCR included increased fat intake, depression, poor dietary restraint, black-and-white thinking, low self-efficacy, greater hunger, poor problem-solving skills, binge eating, evaluating self-worth in terms of shape and weight, unrealistic weight loss goals, more recent weight loss (for less than 2 years) and greater decreases in energy expenditure.

4.15.7 Conclusion

Health professionals need to give as much importance to weight loss maintenance as to weight loss itself. Ensuring that patients are able to maintain weight loss will involve extended care, personal contact and follow-up (suggested in the literature to be between 6 months and 5 years). People wanting to maintain weight loss need to develop the behavioural skills of self-monitoring intake and weight, goal setting, relapse prevention and gaining social support, in addition to the others that have been discussed.

Weight maintenance can be possible, given the right support. Retrospectively, examples such as NWCR indicate that many of the behaviours, diets and levels of physical activity of successful weight loss maintainers are similar to those in successful prospective weight maintenance studies such as WLMRCT, as well as in practice at secondary care setting of the Glasgow and Clyde Weight Management Services (GCWMS). It also seems that, as time goes by, the maintenance of weight loss becomes easier, presumably as new behaviours become more habitual. The method of weight loss, whether via lifestyle changes, pharmacotherapy or bariatric surgery, has implications on how easy individuals are likely to find maintaining their weight, and on the strategies that may be the most effective.

The methods necessary for successful weight maintenance can be categorised in two ways – the first being methods that individuals can use by themselves, such as self-monitoring, and the second being the elements that need to be provided by health professionals or another support system. Individuals in NWCR are a self-selecting group, and their methods of weight loss maintenance cannot be generalised as being possible for every person after weight loss. It is those people who cannot maintain their weight loss alone that need effective interventions to provide the necessary knowledge, skills and support. Both the STOP Regain study and WLMRCT found that personal contact resulted in the least weight regain, followed by technology and, last, by a control (newsletter or self-directed).

4.15.8 Summary box

Key points

- Weight loss maintenance has been defined as a weight change of <3% [1].
- Long-term weight loss maintenance is possible, but requires sustained behaviour changes.
- Face-to-face contact reduces weight regain, compared to Internet/technology-based support.
- Current guidelines recommend a minimum of 30 min of moderate-intensity physical activity a day, which probably is insufficient for weight loss maintenance. About 80 min daily of moderate physical activity is likely to be necessary.
- Weight loss maintenance becomes easier over time. The risk of weight regain reduces after 1 year, and further after 2.5 years of having maintained the lost weight.
- The perceived ease of weight loss maintenance after weight loss varies, depending on the method of weight loss.
- The cost-effectiveness of extended, personal contact in weight maintenance programmes should be evaluated.

References

1. Stevens J, Truesdale KP, McClain JE, Cai J. The definition of weight maintenance. *International Journal of Obesity* 2006; **30**: 391–399.
2. Crawford D, Jeffery RW, French SA. Can anyone successfully control their weight? Findings of a three year community-based study of men and women. *International Journal of Obesity and Related Metabolic Disorders* 2000; **9**(24): 1107–1110.
3. Field AE, Wing RR, Manson JE, Spiegelman DL, Willett WC. Relationship of a large weight loss to long-term weight change among young and middle-aged US women. *International Journal of Obesity and Related Metabolic Disorders* 2001; **25**(8): 1113–1121.
4. Lowe MR, Miller-Kovach K, Phelan S. Weight-loss maintenance in overweight individuals one to five years following successful completion of a commercial weight loss program. *International Journal of Obesity and Related Metabolic Disorders* 2001; **25**(3): 325–331.
5. McGuire MT, Wing RR, Klem ML, Hill JO. Behavioral strategies of individuals who have maintained long-term weight losses. *Obesity Research* 1999; **7**(4): 334–341.
6. McGuire MT, Wing RR, Hill JO. The prevalence of weight loss maintenance among American adults. *International Journal of Obesity and Related Metabolic Disorders* 1999; **23**(12): 1314–1319.
7. Moore LL, Visioni AJ, Wilson PW, D'Agostino RB, Finkle WD, Ellison RC. Can sustained weight loss in overweight individuals reduce the risk of diabetes mellitus? *Epidemiology* 2000; **11**(3): 269–273.
8. Mogul HR, Peterson SJ, Weinstein BI, Li J, Southren AL. Long-term (2–4 year) weight reduction with metformin plus carbohydrate-modified diet in euglycemic, hyperinsulinemic, midlife women (Syndrome W). *Heart Disease* 2003; **5**(6): 384–392.
9. Sarlio-Lähteenkorva S, Rissanen A, Kaprio J. A descriptive study of weight loss maintenance: 6 and 15 year follow-up of initially overweight adults. *International Journal of Obesity and Related Metabolic Disorders* 2000; **24**(1): 116–125.
10. Wadden TA, Anderson DA, Foster GD. Two-year changes in lipids and lipoproteins associated with the maintenance of a 5% to 10% reduction in initial weight: some findings and some questions. *Obesity Research* 1999; **7**(2): 170–178.
11. Wing RR, Hill JO. Successful weight loss maintenance. *Annual Review of Nutrition* 2001; **21**: 323–341.
12. SIGN 115. Management of obesity: A clinical guideline, 2010. Available from: http://www.sign.ac.uk/guidelines/fulltext/115/, accessed on September 2016.
13. Tyson CC, Appel LJ, Vollmer WM, Jerome GJ, Brantley PJ, et al. Impact of 5-year weight change on blood pressure: results from the weight loss maintenance trial. *Journal of Clinical Hypertension* 2013; **15**: 458–464.
14. Lien LF, Haqq AM, Arlotto M, Slentz CA, Muehlbauer MJ, McMahon RL, et al. The STEDMAN project: biophysical, biochemical and metabolic effects of a behavioural weight loss intervention during weight loss, maintenance and re-gain. *OMICS* 2009; **13**: 21–35.
15. Thomas JG, Bond DS, Phelan S, Hill JO, Wing RR. Weight-loss maintenance for 10 years in the National Weight Control Registry. *American Journal of Preventive Medicine* 2014; **46**(1): 17–23.
16. Svetkey LP, Stevens VJ, Brantley PJ, Appel LJ, Hollis JF, et al. Weight Loss Maintenance Collaborative Research Group. Comparison of strategies for sustaining weight loss: the weight loss maintenance randomized controlled trial. *JAMA* 2008; **299**: 1139–1148.
17. Wing RR, Tate DF, Gorin AA, Raynor HA, Fava JL. A self-regulation program for maintenance of weight loss. *The New England Journal of Medicine* 2006; **355**: 1563–1571.
18. Middleton KM, Patidar SM, Perri MG. The impact of extended care on the long-term maintenance of weight loss: a systematic review and meta-analysis. *Obesity Reviews* 2012; **13**: 506–517.
19. Weinsier RL, Hunter GR, Desmond RA, Byrne NM, Zuckerman PA, Darnell BE. Free living activity energy expenditure in women successful and unsuccessful in maintaining a normal body weight. *American Journal of Clinical Nutrition* 2002; **75**: 499–504.
20. Thomas JG, Bond DS, Phelan S, Hill JO, Wing RR. Weight loss maintenance for 10 years in the Nationals Weight Control Registry. *American Journal of Preventive Medicine* 2014; **46**: 17–23.
21. Klem ML, Wing RR, McGuire MT, Seagle HM, Hill JO, et al. A descriptive study of individuals successful at long term maintenance of substantial weight loss. *American Journal of Clinical Nutrition* 1997; **66**: 239–246.

22. Shick SM, Wing RR, Klem ML, McGuire MT, Hill JO, Seagle H. Persons successful at long term weight loss and maintenance continue to consume a low-energy, low fat diet. *Journal of the American Dietetic Association* 1998; **98**: 408–413.

23. Lantz H, Peltonen M, Agren L, Torgerson LS. A dietary and behavioural programme for the treatment of obesity. A 4-year clinical trial and long term post-treatment follow up. *Journal of Internal Medicine* 2003; **253**: 272–279.

24. Klem ML, Wing RR, Lang W, McGuire MT, Hill JO. Does weight loss maintenance become easier over time. *Obesity Research* 2000; **8**: 438–444.

25. Butryn ML, Phelan S, Hill JO, Wing RR. Consistent self-monitoring of weight: a key component of successful weight loss maintenance. *Obesity* 2007; **15**: 3091–3096.

26. Funk KL, Stevens VJ, Appel LJ, Bauck A, Brantley PJ, Champagne CM, et al. Associations of internet website use with weight change in a long-term weight loss maintenance programme. *Journal of Medical Internet Research* 2010; **12**: e29.

27. Logue J, Allardice G, Gillies M, Forde L, Morrison DS. Outcomes of a specialist weight management programme in the UK National Health Service: a prospective study of 1838 patients. *BMJ Open* 2014; **4**: e003747.

28. McLeod H, Anderson F, MacNaughton S, Forde L. Weight maintenance outcomes of patients who have successfully lost weight during an NHS multicomponent weight management programme, ECO poster presentation.

29. Woo J, Sea MM, Tong P, Ko GT, Lee Z, Chan J, Chow FC. Effectiveness of a lifestyle modification programme in weight maintenance in obese subjects after cessation of treatment with Orlistat. *Journal of Evaluation in Clinical Practice* 2007; **13**: 853–859.

30. Vogels N, Westerterp-Plantenga MS. Successful long-term weight maintenance: a 2-year follow up. *Obesity* 2007; **15**: 1258–1266.

31. Johansson K, Neovius M, Hemmingsson E. Effects of anti-obesity drugs, diet and exercise on weight loss maintenance after a very-low-calorie diet or low-calorie diet: a systematic review and meta-analysis of randomised controlled trials. *American Journal of Clinical Nutrition* 2014; **99**: 14–23.

32. LeCheminant JD, Lacobsen DJ, Hall MA, Donnelly JE. A comparison of meal replacements and medication in weight maintenance after weight loss. *Journal of the American College of Nutrition* 2005; **24**: 347–353.

33. McGuire MT, Wing RR, Klem ML, Seagle HM, Hill JO. Long term maintenance of weight loss: do people who lose weight through various weight loss methods use different behaviours to maintain their weight? *International Journal of Obesity and Related Metabolic Disorders* 1998; **22**: 572–577.

34. Bond DS, Phelan S, Leahey TM, Hill JO, Wing RR. Weight loss maintenance in successful weight losers: surgical vs. non-surgical methods. *International Journal of Obesity* (London) 2009; **33**: 173–180.

Chapter 4.16

Economic cost of obesity and the cost-effectiveness of weight management

Louise McCombie and Eleanor Grieve
University of Glasgow, Glasgow, UK

4.16.1 Introduction

Many commentators have noted the impact that obesity is having both on society and health services across the world. The impact is wide ranging, from personal day-to-day issues through to the economic impact on health services and the wider economy. There is now general acceptance that we live in an obesogenic environment, and that the factors behind this are multifactorial and complex. However, a key question concerns the impact of weight management intervention and the cost or cost-effective impact therein. By understanding this in more detail, informed decisions can be made around appropriate funding and commissioning for supporting people who wish to seek weight management interventions.

This chapter aims to outline some key areas of impact being observed with the increasing rate of obesity and the resource burden of severe and complicated obesity. The impact of realistic and achievable weight change is also considered, as well as the cost-effectiveness of currently available interventions for the management of obesity.

4.16.2 The cost burden of obesity

Estimates of the direct costs to the National Health Service (NHS) for treating overweight and obesity and related morbidity in the UK have ranged from

£479.3 million in 1998 [1] to £4.2 billion in 2007 [2]. Estimates of the indirect costs (arising from the impact of obesity on the wider economy, such as loss of productivity) over the same period ranged between £2.6 billion [1] and £15.8 billion [2]. The impact that obesity has imposed on other clinical issues is clear and extensive. Estimates suggest that 80% of the current prevalence of diabetes is due to obesity, and that 4.5% of the UK population is currently diabetic. Diabetes care costs presently account for around 10% of the total NHS spend, for this 4.5% of the population [3]. Other clinical issues such as hypertension, cardiovascular disease, asthma, arthritis-related disability, polycystic ovarian syndrome infertility, many cancers and sleep apnoea are all either caused or exacerbated by excess weight [4].

A number of studies have put more detail around not just the economic impact of excess weight on the NHS in the UK, but indeed the impact of increasing weight within the already obese populations. For a cohort of 8450 patients registered in general practice in the UK, data was collected on general practice appointments, prescribed medications and the presence of clinical conditions. The obese population made significantly more visits to the general practitioner (GP)/family doctor ($P < 0.001$), practice nurse ($P < 0.001$) and to hospitals ($P < 0.034$) [5]. This relationship remained for GP/family doctor and practice nurse attendances after adjustments for age, sex, social deprivation and the number of comorbid conditions (Figure 4.16.1, Table 4.16.1). Also, in the obese population, there

Advanced Nutrition and Dietetics in Obesity, First Edition. Edited by Catherine Hankey.
© 2018 John Wiley & Sons Ltd. Published 2018 by John Wiley & Sons Ltd.

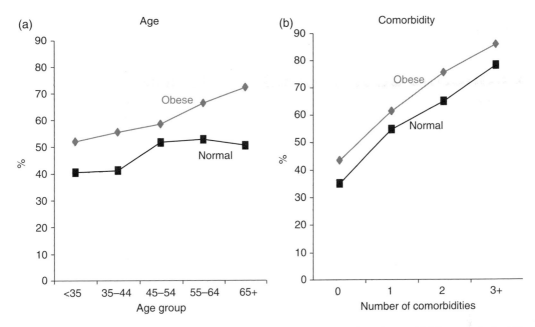

Figure 4.16.1 Frequent GP/family doctor attendance by age group, number of comorbidities and obesity [5]. Panel (a): the frequency of GP/family doctor attendance vs. age is significant among both obese ($P < 0.001$) and normal-weight ($P = 0.004$) patients. The obese group is always above the normal-weight group, demonstrating that the obese make significantly more visits to the GP for any given age group ($P < 0.001$). Panel (b): the frequency of GP/family doctor attendance vs. number of comorbidities is highly significant among both obese ($P < 0.001$) and normal-weight ($P < 0.001$) patients. The obese group is always above the normal-weight group, demonstrating that the obese make significantly more visits to the GP for any given number of comorbidities ($P < 0.001$).

Table 4.16.1 Relationship between frequent GP/family doctor attendance (≥4 appointments/y) and level of obesity [5]

Level of obesity (BMI, kg/m²)	Odds ratio (95% CI)	Odds ratio (95% CI)	Odds ratio (95% CI)
Adjusting for	Age group	Age group	Age group
	Sex	Sex	Sex
	Deprivation	Deprivation	Deprivation
	Country	Country	Country
		Presence of any comorbidity	Number of comorbidities
Normal weight	1 (reference)	1 (reference)	1 (reference)
30–32.49	1.48 (1.24–1.78)	1.36 (1.13–1.64)	1.29 (1.07–1.56)
32.50–34.99	1.58 (1.30–1.92)	1.40 (1.15–1.71)	1.30 (1.06–1.59)
35–37.49	1.63 (1.31–2.02)	1.35 (1.08–1.68)	1.17 (0.94–1.47)
37.50–39.99	2 (1.55–2.58)	1.64 (1.26–2.14)	1.45 (1.11–1.90)
40+	2.08 (1.64–2.65)	1.69 (1.32–2.16)	1.48 (1.15–1.90)
Test for trend within obese	$P < 0.001$	$P < 0.001$	$P = 0.019$
Overall obese vs. normal weight	1.64 (1.38–1.95) $P < 0.001$	1.43 (1.20–1.71) $P < 0.001$	1.30 (1.09–1.56) $P = 0.005$

was an increasing relationship between frequency of GP visits and higher BMI, which again remained significant after adjustments for age, sex, social deprivation and the number of comorbid conditions (Table 4.16.1) [5]. Using the same cohort data on prescribed medications showed that obesity resulted in significantly greater numbers of patients being prescribed drugs from eight of the 15 drug categories; importantly, these eight categories accounted for >87% of the prescribing budget. Further analysis of the actual burden of prescribing using the system of defined daily doses showed that the obese cohort was prescribed two–four times the volume of many commonly used drugs as compared to an age-and-sex-matched normal-weight cohort. Finally, the pattern of increased prescribing was observed in both obese and normal-weight groups with increasing number of comorbidities. However, there was an additional and significant impact of obesity that was also apparent in relation to the number of patients receiving 'polypharmacy' (four or more repeat medications at one time), illustrated by twice the number of obese patients receiving 10 or more drugs as compared to the age-and-sex-matched normal-weight cohort [6].

A further method of assessing the economic burden of obesity is to consider attributable costs – that is, the costs of healthcare resources that can be directly attributed to obesity or overweight, or the costs that would not have to be borne if overweight and obesity did not exist. Analysis on this concluded that up to 23% of the cost of all prescriptions across the UK population could be attributed to obesity. When overweight was also considered, this figure increased to 34% [7]. At the time of this writing, the spend on prescribed medication in the UK is £9.27 billion [8]. In other words, if the overweight and obese population were of normal BMI, then £2.94 billion would not be spent on prescribed medications. These figures appear dramatic and convincing; however, the following two key points need to be considered:

(1) Overweight and obesity exists in the population.
(2) What impacts do realistic weight management interventions have on the overweight and obese population?

These are critical issues, as many previous commentaries have in some ways oversimplified the economic impact of obesity by comparisons to the normal-weight population (BMI 18.5 < 25 kg/m² or in some cases 18.5–22 kg/m²). The currently available weight management interventions will not shift the entire obese population into the 'normal' BMI range; however, weight management interventions with proven evidence of effectiveness/cost analysis will result in health and economic benefits.

4.16.3 The economic impact of realistic weight management interventions

While some individuals will lose enough weight to move into the optimal BMI range of 18.5–25 kg/m², outcomes for weight management interventions tend to fall into the following categories:

- *Lifestyle*: 5–10 kg loss in up to 50% of the protocol-compliant population
- *Lifestyle including a phase of formula diets such as very-low-energy diets*: >15 kg loss in 50% of the compliant population
- *Bariatric surgery*: >15 kg loss in around 80% of the compliant population

This essentially means that, while comparisons between the economic cost of normal-weight and obese populations are interesting, they do not reflect the burden/impact that will result from the available weight management interventions. Additionally, given the recent ongoing trend of increasing obesity, particularly related to the severe and complicated group [9], many commentators speak of cost avoidance as opposed to cost saving. In other words, act now to prevent/reduce/minimise spend in the future.

How cost-effectiveness is measured

Economics can be defined as a discipline concerned with the efficient allocation of scarce resources [10,12,17–21] – *efficient* in the sense of achieving the greatest benefit for a population from the resources available. A key implication is that economics explicitly focusses on choices and trade-offs that need to be made between competing (alternative) uses of resources. The relevance of the idea of finite resources and the consequent necessity of choice is clear in the context of healthcare. And, in line with the earlier definition, health economics is not concerned narrowly with 'saving money', but rather with achieving value for money in ensuring that health benefits are maximised, given the expenditure being made. The concepts of 'value for money', 'cost-effectiveness', 'efficiency' and 'opportunity costs' – in other words, the benefits forgone by choosing one course of action in preference to another – are central to health economics [10–12,16–21]. The use of economic evaluations started to become widespread to aid decision-making in the 1990s [13] for reimbursement agencies, including the National Institute for Health and Care Excellence

(NICE) in England and Wales in order to reconcile the unlimited health demands and the ever-growing variety of health technologies with the realities of an increasingly resource-constrained environment [14,15].

Establishing cost-effectiveness involves weighing up the costs and benefits associated with an intervention to ensure value for money in allocating resources between alternatives [16]. Economic evaluation is thus concerned with the measurement and comparison of the outcomes and costs of two or more alternative interventions in order to establish the incremental difference between those alternatives – in other words, assessing what additional health benefits can be achieved, and finding out what it will additionally cost [17,18]. The different types of methods are briefly outlined in Box 4.16.1. These methods differ according to how health outcomes are defined.

Box 4.16.1 Summary of approaches to economic evaluations in healthcare

Cost minimisation
Cost minimisation seeks to identify which of two or more interventions has the lowest cost. The effects are identical between options, so it is simply about establishing the least costly way of achieving this outcome, with the cheapest being the preferred option [11,17].

Cost consequence analysis
Cost consequence analysis determines the intervention that has the best combination of cost and all outcomes for a given condition. The outcomes are many and listed with no comparable valuation. There is a no decision rule. Hence, in order to identify the cost-effective option, the decision-maker is left to select the most important outcome from the list, or to implicitly value the relative importance of these [11,17,19].

Cost-effectiveness analysis
Cost-effectiveness analysis (CEA) determines the intervention that is the best combination of cost and outcome as measured in natural units. The outcome is a single clinical or health effect common to each alternative. Results are presented as the incremental cost per unit of health gain, known as the *incremental cost-effectiveness ratio* (ICER). Decisions are based upon whether the additional cost is worth the additional benefit, relative to the budget or the decision-maker's willingness-to-pay threshold [11,16–21].

Cost utility analysis
Cost utility analysis (CUA) determines the intervention for any condition that is the best combination of cost and utility. It applies the same principles as CEA, but the unit of the effect is expressed as quality-adjusted life years (QALYs), and the ICER is expressed as the cost per QALY gained. QALYs provide a 'common currency' [22] with which to compare independent treatments instead of a disease-specific outcome. The length of life gained by an individual is weighted against the quality of life that is derived from the individual's preferences for life-states. Different types of tools exist to obtain these values. QALYs are the preferred outcomes for decision-makers as, being generic outcome measures, they enable the comparison of ICERs across different diseases [11,17–21].

Cost-benefit analysis
Cost–benefit analysis (CBA) measures both the costs and consequences of alternatives in monetary units. It differs from CEA and CUA as it can make the case to expand the budget available for an area of need, rather than working to achieve efficiency within the constraints of an existing budget or resources [19].

Regarding costs, the true value of something is regarded not in just financial terms, but as the value of forgone benefits that could be obtained by putting the resources to their next-best alternative use [17]. Costs and resources are also determined according to the perspective from which they are viewed [17].

Trial-based economic evaluations and decision modelling

Economic evaluations are commonly carried out alongside randomised controlled trials [23]. Alternatively, decision-analytic models may be used to synthesise data from multiple sources or to extrapolate to health outcomes beyond the length of a trial, often over a lifetime [24]. For example, outcome measures in a weight management trial may include percentage weight reduction, systolic and diastolic blood pressure, physical activity levels, etc. Since obesity is a risk factor associated with many chronic and other conditions occurring beyond the timeframe of a trial, including coronary heart disease, diabetes, stroke, some cancers and arthritis [25], modelling can be employed to link these short-term outcomes measured within the trial to potential longer-term impacts on health. A recent review [26] found how surrogate measures in weight management evaluations are used to predict long-term health outcomes.

4.16.4 Cost-effectiveness of weight management interventions

NICE, which has significantly contributed to health technology assessment (HTA) around the world, published guidance on obesity in 2006 [25]. Part of this publication included a health economic review of the evidence of cost-effectiveness for weight management interventions. The initial conclusion from this work was that there was no good-quality cost-effectiveness evidence on the identification or assessment of obesity. Therefore, the focus would be on the cost-effectiveness of treatment options. When focussing on non-pharmacological interventions, the literature search yielded four papers, plus one using lifestyle intervention as the control and providing economic data. The authors of the review

then applied economic modelling to studies with sufficient details around interventions, including 12-month outcomes to assess the cost per outcome. The conclusion from this work in terms of the range of cost per QALY was as follows:

* Diet: £174–£2039
* Behavioural treatment: £4360–£10,729
* Physical activity: £9971–£41,149

The key considerations for cost-effectiveness was centred around the duration of the effects of the treatment, or the rate of any weight regain at intervention completion.

Some key publications exploring weight management interventions used in the UK have followed this NICE report. The Counterweight Programme was tested for cost-effectiveness using the model included in the NICE Guidance 2006 [27]. Costings for programme delivery had already been published. Using observed outcome data, the conclusion was that, over a patient lifetime, there would actually be a cost saving – that is, the intervention was dominant. A limitation with this UK assessment of cost-effectiveness cited by other reporters was that it was not a randomised controlled trial. An HTA systematic review found this to be one of only two studies meeting the minimal core inclusion criteria for cost-effectiveness assessment. The second study was based in the USA [28].

Analyses of the cost-effectiveness of a commercial weight management programme, Weight Watchers, concluded that, compared to routine care, and in a population with BMIs of 27–35 kg/m^2, the programme would result in an increased QALY of 0.03 (i.e. 3 life days of perfect health per 100 patients), and at an overall cost saving of AUS\$70 (approximately £38.40) [29]. At the level of contact resulting in the observed weight change outcomes, the authors do note (in a separate but associated publication) that achieving this level of weight change may be beyond the financial reach of a substantial proportion of the population. This may be particularly true for those who need it most, owing to the out-of-pocket costs for additional contacts not funded by healthcare services. (Most frequently healthcare services will routinely fund 12 contacts, as compared to the 36 contacts that those who achieved the published weight change outcomes were provided) and the additional travel expenses [30].

More recently, a review of NICE guidelines on obesity [31] concluded (from the economic modelling of weight management interventions) that, for weight loss maintained for life (i.e. below the normal expected weight trajectory), and compared with what no intervention would achieve, the following results were found:

- A 12-week programme costing £100 or less would be cost-effective where loss of 1 kg is achieved.
- A 24-week programme costing £200 or less would be cost-effective where loss of 1 kg is achieved.

Data was not available to conclude if this was the case in populations with BMIs of >40 kg/m^2.

- For programmes costing £500 or more, a 2 kg differential must be maintained for life.
- For programmes costing £1000 or more, a 3 kg differential must be maintained for life.

Finally, programmes costing more than £100 per head will not be cost-effective if participants regain the lost weight within 2–3 years or less (compared to the expected trajectory – i.e. people returning to normal pattern of weight gain observed in the population, as opposed to keeping the weight off for life; hence, the trajectory is lowered by least 1 kg for life), the key factor being the speed at which weight is regained, rather than the average initial weight loss.

Cost-effectiveness in severe and complicated obesity

Burden of disease studies typically classify individuals with a BMI of >30 kg/m^2 as a single group ('obese'), and make comparisons against those with lower BMIs. A recent systematic review [32] found little data presented in the literature on the economic burden of obesity disaggregated beyond a BMI of 40 kg/m^2, the fastest growing category of obesity, with very little analysis of any measure or gradient of costs beyond 40 kg/m^2. From those studies identified, multiplier effects were derived for costs incurred by the severely obese as compared to those of normal weight. They ranged 1.5–3.9 for direct costs, and 1.7–8 for productivity costs that included workers' compensation claims and number of lost workdays. Given the current practice of grouping people homogenously above a threshold BMI of 30 or 40 kg/m^2, the multiplier effects for those at the

highest end of the spectrum are likely to be underestimated, in turn impacting on the value for money of interventions aimed at the severely obese.

A review of NICE guidelines clinical recommendations advocates increased access to bariatric surgery for those with type 2 diabetes diagnosed within 10 years. Of note is that recognition is made of the studies cited as being of low or very low quality, with potentially serious limitations. As of 2012, bariatric surgery has the most published evidence for the treatment of severe and complicated obesity. However, nonsurgical interventions are also required to address this increasing problem, owing to limitations around the access to and eligibility for bariatric surgery. An initial cost analysis has been conducted to compare the use of bariatric surgery against a programme that involves a phase of total diet replacement followed by stepped food reintroduction and weight loss maintenance. This demonstrated that, for £1 million worth of healthcare service resources, >15 kg weight loss can be achieved in around 110 people using bariatric surgery, as compared to 383 people when using the programme involving a phase of total diet replacement. Therefore, for the same level of resources, three times as many people are likely to achieve >15 kg weight loss in comparison to bariatric surgery [33]. The availability of this type of programme also means that, in a time of healthcare service 'rationing', more people may be able to access a weight management solution that is appropriate for the treatment of severe and complicated obesity. This would not replace the option of bariatric surgery; instead, it would potentially provide a solution for those requiring greater levels of weight loss, but who cannot or will not access bariatric surgery.

4.16.5 Conclusion

The economic burden that obesity places on society and healthcare services is clear and undisputed. However, stating the impact of obesity as compared to a normal-weight population is not reflective of what can or will be achieved with proven solutions for weight management. Evidence around the health and societal benefits of realistic and achievable weight management is building year on year, with new and innovative community-based programmes adding to this evidence base [34]. For positive results, it is essential to have everyone involved, including the participants in weight loss programmes. Patients and staff holding appropriate expectations of what moderate weight loss can bring, in terms of health and well-being. That said, the economic evidence base for weight management remains limited – especially around important issues such as (1) sustaining and maintaining weight loss; and (2) key factors that have a direct bearing upon the cost-effectiveness of interventions – due to the aforementioned challenges in carrying out robust studies. There is a clear need for longer-term studies, with a defined aim of establishing costs and cost-effectiveness. Thereafter, the evidence will equip decision-makers with a clearer vision around short- and longer-term spending and the anticipated consequences on future spending, such as cost avoidance vs. cost saving.

4.16.6 Summary box

Key points

- Obesity has placed a considerable economic burden on healthcare systems and the society in general.
- Estimating the direct cost of obesity is challenging, and estimates of the potential cost benefits in comparison to a normal-weight population is flawed.
- Evidence for clinical and societal benefits of weight loss is increasing, although more evidence is required for the cost benefits from sustained weight loss maintenance.
- Health costs of obesity and the longer-term impact and cost-effectiveness of weight management interventions are required to guide future spending on this disease.

References

1. National Audit Office. *Tackling Obesity in England*. London: The Stationery Office, 2001.
2. Butland B, Jebb S, Kopelman P, et al. Tackling obesities: future choices – *project report*, 2nd edn. London: Foresight Programme of the Government Office for Science, 2007.
3. Diabetes: Facts and Stats. Diabetes UK. Available from: http://www.diabetes.org.uk/Documents/About%20Us/Statistics/Diabetes-key-stats-guidelines-April2014.pdf.
4. SIGN 115. Management of obesity. A national clinical guideline. Edinburgh, Scotland. Scottish Intercollegiate Guideline Network, 2010.
5. Counterweight Project Team. Obesity impacts on general practice appointments. *Obesity Research* 2005; **13**: 1442–1449.
6. Counterweight Project Team. Impact of obesity on drug prescribing in primary care. *British Journal of General Practice* 2005; **55**: 743–749.
7. The Counterweight Project Team. Influence of body mass index on prescribing costs and potential cost savings of a weight management programme in primary care. *Journal of Health Services Research & Policy* 2008; **13**: 158–166.
8. Prescriptions Dispensed in the Community, Statistics for England, 2002–2012. Available from: http://www.hscic.gov.uk/catalogue/PUB20200, last accessed 2 July 2016.
9. The Scottish Government 2010. Scottish Health Survey 2009. Available from: http://www.scotland.gov.uk/Publications/2010/09/23154223/80, last accessed 2 July 2016.
10. Wonderling D, Gruen R, Black N. *Introduction to Health Economics*. Maidenhead: Open University Press, 2009.
11. McDaid D. Outcomes, costs and economic evaluation: Health Technology Assessment Summer School – 2–4 June 2010, European Federation of Neurological Associations (EFNA) and London School of Economics (LSE).
12. Haycox A, Noble E. *What Is Health Economics?* 2nd edn. London: Hayward Medical Communications, 2009.
13. Mathes T, Jacobs E, Morfeld JC, Pieper D. Methods of international health technology assessment agencies for economic evaluations – a comparative analysis. *BMC Health Services Research* 2013; **13**: 371.
14. Sorenson C, Drummond M, Kanavos P. Ensuring value for money in health care: the role of health technology assessment in the European Union. World Health Organisation, 2008.
15. Taylor R, Taylor R. *What Is Health Technology Assessment?* London: Hayward Medical Communications, 2009.
16. Phillips C. *What Is Cost-Effectiveness?* 2nd edn. London: Hayward Medical Communication, 2009.
17. Fox-Rushby, Cairns J. *Economic Evaluation*. Maidenhead: Open University Press, 2009.
18. Elliot R, Payne K. *Essentials of Economic Evaluation in Healthcare*. London: Pharmaceutical Press, 2005.
19. Drummond M, Sculpher M, Torrance G, O'Brien B, Stoddart G. *Methods for the Economic Evaluation of Health Care Programmes*, 3rd edn. Oxford: Oxford University Press, 2005.
20. Muennig, P. *Cost-Effectiveness Analysis in Health: A Practical Approach*, 2nd ed. Wiley, 2007. ISBN: 978-0-7879-9556-0.
21. Guinness L, Wiseman V. *Introduction to Health Economics (Understanding Public Health)*. Maidenhead: Open University Press, 2011.
22. Phillips C. *What Is a QALY?* 2nd edn. London: Hayward Medical Communications, 2009.
23. Petrou S, Gray A. Economic evaluation alongside randomised controlled trials: design, conduct, analysis, and reporting. *BMJ* 2011; **342**: d1548.
24. Petrou S, Gray A. Economic evaluation using decision analytical modelling: design, conduct, analysis, and reporting. *BMJ* 2011; **342**: d1766.
25. NICE CG43 Obesity: full guideline, section 6 – health economics: evidence statements and reviews, 19 November 2007.

26. Griffiths UK, Anigbogu B, Nanchahal K. Economic evaluations of adult weight management interventions: a systematic literature review focusing on methods used for determining health impact. *Applied Health Economics and Health Policy* 2012; **10**: 145–162.

27. Counterweight Project Team, Trueman P. Long-term cost effectiveness of weight management in primary care. *International Journal of Clinical Practice* 2010; **64**: 775–783.

28. Loveman E, Frampton GK, Shepherd J, Picot J, Cooper K, Bryant J, et al. The clinical effectiveness and cost effectiveness of long-term weight management schemes for adults: a systematic review. *Health Technology Assessment* 2011; **15**: 1–182.

29. Fuller NR, Colagiuri S, Schofield D, Olson AD, Shrestha R, Holzapfel C, et al. A within-trial cost-effectiveness analysis of primary care referral to a commercial provider for weight loss treatment, relative to standard care – an international randomised controlled trial. *International Journal of Obesity* 2013; **37**: 828–834.

30. Fuller NR, Carter H, Schofield D, Hauner H, Jebb SA, Colagiuri S, et al. Cost effectiveness of primary care referral to a commercial provider for weight loss treatment, relative to standard care: a modelled lifetime analysis. *International Journal of Obesity* 2014; **38**: 1104–1109.

31. NICE public health guidance 53. Managing overweight and obesity in adults – lifestyle weight management services. NICE. May 2014. Available from: https://www.nice.org.uk/guidance/ph53, last accessed 2 July 2016.

32. Grieve E, Fenwick E, Yang H-C, Lean M. The disproportionate economic burden associated with severe and complicated obesity: a systematic review. *Obesity Reviews* 2013; **14**: 883–894.

33. Lean M, Brosnahan N, McLoone P, McCombie L, Higgs AB, Ross H, et al. Feasibility and indicative results from a 12-month low-energy liquid diet treatment and maintenance programme for severe obesity. *British Journal of General Practice* 2013; **63**: e115–e124.

34. Hunt K, Wyke S, Gray CM, Anderson AS, Brady A, Bunn C, et al. A gender-sensitised weight loss and healthy living programme for overweight and obese men delivered by Scottish Premier League football clubs (FFIT): a pragmatic randomised controlled trial. *Lancet* 2014; **383**: 1211–1221.

Aetiology of obesity in children

Chapter 5.1

Genetics, epigenetics and obesity: focus on studies in children

Thomas Reinehr

University of Witten, Witten, Germany

5.1.1 Introduction

Obesity in childhood is regarded as a multi-causal disease with complex interrelationships between genes, environment and behaviour [1]. The most prevalent consequences of obesity – such as hypertension, dyslipidaemia and disturbed glucose metabolism [2], summarised as the *metabolic syndrome* [3], and determining the morbidity and mortality effects in obesity [4,5] – depend not only on the degree of overweight, but also on the genetic background [6]. Understanding the genetic mechanisms behind obesity and its associated comorbidities will probably allow the development of specific tailored interventions for prevention and treatment of childhood obesity in future.

5.1.2 The impact of genes on weight status

It is widely accepted that obesity is a polygenetic disease with environment–gene interactions [7]. Studies have clearly demonstrated that the genetic predisposition to obesity determines 50–70% of body mass index (BMI) variance [7,8].

Monogenic forms

There are a small number of monogenic forms of obesity, such as melanocortin 4 receptor gene (*MC4R*) or proopiomelanocortin gene (*POMC*)

mutations, leptin receptor insufficiency or leptin deficiency [7,9,10]. All these mutations are located in the leptin pathway. Leptin is a hormone predominantly released by adipocytes, circulating at levels proportional to the body's adiposity. More than a decade ago, research showed that the ob gene in mice and humans expresses the hormone leptin that is crucial for weight control [18]. Leptin stimulates the leptin receptor in the hypothalamus, activating melanocortin 4 (*MC4*) via the stimulation of proopiomelanocortin (*POMC*). Activation of the *MC4R* results in satiety. This pathway is the strongest satiety signal known so far. Mutations in this pathway are characterised by a major effect of the respective mutation on the development of obesity. Detecting these mutations has helped us understand the regulation of satiety in humans.

Studies in mice and humans have pointed out the critical importance of the central melanocortinergic pathway in the control of energy homeostasis, particularly the pivotal role of the *MC4R* gene. Previous studies in humans have shown that the prevalence of functionally relevant *MC4R* mutations ranges from 0.5 to 5.8% in obese children and adolescents [11]. More than 90 different obesity-associated mutations in the *MC4R*, most of which are non-synonymous mutations leading to either total or partial loss of function, have so far been reported [12–15]. These mutations within the coding region are assumed to have a major effect on BMI, averaging approximately 4.5 kg/m^2 and 9 kg/m^2 in adult males and females, respectively [11]. The presence of *MC4R*

Advanced Nutrition and Dietetics in Obesity, First Edition. Edited by Catherine Hankey.
© 2018 John Wiley & Sons Ltd. Published 2018 by John Wiley & Sons Ltd.

mutations also influence the outcomes in lifestyle interventions in obese children. Children with functionally relevant *MC4R* mutations demonstrated a similar degree of overweight 1 year after the end of lifestyle interventions, as they had lost weight through the 1-year intervention at baseline too, while children without these mutations were able to maintain the degree of weight loss achieved in the intervention [16,17].

The extremely rare autosomal recessive genetic disorders, such as leptin and leptin receptor deficiency, are further well-established monogenic causes of obesity [7,10,18,19]. Two copies of the gene must be mutated for a person to be affected by an autosomal recessive disorder. An affected person usually has unaffected parents who each carry a single copy of the mutated gene (and are referred to as 'carriers'). Interestingly, leptin deficiency due to mutations in the leptin receptor gene has been associated with central hypothyroidism and hypogonadotropic hypogonadism in humans, since leptin innervates hypophysiotropic TRH and LHRH neurons [20].

Polymorphisms

Genetic polymorphism is the simultaneous occurrence in the same locality of two or more discontinuous forms in such proportions that the rarest of them cannot be maintained just by recurrent mutation or immigration. Large genome-wide association studies (GWASs), conducted in hundreds of thousands of adults and children, have identified >30 human single nucleotide polymorphisms (SNPs) so far associated with increased BMI (see Table 5.1.1) [7,21–23]. Polymorphisms are genetic variants that occur in more than 1% of the population, in contrast to monogenetic defects. SNPs are DNA sequence variations that occur when a single nucleotide (A, T, C or G) in the genome sequence is altered. SNPs make up approximately 90% of all human genetic variation. They appear once every 100–300 bases along the 3-billion-base human genome, and can occur in the coding (gene) and non-coding regions of the genome. Many SNPs have no (direct) effect on function, but could predispose individuals to disease or influence their response to a drug.

The SNPs summarised in Table 5.1.1 have a relatively small effect size on body weight (usually below 1 kg for an individual), but they are frequent, and thus relevant in a substantial number of obese individuals. SNPs are associated not only with weight gain. For example, two polymorphisms in the *MC4R* gene, Val103Ile and Ile251Leu, which occur in 1–3% of the examined populations, respectively, are both associated with a slightly decreased BMI [13].

The function of most SNPs associated with obesity are unknown, but some loci (*MC4R, POMC, SH2B1, BDNF*) map near key hypothalamic regulators of energy balance, and one is near GIPR, an incretin receptor. The biological function of the SNPs with the greatest impact on weight (*FTO* and *INSIG2*) is largely unknown. A relationship between polymorphisms at the *FTO* and physical activity levels have been reported [24]. Furthermore, *FTO* is expressed in multiple tissues throughout the brain and the periphery, with high expression in the pituitary and adrenal glands and the hypothalamus. It has thus been suggested that *FTO* might play a role in the hypothalamic–pituitary–adrenal axis. Recently, a knock-out mouse model for *FTO* showed that the lack of FTO protects from obesity [25]. The leanness of FTO-deficient mice developed because of increased energy expenditure and systemic sympathetic activation, despite decreased spontaneous locomotor activity and relative hyperphagia. Additionally, the allelic variation of *FTO* has been shown to be associated with a reduced cerebrocortical insulin response [26].

The mechanisms by which *INSIG2* influences body weight are also unclear. *INSIG2* encodes a protein of the endoplasmic reticulum (ER) that blocks proteolytic activation of sterol regulatory element-binding proteins and membrane-bound transcription factors that activate synthesis of cholesterol and fatty acids in animal cells [27,28]. These proteins also restrict lipogenesis in mature adipocytes and block the differentiation of preadipocytes.

The impact of polymorphisms on weight has been studied not only in cross-sectional studies but also in longitudinal research. The Cardiovascular Risk in Young Finns Study, which analysed the 27-year follow-up of 2119 children, demonstrated that

Table 5.1.1 Variants with a polygenic effect on human body weight [44,45]

Nearest gene	Chromosome nearest gene	Effect on BMI
Insulin-induced gene-2 (*INSIG2*)*	2q14.2	+1.0 kg/m^2 for CC genotype
Fat mass and obesity–associated gene (*FTO*)	16q12.2	+0.40 kg/m^2 per A allele
Melanocortin 4 receptor (*MC4R*)	18q21.32	+0.23 kg/m^2 per A allele
Transmembrane protein 18 gene (*TMEM 18*)	2p25.3	+0.37 kg/m^2 per T allele
Serologically defined colon cancer antigen 8 (*SDCCAG8*)*	1q43–q44	+0.04 kg/m^2 per T allele
Tankyrase (TNKS) methionine sulfoxide reductase A (*MSRA*)*	8p23.1	−0.12 kg/m^2 per A allele
Glucosamine-6-phosphate deaminase 2 (*GNPDA2*)	4p12	+0.18 kg/m^2 per G allele
Brain-derived neurotrophic factor (*BDNF*)	11p13	+0.19 kg/m^2 per A allele
Neuronal growth regulator 1 (*NEGR1*)	1p31.1	+0.13 kg/m^2 per A allele
SH2B adaptor protein 1 (*SH2B1*)	16p11.2	+0.15 kg/m^2 per T allele
ETS variant 5 (*ETV5*)	3	+0.14 kg/m^2 per T allele
Mitochondrial carrier 2 (*MTCH2*)	11p11.2	+0.06 kg/m^2 per T allele
Potassium channel tetramerisation domain 15 (*KCTD15*)	19q13.11	+0.06 kg/m^2 per G allele
SEC16 homolog B (*SEC16B*)	1q25.2	+0.22 kg/m^2 per G allele
Transcription factor AP-2 beta (*TFAP2B*)	*6q12*	+0.13 kg/m^2 per G allele
Fas apoptotic inhibitory molecule 2 (*FAIM2*)	*12q13*	+0.12 kg/m^2 per T allele
Neurexin (*NRXN3*)	*14q31*	+0.13 kg/m^2 per T allele
Rab and DnaJ domain-containing protein A (*RBJ*)	2q23.3	+0.14 kg/m^2 per C allele
CNV near G protein-coupled receptor (*GPR*) *C5B*	*16q12*	+0.17 kg/m^2 per C allele
Mitogen-activated protein kinase kinase 5 (*MAP2K5*)	*15q23*	+0.13 kg/m^2 per G allele
Glutaminyl-peptide cyclotransferase-like (*QPCTL*)	*19q13.23*	+0.15 kg/m^2 per C allele
TNNI3 interacting kinase (*TNNI3K*)	*1q31.1*	+0.07 kg/m^2 per A allele
Solute carrier family 39 (zinc), member 8 (*SLC39A8*)	4q22–q24	+0.19 kg/m^2 per T allele
POC5 centriolar protein homolog (*FLJ35779*)	5q13.3	+0.10 kg/m^2 per T allele
Leucine-rich repeat neuronal 6C (*LRRN6C*)	9p21.2	+0.11 kg/m^2 per G allele
Transmembrane protein 160 (*TMEM160*)	19q13.32	+0.09 kg/m^2 per A allele
Fanconi anaemia, complementation group L (*FANCL*)	2p16.1	+0.10 kg/m^2 per T allele
Cell adhesion molecule 2 (*CADM2*)	3p12.1	+0.10 kg/m^2 per G allele
Protein kinase D1 (*PRKD1*)	*14q11*	+0.17 kg/m^2 per T allele
Low-density lipoprotein receptor-protein 1B (*LRP1B*)	2q21.2	+0.09 kg/m^2 per C allele
Polypyrimidine tract binding protein 2 (*PTBP2*)	*1q21.3*	+0.06 kg/m^2 per C allele
Mitochondrial translational initiation factor 3 (*MTIF3*)	*13q12.2*	+0.09 kg/m^2 per G allele
Zinc finger protein 608 (*ZNF608*)	*5q23.3*	+0.07 kg/m^2 per A allele
Ribosomal protein L27a (*RPL27A*)	*11q15*	+0.06 kg/m^2 per C allele
Nucleoside diphosphate moiety X-type motif 3 (*NUDT3*)	*6q21.2*	+0.06 kg/m^2 per G allele

* not confirmed in [23].

polymorphisms near genes *FLJ35779*, *TFAP2B* and *LRRN6C* are independently related with adulthood obesity [29]. However, genetic risk markers only marginally improve the prediction of obesity in adulthood. Childhood BMI, family income (inversely) and mother's BMI were much stronger predictive factors, suggesting that polymorphisms have only a low impact on BMI.

The outcome of a lifestyle intervention for obese children was also influenced by polymorphisms. For example, the carriers of the risk alleles in *INSIG2* lose less weight as compared to the carrier of the wild gene [30]. The difference was nearly 0.5 BMI points. Children homozygous for the obesity risk-A-allele in *FTO* lost weight in the intervention, but to a less degree than children heterozygous or homozygous for the wild-type allele [31]. However, after adjusting for age, gender, baseline BMI and the analysed gene polymorphisms, this association between *FTO* and BMI change was not significant.

Interestingly the combination of the risk alleles in *INSIG2* and *FTO* was significantly associated with the lowest degree of overweight reduction in a lifestyle intervention [32]. In concordance, a study in adults showed that homozygosity for both polymorphisms in *FTO* and *INSIG2*, as well as the combination of *FTO/INSIG2* homozygosity/heterozygosity, leads to an increased BMI (nearly 0.75 BMI points) [33]. These findings suggest that the effects of *INSIG2* and *FTO* aggravate each other and hint towards gene–gene interactions.

Copy number variants

CNVs – a form of structural variation – are alterations of the DNA of a genome that results in the cell having an abnormal number of copies of one or more sections of the DNA. The search for CNVs in large, rare chromosomal deletions associated with severe early-onset obesity is a new genetic strategy. For example, Bochukova et al. showed that rare CNVs are associated with severe early-onset obesity [34]: a deletion of 16p11.2 was associated with highly penetrant familial severe early-onset obesity. Furthermore, deletion carriers exhibited hyperphagia and severe insulin resistance disproportionate to the degree of obesity. The data of this study suggest that the phenotype is consistent with a role for the Src homology 2 domain-containing adapter protein 1 (*SH2B1*) in human energy homeostasis and glucose metabolism. The prevalence of the *SH2B1*-containing deletion in patients with severe early-onset obesity was significantly greater than in controls. *SH2B1* encodes an adaptor protein involved in leptin and insulin signalling. Based on this observation, 19 similar deletions were identified from GWAS data in >16,000 children and adults from eight European cohorts [35]. These deletions were absent from healthy normal-weight controls, and accounted for 0.7% of the morbid obesity cases (BMI ≥ 40 or BMI-SDS ≥ 4).

Epigenetics

Epigenetics describes the phenomena of inherited changes in gene function that occur independently of the changes in the nucleotide sequence. Epigenetic studies are new promising genetic diagnostic approaches since obesity is the consequence of environment–gene interactions [36]. The underlying genetic mechanisms likely involve a combination of epigenetic and transcriptional modifications (Figure 5.1.1). Initially, it was believed that epigenetic modifications were unidirectional, but recent studies have demonstrated that the epigenome is in fact highly dynamic, changing in response to nutrient availability, physical exercise and aging, among other exposures of changes in the nucleotide sequence [36]. While nearly all cells in the body have the same nuclear genome, different cell types have their own epigenomes, a characteristic essential for the development of cell-specific phenotypes. Early-life nutrition represents an intriguing example of how environmentally augmented epigenetic events might affect an individual's response to metabolic load and disease susceptibility in adulthood, with numerous studies lending weight to this hypothesis [36].

Epigenetics could also help explain individual differences in weight loss after an energy-restriction intervention [37]: a hypocaloric-diet-induced weight loss in humans altered DNA methylation status of specific genes (ATP10A and CD44 genes). Furthermore, DNA methylation levels in several CpGs located in these genes showed statistical baseline differences, depending on the weight-loss outcome. The authors conclude that baseline DNA methylation patterns may be used as epigenetic markers that could help predict weight loss [37]. Nevertheless, our understanding of how epigenetic events early in life influence the development of obesity and its comorbidities remains rudimentary.

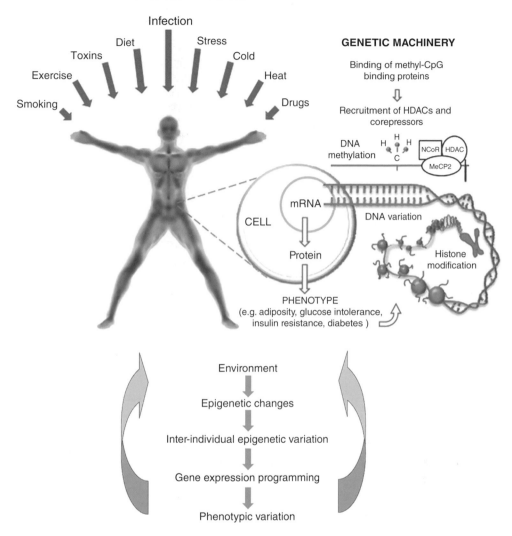

Figure 5.1.1   Postulated mechanisms that underlie observations of gene–environment interactions (adapted from reference [36]).
HDAC, histone deacetylase; NCor, nuclear receptor corepressor; MeCP2, methyl-CpG-binding protein 2.

5.1.3 Impact of genes on cardiovascular risk factors

Not only obesity but also the prevalence of cardiovascular risk factors in obesity is influenced by the genetic background of the individual. For example, one of the most important factors influencing insulin sensitivity and resistance are variations in *TCF7L2* [38]. *TCF7L2* encodes a transcription factor and thereby regulates blood glucose homeostasis through the regulation of proglucagon gene expression. The SNP rs7903146 in *TCF7L2* is associated with an increased risk of type 2 diabetes and a slightly reduced risk for obesity, affecting nearly 7% of all obese persons. Furthermore, the T-allele at rs7903146 in *TCF7L2* was associated with a significant negative dosage effect per allele on the improvement of insulin resistance and sensitivity indices such as HOMA-IR and QUICKI after a lifestyle intervention, independently of the degree of weight loss, age and gender [39]. This finding is in line with the longitudinal study by Florez et al., demonstrating that the T-allele at rs7903146 is associated with impaired β-cell function [33].

Another example is the polymorphisms (SNP rs10830963) in *MTNR1B* (melatonin receptor 1B gene), which is also associated with type 2 diabetes but not to insulin sensitivity or resistance [40]. Interestingly, in weight loss of >2 BMI points, glucose levels remained stable in individuals with the high-risk allele [40].

Other examples of a genetic background of cardiovascular risk factors are polymorphisms in the low-density lipoprotein receptor gene (LDLR). Linsel-Nitschke and colleagues found that each copy of the minor T allele of the SNP rs2228671 within LDLR (frequency 11%) was related to a decrease of LDL cholesterol levels [41]. In parallel, the T allele of rs2228671 was associated with a significantly lower risk of coronary artery disease. Also, another SNP rs599839 located at chromosome 1p13.3 has been demonstrated to be associated with the risk of coronary artery disease and with serum levels of LDL cholesterol [42].

Non-alcoholic fatty liver disease (NAFLD) is a spectrum of diseases that ranges from steatosis to steatohepatitis, affecting up 10% of all obese children, with a male predominance [43]. Speliotes et al. demonstrated by GWAS in 7176 individuals that nearly 26% of the variation in hepatic steatosis is heritable [44]. They identified three variants near patatin-like phospholipase domain-containing protein 3 (*PNPLA3*), neurocan (*NCAN*) and protein phosphatase 1 regulatory subunit 3b (*PPP1R3B*) that associated with hepatic steatosis, and showed that variants in or near *NCAN*, glucokinase regulatory protein (*GCKR*), lysophospholipase-like 1 (*LYPLAL1*) and *PNPLA3*, but not *PPP1R3B*, associated with histologic lobular inflammation/fibrosis.

5.1.4 Summary

Monogenetic disorders are rare in obesity, but are helpful for understanding the regulation of body weight in humans. The most prevalent monogenetic diseases in obesity are *MC4R* mutations, occurring in 3–5% of all obese children. Since carriers of the *MC4R* mutations can lose body weight but have difficulties in maintaining this weight loss, very long lifestyle interventions seem to be necessary for these children.

SNPs associated with obesity are much more prevalent than monogenetic disorders but have only low impact on weight status (usually below 1 kg). However, all these SNPs only explain up to 4% of the variance of BMI. Therefore, this research approach will not succeed in explaining childhood obesity, or the high heritability of BMI.

A new promising strategy for identifying missing heritability in obesity are cohorts with extreme phenotypes that are likely to be enriched for rare variants, which improve the power for their discovery. The loci identified by this strategy may be subsequently analysed to reveal additional rare variants that further contribute to the missing heritability. It seems to be a very ingenious approach to combine 'the power of the extreme' in small, well-phenotyped cohorts, with targeted follow-up in case-control and population cohorts.

Epigenetic studies reflecting the hypotheses of gene–environment interactions is another new and promising genetic approach. However, further experimental and longitudinal studies are necessary to clarify the role of epigenetics in human obesity.

In summary, obesity and its comorbidities have a high heritability, and even the weight loss and cardiovascular risk factor improvements achievable through lifestyle interventions depend partly on genetic backgrounds. Therefore, obesity and weight loss in lifestyle interventions are not attributable only to eating and exercise behaviours. In conclusion, we need to be very cautious not to blame obese children, or children in whom lifestyle interventions have been unsuccessful, of having 'unhealthy' lifestyles, which maybe not very different from those of lean children with more favourable genetic backgrounds.

5.1.5 Summary box

Key points

- Monogenetic disorders are rare in obesity; the most prevalent monogenetic diseases in obesity occur in 3–5% of all obese children.
- A carrier of the *MC4R* mutation (3–5% obese children) can lose body weight but have difficulties in maintaining weight loss.
- SNPs do not adequately explain childhood obesity, or the high heritability of BMI. They are more prevalent than monogenetic disorders but have only a low impact on weight status (usually below 1 kg) and explain ≥4% of BMI variance.
- Epigenetic studies reflecting the hypotheses of gene–environment interactions are promising, but further research is necessary to clarify the role of epigenetics in human obesity.
- Some obese children, or children in whom lifestyle interventions have been unsuccessful, may have less favourable genetic backgrounds than those who are lean.

References

1. Hebebrand J, Sommerlad C, Geller F, Gorg T, Hinney A. The genetics of obesity: practical implications. *International Journal of Obesity and Related Metabolic Disorders* 2001; **25**(1): S10–S18.
2. l'Allemand D, Wiegand S, Reinehr T, et al. Cardiovascular risk in 26,008 European overweight children as established by a multicenter database. *Obesity* (Silver Spring) 2008; **16**(7): 1672–1679.
3. Alberti KG, Zimmet P, Shaw J. Metabolic syndrome – a new world-wide definition. A consensus statement from the International Diabetes Federation. *Diabetic Medicine* 2006; **23**(5): 469–480.
4. Baker JL, Olsen LW, Sorensen TI. Childhood body-mass index and the risk of coronary heart disease in adulthood. *The New England Journal of Medicine* 2007; **357**(23): 2329–2337.
5. Franks PW, Hanson RL, Knowler WC, Sievers ML, Bennett PH, Looker HC. Childhood obesity, other cardiovascular risk factors, and premature death. *The New England Journal of Medicine* 2010; **362**(6): 485–493.
6. Alisi A, Cianfarani S, Manco M, Agostoni C, Nobili V. Non-alcoholic fatty liver disease and metabolic syndrome in adolescents: pathogenetic role of genetic background and intrauterine environment. *Annals of Medicine* 2012; **44**(1): 29–40.
7. Hinney A, Vogel CI, Hebebrand J. From monogenic to polygenic obesity: recent advances. *European Child & Adolescent Psychiatry* 2010; **19**(3): 297–310.
8. Farooqi IS, O'Rahilly S. Recent advances in the genetics of severe childhood obesity. *Archives of Disease in Childhood* 2000; **83**(1): 31–34.
9. Hinney A, Bettecken T, Tarnow P, et al. Prevalence, spectrum, and functional characterization of melanocortin-4 receptor gene mutations in a representative population-based sample and obese adults from Germany. *Journal of Clinical Endocrinology and Metabolism* 2006; **91**(5): 1761–1769.
10. Farooqi IS, O'Rahilly S. Monogenic human obesity syndromes. *Recent Progress in Hormone Research* 2004; **59**: 409–424.
11. Dempfle A, Hinney A, Heinzel-Gutenbrunner M, et al. Large quantitative effect of melanocortin-4 receptor gene mutations on body mass index. *Journal of Medical Genetics* 2004; **41**(10): 795–800.
12. Heid IM, Vollmert C, Kronenberg F, et al. Association of the MC4R V103I polymorphism with the metabolic syndrome: the KORA Study. *Obesity* (Silver Spring) 2008; **16**(2): 369–376.
13. Geller F, Reichwald K, Dempfle A, et al. Melanocortin-4 receptor gene variant I103 is negatively associated with obesity. *American Journal of Human Genetics* 2004; **74**(3): 572–581.
14. Chambers JC, Elliott P, Zabaneh D, et al. Common genetic variation near MC4R is associated with waist circumference and insulin resistance. *Nature Genetics* 2008; **40**(6): 716–718.
15. Loos RJ, Lindgren CM, Li S, et al. Common variants near MC4R are associated with fat mass, weight and risk of obesity. *Nature Genetics* 2008; **40**(6): 768–775.
16. Reinehr T, Hebebrand J, Friedel S, et al. Lifestyle intervention in obese children with variations in the melanocortin 4 receptor gene. *Obesity* (Silver Spring) 2009; **17**(2): 382–389.
17. Hainerova I, Larsen LH, Holst B, et al. Melanocortin 4 receptor mutations in obese Czech children: studies of prevalence, phenotype development, weight reduction response, and functional analysis. *Journal of Clinical Endocrinology and Metabolism* 2007; **92**(9): 3689–3696.
18. Clement K, Vaisse C, Lahlou N, et al. A mutation in the human leptin receptor gene causes obesity and pituitary dysfunction. *Nature* 1998; **392**(6674): 398–401.
19. Zhang Y, Proenca R, Maffei M, Barone M, Leopold L, Friedman JM. Positional cloning of the mouse obese gene and its human homologue. *Nature* 1994; **372**(6505): 425–432.
20. Ortiga-Carvalho TM, Oliveira KJ, Soares BA, Pazos-Moura CC. The role of leptin in the regulation of TSH secretion in the fed state: in vivo and in vitro studies. *Journal of Endocrinology* 2002; **174**(1): 121–125.
21. Krude H, Biebermann H, Gruters A. Mutations in the human proopiomelanocortin gene. *Annals of the New York Academy of Sciences* 2003; **994**: 233–239.
22. Krude H, Biebermann H, Schnabel D, et al. Obesity due to proopiomelanocortin deficiency: three new cases and treatment trials with thyroid hormone and ACTH4-10. *Journal of Clinical Endocrinology and Metabolism* 2003; **88**(10): 4633–4640.

23. Speliotes EK, Willer CJ, Berndt SI, et al. Association analyses of 249,796 individuals reveal 18 new loci associated with body mass index. *Nature Genetics* 2010; **42**(11): 937–948.

24. Andreasen CH, Stender-Petersen KL, Mogensen MS, et al. Low physical activity accentuates the effect of the FTO rs9939609 polymorphism on body fat accumulation. *Diabetes* 2008; **57**(1): 95–101.

25. Fischer J, Koch L, Emmerling C, et al. Inactivation of the *FTO* gene protects from obesity. *Nature* 2009; **458**: 894–898.

26. Hinney A, Nguyen TT, Scherag A, et al. Genome wide association (GWA) study for early onset extreme obesity supports the role of fat mass and obesity associated gene (*FTO*) variants. *PLoS ONE* 2007; **2**(12): e1361.

27. Lyon HN, Emilsson V, Hinney A, et al. The association of a SNP upstream of INSIG2 with body mass index is reproduced in several but not all cohorts. *PLoS Genetics* 2007; **3**(4): e61.

28. Gong Y, Lee JN, Brown MS, Goldstein JL, Ye J. Juxtamembranous aspartic acid in Insig-1 and Insig-2 is required for cholesterol homeostasis. *Proceedings of the National Academy of Sciences USA* 2006; **103**(16): 6154–6159.

29. Juonala M, Juhola J, Magnussen CG, et al. Childhood environmental and genetic predictors of adulthood obesity: the cardiovascular risk in Young Finns study. *Journal of Clinical Endocrinology and Metabolism* 2011; **96**(9): E1542–E1549.

30. Reinehr T, Hinney A, Nguyen TT, Hebebrand J. Evidence of an influence of a polymorphism near the INSIG2 on weight loss during a lifestyle intervention in obese children and adolescents. *Diabetes* 2008; **57**(3): 623–626.

31. Muller TD, Hinney A, Scherag A, et al. 'Fat mass and obesity associated' gene (FTO): no significant association of variant rs9939609 with weight loss in a lifestyle intervention and lipid metabolism markers in German obese children and adolescents. *BMC Medical Genetics* 2008; **9**: 85.

32. Reinehr T, Hinney A, Toschke AM, Hebebrand J. Aggravating effect of INSIG2 and FTO on overweight reduction in a one-year lifestyle intervention. *Archives of Disease in Childhood* 2009; **94**(12): 965–967.

33. Florez JC, Jablonski KA, Bayley N, et al. TCF7L2 polymorphisms and progression to diabetes in the Diabetes Prevention Program. *The New England Journal of Medicine* 2006; **355**(3): 241–250.

34. Bochukova EG, Huang N, Keogh J, et al. Large, rare chromosomal deletions associated with severe early-onset obesity. *Nature* 2010; **463**(7281): 666–670.

35. Walters RG, Jacquemont S, Valsesia A, et al. A new highly penetrant form of obesity due to deletions on chromosome 16p11.2. *Nature* 2010; **463**(7281): 671–675.

36. Franks PW, Ling C. Epigenetics and obesity: the devil is in the details. *BMC Medicine* 2010; **8**: 88.

37. Milagro FI, Campion J, Cordero P et al. A dual epigenomic approach for the search of obesity biomarkers: DNA methylation in relation to diet-induced weight loss. *The FASEB Journal* 2011; **25**(4): 1378–1389.

38. Grant SF, Thorleifsson G, Reynisdottir I, et al. Variant of transcription factor 7-like 2 (TCF7L2) gene confers risk of type 2 diabetes. *Nature Genetics* 2006; **38**(3): 320–323.

39. Reinehr T, Friedel S, Mueller TD, Toschke AM, Hebebrand J, Hinney A. Evidence for an influence of TCF7L2 polymorphism rs7903146 on insulin resistance and sensitivity indices in overweight children and adolescents during a lifestyle intervention. *International Journal of Obesity* (London) 2008; **32**(10): 1521–1524.

40. Reinehr T, Scherag A, Wang HJ, et al. Relationship between MTNR1B (melatonin receptor 1B gene) polymorphism rs10830963 and glucose levels in overweight children and adolescents. *Pediatric Diabetes* 2011; **12**: 435–441.

41. Linsel-Nitschke P, Gotz A, Erdmann J, et al. Lifelong reduction of LDL-cholesterol related to a common variant in the LDL-receptor gene decreases the risk of coronary artery disease – a Mendelian Randomisation study. *PLoS ONE* 2008; **3**(8): e2986.

42. Linsel-Nitschke P, Heeren J, Aherrahrou Z, et al. Genetic variation at chromosome 1p13.3 affects sortilin mRNA expression, cellular LDL-uptake and serum LDL levels which translates to the risk of coronary artery disease. *Atherosclerosis* 2010; **208**(1): 183–189.

43. Wiegand S, Keller KM, Robl M, et al. Obese boys at increased risk for nonalcoholic liver disease: evaluation of 16 390 overweight or obese children and adolescents. *International Journal of Obesity* (London) 2010; **34**(10): 1468–1474.

44. Speliotes EK, Yerges-Armstrong LM, Wu J, et al. Genome-wide association analysis identifies variants associated with nonalcoholic fatty liver disease that have distinct effects on metabolic traits. *PLoS Genetics* 2011; **7**(3): e1001324.

45. Hebebrand J, Friedel S, Schauble N, Geller F, Hinney A. Perspectives: molecular genetic research in human obesity. *Obesity Reviews* 2003; **4**(3): 139–146.

Chapter 5.2

Food intake, eating behaviour and obesity in children

Marion Hetherington, Chandani Nekitsing, Janet McNally and Netalie Shloim
University of Leeds, Leeds, UK

5.2.1 Introduction

Overweight and obesity in childhood are more evident now than ever before. Obesity in early life, which was once rare even in urbanised and developed economies, is now commonplace, with international surveys showing that childhood obesity is a global problem [1]. Estimates for obesity in school-age children range from 5 to 10% in Europe and the Americas, respectively, and for overweight the range is from 25.5 to 27.7% in these same regions [1]. Early life is a critical period for the development of obesity [2], since obesity in childhood appears to track into later life [3,4]. This suggests that patterns of eating and activity acquired from an early age are relatively stable. During infancy, mothers provide their infants with milk, and then, at around 6 months, introduce them to the family diet. (*Note*: It is recognised that 'caregivers' can be mothers, fathers or guardians; however, for the purposes of this chapter, we shall refer to mothers, since most research has focussed on the role of mothers in infant feeding.) The decision to breastfeed or use formula, the time at which solids are introduced and the feeding practices employed by parents are thought to affect later obesity risk. Therefore, in this chapter, the evidence on how food habits are formed in early life will be explored, as will the proposition that infant feeding sets the foundation for self-regulation and appetite control, promoting healthy weight gain and growth.

Of course, the corollary of this proposition is that early life might also sow the seeds for later overeating and poor appetite expression; therefore, the research that links feeding practices and eating habits to later obesity risk will be evaluated in parallel.

5.2.2 Exposure starts early

The earliest exposure to odour, flavour and food occurs before birth. Around the end of the third trimester, the foetus swallows up to 1 litre of amniotic fluid per day. The foetus is therefore exposed to the sensory features of the maternal diet – specifically, chemicals that are transmitted through the placenta to the amniotic fluid [5]. For example, mothers who consume foods containing volatile compounds such as those found in garlic or fennel share the flavour of these foods with the developing foetus. It is known from research by Mennella et al. [6] that amniotic fluid carries odour and flavour. They demonstrated that flavour can be transmitted by the mother to the foetus. In this study, 10 mothers were assigned to receive either a flavourless or a garlic-flavoured capsule. Then, 13 sensory panellists rated the strength of odour of five paired samples of amniotic fluid (garlic present or absent). A significant effect was found for all but one pair, indicating that the panellists could detect the presence of garlic accurately. Studies on newborn babies indicate that those exposed to garlic during pregnancy show preference for milk containing garlic compared to milk that does not. Newborn babies orient and make mouthing movements towards odours and flavours that are familiar and complex; thus, they have learned through exposure and experience to prefer components of the maternal diet. However, familiarity is not enough, since infants who are formula-fed prefer human breast milk [7]. Thus, the rich chemosensory medium of human milk is preferred over formula, which is rather bland and no longer permitted to have added flavour. Interestingly, adults who, as infants, had been exposed to vanillin-flavoured formula milk (when this was permitted) showed a preference for ketchup containing vanillin, as compared to plain ketchup [8]. This suggests that experience with vanillin in early life shapes flavour preference during adulthood.

Breastfeeding provides a powerful medium through which infants experience flavour. Research on weaning-age infants has demonstrated that breastfed babies are more willing to accept new foods, including green vegetables, as compared to formula-fed babies [9]. This may be due to the greater flavour experience and sensory complexity of breast milk as compared to formula milk, or it could be due to the other psychological benefits of breastfeeding. However, for now, the initial premise is that the flavour experience begins during pregnancy and continues with the decisions that mothers make about feeding, including breastfeeding. This flavour experience may guide preference and choice in later life too.

The importance of weaning

The introduction to solid foods, complementary feeding or 'weaning' is the next important step in the development of food preferences and appetite entrainment. Infants are born as 'univores', perfectly adapted to consuming breast milk, which is sweet in taste. Experiments with newborn babies confirm that infants have an innate, unlearned preference for sweet tastes. Thus, Steiner [10] – who filmed the gusto-facial response of babies to basic tastes (sour, sweet, salty and bitter) compared to water – found that, before the babies had been fed

their first milk meal, they showed a positive affective response to sweetness and a negative, aversive response to bitterness. However, infants must make the transition from being univores to omnivores at around 6 months of age. For all infants, the weaning period is a critical time during which family foods are presented – perhaps at first as purees before systematic exposure to lumps, and then to foods in solid form.

In recent years, some parents have adopted a 'baby-led' method, rather than a spoon-feeding approach, to infant weaning. Baby-led weaning (BLW) involves infants feeding themselves at around 6 months of age. At this stage, babies are able to support themselves, grasp food and move it to the mouth. Proponents of the practice suggest that it enables infants to regulate their intake, as they are able to control consumption, as well as the pace and duration of eating [11].

The research literature in relation to BLW is scant so far; however, there are preliminary indications that such an approach may contribute to the development of healthy appetite regulation. In a questionnaire-based study, Brown and Lee [11] found that the use of the BLW approach in infancy was associated with greater responsiveness to satiety in toddlers. Meanwhile, another questionnaire-based study by Townsend and Pitchford [12] found that children weaned using the BLW approach had a lower BMI and preferences for healthier foods (complex carbohydrates) in comparison to spoon-fed infants. Such findings may arise from associations between BLW and additional factors that support appetite regulation, such as breastfeeding [11]. Furthermore, as noted earlier, BLW is associated with greater infant control in feeding or a more responsive feeding style by parents [13]. Such feeding styles appear to assist in developing appetite regulation and in lowering obesity risk [14]. The BLW approach presupposes that infants are capable of choosing which foods to eat to support good health and development, and how much. The classic studies by Clara Davis [15,16] demonstrated that young children can indeed select foods that are not merely their favourite or sweet foods. These longitudinal observational studies showed that, if given an array of raw and processed foods, infants select a varied, healthy diet. This may be interpreted as an innate 'nutritional wisdom', but evidence suggests that infants learn to consume foods that provide benefits to them – for example, an infant preferentially selected cod liver oil when vitamin D deficient. In this case, despite the aversive taste of the oil, it was selected and consumed, thereby reversing the early symptoms of rickets.

Clearly then, at weaning, babies are willing to accept even rather unusual foods, or those that adults might find disagreeable. Since they have an innate preference for sweet tastes, they do not need to learn to like sweetness. However, developing a liking for bitter foods, such as vegetables, takes several exposures. Caregivers may decide to give up after only a few exposures, since facial responses may be interpreted as dislike; however, it generally takes 5–10 exposures for acceptance of an unfamiliar food or texture [17].

In the first year of life, infants are willing to try new foods, but older children are less amenable to novelty. By the age of 24 months or so, neophobia begins. This means that, as children become more mobile and independent, they also become more wary about new foods, and even refuse previously liked foods. Parents have a window of opportunity in the first years of the infant's life, before neophobia begins, to introduce foods such as vegetables. Studies of school-age children show that interventions to encourage intake of fruit and vegetables are selectively successful for fruit but have no or little effect on vegetables [18]. Therefore, in school-age children, it is much more challenging to encourage vegetable intake compared to weaning- and pre-school-age children.

5.2.3 Eating traits

In order to understand the feeding interactions between mothers and their infants, it is important to know to what extent eating traits are heritable, and what is learned. Thus, mothers are often able to say, even in the early weeks of life, that they have a 'hungry' or a 'fussy' baby [19,20]. Mothers who identify their babies as hungry are more likely to introduce solid foods earlier than 6 months [20,21], and, in so

doing, increase the risk of exposing their infants to higher-energy-density diets and more rapid infant weight gain [22].

How then do mothers recognise hunger, appetite and satiety in their babies and infants? Studies indicate that mothers use a range of cues in responding to their infants' hunger and satiety. Commonly identified hunger cues include rooting, sucking fingers, licking the lips and reaching for food [23]. Meanwhile, cues such as pulling/pushing away, spitting food, refusal to open the mouth or withdrawal from the nipple are taken as indications of satiety [23]. Crying and fussing have been reported both as an indication of hunger and of satiety. Where crying has been identified as a hunger cue, some mothers have reported their babies as having a distinct 'hungry cry' [19]. On further examination though, it would appear that mothers tend to use external cues such as time of day or time since the last feed to determine which cries indicate hunger and which indicate distress [19]. As might be expected, there are indications that the specificity and clarity of hunger and satiety cues increase with age, and that parents are therefore more able to recognise and respond to the cues of older infants [24].

In order to identify eating traits in babies and infants, interviews and focus groups have been conducted with mothers to map out the qualitative dimensions of these traits. However, this approach is very time consuming and highly specialised. A more quantitative approach might involve asking mothers to complete questionnaires that measure a variety of eating behaviours associated with risk of obesity, such as avid appetite, low satiety responsiveness and rapid eating. For example, the Baby Eating Behaviour Questionnaire (BEBQ) [25] has been developed to characterise infant appetite during the milk-feeding phase. The BEBQ was adapted and developed from the Child Eating Behaviour Questionnaire (CEBQ) [26]. This was originally developed and validated with 3–8-year-old children; contains 35 questions to assess a range of eating traits; is widely used; and has been translated into many different languages. The CEBQ characterises key components of eating styles thought to impact on the types and quantities of foods consumed by children [27]. These relate to how responsive children are to the presence and availability of foods, to internal cues of hunger and satiety, and to the rate of eating. The items relate to eight key factors: food enjoyment, food responsiveness, satiety responsiveness, emotional overeating, emotional undereating, food fussiness, slowness in eating and the desire to drink.

Evidence from twin studies shows that features of appetite expression such as satiety responsiveness, enjoyment of food and responsiveness to the presence of palatable foods are heritable and relate to adiposity [27]. Thus, the tendency to overeat relative to energy expenditure may form part of a behavioural phenotype, increasing susceptibility to the development of overweight and obesity.

5.2.4 Self-regulation

Children who respond accurately and immediately in the short term to energy-dense foods are said to demonstrate good self-regulation [28] – a quality that facilitates energy balance. Young children, in particular, appear to show good self-regulation – for example, by adapting to variations in the energy density of formula milk and adjusting food intake in line with the energy content of a preload. Preschool children show compensation of around 50–80% of the energy content of a fixed energy load given prior to a test meal [29–31]; however, as children get older, their capacity to regulate accurately in the short-term decreases [29]. The capacity to compensate for the energy content of a fixed amount of food (preload), sometimes called the 'compensation index' (COMPX), may reflect responsiveness to the internal cues of satiation and satiety. COMPX may be linked to a specific genotype [32], or may be acquired through experience.

In contrast, eating when not hungry or eating in response to the presence of high-energy-density, palatable foods may reflect weak responsiveness to internal cues of hunger and satiety. The tendency to eat when not hungry or when faced with appealing, palatable foods is known as 'disinhibition' in adults. Disinhibition strongly and consistently differentiates obese and non-obese adults. In children, eating in the absence of hunger (EAH) is considered a precursor to disinhibited eating, and is linked to

obesity risk [33,34]. EAH is influenced by restrictive feeding practices [34], although it appears that mothers' concerns about children's weight mediates restriction over food rather than causing weight gain [35]. EAH may reflect poor self-regulation, since food intake is driven more by the mere presence and availability of palatable foods than by any underlying biological need. Indeed, proximity to snack foods can encourage children to eat, regardless of whether the food is high or low in energy density [36].

Mealtime interaction

Eating behaviours should also be considered by the complexity of early mealtime interactions. As such, early experiences of feeding are important for setting the foundation of healthy eating later in life [37]. Thus, although infants are born with the ability to self-regulate energy intake, some parents do not find recognising hunger and satiety cues as a straightforward process, potentially resulting in mothers over-feeding their infants, thus reducing their ability to self-regulate [38].

In addition, excessive parental control on feeding may be adversely associated with under- or over-feeding [39], or with slower weight gain [40]. The infants of parents who use such feeding behaviours might therefore have lower levels of awareness to their own hunger and satiety cues. Thus, parental control may reflect responsiveness to their child, but in a oppositional rather than supportive direction. Given the influence of eating traits on the risk of obesity, and the role of parents in responding to these characteristics, mealtimes may hold the key to understanding the dynamic nature of the parent–child interaction in determining food intake and the development of appetite control.

5.2.5 Conclusion

In conclusion, the prevalence of childhood obesity is increasing, and healthy eating habits should therefore be adopted early in life. Research has shown that breastfed infants, who are exposed to components of maternal diet, experience different flavours and accept novel foods during weaning. For all infants introduction of solid foods, and repeatedly exposing infants to novel/disliked foods, encourages the consumption of such foods.

Nevertheless, healthy eating habits are not solely regarded via the types of food, but also through maternal responsiveness and mealtime interactions. Given that infants are born with the ability to self-regulate and know when they are full, mothers should recognise the hunger and satiety cues of their babies. Feeding responsively will promote self-regulation and reduce the likelihood of overfeeding. Thus, maternal feeding styles, including maternal control and interactions during mealtime, contribute to the development of infants' eating habits.

5.2.6 Summary box

Key points

- Childhood obesity is a global concern, and early infant feeding influences obesity risk.
- Babies are able to regulate energy intake and prefer sweetness from birth, but must learn to like other tastes as well.
- Breastfeeding encourages healthy eating through exposure to complex tastes.
- Weaning is a critical period for the acceptance of novel foods with bitter tastes, such as vegetables.
- Eating traits such as enjoyment of food and avid appetite facilitate overconsumption.
- Parental sensitivity to infant hunger and satiety cues may enhance self-regulation and prevent overeating.

References

1. Wang Y, Lobstein T. Worldwide trends in childhood overweight and obesity. *International Journal of Pediatric Obesity* 2006; **1**: 11–25.
2. Dietz W. Critical periods in childhood for the development of obesity. *American Journal of Clinical Nutrition* 1994; **59**: 955–959.
3. Wright CM, Emmett PM, Ness AR, Reilly JJ, Sherriff A. Tracking of obesity and body fatness through mid-childhood. *Archives of Disease in Childhood* 2010; **95**: 612–617.
4. Singh AS, Mulder C, Twisk JWR, Van Mechelen W, Chinapaw MJM. Tracking of childhood overweight into adulthood: a systematic review of the literature. *Obesity Reviews* 2008; **9**: 474–488.

5. Mennella JA. Ontogeny of taste preferences: basic biology and implications for health. *American Journal of Clinical Nutrition* 2014; **99**(3): 704S–711S. doi: 10.3945/ajcn.113.067694.
6. Mennella JA, Johnson A, Beauchamp GK. Garlic ingestion by pregnant women alters the odor of amniotic fluid. *Chemical Senses* 1995; **20**: 207–209.
7. Marlier L, Schaal B. Human newborns prefer human milk: conspecific milk odor is attractive without postnatal exposure. *Child Development* 2005; **76**: 155–168.
8. Haller R, Rummel C, Henneberg S, Pollmer U, Koster EP. The influence of early experience with vanillin on food preference later in life. *Chemical Senses* 1999; **24**: 465–467.
9. Sullivan SA, Birch LL. Infant dietary experience and acceptance of solid foods. *Pediatrics* 1994; **93**: 271–277.
10. Steiner JE. Facial expressions of the neonate infant indicating the hedonics of food-related chemical stimuli. In: Weiffenbach JM (ed) *Taste and Development: The Genesis of Sweet Preference*. Washington, DC: US Government Printing Office, 1977.
11. Brown A, Lee MD. Early influences on child satiety-responsiveness: the role of weaning style. *Pediatric Obesity* 2015; **10**(1): 57–66. doi: 10.1111/j.2047-6310.2013.00207.x.
12. Townsend E, Pitchford N. Baby knows best? The impact of weaning style on food preferences and body mass index in early childhood in a case-controlled sample. *BMJ Open* 2012; **2**(1): e000298. doi: 10.1136/bmjopen-2011-000298.
13. Brown A, Lee M. Maternal child-feeding style during the weaning period: association with infant weight and maternal eating style. *Eating Behaviors* 2011; **12**: 108–111.
14. DiSantis K, Hodges E, Johnson S, Fisher J. The role of responsive feeding in overweight during infancy and toddlerhood: a systematic review. *International Journal of Obesity* 2011; **35**: 480–492.
15. Davis C. Self selection of diet by newly weaned infants: an experimental study. *American Journal of Diseases of Children* 1928; **36**: 651–679.
16. Davis C. Results of the self-selection of diets by young children. *Canadian Medical Association Journal* 1939; **41**: 257–261.
17. Caton SJ, Blundell P, Ahern SM, et al. Learning to eat vegetables in early life: the role of timing, age and individual eating traits. *PLoS ONE* 2014; **9**(5): e97609. doi: 10.1371/journal.pone.0097609
18. Evans CE, Christian MS, Cleghorn CL, Greenwood DC, Cade JE. Systematic review and meta-analysis of school-based interventions to improve daily fruit and vegetable intake in children aged 5 to 12 y. *American Journal of Clinical Nutrition* 2012; **96**: 889–901.
19. Anderson AS, Guthrie CA, Alder EM, Forsyth S, Howie PW, Williams FLR. Rattling the plate – reasons and rationales for early weaning. *Health Education Research* 2001; **16**: 471–479.
20. Wright CM, Parkinson KN, Drewett RF. Why are babies weaned early? Data from a prospective population based cohort study. *Archives of Disease in Childhood* 2004; **89**: 813–816.
21. Alder EM, Williams FLR, Anderson AS, Forsyth S, Florey CdV, van der Velde P. What influences the timing of the introduction of solid food to infants? *British Journal of Nutrition* 2004; **92**: 527–531.

22. Ong KK, Emmett PM, Noble S, Ness A, Dunger DB. Dietary energy intake at the age of 4 months predicts postnatal weight gain and childhood body mass index. *Pediatrics* 2006; **117**: e503–e508.
23. Hodges EA, Hughes SO, Hopkinson J, Fisher JO. Maternal decisions about the initiation and termination of infant feeding. *Appetite* 2008; **50**: 333–339.
24. Hodges EA, Johnson SL, Hughes SO, Hopkinson JM, Butte NF, Fisher JO. Development of the responsiveness to child feeding cues scale. *Appetite* 2013; **65**: 210–219.
25. Llewellyn CH, van Jaarsveld CH, Johnson L, Carnell S, Wardle J. Development and factor structure of the Baby Eating Behaviour Questionnaire in the Gemini birth cohort. *Appetite* 2011; **57**(2, Oct): 388–396.
26. Wardle J, Guthrie CA, Sanderson S, Rapoport L. Development of the children's eating behaviour questionnaire. *Journal of Child Psychology and Psychiatry* 2001; **42**: 963–970.
27. Wardle J, Carnell S. Appetite is a heritable phenotype associated with adiposity. *Annals of Behavioral Medicine* 2009; **38**: 25–30.
28. Cecil JE, Tavendale R, Watt P, Hetherington MM, Palmer CNA. An obesity-associated FTO gene variant and increased energy intake in children. *The New England Journal of Medicine* 2008; **359**: 2558–2566.
29. Hetherington MM, Wood C, Lyburn SC. Response to energy dilution in the short-term: evidence of nutritional wisdom in young children? *Nutritional Neuroscience* 2000; **3**: 321–329.
30. Birch LL, McPhee L, Sullivan S, Johnson S. Conditioned meal initiation in young children. *Appetite* 1989; **13**: 105–113.
31. Birch LL, McPhee LS, Bryant JL, Johnson SL. Children's lunch intake: effects of midmorning snacks varying in energy density and fat content. *Appetite* 1993; **20**: 83–94.
32. Cecil JE, Palmer CN, Wrieden W, et al. Energy intakes of children after preloads: adjustment, not compensation. *American Journal of Clinical Nutrition* 2005; **82**: 302–308.
33. Kral TVE, Faith MS. Influences on child eating and weight development from a behavioral genetics perspective. *Journal of Pediatric Psychology* 2009; **34**: 596–605.
34. Fisher JO, Birch LL. Eating in the absence of hunger and overweight in girls from 5 to 7 y of age. *American Journal of Clinical Nutrition* 2002; **76**: 226–231.
35. Webber L, Cooke L, Hill C, Wardle J. Associations between children's appetitive traits and maternal feeding practices. *Journal of the American Dietetic Association* 2010; **110**: 1718–1722.
36. Musher-Eizenman DR, Young KM, Laurene K, Galliger C, Hauser J, Wagner Oehlhof M. Children's sensitivity to external food cues: how distance to serving bowl influences children's consumption. *Health Education & Behavior* 2010; **37**: 186–192.
37. Nicklaus S, Remy E. Early origins of overeating: tracking between early food habits and later eating patterns. *Current Obesity Reports* 2013; **2**: 179–184.
38. Li R, Fein SB, Grummer-Strawn LM. Do infants fed from bottles lack self-regulation of milk intake compared with directly breastfed infants? *Pediatrics* 2010; **125**: e1386–e1393.
39. Birch LL, Fisher JO. Development of eating behaviors among children and adolescents. *Pediatrics* 1998; **101**: 539–549.
40. Farrow C, Blissett J. Does maternal control during feeding moderate early infant weight gain? *Pediatrics* 2006; **118**: e293–e298.

Chapter 5.3

Physical activity and inactivity in the aetiology of obesity in children

Ulf Ekelund
Norwegian School of Sport Sciences, Oslo, Norway

5.3.1 Introduction

The specific causes of overweight and obesity are varied and complex but, including intra-uterine and early-life exposures, the genetic, biological, socio-cultural and environmental components, at a population level, are consistent with sustained positive energy balance. A sedentary lifestyle and low levels of physical activity (PA) participation have therefore been implicated in this trend.

This chapter aims to describe population levels of PA in children and discuss the strength of evidence underlying the assertion that there is a secular decline in population levels of PA, which occurred in parallel with the increase in obesity prevalence. The aim is also to discuss whether higher levels of PA prevent weight gain, and whether sedentary behaviour and physical inactivity induces weight gain in children. The issue of reverse or bidirectional causality for the association between physical inactivity with body weight gain will be discussed, Finally, public health guidelines for PA will be summarised. To understand these complex relationships, the chapter will provide a brief overview of some of the methods used for assessing population levels of PA in youth defined as those less than 18 years of age. A glossary of specific terms is provided in Box 5.3.1.

5.3.2 Assessment of physical activity in children

Population assessment of PA includes self-reporting and objective monitoring of PA, either by direct measurement of body movement (e.g. by accelerometry), by a physiological response (e.g. heart rate) to body movement or a combination of both (e.g. combined heart rate and movement sensing) (www.mrc-toolkit.ac.uk).

Self-reported physical activity

The accuracy of self-reports is influenced by the ability of the respondent to accurately recall all relevant activities retrospectively. Therefore, self-report methods are subject to recall bias. This can either be intentional or accidental false recall, missed recall or differential reporting accuracy of different intensities, dimensions and domains of activity. The age of the respondent is another important variable in determining the method of administration. Accurate self-report data are particularly problematic in children younger than 12 years [1]. Therefore, parental and teacher-reported questionnaires or proxy-reports are often used. However, recall of children's PA is also difficult for adults, and unique limitations and errors are associated with this method.

Advanced Nutrition and Dietetics in Obesity, First Edition. Edited by Catherine Hankey.
© 2018 John Wiley & Sons Ltd. Published 2018 by John Wiley & Sons Ltd.

Box 5.3.1 Glossary of definitions used in physical activity research and practice

Confounder

A variable (e.g. energy intake) that is associated with both the exposure (e.g. PA) and the outcome (e.g. obesity).

Energy balance

Energy balance is achieved when energy intake equals energy expenditure (external work, internal work, growth and repair, and heat production), and is usually tightly regulated by neuro-endocrine feedback systems. In theory, energy balance and, therefore, a stable body weight can be maintained at various levels of energy intake and expenditure (i.e. 'energy flux'). Although direct evidence is lacking, it is likely that a stable body weight is more easily maintained at high energy flux. An increase in total daily energy expenditure (TEE) is possible either through an increase in overall PA or a gain in body weight due to a positive energy balance. In the latter case, body weight will increase until a new and higher level of energy balance is established.

Energy gap

The term 'energy gap' has been used to characterise different aspects of weight gain. Some have defined energy gap as the difference in energy intake or expenditure between normal-weight individuals and individuals at various levels of excess weight when weight stability is present [6]. Using this approach, when comparing normal-weight individuals with obese individuals, the energy gap is estimated to be approximately 300–400 kcal per day. These estimates are considerably larger than the often-quoted energy gap of 50–100 kcal per day based on an average population weight gain between two time points [7].

Others [8] have defined the positive energy balance needed to create weight gain over a period of time as the 'energy imbalance gap'. However, they extended their model and also considered that, in order for energy imbalance to drive the gain in body weight over time, energy intake needs to keep rising, because TEE is continuously rising due to a higher body weight, which increases resting energy expenditure (REE) and possibly also PA energy expenditure (PAEE). The latter is explained by the increased energy required to move a larger body, but does not indicate higher levels of body movement per se. Eventually, energy intake and expenditure (i.e. energy flux) are higher than before weight gain. The 'energy maintenance gap' has been estimated to be about 350 kcal per day in US children [8]. This amount is substantial, and equates approximately to more than 100 min of moderate-intensity PA per day for a child with a body weight of 50 kg, suggesting that it is unlikely that small increases in PA will be sufficient to reverse the obesity epidemic.

Metabolic energy turnover (MET)

MET is usually used to quantify the intensity of activities in absolute values, with 1 MET corresponding to the resting metabolic rate (RMR). Originally, 1 MET was defined as 3.5 mL O_2/kg/min in adults. RMR in relation to body weight is higher in young children, and decreasing with age. For example, in a 6-year-old child, RMR is likely to be 6–8 mL O_2/kg/min, and thereafter steadily decrease throughout puberty.

Physical activity (PA)

PA has been defined as 'any bodily movement produced by skeletal muscles that increase energy expenditure above the resting level'. This definition recognises PA as dynamic body movement, takes all types and domains of activity into account and provides a platform for how to measure PA.

Physically active

Individuals who meet established guidelines for PA are categorised as physically active.

Physical activity guidelines

Most health authorities agree that children and adolescents should accumulate at least 60 min of moderate- and vigorous-intensity PA each day. 'Moderate intensity' is defined as an intensity of PA that increases energy expenditure three–four times above the resting levels – for example, brisk walking.

Physical inactivity
The absence of PA, usually a reflection of the proportion of time spent below the threshold for moderate intensity PA, and therefore not meeting established guidelines.

Reverse causality
In epidemiological terms, this refers to a process when the direction of association is opposite to the expected (e.g. 'Does lower levels of PA cause obesity, or does obesity induce lower levels of PA?').

Sedentary behaviour
Sedentary behaviour defines those behaviours that involve sitting or lounging, very low levels of muscle contractions and activities for which energy expenditure is low. Sedentary behaviours are generally defined as physical activities of intensity between 1 and 1.5 METs.

Physical activity questionnaires

Most questionnaires developed for use in children consider specific types of activity, such as duration and frequency of sport and exercise, and recreational PA [2–4], which may be more accurately recalled as compared to habitual activity, as the individual has made a conscious decision to carry out that activity in a defined period. The correlation between any self-report and an objective instrument is low to moderate, at best. This is not surprising, given the limitations of self-reports to assess the intermittent nature of children's PA [5]. Self-report instruments usually overestimate the intensities and durations of different types of sports. This is because many sports are intermittent in nature, and a child who (accurately) reports practicing or playing football, usually coded as vigorous intensity, for 1 hour may only be physically active at vigorous intensity for a limited period of that hour. Therefore, most researchers agree that objective methods are preferable when measuring sedentary time and PA in children.

Objective measurement of physical activity by accelerometry

Accelerometry is currently the most commonly used objective method for measuring PA. The development of these devices has substantially increased our ability to obtain accurate measurements of the volume, pattern, frequency, intensity and duration of children's PA and sedentary behaviours [6–10]. Furthermore, strong and consistent associations have been identified between objectively measured PA and health outcomes [11]. Newer versions of accelerometers measure the acceleration of the body

or different parts of body in one, two or three dimensions in its raw format. This information can subsequently be converted into a specific, predefined period (epoch). Accelerometry has been used to assess free-living PA in many relatively large-scale observational studies ($N > 1000$ children). Data from these studies pooled in large datasets have enabled more detailed analyses of the patterns and trends of PA, and any associations with health outcomes [12].

However, the interpretation of PA data from accelerometry is a challenge, and specific issues associated with data interpretation need consideration. The most imminent issue relates to the definition of intensity categories for the amount of time spent sedentary, and in light-, moderate- and vigorous-intensity PA. Unfortunately, no consensus has been reached on the most appropriate intensity cut-points to use in children, and the interpretation of accelerometer data is therefore influenced by the cut-points employed. For example, intensity thresholds for one of the most commonly used accelerometers, Actigraph (www.actigraph.com), vary between 100 counts per min (cpm) and 1100 cpm for time spent sedentary, and 615–3600 cmp for time spent in moderate–vigorous-intensity PA (MVPA). This variability in intensity thresholds influences the estimates for the prevalence of children active children, when judged according to public health guidelines [13].

Objective measurement of physical activity by heart rate and movement sensing

Accelerometry is limited in its ability to assess the increased energy expenditure associated with specific activities such as cycling, walking up stairs and carrying loads. Limitations with estimating energy expenditure from the heart rate include the increase in heart rate due to environmental and emotional factors. However, these errors are uncorrelated, and combining information from one physiological measure (e.g. heart rate) with body movement by accelerometry may overcome the limitations with either method used alone. Unfortunately, the high cost of these monitors may prohibit their use in population-based research. Nevertheless, these sensors provide interesting information on the various sub-components of PA that may particularly applicable to children. Prediction equations for estimating PA energy expenditure (PAEE) from acceleration and heart rate measures combined in branched equation modelling reduces the error of predicted PAEE in children [14]. However, additional research during free-living conditions is required to determine whether the increased accuracy of this method outweighs the increased cost of measurement.

Given the limitations with self-reports, particularly in children younger than 12 years of age, the use of an objective assessment method is recommended, both in clinical and research settings. Accelerometry is widely used, simple and provide useful information on both overall activity levels and times spent sedentary, and in different intensity levels of PA. Practitioners without any experience in objective monitoring of PA who want to use this method may contact an academic institution for further advice.

5.3.3 Current levels of physical activity among young people

Most public health authorities (e.g. Centres for Disease Control and Prevention, USA; Department of Health, UK; Public Health Agency of Canada/ Canadian Society for Exercise Physiology, Canada) agree that young people (<18 years) should accumulate at least 60 min of MVPA on at least 5 days per week. In addition, the benefits of vigorous-intensity activity are acknowledged. Although the underlying evidence for these recommendations may be considered weak, they provide a framework when evaluating population levels of PA in the youth.

Data on self-reported PA from the Health Behaviour in School-aged Children study, the Youth Risk Behaviour Surveillance System and the World Health Organisation's Global school-based student health survey suggest that approximately 25–30% of school-aged children are physically active according to the current recommendations [15,16]. Although these estimates should be interpreted with some caution, owing to the limitations associated with self-reported PA, they suggest that a substantial proportion of children worldwide can be considered as physically inactive.

Data on the prevalence of physically inactive children vary considerably when PA has been measured by using accelerometry, owing to the different definitions of intensity levels. Table 5.3.1 summarises the data on sufficiently active children in cohort studies including more than 1000 participants [17–24]. These results clearly highlight that the inconsistent use of intensity thresholds is a major issue when trying to quantify the prevalence of sufficiently active young people by using accelerometry, with prevalence estimates ranging from 0.4 to >98% across studies. Despite the difficulty in interpreting the prevalence of physically active children from these data, two patterns are consistent: PA levels decline by age, and boys are more active than girls.

Secular decline in physical activity among young people

Unfortunately, neither direct measurements of free-living PA nor population-level information on self-reported PA in children are available during the period preceding the worldwide increase in the prevalence of obesity. We are therefore left with uncertainty as to what the population trends in the overall levels of PA were in children of all ages before the obesity epidemic.

Data on self-reported PA collected since the early 1990s do not support the notion that PA levels have declined in children during this period. However, the available information is limited to those participating in sports, physical education and more vigorous-intensity exercises, and it is likely that activity levels have declined in other domains – for example, transport-related PA and outdoor play. A few studies have examined the time trends in PA using accelerometry

Table 5.3.1 Prevalence of young people accumulating 60 min or more of moderate- and vigorous-intensity PA/day, measured using accelerometry in studies with more than 1000 participants

Reference	Design	Country	Age	MVPA threshold	MVPA definition	Prevalence sufficiently active
Riddoch et al. [23]	Cross-sectional (N=2185)	Denmark, Estonia, Norway, Portugal	9 and 15 years	9 years: 1000 cpm 15 years: 1500 cpm	≥3 METs	9 years: boys, 97.4%; girls, 97.6% 15 years: boys, 81.9%; girls, 62%
Nader et al. [24]	Longitudinal (N=1032)	USA	9–15 years	Age dependent*	≥3 METs	9 and 11 years: >96% (weekdays) 12 years: 83.4% (weekdays) 15 years: 30.6% (weekdays)
Troiano et al. [25]	Cross-sectional (N=1778)	USA	6–19 years	Age dependent*	≥4 METs	6–11 years: boys, 48.9%; girls, 34.7% 12–15 years: boys, 11.9%; girls, 3.4% 16–19 years: boys, 10%; girls, 5.4%
Riddoch et al. [26]	Cross-sectional (N=5595)	UK	12 years	3600 cpm	≥4 METs	Boys: 5.1% Girls: 0.4%
Steele et al. [27]	Cross-sectional (N=1862)	UK	10 years	2000 cpm	NA	Boys: 81.5% Girls: 59.4%
Thompson et al. [28]	Cross-sectional (N=1730 and N=2341)	Canada	8–16 years	NA	NA	2001–2002 8 years: boys, 89.7%; girls, 92.3% 12 years: boys, 44.9%; girls, 29.4% 16 years: boys, 7.9%; girls, 5.5% 2005–2006 8 years: boys, 80.5%; girls, 82.6% 12 years: boys, 36.2%; girls, 20.5% 16 years: boys, 7.7%; girls, 0.3%
Owen et al. [29]	Cross-sectional (N=2071)	UK	10 years	2000 cpm	NA	Boys: 76% Girls: 53%
Baptista et al. [30]	Cross-sectional (N=2714)	Portugal	10–17 years	Age dependent*	≥4 METs	10–11 years: boys, 66%; girls, 55% 12–13 years: boys, 50%; girls, 34% 14–15 years: boys, 40%; girls, 30% 16–17 years: boys, 30%; girls, 20%**

MET: metabolic equivalents

* Age-dependent equation: METs = 2.757 + (0.0015 × counts/min) − (0.08957 × age [years]) − (0.000038 × counts/min × age [years]) [23]

** Results extracted from reference [24]

or other objective assessment methods, albeit with inconsistent results [16,22]. Another approach to address whether young people's PA has declined is to compare children living in a 'traditional' lifestyle, owing to religious beliefs (i.e. Old Order Amish and Old Order Mennonite), against those living in a more 'contemporary' lifestyle. Children living in traditional lifestyles appear to be more active than contemporary-lifestyle children (about 80 min vs. 55 min of MVPA/day, respectively), and this difference is primarily due to higher habitual activity levels in those children living in traditional lifestyles, even despite not participating in organised sports and physical education [25].

In summary, more information obtained by implementing objective measurements of PA in repeated surveys in population-representative samples of youth are needed to understand PA time trends. This approach has been adopted by the National Health and Nutrition Examination Survey (NHANES) in the USA and the Health Survey in the UK.

5.3.4 Physical activity and adiposity in children

There is compelling evidence of strong inverse cross-sectional associations between PA and body weight, fat mass and obesity in children and youth [26,27]. Furthermore, obese youth are less physically active as measured by accelerometry – that is, they move less than matched normal-weight controls, although the absolute energy expenditure due to PA does not differ between groups [28]. Figure 5.3.1 displays the difference in the average daily intensity of PA between normal-weight and obese adolescents (Figure 5.3.1a), and the similarity in absolute PA energy expenditure (PAEE, MJ per day) between groups (Figure 5.3.1b).

Does physical activity prevent unhealthy weight gain and obesity?

Cross-sectional and case-control studies cannot be used to infer causality and to determine the direction of association. Prospective observational cohort studies, in which PA and body weight or body composition are measured at baseline and body weight

or body composition are measured again at follow-up, and randomised controlled trials are better placed to suggest a causal direction of association. However, it is unlikely that population-based randomised controlled trials on habitual PA in children can be conducted for practical and ethical reasons.

The possibility to observe a prospective or longitudinal association between PA and subsequent gain in body weight and adiposity depends on the measurement precision of the exposure variable (i.e. PA), the precision and definition of the outcome variable, the sample size and follow-up time. It is generally considered that objective methods for assessing PA are more precise as compared to self-reports, owing to misclassification from self-reports, which is even more pronounced in children as compared to adults. The measurement of the outcome variable (e.g. body weight or body composition) offers another challenge, as these variables also change by time due to growth and maturation. The use of standardised standard deviation (SD) scores, based on the baseline distribution of body weight or body composition, and statistical adjustment for confounding of maturity may, to some extent, overcome these analytical issues. Therefore, a measure of biological or sexual maturity, such as the Tanner scale [29], is recommended when conducting research in youths, as this variable can be controlled for in subsequent analyses on the associations between activity and body weight and composition.

When summarising the available evidence for a prospective association between higher levels of objectively measured baseline PA and excessive weight or body fat gain, recent reviews have usually found weak evidence or no evidence of the more physically active members of the population gaining less excess body weight or adiposity than those who are less physically active [30]. Unfortunately, neither of these reviews could synthesise the results in the form of a meta-analysis, owing to the marked heterogeneity in exposure and outcome measurements.

Does sedentary behaviour predict obesity in young people?

Recent data from the NHANES on Americans between 6 and 60 years of age suggest that most their time awake (55%) was spent sedentary [31].

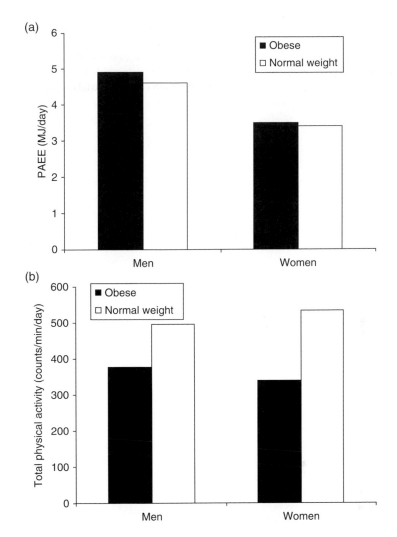

Figure 5.3.1 PA energy expenditure (MJ/day, Figure 5.3.1a) measured by the doubly labelled water method, and total PA (counts/min per day, Figure 5.3.1b) measured by accelerometry in obese and normal-weight men and women. Total PA by accelerometry was significantly different between groups ($P<0.01$). Data extracted from reference [34].

Many health authorities and organisations have also recognised the potentially detrimental effects of prolonged time spent sedentary, and have consequently compiled guidelines for reducing the amount of sedentary time, especially TV viewing.

In large-scale cohort studies, self-reported time spent watching TV is usually used as a proxy marker of sedentary behaviour. Two recent reviews [32,33] observed significant associations between TV viewing and body fat, although one of these reported that this association was not likely to be clinically relevant [32]. Further cross-sectional studies that used an objective measure of sedentary behaviour and more sensitive measures of body fat found positive associations and greater risks of being obese with sedentary behaviour [34,35]. Interestingly, both studies also reported that the magnitude of association between moderate and vigorous PA and obesity was stronger than the association between sedentary behaviour and obesity.

Few prospective observational studies are available that report on the association between baseline sedentary behaviour (i.e. TV viewing) and a measure of obesity later in time. In a well-conducted study in a New Zealand birth cohort ($N=1019$), it was observed that parental- and self-reported TV viewing between 5 and 15 years predicted BMI at age 26 years, independent of childhood BMI, self-reported PA and other confounders [36]. Another study reported that each additional hour of watching TV at age 5 years was associated with a 7% increased risk of obesity at age 30 years [37].

The observed positive association between TV viewing and gain in body weight or development of obesity may be mediated by other behaviours, such as unconscious snacking while watching TV, a reduction in PA or both. Although studies attempt to adjust their analyses for PA and dietary intake, residual confounding may persist, owing to the imprecise measures of these confounders. Only randomisation within a trial can perfectly deal with confounding. Epstein et al. [38] examined the effect of experimentally induced changes in sedentary behaviour in 12–16-year-old normal-weight adolescents ($N=16$). The authors applied a within-individual cross-over design, with three phases, each of 3-week duration: the baseline, increase and decrease phases (25–50% of self-reported baseline values) in sedentary time. The time spent sedentary was significantly lower for the decrease phase as compared to baseline. When sedentary time was experimentally decreased, the energy intake decreased and PA increased. In contrast, when the researchers experimentally increased sedentary time over 3 weeks, there were no effects on either energy intake or PA. The authors concluded that decreasing sedentary behaviour can decrease energy intake, and that sedentary behaviour should hence be considered as an important component of interventions to prevent body weight gain.

5.3.5 The issue of reverse or bidirectional causality

It is possible that heavier individuals are less likely to adhere to PA between two time points in an observational study. Studies in adults have suggested that PA at baseline was unrelated to weight gain, but the converse was true, since a higher body weight or BMI at baseline was significantly related to an increased risk of becoming sedentary at follow-up, suggesting reverse causality.

However, it is difficult to determine the direction of association in any observational study when the exposure and the outcome are measured with different degrees of precision. There is a marked difference in measurement precision between the measure of body weight and that of PA or sedentary behaviour. When the more imprecise variable (PA) is used as the outcome, the magnitude of effect is estimated accurately, but with error. When the more imprecise variable is used as the exposure, the measure of effect is attenuated. Because PA and sedentary behaviour usually are measured with self-reports, which is much less precise than is the measure of body weight, it is not surprising that baseline body weight predicts follow-up PA (or sedentary time), whereas, because of measurement error, the reverse may not be detectable.

In an attempt to overcome this, Kwon et al. [39] examined the associations between objectively measured time in MVPA by accelerometry, with gain in fat mass in 326 children aged 5–11 years, in which objectively measured PA and fat mass were available at three time points (5 years, 8 years and 11 years). Time spent in MVPA did not predict fat mass at follow-up. In contrast, baseline fat mass significantly predicted decreased time in MVPA at follow-up, suggesting that adiposity level may be a determinant of PA. Similar observations were made in a large pooled analysis of the prospective associations between objectively measured MVPA, sedentary time and cardio-metabolic risk factors in more than 20,000 youth (mean age 12.8 years) [40]. In this study, baseline sedentary time did not predict abdominal obesity (waist circumference) at follow-up, whereas greater waist circumference at baseline predicted an increase in sedentary time [40].

Taken together, these studies suggest that the nature of the complex relationships between PA, sedentary behaviour and gain in body weight may be either reverse or bidirectional. It may be that the direction of association between PA and sedentary behaviour with change in body weight differs by age, by the baseline prevalence of obesity in the population and by whether the population examined is in energy balance or in a state of positive energy balance during the follow-up period. Furthermore, the association is even more complicated by the impact of energy intake on energy balance, an exposure even more difficult to accurately measure than PA in observational cohort studies.

The association between PA, sedentary behaviour and obesity is of public health importance. Therefore, future longitudinal studies including multiple, repeated and precise measurements of the exposure and outcome from an early age (before the amount of fat accumulated may hinder PA) are more likely to be able to address the issue of bidirectional or reverse causality. Furthermore, well-conducted studies are warranted that control for the confounding effect of dietary intake and change in sexual maturity during adolescence.

5.3.6 Summary box

Key points

- Self-reported PA is associated with substantial measurement error. Therefore, objective methods are recommended when assessing young peoples' PA.
- Current data suggest that a substantial proportion of youth do not achieve the recommended levels of 60 min of daily moderate-to-vigorous-intensity PA.
- The prospective association between baseline levels of PA and gain in body weight, fat mass or development of obesity is weak, and possibly bi-directional.
- Higher levels of sedentary behaviour, defined as amount of TV viewing, may predict weight gain. However, whether this association is mediated by lower levels of overall PA or dietary intake needs further examination.
- Observational studies with a repeated measurement design using state-of-the-art methods for measuring PA and body fat are needed to inform public health guidelines.

Useful web links

1. http://dapa-toolkit.mrc.ac.uk/
2. https://sites.google.com/site/compendiumofphysicalactivities/
3. http://www.parcph.org/mission.aspx

References

1. Sallis JF. Self-report measures of children's physical activity. *Journal of School Health* 1991; **61**: 215–219.
2. Corder K, Ekelund U, Steele R, Wareham N, Brage S. Assessment of physical activity in youth. *Journal of Applied Physiology* 2008; **105**: 977–987.
3. Adamo K, Prince SA, Tricco AC, Conner-Gorber S, Tremblay M. A comparison of indirect versus direct measures for assessing physical activity in the pediatric population: a systematic review. *International Journal of Pediatric Obesity* 2009; **4**: 2–27.
4. Chinapaw MJM, Mokkink LB, van Poppel MNM, van Mechelen W, Terwee CB. Physical activity questionnaires for youth: a systematic review of measurement properties. *Sports Medicine* 2010; **40**: 539–563.
5. Baquet G, Stratton G, Van Praagh E, Berthoin S. Improving physical activity assessment in prepubertal children with high-frequency accelerometry monitoring: a methodological issue. *Preventive Medicine* 2007; **44**: 143–147.
6. Kohl HW, Fulton JE, Caspersen CJ. Assessment of physical activity among children and adolescents: a review and synthesis. *Preventive Medicine* 2000; **31**: 54–76.
7. Trost SG. Measurement of physical activity in children and adolescents. *American Journal of Lifestyle Medicine* 2007; **1**: 299–314.
8. Reilly JJ, Penpraze V, Hislop J, Davies G, Grant S, Paton JY. Objective measurement of physical activity and sedentary behaviour: review with new data. *Archives of Disease in Childhood* 2008; **93**: 614–619.
9. Rowlands A. Accelerometer assessment of physical activity in children: an update. *Pediatric Exercise Science* 2007; **19**: 252–266.
10. Oliver M, Schofield G, Kolt G. Physical activity in preschoolers. Understanding prevalence and measurement issues. *Sports Medicine* 2007; **37**: 1045–1070.
11. Steele R, Brage S, Corder K, Wareham NJ, Ekelund U. Physical activity, cardiorespiratory fitness and the metabolic syndrome in youth. *Journal of Applied Physiology* 2008; **105**: 342–351.
12. Sherar LB, Griew P, Esliger DW, Cooper AR, Ekelund U, Judge K, Riddoch C. International Children's Accelerometry Database (ICAD): design and methods. *BMC Public Health* 2011; **11**: 485.
13. Ekelund U, Tomkinson G, Armstrong N. What proportion of youth are physically active? Measurement issues, levels and recent time trends. *British Journal of Sports Medicine* 2011; **45**: 859–865.
14. Corder K, Ekelund U, Steele R, Wareham N, Brage S. Assessment of physical activity in youth. *Journal of Applied Physiology* 2008; **105**: 977–987.
15. Roberts C, Tynjaka J, Komkov A. Physical activity. In: Currie C, Roberts C, Morgan A, Smith R, Settertobulte W, Samdal O, Barnekow Rasmussen V (eds) *Young People's Health in Context. Health Behaviour in School-Aged Children (HBSC) Study: International Report from the 2001–2002 Survey.* Copenhagen: World Health Organization, 2004, pp. 90–97.
16. Li S, Treuth MS, Wang Y. How active are American adolescents and have they become less active? *Obesity Reviews* 2010; **11**: 847–862.

17. Riddoch CJ, Andersen LB, Wedderkopp N, Harro M, Klasson-Heggebö L, Sardinha L, et al. Physical activity levels and patterns of 9- and 15-year-old European children. *Medicine & Science in Sports & Exercise* 2004; **36**: 86–92.

18. Nader PR, Bradley RH, Houts RM, McRitchie SL, O'Brien M. Moderate-to-vigorous physical activity from ages 9 to 15 years. *JAMA* 2008; **300**: 295–305.

19. Troiano RP, Berrigan D, Dodd KW, Mâsse LC, Tilert T, McDowell M. Physical activity in the United States measured by accelerometer. *Medicine & Science in Sports & Exercise* 2008; **40**: 181–188.

20. Riddoch CJ, Mattocks C, Deere K, Saunders J, Kirkby J, Tilling K, Leary SD, Blair SN, Ness AR. Objective measurement of levels and patterns of physical activity. *Archives of Disease in Childhood* 2007; **92**: 963–969.

21. Steele R, van Sluijs EMF, Cassidy A, Griffin SJ, Ekelund U. Targeting sedentary time or moderate- and vigorous intensity activity: independent relations with adiposity in a population-based sample of 10-y-old British children. *American Journal of Clinical Nutrition* 2009; **90**: 1185–1192.

22. Thompson AM, McHugh MC, Blanchard CM, Campagna PD, Durant MA; Rehman LA; Murphy RJL, Wadsworth LA. Physical activity in children and youth in Nova Scotia from 2001/02 and 2005/06. *Preventive Medicine* 2009; **49**: 407–409.

23. Owen CG, Nightingale CM, Rudnicka AR, Cook DG, Ekelund U, Whincup P. Ethnic and gender differences in physical activity levels among 9–10-year-old children of white European, South East Asian, and African–Caribbean origin: the Child Health Heart Study in England (CHASE). *International Journal of Epidemiology* 2009; **38**: 1082–1093.

24. Baptista F, Santos DA, Silva AM, Mota J, Santos R, Vale S, Ferreira JP, Raimundo AM, Moreira H, Sardinha LB. Prevalence of Portuguese population attaining sufficient physical activity. *Medicine and Science in Sports and Exercise* 2012; **44**: 466–473.

25. Esliger DW, Tremblay MS, Copeland JL, Barnes JD, Huntington GE, Bassett DR Jr. Physical activity profile of Old Order Amish, Mennonite, and contemporary children. *Medicine and Science in Sports and Exercise* 2010; **42**: 296–303.

26. Jimenez-Pavon D, Kelly J, Reilly JJ. Associations between objectively measured habitual physical activity and adiposity in children and adolescents: Systematic review. *International Journal of Pediatric Obesity* 2010; **5**: 3–18.

27. Sijtsma A, Sauer PJJ, Stolk RP, Corpeleijn. Is directly measured physical activity related to adiposity in preschool children? *International Journal of Pediatric Obesity* 2011; **6**: 389–400.

28. Ekelund U, Åman J, Yngve A, Renman C, Westerterp K, Sjöström M. Physical activity but not energy expenditure is reduced in obese adolescents: a case – control study. *American Journal of Clinical Nutrition* 2002; **76**: 935–941.

29. Tanner J. *Growth at Adolescence*, 2nd edn. Oxford: Blackwell Scientific, 1962.

30. Wilks DC, Besson H, Lindroos AK, Ekelund U. Objectively measured physical activity and obesity prevention in children, adolescents and adults: a systematic review of prospective studies. *Obesity Reviews* 2010; **12**: e119–e129.

31. Matthews CE, Chen KY, Freedson PS, Buchowski MS, Beech BM, Pate RR, Troiano RP. Amount of time spent in sedentary behaviours in the United States 2003–2004. *American Journal of Epidemiology* 2008; **167**: 875–881.

32. Marshall SJ, Biddle SJH, Gorely T, Cameron N, Murdey I. Relationships between media use, body fatness and physical activity in children and youth: a meta-analysis. *International Journal of Obesity* 2004; **28**: 1238–1246.

33. Rey-Lopez JP, Vicente-Rodriguez G, Biosca M, Moreno LA. Sedentary behaviour and obesity development in children and adolescents. *Nutrition Metabolism and Cardiovascular Diseases* 2008; **18**: 242–251.

34. Steele RM, van Sluijs EMF, Cassidy A, Griffin SJ, Ekelund U. Targeting sedentary time or moderate- and vigorous-intensity activity: independent relations with adiposity in a population-based sample of 10-y-old British children. *American Journal of Clinical Nutrition* 2009; **90**: 1185–1192.

35. Mitchell JA, Mattocks C, Ness AR, Leary SD, Pate RR, Dowda M, et al. Sedentary behavior and obesity in a large cohort of children. *Obesity* 2009; **17**: 1596–1602.

36. Hancox RJ, Milne BJ, Paulton R. Association between child and adolescent television viewing and adult health: a longitudinal study. *Lancet* 2004; **364**: 257–262.

37. Viner RM, Cole TJ. Television viewing in early childhood predicts adult body mass index. *Journal of Pediatrics* 2005; **147**: 429–435.

38. Epstein LH, Roemmich JN, Paluch RA, Raynor HA. Influence of changes in sedentary behavior on energy and macronutrient intake in youth. *American Journal of Clinical Nutrition* 2005; **81**: 361–366.

39. Kwon S, Janz KF, Burns TL, Levy SM. Effects of adiposity on physical activity in childhood: Iowa Bone Development Study. *Medicine and Science in Sports and Exercise* 2011; **43**: 443–448.

40. Ekelund U, Luan J, Sherar LB, Esliger DW, Griew P, Cooper A. Moderate to vigorous physical activity and sedentary time and cardiometabolic risk factors in children and adolescents. *JAMA* 2012; **307**: 704–712.

SECTION 6

Weight management in children

Chapter 6.1

Diet in the management of weight loss in childhood obesity

Laura Stewart

Perth Royal Infirmary, Perth, UK

6.1.1 Introduction

There is a recognition that the prevalence of childhood obesity increased dramatically in the early 1990s [1]. The causes of childhood obesity are, without doubt, complex and multifactorial [2]. However, there is agreement that the modern environment and lifestyle has led to chronic positive energy imbalance [3]. The term 'obesogenic environment' has been used to describe this, which denotes a setting that encourages the consumption of foods high in energy density but low in nutrients, in combination with decreased physical activity and high levels of sedentary behaviours, such as watching TV and computer use [4–7]. Management of childhood obesity therefore requires tackling both sides of the energy balance, and must address decreasing total dietary energy intake, increasing physical activity and decreasing sedentary behaviours (screen time) [8–11]. While this chapter focuses on the dietary aspects of childhood weight management, any dietary manipulation must be viewed in the context of both sides of the energy balance, along with physical activity and sedentary behaviours (screen time), which are discussed elsewhere in this book.

6.1.2 Dietary intake in children

Before considering the areas of change to be explored when managing childhood obesity, it is useful to discuss the impact of modern dietary eating patterns on excessive energy intake.

Fat and sugar intakes

There is evidence to show that the overall proportion of fat has increased over the last 50 years [6,12]. Trends show increased consumption of foods that are particularly high in fat and energy density, such as convenience foods used in the home and 'takeaway' meals [6]. High-fat foods influence the overall energy intake, as these foods are more energy dense – that is, more energy per gram of food is consumed than in the case of lower-fat foods.

The increased consumption of sugar-sweetened beverages, with their ubiquitous availability in vending machines, has also been associated with childhood obesity and the obesogenic environment [6,7,13]. Ludwig et al. [14] reported an observational prospective study in school-aged children with the odds ratio of becoming obese increasing by 1.6 for each can or glass of sugary beverages consumed. This study concluded that the baseline intake of sugary beverages and an increase in the quantity of sugary beverages consumed are both independent predictors of increases in BMI [4,12,14]. Additionally, intervention studies that have focused on reduction in the consumption of sugar-sweetened beverages have suggested that reduced consumption might be helpful in the prevention of childhood obesity [15].

There is a school of thought that TV viewing encourages an increased intake of high-sugar and high-fat energy-dense snacks by an association with eating while watching. There is a continuing worldwide debate on the influence of TV advertising of

Advanced Nutrition and Dietetics in Obesity, First Edition. Edited by Catherine Hankey.
© 2018 John Wiley & Sons Ltd. Published 2018 by John Wiley & Sons Ltd.

high-fat, high-energy snacks/fast foods and sugar-sweetened beverages on children's choices of foods [16–20].

Portion sizes

There has been a trend of increasing food portion sizes over the last few decades, particularly in foods eaten outside the home [6,7]. For example, French et al. [6] report that, in the USA, a 12-oz soft drink portion is now sold as a 'child'-sized drink, while in the 1950s this same size was considered an adult 'king' size. Bagels and muffins, which were once sold at a standard portion size of 2–3 oz, are now sold at sizes of 4–7 oz. Hill talks of a growing trend in 'super sizing' portions in fast-food restaurants [4]. French and colleagues suggest that these larger portions eaten outside of the home influence overall eating habits, as the larger portion sizes are now served and eaten when families cook at home. Indeed, as a population, there is limited awareness of what constitutes a 'normal' portion, and parents frequently underestimate the portions they give to their children [6]. Included in this tendency to larger portions is the trend of large plate sizes, and Wansink et al. have shown that there is a tendency to eat to the size of the plate and spoon; thus, larger plates and bowls lead to having larger meal sizes [21]. Work by Fisher et al. has demonstrated that offering larger portion sizes to young children can affect both their total energy intakes and their reactions to satiety [22]. They suggest that being given larger portion sizes than they can consume can override the natural satiety sensors in children as young as 2 years of age.

6.1.3 Changing childhood eating behaviour

Establishing current eating behaviours

An important first step is for the healthcare professional, as well as the child and parents, to understand current eating patterns and behaviours. The use of a lifestyle diary [23] corresponds with the behavioural change techniques recommended for use in childhood obesity [8,9] (Box 6.1.1), and is

---

Box 6.1.1   Behavioural change tools that should be utilised in childhood obesity weight management

- Stimulus control
- Self-monitoring
- Goal setting
- Non-dietary rewards for reaching goals
- Problem-solving [8,9]
- Although not strictly behavioural techniques, giving praise and encouraging parents to become role models for the desired behaviours [9]

---

effective in developing a rapport with the child and family [24,25]. Information will be exchanged over a number of sessions as a relationship and rapport is developed, enabling the health professional to hone into that individual child and family's main areas requiring exploration and advice. However, experience and good practice informs us that the health professional should particularly look for patterns around the following:

- High-fat and high-sugary snacks intake (e.g. sweets, crisps), as well as where eaten and the frequency
- Typical number of meals per day – for example, if breakfast or supper is taken on a regular basis
- Use and frequency of convenience foods at meal times
- Use and frequency of carry-out meals – for example, chip shop, Indian/Chinese, burger meals, pizza takeaways
- Use of sugar-sweetened beverages – for example, cola, sport drinks, sugary flavoured water
- Portion sizes for the child and the whole family
- Whether the child eats fruit and/or vegetables on a regular basis
- Whether food is used as a reward/treat after physical activity
- Whether visiting particular relatives or family friends (e.g. grandparents) leads to an increased intake of high-energy foods
- Whether there are particular times of the day when the child snacks more (e.g. after school, during the evening)
- Whether the child eats due to boredom or for comfort
- The types of behaviours concerning food and eating patterns that the parents are modelling to the child

Dietary advice

For an overweight or obese child to get his or her body weight under control, the child and the whole family are required to reduce their total energy intake, while at the same time ensuring a balanced intake of essential nutrients. While the aim of diet therapy is to reduce the total energy intake, energy/calorie counting *per se* is not typically used with children [26]. An earlier systematic review by Collins et al. [27] concluded that overall energy reduction was important, while no type of dietary manipulation (e.g. low carbohydrate, high protein) was particularly more effective in childhood obesity. They did find that the most frequently used 'regime' for educating families on energy restriction was the traffic light scheme, as used by Epstein and others. Traffic light regimes categorises foods into red (high in sugar and fat), amber (mainly protein and carbohydrates, with attention to portion size) and green (lower in energy, primarily fruit and vegetables) [23,27–30].

Although there are common themes in the advice given to overweight or obese children and their families, healthcare professionals should approach each child as an individual and tailor their advice for the child and his or her family's particular circumstances [9]. The meta-analysis in the Cochrane review on the treatment of childhood obesity showed that the most effective treatments were those that combined diet and lifestyle changes [11]. A systematic review by Ho et al. showed that dietary modification combined with exercise was effective in reducing metabolic risk, with particular reference to high-density-lipoprotein cholesterol and fasting insulin in the short term [31]. Therefore, the advice outlined in the following text should be given in the context of the individual child's energy balance, and delivered with the utilisation of behavioural change tools (Box 6.1.1) [8,9,11].

In childhood and adolescence, it is essential to ensure that normal height growth continues when dietary energy intake is restricted. As discussed in Chapter 1.5 in this book (titled 'Diagnostic criteria and assessment of obesity in children'), this should be done by plotting the weight, height and body mass index (BMI) on national growth charts; in the UK, BMI should be plotted on the UK 1990 data

---

Box 6.1.2 Intakes from food groups

Milk and dairy – aim to give 300 ml daily, with a maximum of 600 ml. Semi-skimmed or skimmed milk can be used. Low-fat/low-sugar yoghurts, cheese, low-fat hard cheese can be used.

Meat, fish, poultry, egg, cheese, beans and lentils – two portions should be given from this group daily; all should be grilled, boiled or baked, not fried. Low-fat meats should be used where possible.

Cereal foods – breakfast cereal, bread, rice, pasta and crackers – at least one portion should be included at each meal; avoid adding extra fat and sugar.

Vegetables and fruit – aim for five age-appropriate portions daily (only one 120 ml glass to be unsweetened fruit juice).

---

centile charts (available from Harlow Printing Ltd) [8]. A balanced diet (Box 6.1.2) should ensure age-appropriate quantities of proteins, vitamins and minerals. However, children who refuse to eat certain foods or food groups may require vitamin and/or mineral supplements such as iron, calcium or multivitamins [26].

Reducing high-energy foods and drinks

Although evidence and guidelines inform that the total energy intake must be reduced, they do not give practical advice on how this should be achieved. Therefore, this section is based around current good practices to help the children and their families to reduce the frequency and portion size of foods high in sugar and fat, and, where possible, to replace them with foods lower in energy, such as fruit and vegetables [8,10]. The general health message of 'five portions of fruit and vegetables per day' can be utilised in childhood weight management to encourage the increase use of these foods as snacks to replace high-energy-dense snacks. Although fruit and vegetables are particularly low in energy, it should be kept in mind that fruit and vegetables do have an energy value, with a small glass (120 ml) of fruit juice counting as one of the five portions of fruit and vegetables per day – for example, 120 ml of fresh orange juice gives 46 kcals. Children should be encouraged to replace the consumption of sugary drinks, including fruit juice, with plain water. In the traffic light scheme, red foods and drinks are those particularly high in sugar and fat, and the green foods are those lower in energy, such as fruit and vegetables. There is a concerted effort to guide children and their families to reduce intake of red foods and increase the consumption of green foods [23,28]. Consideration should always be given to ensuring that a balance of foods, with age-appropriate portions, is consumed daily (Box 6.1.2).

Carry-out or takeaway meals, which may be ubiquitous in family food intake, can be particularly high in sugar and fat. Therefore, the frequency of carry-out meals needs to be explored, and consideration given to finding ways to minimise consumption. Children and young people often spend their pocket money on high-energy snacks and drinks, indeed often as replacements for main meals. Thus, pocket money and the question of foods eaten outside of the home and beyond the parents' influence, including school lunchtimes, ought to be explored, and solutions discussed. For senior pupils, the pull of peer pressure to eat the same as others at lunch time can often make this a difficult area to make changes, and goals for change require to be carefully explored. Although some parents of younger children feel more 'in control' by providing a packed lunch, the quantities and types of foods included in the packed lunch still require to be explored and discussed.

Portion sizes

Discussions around family portion sizes and age-appropriate portions are exceedingly important during any childhood weight management consultation. As discussed in the preceding text, many parents and families are unaware of the size of age-appropriate portions. In many families, parents and children eat similar portion sizes. The role of the healthcare professional is often to help educate the parent and child about the correct and appropriate portions for age. In the UK, both the Caroline Walker Trust's 'Children Eating Well' (CHEW) programme and Nutrition and Diet Resources UK (NDR-UK) currently give very helpful advice in a pictorial manner on portion sizes for children of

different age groups. Using food models can also help make sessions on portion sizes more interactive. Advice can be given to parents to help them control portion size at meal times/snacks – such as using smaller plates; the parent/carer serving meals instead of letting the family members serve themselves; cooking only the required food quantity; using the simple fist or palm of the hand to estimate portions, etc.

Slimming foods and meal replacements

There is currently no evidence to support the use of special 'slimming foods' and drinks as meal replacements in children and adolescents; therefore, these are not recommended for use in this age group [8,32].

Written advice

As with all diet therapy, written information should be given to the parents/carers and children. The age of the child will determine whether the written leaflets are aimed directly at the child, the parent or both. Therefore, materials need to be age-appropriate as well as appealing to children and young people. Written information on reading food labels (e.g. British Heart Foundation) can be very helpful for families.

6.1.4 Weight maintenance

As discussed in other resources, BMI will decrease over time if the child's weight remains stable while the height continues to increase [8,9,33]. For those adolescents in the very severe BMI range (≥3.5 SD), a weight loss of around 1–2 kg per month is acceptable [8]. Data on long-term maintenance in childhood obesity remains scant; however, a study following up children who had completed treatment programmes showed that the decrease in BMI was maintained only while the family continued with regular reviews [34]. This suggests that some post-programme monitoring may be essential for maintaining family lifestyle changes and control of BMI.

6.1.5 Summary box

Key points

- Dietary advice to reduce energy intake must be provided, and implementation should be guided by negotiation to alter children's usual eating patterns.
- Meal replacement – slimming meals are not advocated for use in children to challenge excess weight gain.
- Takeaway meals must be minimised – as they are known to be high-energy sources.
- Parental involvement is essential to maximise the chance of family-based dietary changes.
- Weight maintenance is key – and evidence indicates that follow-up monitoring post intervention is justified.

Useful resources

1. Harlow Printing Ltd for UK Body Mass Index centile charts
2. British Heart Foundation: www.bhf.org.uk
3. Nutrition and Diet Resources UK: www.ndr-uk.org
4. Caroline Walker Trust CHEW resources: www.cwt-chew.org.uk

References

1. Reilly JJ, Dorosty AR. Epidemic of obesity in UK children. *The Lancet* 1999; **354**(9193): 1874–1875.
2. Foresight. Tackling obesity: future choices – project report, 2007. Government Office for Science.
3. Lobstein T, Baur L, Uauy R, for the IASO International Obesity Task Force. Obesity in children and young people: a crisis in public health. *Obesity Reviews* 2004; **5**(1, May): 4–85.
4. Hill JO, Peters JC. Environmental contributions to the obesity epidemic. *Science* 1998; **280**(5368): 1371–1374.
5. Swinburn B, Egger G. The runaway weight gain train: too many accelerators, not enough brakes. *BMJ* 2004; **329**: 736–739.
6. French SA, Story MT, Jeffery RW. Environmental influences on eating and physical activity. *Annual Review of Public Health* 2001; **22**: 309–335.
7. Swinburn B, Egger G. Preventive strategies against weight gain and obesity. *Obesity Reviews* 2002; **3**: 289–301.
8. Scottish Intercollegiate Guideline Network (SIGN). *Management of Obesity: A National Clinical Guideline*. Edinburgh: SIGN 115, 2010.
9. National Institute for Health and Clinical Excellence. Obesity guidance on the prevention, identification, assessment and management of overweight and obesity in adults and children. NICE Clinical Guidelines 43, 2006.
10. Barlow SE, Expert Committee. Expert committee recommendations regarding the prevention, assessment and treatment of child and adolescent overweight and obesity: summary report. *Pediatrics* 2007; **120**: S164–S192.
11. Luttikhuis HO, Baur L, Jansen H, Shrewsbury VA, O'Malley C, Stolk RP, et al. Interventions for treating obesity in children. *Cochrane Database of Systematic Reviews* 2008; **3**: 1–57.
12. Prentice AM, Jebb SA. Obesity in Britain: gluttony or sloth? *BMJ* 1995; **311**(7002): 437–439.
13. Whitaker RC. Obesity prevention in pediatric primary care. Four behaviors to target. *Archives of Pediatrics and Adolescent Medicine* 2003; **157**: 725–727.
14. Ludwig DS, Peterson KE, Gortmaker SL. Relation between consumption of sugar-sweetened drinks and childhood obesity: a prospective, observational study. *The Lancet* 2001; **357**: 505–508.
15. James J, Thomas P, Cavan D, Kerr D. Preventing childhood obesity by reducing consumption of carbonated drinks: cluster randomised controlled trial. *BMJ* 2004; **328**: 1237.
16. Dietz WH. The obesity epidemic in young children. *BMJ* 2001; **322**: 313–314.
17. Dietz WH, Gortmaker SL. Do we fatten our children at the television set? Obesity and television viewing in children and adolescents. *Pediatrics* 1985; **75**(5): 807–812.
18. Ludwig DS, Gortmaker SL. Programming obesity in childhood. *The Lancet* 2004; **364**: 226–227.
19. Wiecha JL, Peterson KE, Ludwig DS, Kim J, Sobol A, Gortmaker SL. When children eat what they watch: impact of television viewing on dietary intake in youth. *Archives of Pediatrics and Adolescent Medicine* 2006; **160**:436–442.
20. Lobstein T, Dibb S. Evidence of a possible link between obesogenic food advertising and child overweight. *Obesity Reviews* 2005; **6**: 203–208.
21. Wansink B, van Ittersum K, Painter JE. Ice cream illusions. Bowls, spoons and self-service portions sizes. *American Journal of Preventive Medicine* 2006; **3**: 240–243.
22. Fisher JO, Kral TVE. Super-size me: portion size effects on young children's eating. *Physiology & Behavior* 2008; **93**: 39–47.
23. Stewart L, Houghton J, Hughes AR, Pearson D, Reilly JJ. Dietetic management of pediatric overweight: development of a practical and evidence-based behavioral approach. *JADA* 2005; **105**(Nov): 1810–1815.
24. Stewart L, Chapple J, Hughes AR, Poustie V, Reilly JJ. The use of behavioural change techniques in the treatment of paediatric obesity: qualitative evaluation of parental perspectives on treatment. *JHND* 2008; **21**(5): 464–473.
25. Sahota P, Wordley J, Woodward J. Health behaviour change models and approaches for families and young people to support HEAT 3: Child Healthy Weight Programmes. Edinburgh, NHS Health Scotland: Woodburn House, 2010.
26. Stewart L. Obesity. In: Shaw V (ed) *Clinical Paediatric Dietetics*, 3rd edn. Oxford: Blackwell Publishing Ltd., 2008.
27. Collins CE, Warren J, McCoy P, Stokes BJ. Measuring effectiveness of dietetic interventions in child obesity: a systematic review of randomized trials. *Applied Physiology Nutrition and Metabolism* 2006; **160**(9): 906–922.

28. Epstein LH, Wing RR, Valoski AM. Childhood obesity. *Pediatric Clinics of North America* 1985; **32**(2): 363–379.

29. Reinehr T. Clinical presentation of type 2 diabetes mellitus in children and adolescents. *IJO* 2005; **29**: S105–S110.

30. Reinehr T, Schaefer A, Winkel K, Finne E, Toschke AM, Kolip P. An effective lifestyle intervention in overweight children: Findings from a randomized controlled trial on 'Obeldicks light'. *Clinical Nutrition* 2010; **29**: 331–336.

31. Ho M, Garnett SP, Baur L, Burrows T, Stewart L, Neve M, et al. Impact of dietary and exercise interventions on weight change and metabolic outcomes in obese children and adolescents. A systematic review and meta-analysis of randomized trials. *JAMA Pediatrics* 2013; **167**(8): 759–768.

32. Stewart L. Childhood obesity. *Medicine* 2011; **39**(1): 42–44.

33. Reinehr T. Effectiveness of lifestyle interventions in overweight children. *Proceedings of the Nutrition Society* 2011; **70**(4): 494–505.

34. Wilfey DE, Stein RI, Saelens BE, Mockus DS, Matt GE, Hayden-Wade HA, et al. Efficacy of maintenance treatment approaches for childhood overweight. *JAMA* 2007; **298**(14): 1661–1673.

Chapter 6.2

Physical activity in the management of weight loss in childhood obesity

Louise A Kelly

California Lutheran University, Thousand Oaks, CA, USA

6.2.1 Defining 'physical activity'

There is substantial evidence to support the importance of regular participation in physical activity in order to maintain health, decrease risk of chronic diseases and increase longevity. As a result, many worldwide expert panels have produced physical activity guidelines. However, the epidemiological definition of 'physical activity' still causes confusion. 'Physical activity', 'sport' and 'physical fitness' are, in fact, very distinct concepts. These have been used interchangeably in both specialist and layman's literature, adding to the confusion, and thus highlighting the need for a consensus statement on how 'physical activity' is defined. The terminology has gradually been clarified, and a broad consensus reached on how the various terms should best be defined [1–4].

As a consequence, 'physical activity' is defined as bodily movement produced by the contraction of skeletal muscles that increases energy expenditure (EE) above the basal level [1–4]. 'Exercise' is a subcategory of physical activity, which is repetitive, structured and purposive, in the sense that improved maintenance of physical fitness is an objective [1]. 'Sport' is another subset of physical activity, and involves structured physical activities in competitive situations. 'Physical fitness' is the ability to carry out daily tasks without undue fatigue, and with vigour, alertness and ample energy to enjoy leisure-time pursuits and meet unforeseen circumstances. It can be seen from these now widely accepted definitions that physical activity is a very broad construct that includes all kinds of movement, while exercise is more narrowly defined. Finally, 'sedentary behaviour' is defined as a state in which bodily movement is minimal [5]. In terms of EE, sedentary behaviour represents a state where EE approximates to the resting metabolic rate [5].

Physical activity programmes should be part of a multidisciplinary approach for the treatment of paediatric obesity. Increasing physical activity has many benefits, such as loss of fat mass (particularly visceral fat); increase in lean body mass (through fat oxidation in the skeletal muscle); increased EE; improving the metabolic profile; and improving quality of life and life expectancy. Despite its tremendous benefits, the process of increasing physical activity and maintaining the increase, particularly in the paediatric population, remains an arduous task.

6.2.2 Physical activity as a component of energy expenditure

The laws of thermodynamics dictate that the energy entering a system minus the energy leaving equals the energy stored in the system. When the laws thermodynamics are applied to humans, it means that the energy taken in as food must be expended, or the excess will be stored, largely as body fat [6].

Advanced Nutrition and Dietetics in Obesity, First Edition. Edited by Catherine Hankey.
© 2018 John Wiley & Sons Ltd. Published 2018 by John Wiley & Sons Ltd.

A mismatch in this equation between intake and expenditure results in underweight or overweight and obesity. DeLany et al. (1998) noted that obesity is the result of sustained positive energy balance, owing to increased energy intake and/or decreased total EE [7].

Three components of EE have been identified in humans: (1) basal metabolic rate (BMR), which typically represents about 60–70% of the total EE; (2) diet-induced thermogenesis (DIT), which typically represents about 10% of the energy content of food eaten [4]; and (3) the energetic cost of physical activity (PA), which accounts for the remaining 20–30% of EE in typical humans living in Western societies [4]. The latter may vary strongly, depending on the rate of voluntary activity [4]. EE during activity varies enormously during an average day, from close to BMR while at rest in bed to more than 10 times the BMR during vigorous exercise. The energy expended through physical activity is the most variable component of total EE within and between individuals [8].

6.2.3 Physical activity in children

Until recently, little was known about the physical activity levels of young children [9–11]. Most existing data have been obtained from older children/ adolescents, or from studies before the obesity epidemic. It has been argued that physical activity in young children and preschool children is typically performed in short bursts, instead of sustained periods of movement [12,13]; that is, activity patterns are intermittent in nature. Young children are thought to be spontaneously active, with frequent bouts of brief physical activity, and rapid transitions between high- and low-intensity physical activities. This physical activity is obtained through exercise play, rough and tumble play, pretend play and imaginary play [13].

Play is the most natural way for young children to be active [14]. While there is concern that the activity levels in youngsters gradually decline through the adolescent years as children are habituated to

sedentary living [14], current research suggests that young children spend a considerable amount of time engaged in sedentary behaviours [15–19]. The adult lifestyle (which probably directly influences the child) is organised in such a way as to reduce physical activity [14]. Houses contain appliances to 'make our lives easier', thus reducing our activity levels and encouraging sedentary behaviour. Children are increasingly kept indoors – at school, and at home to do homework. TV programmes are produced to capture their attention. As the number of hours spent watching TV has increased [20–22], the activity level of children has decreased, and the level of sedentary behaviour has probably increased [15,17].

Sallis et al. (2000), in an extensive review of the correlates of physical activity levels in children, evaluated 102 published studies [10], of which 54 studies were in children aged 3–12 years. Unfortunately, there were very little data on preschool-aged children. Over 80% of the studies were conducted in the USA. Of the 12 studies included in this review, five found that boys were more active than girls even at the preschool age, and the time spent outdoors resulted in higher-than-average activity levels [23]. Trost et al. (2002) also reported a rapid decline in physical activity during childhood and adolescence [24].

Furthermore, Gavarry et al. (2003), while investigating habitual physical activity during school time and free time in 82 children using heart rates and questionnaires to assess physical activity, concluded that children, irrespective of gender, were more sedentary during free days than during school, presumably because they spend more time engaging in sedentary behaviours on free days [25]. Sleap and Warburton (1996) observed that free time periods at school were associated with more intense physical activity than free time periods out of school (evenings, weekends and holidays) in 5–11 year olds in the UK [26]. However, no differences in habitual physical activity between weekdays and weekends have been observed in other samples of European preschoolers and primary one school children [27].

A few studies have reported seasonal differences in activity levels. Fulton et al. (2001) found that sedentary behaviour was higher in winter than in summer [28]. In a review by Sallis et al. (2000), the variables that were statistically and positively associated with children's physical activity consistently were sex (male), parental overweight status, physical activity preferences, intention to be active, perceived barriers (inverse), previous physical activity, healthy diet, programme/facilities access and time spent outdoors [10]. Sallis et al. (2000) suggested that additional studies were needed to confirm the findings and explore the additional factors that may influence a child's activity behaviour [10]. While investigating the factors associated with physical activity in young children, Finn et al. (2002) found that sex, history of preterm birth, childcare centre and the father's BMI were the biggest influences on the daily physical activity of young children [29]. The childcare centre was the strongest predictor of activity levels. This finding was in line with the findings of Pate et al. (2004), who, using the accelerometer, investigated the demographic factors that might be associated with physical activity in 281 US preschool children [30].

To date, a relatively small number of studies have examined the tendency of physical activity behaviour to continue from childhood to adolescence and adulthood. These studies vary considerably with respect to the length of follow-up, the population studied, the methods of assessing physical activity and the analytical method used to assess tracking [31]. Yet, despite these variations, evidence suggests that, over a relatively short interval (3–5 years), physical activity behaviour, to some extent, remains constant over time [32]. Data from several longitudinal studies indicate that youth at the extremes of the physical activity distribution (i.e. those with the lowest and highest levels of physical activity) tend to retain their ranking with respect to physical activity over time [33,19]. In a review article on the tracking of physical activity, Malina (1996) reported low to moderate tracking of participation in physical activity and sports from childhood into adulthood [34]. Despite this extensive review, the age span of the participants in the ranking studies were diverse, with ages ranging from 3 years [33] to 23 years [35].

6.2.4 Physical activity and exercise recommendations

No evidence-based guidelines currently exist for the levels of physical activity necessary to reduce overweight or obesity in children. However, published guidelines from the Centers for Disease Control and Prevention (CDC) and the American College of Sports Medicine (ACSM) do exist. These guidelines suggest that children older than 6 years of age should engage in 60 min or more of aerobic exercise of moderate intensity each day of the week, and vigorous-intensity activity on at least 3 days in a week. Activities to increase muscular strength (e.g. push-ups or gymnastics) and bone strength (e.g. running, jumping rope) are recommended at least 3 days a week as part of the child's 60+ minutes of activity [36,37].

Levels of obesity vary greatly in children, as do the levels of adiposity, distribution of body fat, duration of obesity, previous levels of physical activity, fitness, motor skills, muscular strength, complications and comorbidities. Therefore, each child should be treated on an individual basis. Most typical 'weight management' programmes for youth use energy-restrictive diets, behaviour modification techniques, physical activity and/or drugs, but these approaches have generally not been successful.

With regards to aerobic exercise, a general rule of thumb is to engage the overweight/obese child in aerobic exercise at intensities lower than 60% of maximum heart rate, or VO_2 max, for at least 30 min, repeated at a frequency of 3 days/week. At this intensity and duration, the aim is to avoid stimulating appetite or inducing conflicting post-exercise rest. The modality of exercise is trivial; at this dose and duration of exercise, the modalities are comparable, and it is the depletion of fat stores that is important [38].

There are very few clinical research studies that have demonstrated the efficacy of specific interventions for improving obesity status in children. A number of physical activity initiatives (with and without dietary changes) have been used to treat obesity in boys and girls by increasing EE to support weight loss [39–41]. However, even the most intensive aerobic exercise interventions have led to only small reductions in body fat, with uncertain impact on metabolic risk [42,43].

Evidence from adults suggests that incorporation of strength training may be important for improving body composition (increased muscle mass and decreased fat mass) and fat redistribution (reduced visceral fat and intramuscular lipid) [44–47]. Strength training has also been shown to improve insulin sensitivity and glucose regulation in adults with impaired glucose tolerance or type 2 diabetes [48–50]. However, further studies are needed to identify whether these effects are mediated through changes in body composition or other mechanisms. Several organisations have recently endorsed resistance training as a safe activity for children and adolescents as a means of improving strength and decreasing risk of sports-related injuries, provided appropriate supervision and instruction are given [51,52]. However, to date, most resistance training studies in younger populations have focused on safety, strength improvements and musculature changes [53,54]. One prior study examined a 6-week program that combined a dietary intervention (low energy, 20–25% energy from fat, high in complex carbohydrate) with strength training in obese children, and showed a 6% improvement in cholesterol [55]. Treuth et al. conducted a resistance training trial with 12 overweight Caucasian girls, and showed that resistance training (20-min sessions, 3 days/week for 5 months) led to increased strength and improvement in visceral fat. Small improvements in glucose tolerance and insulin levels (determined using an oral glucose tolerance test) were noted, but these changes did not achieve statistical significance [56,44]. However, the small sample sizes in these studies are a limitation of these findings.

Whatever the physical activity/exercise chosen, programmes need to progress slowly, preceded and followed by gradual warm-up and cool-down periods, respectively. Fun, enthusiastic leadership, group activities, and parental support and participation are strong motivating factors in children, and should be incorporated into every exercise programme [57]. Individual exercises and sports events must be chosen carefully to avoid overweight/obese children feeling unable to complete the activity, and the subsequent failure, increases the likelihood of them giving up the programme.

6.2.5 Summary box

Key points

- *Physical activity* is defined as bodily movement that increases energy expenditure (EE) above the basal level. *Exercise* is a subcategory of physical activity, and is repetitive, structured and purposive.
- Currently, 60 min or more of daily aerobic exercise of moderate intensity and vigorous-intensity activity on at least 3 days in a week is advocated for children above 6 years of age.
- Activities to increase muscular strength (e.g. push-ups or gymnastics) and bone strength (e.g. running, jumping rope) are recommended for at least 3 days a week as part of a child's 60+ min of activity.
- Interventions should not increase appetite; also, periods of sedentary rest should not be advocated post activity.
- Providing motivation to children who follow carefully planned exercise regimes is essential for maximising the chances of these being sustained.
- Most intensive aerobic exercise interventions have achieved only small reductions in body fat, with an uncertain impact on metabolic risk.

References

1. Casperson CJ, Powell KE, Christenson GM. Physical activity, exercise, and physical fitness: definitions and distinctions for health-related research. *Public Health Reports* 1985; **100**: 126–131.
2. Casperson CJ. Physical activity epidemiology: concepts, methods, and applications to exercise science. *Exercise and Sport Sciences Reviews* 1989; **17**: 423–473.
3. Casperson CJ, Nixon PA, DuRant RH. Physical activity epidemiology applied to children and adolescents. *Exercise and Sport Sciences Reviews* 1998; **26**: 341–403.
4. Powers SK, Howley ET. *Exercise Physiology: Theory and Applications to Fitness and Performance*. Dubuque, IA: Wm. C. Brown, 1990.
5. Dietz WH. The role of lifestyle in health: the epidemiology and consequences of inactivity. *Proceedings of the Nutrition Society* 1996; **55**: 829–840.
6. Rowland TW. Obesity and physical activity. *Exercise and Children's Health*. Champaign, IL, England: Human Kinetics, 1990.
7. DeLany JP. Roles of energy expenditure in the development of pediatric obesity. *American Journal of Clinical Nutrition* 1998; **68**: S950–S955.

8. Goran MI, Carpenter WH, Poehlman ET. Total energy expenditure in 4 to 6-yr-old children. *American Journal of Physiology, Endocrinology and Metabolism* 1993; **264**(5 Pt 1): E706–E711.
9. Kohl HW, Hobbs KE. Development of physical activity behaviors among children and adolescents. *Pediatrics* 1998; **101**: 549.
10. Sallis JF, Prochaska JJ, Taylor WC. A review of correlates of physical activity of children and adolescents. *Medicine and Science in Sports and Exercise* 2000; **32**: 963–975.
11. Livingstone MBE, McKinley MC, Robson PJ, Wallace JMW. How active are we? Levels of routine physical activity in children and adults. *Proceedings of the Nutrition Society* 2003; **62**: 681–701.
12. Bailey R, Olson J, Pepper S, Proszasz J, Barstow T, Cooper D. The level and tempo of children's physical activities: an observational study. *Medicine and Science in Sports and Exercise* 1995; **27**: 1033–1041.
13. Pellegrini AD, Smith PK. Physical activity play: the nature and function of a neglected aspect of play. *Child Development* 1998; **69**: 577–598.
14. Riddoch CJ, Boreham AG. The health related physical activity of children. *Sports Medicine* 1995; **19**: 86–102.
15. Reilly JJ, Jackson DM, Montgomery C, Kelly LA, Slater C, Grant S, et al. Levels of total energy expenditure and physical activity in modern children. *Lancet* 2004; **363**: 211–212.
16. Montgomery C, Reilly JJ, Jackson DM, Kelly LA, Slater C, Paton JY, et al. Relation between physical activity and energy expenditure in a representative sample of young children. *American Journal of Clinical Nutrition* 2004; **80**: 591–596.
17. Chinapaw M, Altenburg T, Brug J. Sedentary behaviour and health in children – evaluating the evidence. *Preventive Medicine* 2015; **70**: 1–2.
18. Kelly LA, Reilly JJ, Fisher A, Montgomery C, Williamson A, McColl JH, et al. Effect of socio-economic status on objectively measured physical activity. *Archives of Disease in Childhood* 2006; **9**: 35–38.
19. Kelly LA, Reilly JJ, Jackson DM, Montgomery CS, Grant JY Paton. Tracking of physical activity and sedentary behavior in young children. *Pediatric Exercise Science* 2007; **19**: 51–60.
20. Durant RH, Baranowski T, Johnson M, Thompson WO. Relationship among television watching, physical activity, and body composition of young children. *Pediatrics* 1994; **94**: 449–455.
21. Gortmaker SL, Must A, Sobol AM, Peterson K, Colditz GA, Dietz WH. Television viewing as a cause of increasing obesity among children in the United States. *Archives of Pediatrics and Adolescent Medicine* 1996; **150**: 356–362.
22. Reilly JJ, Dick S, McNeill G, Tremblay MS. Results from Scotland's 2013 report card on physical activity for children and youth. *Journal of Physical Activity and Health* 2014; **11**(1): S93–S97.
23. Pate RR, Pratt M, Blair SN, Haskell WL, Macera CA, et al. Physical activity and health. A recommendation from the Centers for Disease Control and Prevention and the American College of Sports Medicine. *JAMA* 1995; **273**: 402–407.
24. Trost SG, Pate RR, Sallis SF, Freedson PS, Taylor WC, Dowda M, et al. Age and gender differences in objectively measured physical activity in youth. *Medicine & Science in Sports & Exercise* 2002; **34**: 350–355.
25. Gavarry O, Giacomoni M, Bernard T, Seymat M, Falgairette G. Habitual physical activity in children and adolescents during school and free days. *Medicine & Science in Sports & Exercise* 2003; **35**: 525–531.
26. Sleap M, Warburton P. Physical activity levels of 5–11-year-old children in England: cumulative evidence from three direct observations studies. *International Journal of Sports Medicine* 1996; **17**: 248–253.
27. Jackson D, Reilly JJ, Kelly LA, Montgomery C, Grant S, Paton JY. Objectively measured physical activity and inactivity in 3–4 year olds. *Obesity Research* 2003; **11**: 420–425.
28. Fulton JE, McGuire MT, Caspersen CJ, Dietz WH. Interventions for weight loss and weight gain prevention among youth: current issues. *Sports Medicine* 2001; **31**(3): 153–165.
29. Finn K, Johannsen N, Specker B. Factors associated with physical activity in preschool children. *Journal of Pediatrics* 2002; **140**: 81–85.
30. Pate RR, Pfeiffer KA, Trost SG, Ziegler P, Dowda M. Physical activity among children attending preschools. *Pediatrics* 2004; **114**(5, Nov): 1258–1263.
31. Pate RR, Dowda M, O'Neill JR, Ward DS. Change in physical activity participation among adolescent girls from 8th to 12th grade. *Journal of Physical Activity and Health* 2007; **4**(1): 3–16.
32. Sallis JF, Berry CC, Broyles SL, McKenzie TL, Nader PR. Variability and tracking of physical activity over 2 yr in young children. *Medicine & Science in Sports & Exercise* 1995; **27**: 1049.
33. Raitakari, OT, Prkka, KVK, Taimela S, Telama R, Räsänen L, Viíkarí JSA. Effects of persistent physical activity and inactivity on coronary risk factors in children and young adults the cardiovascular risk in Young Finns. *American Journal of Epidemiology* 1994; **140**: 195–205.
34. Malina, R. Tracking of physical activity and physical fitness across a lifespan. *Research Quarterly for Exercise and Sport* 1996; **67**: 48–57.
35. Kuh DH, Cooper C. Physical activity at 36 years: patterns and childhood predictors in a longitudinal study. *Journal of Epidemiology and Community Health* 1992;**46**:114–119.
36. Centres for disease control. Health United States for Young Adults, 2008. Available from: http://www.cdc.gov/nchs/data/hus/hus08.pdf, accessed October 2016.
37. U.S. Department of Health and Human Services (DHHS). Physical Activity Guidelines for Americans, 2008. Washington, DC: U.S. Government Printing Office, 2008.
38. Ainsworth BE, Haskell WI, Leon AS, Jacobs DR, Montoye HJ, Sallis JF, et al. Compendium of physical activities: classification of exercise costs of human physical activities. *Medicine & Science in Sports & Exercise* 1993; **25**: 71–80.
39. Becque MD, Katch VL, Rocchini AP, Marks CR, Moorehead C. Coronary risk incidence of obese adolescents: reduction by exercise plus diet intervention. *Pediatrics* 1988; **81**: 605–612.
40. Epstein LM, Wing RR, Penner BC, Kress MJ. Effect of diet and controlled exercise on weight loss in obese children. *Journal of Pediatrics* 1985; **107**: 358–361.
41. Epstein LM, Wing RR, Koeske R, Ossip DJ, Beck S. A comparison of lifestyle change and programmed aerobic exercise on weight and fitness changes in obese children. *Behavior Therapy* 1982; **13**: 651–665.

42. Gutin B, Barbeau P, Owens S, Lemmon CR, Bauman M, Allison J, et al. Effects of exercise intensity on cardiovascular fitness, total body composition, and visceral adiposity of obese adolescents. *American Journal of Clinical Nutrition* 2002; **75**: 818–826.

43. Gutin B, Owens S, Okuyama T, Riggs S, Ferguson M, Litaker M. Effect of physical training and its cessation on percent fat and bone density of children with obesity. *Obesity Research* 1999; **7**: 208–214.

44. Treuth MS, Hunter GR, Kekes-SzaboT, Weinsier RL, Goran MI, Berland L. Reduction in intra-abdominal adipose tissue after strength training in older women. *Journal of Applied Physiology* 1995; **78**: 1425–1431.

45. Ryan AS, Pratley RE, Elahi D, Goldberg AP. Resistive training increases fat-free mass and maintains RMR despite weight loss in postmenopausal women. *Journal of Applied Physiology* 1995; **79**: 818–823.

46. Campbell WW, Crim MC, Young VR, Evans WJ. Increased energy requirements and changes in body composition with resistance training in older adults. *American Journal of Clinical Nutrition* 1994; **60**: 167–175.

47. Campbell WW, Crim MC, Young VR, Joseph U, Evans WJ. Effects of resistance training and dietary protein intake on protein metabolism in older adults. *American Journal of Physiology, Endocrinology and Metabolism* 1995; **268**: E1143–E1153.

48. Smutok MA, Kokkinos PF, Farmer C, Dawson P, Shulman R, DeVane-Bell J, et al. Aerobic versus strength training for risk factor intervention in middle-aged men at high risk for coronary heart disease. *Metabolism* 1993; **42**: 177–184.

49. Cuff DJ, Meneilly GS, Martin A, Ignaszewski A, Tildesley HD, Frohlich JJ. Effective exercise modality to reduce insulin resistance in women with type 2 diabetes. *Diabetes Care* 2003; **26**: 2977–2982.

50. Dunstan DW, Daly RM, Owen N, Jolley D, De Courten M, Shaw J, et al. High-intensity resistance training improves glycemic control in older patients with type 2 diabetes. *Diabetes Care* 2002; **25**: 1729–1736.

51. American Academy of Pediatrics. Strength training by children and adolescents. 2001. Available from: http://pediatrics.aappublications.org/content/pediatrics/107/6/1470.full.pdf, accessed October 2016.

52. Faigenbaum AD, Kraemer WJ, Cahill B, Chandler J, Dziados J, Elfrink LD, et al. Youth resistance training: position statement paper and literature review. *Journal of Strength and Conditioning Research* 1996; **18**: 62–76.

53. Faigenbaum A, Westcott W, Loud R, Long C. The effects of different resistance training protocols on muscular strength and endurance development in children. *Pediatrics* 1999; **104**: 97.

54. Faigenbaum AD, Loud RL, O'Connell J, Glover S, O'Connell J, Westcott WL. Effects of different resistance training protocols on upper-body strength and endurance development in children. *Journal of Strength and Conditioning Research* 2001; **15**: 459–465.

55. Sung RY, Yu CW, Chang SK, Mo SW, Woo KS, Lam CW. Effects of dietary intervention and strength training on blood lipid level in obese children. *Archives of Disease in Childhood* 2002; **86**: 407–410.

56. Treuth MS, Ryan RE, Pratley RE, Rubin MA, Miller JP, Nicklas BJ, et al. Effects of strength training on total and regional body composition in older men. *Journal of Applied Physiology* 1994; **77**: 614–620.

57. Jopling RR. Health-related fitness as preventive medicine. *Pediatrics in Review* 1988; **10**: 141–148.

Chapter 6.3

Psychological and behavioural interventions in childhood obesity

Helen Croker
University College London, London, UK

6.3.1 Background

Many studies have now reported the outcomes from psychological interventions, and, outcomes from randomised controlled trials (RCTs) have been increasingly reported in recent years. For the purposes of this chapter, studies including any behaviour change strategies or with any psychological theory underpinning the intervention will be considered as 'psychological'. These types of interventions are also referred to as 'behavioural', a broad term including interventions based on a defined psychological theory or approach, as well as those using behaviour change strategies in a less structured way. Although such approaches are now the accepted norm for treatment, historically, weight management interventions focused on restricting energy intake, with support for behaviour change only emerging in the 1970s. Early behavioural treatments for obese children tended to target the child directly (often being school-based), with little acknowledgement of the importance of the family. Unsurprisingly, these had limited success, which led to the development of treatments that involved the family to facilitate child behaviour change. These early family-based treatments used behavioural therapy (BT) or cognitive-behavioural therapy (CBT) and achieved better outcomes than the child-directed approaches [1] (see the following text for definitions). These two approaches have remained the mainstay of treatment for many years, although more recent developments propose an even stronger family focus [2].

Systematic reviews of behavioural interventions

Systematic reviews of RCTs have typically found significant but modest benefits for children participating in lifestyle/behavioural treatments as compared to those receiving no or minimal input [3–5]. For example, meta-analyses have revealed body mass index standard deviation score (BMI-SDS) differences of −0.06 [4] and −0.10 [3] in favour of treatment. However, due to the heterogeneous nature of interventions, these reviews provide only limited information regarding the relative effectiveness of different approaches. Other reviews have attempted to unpick whether particular aspects of treatment confer greater success, but the only consistent findings have been that outcomes tend to be better when targeting the family [6] and using multi-component approaches [7]. One review attempted to deconstruct the specific behaviour change techniques used in treatment and found hints that the following could be helpful: personalised feedback about consequences of not changing; environmental restructuring; encouraging the family to practice behaviour changes; encouraging the child to role-model new behaviours; supporting the management of emotional triggers; and teaching general communication skills (e.g. assertiveness) [8]. However, this

Advanced Nutrition and Dietetics in Obesity, First Edition. Edited by Catherine Hankey.
© 2018 John Wiley & Sons Ltd. Published 2018 by John Wiley & Sons Ltd.

was not quantitatively examined and included only a limited number of studies. Another review of primary care interventions found that effective treatments often included techniques for motivational enhancement [9].

Clinical guidelines of behavioural interventions

The findings from systematic reviews are reflected in the clinical guidelines published in a number of countries. All have recommended that interventions be family based, and most promote the use of behavioural modification strategies [10–12]. The US guidelines additionally recommend a stepped-care approach, and advise that motivational interviewing (MI) approaches may be useful [12]. The guidelines have also made recommendations for appropriate dietary and activity changes, and these are covered in the other chapters.

As suggested in the preceding text, psychological treatments typically fall under the umbrella terms 'behavioural' or 'lifestyle', and since they are commonly examined together in reviews, evaluating the effects of different treatment approaches is difficult. The remainder of this chapter will look in more detail at some of the more commonly used approaches and their outcomes. The studies will be confined to RCTs, and will focus on contemporary studies where possible.

6.3.2 Treatment approaches of psychological interventions

A number of psychological interventions have been described, and these are typically delivered in outpatient and community settings. The characteristics of participating children vary (e.g. age and level of overweight), and studies have used a number of different formats (e.g. group vs. one-to-one, differing levels of parental involvement) and varying psychological approaches. Psychological interventions most commonly use the therapeutic approaches BT and CBT, with solution-focused therapy (SFT) and parenting programmes more recently evaluated. While some studies have used such defined therapeu-

tic approaches, others have used behaviour change strategies drawn from models of behaviour change (informed by health psychology) and/or used behavioural strategies from psychological approaches in a less structured way, and some have combined approaches.

Specific psychological approaches and models of behaviour change used to inform childhood obesity interventions include:

Behavioural therapy: This is designed to change children's eating and activity behaviours by providing training for children and parents in behavioural methods [13]. It is based on learning theory, which proposes that, since behaviours are learnt, they can also be 'unlearnt', and treatment aims to shape obesity-related behaviours in order to change energy balance. Strategies include self-monitoring, stimulus control and contractual reinforcement.

CBT: This is based on the theory that a problem (i.e. obesity) is maintained by dysfunctional or 'unhelpful' thoughts and beliefs [14]. CBT uses techniques from BT as well as cognitive strategies aiming to identify and restructure unhelpful thoughts.

Solution-Focused Therapy: The focus is to identify solutions rather than problems [15]. It is a collaborative counselling approach which assumes that clients are experts in solving their problems and have the resources to change, so can be supported to find solutions.

Parenting programmes: The 'Triple P' parenting programme is typically used, and is commonly cited as based on child development theory [17]. It is based on a generic parenting programme and aims to help parents better manage their child's behaviour in relation to weight [16,17].

Social cognitive theory (SCT): Interventions based on this theory aim to increase participants' self-efficacy (confidence in one's ability to carry out the behaviour in question) and address barriers to change [18].

The key strategies taught in behavioural and parenting interventions are briefly outlined in Table 6.3.1; they have been described in detail elsewhere [13,19].

Table 6.3.1 Brief description of behavioural and parenting strategies commonly used in psychologically based programmes

Behavioural strategies	
Self-monitoring	Self-monitoring is a key component in BT, and is essential for setting goals, assessing progress with goals and providing feedback, and rewarding successful goal attainment. Additionally, it can itself result in behaviour change (at least in the short term). Self-monitoring can be about a number of behaviours (e.g. eating and activity) or weight.
Goal setting	Behaviour changes are typically planned using goals, and generally goals are introduced gradually, one behaviour at a time. The acronym 'SMART' (which stands for *s*pecific, *m*easureable, *a*chievable, *r*elevant and *t*ime-limited) is often used to teach the concept of setting specific goals that have the greatest likelihood of being achieved.
Contracting	Families are encouraged to choose appropriate rewards for goal attainment (e.g. non-food and inexpensive). Parents must be in agreement with reward choices, and, for maximum effect, the rewards should be given soon after the goals are achieved. Rewards can include a family activity or time with a parent, which can also improve family relationships.
Stimulus control	This aims to create environments that encourage healthy eating and activity behaviours, and includes reducing triggers for unhealthy behaviours and increasing triggers for healthy behaviours. Examples of reducing triggers for unhealthy eating include not bringing 'unhealthy' foods into the house, and avoiding serving food at the table to reduce the likelihood of having second helpings; for inactivity, examples of reducing triggers include limiting access to computer games, and removing TVs from children's bedrooms. Examples of increasing triggers for healthy eating include having a fruit bowl, and bringing healthy foods into the house; for physical activity, examples of increasing triggers include having clothes and equipment for activity accessible, and establishing routines that incorporate activity (e.g. an after-school club, family walks, and walking or cycling to school).
Relapse prevention	These are strategies for preventing lapses in newly instigated behaviours. Examples include problem-solving, so that families can deal with new challenging situations that arise, and planning ahead for potentially difficult situations (e.g. holidays, Christmas, routine changing). Families can also continue some form of monitoring and, if lapses occur, behaviour changes made in treatment can be reintroduced.
Parenting strategies	
Praise	Parents are instructed in giving praise effectively; this includes being consistent, specific and giving it immediately after the child's behaviour is observed.
Modelling of positive behaviours	Parents are often asked to follow the dietary and activity guidelines in a programme themselves, and are given guidance about the importance of setting a good example to their child.
Other	Consistency, being observant of child behaviour (so that rewards and praise can be used effectively) and limit setting (i.e. saying 'no') can also be useful.

6.3.3 Evidence review

Behavioural therapy

BT is the most extensively evaluated treatment for childhood obesity, and the most widely cited intervention is Len Epstein's 'family-based behavioural treatment' (FBBT) [4]. Epstein's programme has achieved substantial reductions in adiposity, significantly greater than in a control group, but trial evidence is limited [20]. Other evaluations of this treatment have shown significant reductions in children's adiposity over treatment [21], although comparisons with control groups have produced inconsistent results; positive treatment effects have been seen in some studies [22] but not others [21]. Other BT interventions have also achieved significant reductions in adiposity for those undertaking treatment, which have typically been greater than experienced by control groups [23,24]. Studies comparing BT delivered to parents vs. parents and children have shown little difference in outcomes [24]. BT also has the potential to be delivered online, with one study in adolescents showing a greater reduction in body fat over 6 months as compared to a simple education programme [25]. Children undergoing treatment tend to experience reductions in adiposity. Absolute adiposity changes are not always reported, but have been in the order of approximately −0.1 BMI-SDS [21,24] and −0.7 BMI [22] for those attending treatment.

BT is typically delivered over 4–6 months, and most often to 8–12-year-olds [21,22], although programmes sometimes include wider age ranges [24]. Participating children's average adiposity has varied from approximately 2 BMI-SDS [24] to 3 BMI-SDS [21]. They are typically delivered in group formats and target both children and parents, although they may be seen separately [20]. Although older studies have tended to report limited demographic data, more contemporary studies appear to indicate that these programmes are acceptable to families from a range of ethnic and socioeconomic backgrounds [21,23].

Cognitive behavioural therapy

CBT has also produced significant reductions in children's adiposity, and while evidence from RCTs is not conclusive, studies have tended to find benefits for those in treatment as compared to control groups. This has been observed in children [26,27] and adolescents [14]. Other trials have compared CBT delivered to parents vs. parents and children; results varied, with one finding a greater reduction in children's level of overweight when treatment was delivered to parents alone [28], and others finding no group differences [29]. Where reported, absolute adiposity changes for children and adolescents participating in treatment has varied from −1.3 BMI [14] to −2.1 BMI [26].

CBT treatments are usually delivered over 4–6 months to children/adolescents and parents (although they may be seen separately), and most use group formats (although individual formats too have been used) [14]. They have typically targeted children aged 8–12 years, or adolescents [14], and their level of overweight has varied. Although often poorly

reported, the ethnicity and socioeconomic status of families appear to be varied, with treatments seemingly acceptable to families from a range of backgrounds. In fact, in one study, outcomes were better in families of lower socioeconomic status [27].

Solution-Focused Therapy

SFT is a less established treatment, but there is some evidence to support its use. Significant benefits have been shown in those receiving treatment, as compared to controls, [30] although this is not a universal result [31]. Interventions incorporating this approach also appear to be more effective than physical activity interventions [32]. BMI-SDS changes over 6 months of up to −0.3 have been observed for those in treatment [30,32], although studies of less intensive interventions have shown minimal change [31]. These trials have typically included children aged 12 years or younger with 'moderate' obesity (BMI-SDS ≤ 2, approximately). The formats and targets have varied; most have targeted parents and children, although some have included parents alone [32]. Some were delivered in groups [30], and others to families individually [31]. The socioeconomic status of samples in the trials discussed here appears mixed [31], although samples have been predominantly white where ethnicity has been reported [30].

Parenting programmes

Another more recent development in treating childhood obesity is the use of parenting programmes, and children tend to experience significant reductions in the level of overweight across treatment. Results from RCTs have been mixed, however, with studies showing significant [16] and non-significant [17] differences between treatment and control groups. It is not clear whether this approach is more effective with additional 'lifestyle skills training' [17]. Where reported, absolute change over treatment lasting 6–12 months has been in the order of −0.25 BMI-SDS [17]. These approaches tended to target younger children (4–11 years of age) with BMI-SDS < 3; treatments are typically delivered in groups and attended by parents only [16,17]. Samples have generally been predominantly white, and tended to be of above-average socioeconomic status.

Programmes using other models of behaviour change or behavioural strategies less formally

Some interventions are based on other models of behaviour change drawn from health psychology or have used some behavioural techniques. RCTs indicate that such interventions can achieve significant reductions in adiposity, with greater reductions seen with treatment as compared to controls comprising waiting list [33] or self-help [34] in some studies, but no differences in other studies [35]. All of these studies used some of the behavioural techniques from BT and CBT (e.g. goal setting, self-monitoring, stimulus control, and appropriate use of rewards; see Table 6.3.1). Studies have also used SCT to inform interventions [33]. It is difficult to judge how the techniques in these types of studies have been delivered, since they have not been guided by a specific treatment format, although one of the studies included an independent evaluation of the delivery of the behavioural techniques and found that the dietitians carrying out treatment were highly skilled, indicating that the techniques were correctly implemented [35]. The absolute levels of BMI-SDS changes observed with treatment varies, ranging between approximately −0.1 [35], −0.16 [34] and −0.3 [33] over 6 months.

Most treatments have been delivered to both parents and children in groups, an exception being a treatment delivered on an individual basis [35]. Typically, children have been aged 7–12 years [33], although some studies included older [34] or younger children [35]. Children have tended to be overweight [34] or moderately obese, with an average BMI-SDS of 2–3 [33]; a notable exception was a study in which the average BMI-SDS was 3.2 [35]. Families' ethnicity and socioeconomic status have tended to be more diverse than other treatments, with several of the studies including a sizeable proportion of children from low socioeconomic status or non-white families [33–35].

Novel approaches

Results have varied, but promising approaches include BT with additional self-regulation training (a portable weighing scale, on which the child's plate is placed during mealtimes, generating 'real-time' feedback about the eating rate) [36]; MI [37]; CBT with 'peer-enhanced adventure therapy' (comprising group activities to develop social and problem-solving skills and increase self-confidence) [38]; and 'multi-systemic therapy' [39]. The latter targeted the systems in which adolescents with serious problems are embedded. It integrates cognitive and behavioural weight loss strategies with measures to address family, peer and school factors. These approaches have tended to target older children and adolescents, although the MI intervention targets children aged 2–6 years.

Longer-term outcomes

Most trials that have reported longer-term adiposity outcomes have observed good maintenance effects at 3–18-month follow-up. However, since few trials with no input or usual care control groups have reported follow-up outcomes, it is difficult to judge longer-term treatment efficacy. Trials have reported differing outcomes, with some finding better adiposity outcomes at follow-up in treatment vs. control groups [24,26], and others finding no difference [22,25,35].

Other outcomes

Families experience many benefits from participating in treatment, in addition to adiposity reduction. For example, a systematic review demonstrated benefits for lipid profile, fasting insulin and blood pressure for children participating in 'lifestyle' treatments as compared to no- or minimal-input interventions [3]. For other outcomes, improvements have been demonstrated, but achieving significant group differences is more difficult. For example, studies have found improved child behaviours, but significant group differences were only observed in some trials for physical activity [33,35,37] and diet [14]. Likewise, for parenting skills, studies often find improvements, but group differences are rare [16]. For child psychosocial outcomes, quality of life and self-esteem are most commonly reported, and a review concluded that improvements have typically been seen [40]. However, it is less clear whether treatment groups experience greater benefits than control groups, with only a limited number of studies finding significant between-group differences for quality of life [22] or self-esteem [33]. Eating disorder symptoms are rarely reported in RCTs, and these have tended to find no change or improvements [21,27], but a few have shown significant between-group differences [27].

6.3.4 Conclusion

The most commonly evaluated psychologically based programmes are BT and CBT delivered in outpatient or community settings. These can bring substantial adiposity reductions over treatment and follow-up, but there have been fewer well-reported RCTs. Despite this, the literature points to children in intervention groups experiencing significantly greater reductions in adiposity as compared to control groups, especially for BT. These programmes typically target moderately or substantially obese children and appear acceptable to children from low as well as high socioeconomic status. Less formalised BT and CBT, generally delivered by less specialised practitioners, also seem to bring about reductions in adiposity over treatment and relatively short-term follow-up, although long-term trial data are lacking. These typically target overweight or modestly obese children, and appear equally acceptable to low- and high-socioeconomic-status families. In fact, these treatments appear to have been studied in more diverse groups than other approaches. There is preliminary evidence that BT can be delivered online, but these appear less effective over the long term, and more work is needed to improve outcomes. These may offer an alternative approach for older children and adolescents (who may be more difficult to engage in treatment).

There are a number of newer approaches being evaluated. SFT and parenting programmes have achieved significant reductions in children's adiposity across treatments, but data regarding treatment effectiveness in comparison with control groups are inconclusive, and there are limited trial data over the longer term. These data therefore only provide preliminary evidence of efficacy.

Such programmes have typically targeted modestly obese children (and younger and overweight children in the case of parenting programmes), and samples have been of mixed socioeconomic status, but predominantly white. A number of other more novel treatment approaches have been evaluated, including those based on self-regulation, peer-based activity, tackling the systems in which young people live, and motivational interviewing. More work is needed to test these thoroughly (especially in more diverse populations), but they offer promising alternative approaches, especially for older children and adolescents.

RCTs focus on reporting group differences after treatment, but the magnitude of adiposity change for those attending treatment has also been discussed in this chapter. Some investigators have reported that BMI-SDS changes of at least −0.25 are required for a clinically significant impact [41]. It is clear that many of the studies discussed here do not achieve this level of change, although improvements in health and psychosocial outcomes have been observed with even modest adiposity change.

A lack of trial data has been problematic in making treatment recommendations, but it is clear that RCT outcomes have been increasingly reported in recent years. There are several problems with the literature as a whole. The Cochrane review noted that studies were often underpowered, did not report power calculations and did not carry out intention-to-treat (ITT) analyses – the latter potentially resulting in overestimation of treatment effects [4]. Despite the increase in RCTs published, many have not reported ITT analyses. Even when they have reported ITT analyses, these have often only included children who attended follow-up. Other problems include the use of differing measures of child adiposity (although contemporary trials tend to report BMI-SDS outcomes) and the plethora of comparison groups (e.g. waiting list control, usual care, different types of treatment, treatment target), making it difficult to draw conclusions about treatment efficacy and relative treatment effectiveness. Questions remain over the optimum treatment content, length and intensity of treatment (although 6 months is typically considered the minimum required to instil sustainable behaviour change), treatment format (groups vs. individual) and the target of treatment (parents vs. children vs. parents and children), but it is clear that parental involvement is essential. A review of systematic reviews of interventions found that they provided limited information of use for clinical practice, thus limiting the application of evidence [42]. The reporting of ethnicity and socioeconomic status data has been poor in the past, but is improving. Future studies should ensure clarity and should also seek to include families from diverse backgrounds.

6.3.5 Summary box

Key points

- The most commonly evaluated psychologically based programmes are BT and CBT, delivered in outpatient or community settings.
- Programmes can bring substantial adiposity reductions over treatment and follow-up, but there have been a few well-reported RCTs with successful outcomes.
- Moderately or substantially obese children of low as well as high socioeconomic status have participated in these programmes.
- Less formalised BT and CBT seem to bring about reductions in adiposity over treatment and relatively short-term follow-up, although long-term trial data are lacking.
- There is preliminary evidence that BT can be delivered online, but these appear less effective over the long term, although more work is needed to improve outcomes.
- Several novel treatment approaches have been evaluated, including those based on self-regulation, peer-based activity, motivational interviewing and tackling the systems in which young people live. More work is needed to test these thoroughly, but they do offer promising alternative approaches, especially for older children and adolescents.
- Some investigators have reported that BMI-SDS changes of at least −0.25 are required for a clinically significant impact – something not achieved in most studies discussed.
- Questions remain over the optimum treatment content, length and intensity of treatment, treatment format (groups vs. individual) and the target of treatment (parents vs. children vs. parents and children), but it is clear that parental involvement is essential.
- Future studies should ensure clarity, and should also seek to include families from diverse backgrounds.

References

1. Coates TJ, Thoresen CE. Treating obesity in children and adolescents: a review. *American Journal of Public Health* 1978; **68**: 143–151.
2. Sung-Chan P, Sung YW, Zhao X, Brownson RC. Family-based models for childhood-obesity intervention: a systematic review of randomized controlled trials. *Obesity Reviews* 2012; **14**: 265–278.
3. Ho M, Garnett SP, Baur L, Burrows T, Stewart L, Neve M, et al. Effectiveness of lifestyle interventions in child obesity: systematic review with meta-analysis. *Pediatrics* 2012; **130**: e1647–e1671.
4. Oude Luttikhuis H, Baur L, Jansen H, Shrewsbury VA, O'Malley C, Stolk RP, Summerbell CD. Interventions for treating obesity in children. *Cochrane Database Systematic Review* 2009; **3**: 1–57.
5. Sbruzzi G, Eibel B, Barbiero SM, Petkowicz RO, Ribeiro RA, Cesa CC, et al. Educational interventions in childhood obesity: a systematic review with meta-analysis of randomized clinical trials. *Preventive Medicine* 2013; **56**: 254–264.
6. McGovern L, Johnson JN, Paulo R, Hettinger A, Singhal V, Kamath C, et al. Treatment of pediatric obesity: a systematic review and meta-analysis of randomized trials. *Journal of Clinical Endocrinology and Metabolism* 2008; **93**: 4600–4605.
7. Staniford LJ, Breckon JD, Copeland RJ. Treatment of childhood obesity: a systematic review. *Journal of Child and Family Studies* 2012; **21**: 545–564.
8. Martin J, Chater A, Lorencatto F. Effective behavior change techniques in the prevention and management of childhood obesity. *International Journal of Obesity* 2013; **37**(10): 1287–1294. doi:10.1038/ijo.2013.107.
9. Sargent GM, Pilotto, LS, Baur, LA. Components of primary care interventions to treat childhood overweight and obesity: a systematic review of effect. *Obesity Management*, 2010; **12**: 219–235.
10. National Institute for Health and Clinical Excellence (NICE). Obesity. Guidance on the prevention, identification, assessment and management of overweight and obesity in adults and children. NICE Clinical Guidelines, 2006.
11. Scottish Intercollegiate Guidelines Network (SIGN). Management of obesity. SIGN Guidelines 2010.
12. Barlow SE, the Expert Committee. Expert committee recommendations regarding the prevention, assessment, and treatment of child and adolescent overweight and obesity: summary report. *Pediatrics* 2007; **120**: 164–192.
13. Epstein LH. Family-based behavioural treatment for obese children. *International Journal of Obesity* 1996; **20**: 14–21.
14. Tsiros MD, Sinn N, Brennan L, Coates AM, Walkley JW, Petkov J, Howe PR, Buckley JD. Cognitive behavioral therapy improves diet and body composition in overweight and obese adolescents. *American Journal of Clinical Nutrition* 2008; **87**: 1134–1140.
15. Greenberg G, Ganshorn K, Danilkewich A. Solution-focused therapy. Counseling model for busy family physicians. *Canadian Family Physician* 2001; **47**: 2289–2295.
16. West F, Sanders MR, Cleghorn GJ, Davies PS. Randomised clinical trial of a family-based lifestyle intervention for childhood obesity involving parents as the exclusive agents of change. *Behaviour Research and Therapy* 2010; **48**: 1170–1179.

17. Golley RK, Magarey AM, Baur LA, Steinbeck KS, Daniels LA. Twelve-month effectiveness of a parent-led, family-focused weight-management program for prepubertal children: a randomized, controlled trial. *Pediatrics* 2007; **119**: 517–525.

18. Bandura A. Health promotion from the perspective of social cognitive theory. *Psychology & Health* 1998; **13**: 623–649.

19. Robinson TN. Behavioural treatment of childhood and adolescent obesity. *International Journal of Obesity* 1999; **23**: 52–57.

20. Epstein LH, Wing RR, Koeske R, Valoski A. Effect of diet plus exercise on weight change in parents and children. *Journal of Consulting and Clinical Psychology* 1984; **52**: 429–437.

21. Croker H, Viner RM, Nicholls D, Haroun D, Chadwick P, Edwards C, Wells JC, Wardle J. Family-based behavioural treatment of childhood obesity in a UK national health service setting: randomized controlled trial. *International Journal of Obesity* 2011; **36**: 16–26.

22. Kalarchian MA, Levine MD, Arslanian SA, Ewing LJ, Houk PR, Cheng Y, Ringham RM, Sheets CA, Marcus MD. Family-based treatment of severe pediatric obesity: a randomized controlled trial. *Pediatrics* 2009; **124**: 1060–1068.

23. Boutelle KN, Norman GJ, Rock CL, Rhee KE, Crow SJ. Guided self-help for the treatment of pediatric obesity. *Pediatrics* 2013; **131**: e1435–e1442.

24. Janicke DM, Sallinen BJ, Perri MG, Lutes LD, Huerta M, Silverstein JH, Brumback B. Comparison of parent-only vs. family-based interventions for overweight children in underserved rural settings: outcomes from project STORY. *Archives of Pediatrics and Adolescent Medicine* 2008; **162**: 1119–1125.

25. Williamson DA, Walden HM, White MA, York-Crowe E, Newton RL Jr, Alfonso A, Gordon S, Ryan D. Two-year internet-based randomized controlled trial for weight loss in African-American girls. *Obesity* 2006; **14**: 1231–1243.

26. Savoye M, Shaw M, Dziura J, Tamborlane WV, Rose P, Guandalini C, Goldberg-Gell R, Burgert TS, Cali AMG, Weiss R, Caprio S. Effects of a weight management program on body composition and metabolic parameters in overweight children: a randomized controlled trial. *JAMA* 2007; **297**: 2697–2704.

27. Jansen E, Mulkens S, Jansen A. Tackling childhood overweight: treating parents exclusively is effective. *International Journal of Obesity* 2011; **35**: 501–509.

28. Golan M, Kaufman V, Shahar DR. Childhood obesity treatment: targeting parents exclusively v. parents and children. *British Journal of Nutrition* 2006; **95**: 1008–1015.

29. Bathrellou E, Yannakoulia M, Papanikolaou K, Pehlivanidis A, Pervanidou P, Kanaka-Gantenbein C, Tokou I, Tsiantis J, Chrousos GP, Sidossis LS. Parental involvement does not augment the effectiveness of an intense behavioral program for the treatment of childhood obesity. *Hormones* 2010; **9**: 171–175.

30. Reinehr T, Schaefer A, Winkel K, Finne E, Toschke AM, Kolip P. An effective lifestyle intervention in overweight children: findings from a randomized controlled trial on 'Obeldicks light'. *Clinical Nutrition* 2010; **29**: 331–336.

31. Wake M, Lycett K, Clifford SA, Sabin MA, Gunn J, Gibbons K, et al. Shared care obesity management in 3–10 year old children: 12 month outcomes of HopSCOTCH randomised trial. *BMJ* 2013; **346**: f3092.

32. Okely AD, Collins CE, Morgan PJ, Jones RA, Warren JM, Cliff DP, Burrows TL, Colyvas K, Steele JR, Baur LA. Multi-site randomized controlled trial of a child-centered physical activity program, a parent-centered dietary-modification program, or both in overweight children: the HIKCUPS study. *Journal of Pediatrics* 2010; **157**: 388–394.

33. Sacher PM, Kolotourou M, Chadwick PM, Cole TJ, Lawson MS, Lucas A, Singhal A. Randomized controlled trial of the MEND program: a family-based community intervention for childhood obesity. *Obesity* 2010; **18**: S62–S68.

34. Johnston CA, Tyler C, McFarlin BK, Poston WS, Haddock CK, Reeves R, Foreyt JP. Weight loss in overweight Mexican American children: a randomized, controlled trial. *Pediatrics* 2007; **120**: e1450–1457.

35. Hughes AR, Stewart L, Chapple J, McColl JH, Donaldson MDC, Kelnar CJH, Zabihollah M, Ahmed F, Reilly JJ. Randomized, controlled trial of a best-practice individualized behavioral program for treatment of childhood overweight: Scottish Childhood Overweight Treatment Trial (SCOTT). *Pediatrics* 2008; **121**: e539–e546.

36. Ford AL, Bergh C, Sodersten P, Sabin MA, Hollinghurst S, Hunt LP, Shield JPH. Treatment of childhood obesity by retraining eating behaviour: randomised controlled trial. *BMJ* 2010; **340**: b5388.

37. Taveras EM, Gortmaker SL, Hohman KH, Horan CM, Kleinman KP, Mitchell K, Price S, Prosser LA, Rifas-Shiman SL, Gillman MW. Randomized controlled trial to improve primary care to prevent and manage childhood obesity: the high five for kids study. *Archives of Pediatrics and Adolescent Medicine* 2011; **165**: 714–722.

38. Jelalian E, Mehlenbeck R, Lloyd-Richardson EE, Birmaher V, Wing RR. 'Adventure therapy' combined with cognitive-behavioral treatment for overweight adolescents. *International Journal of Obesity* 2006; **30**: 31–39.

39. Naar-King S, Ellis D, Kolmodin K, Cunningham P, Jen KL, Saelens B, Brogan K. A randomized pilot study of multisystemic therapy targeting obesity in African-American adolescents. *Journal of Adolescent Health* 2009; **45**: 417–419.

40. Lowry KW, Sallinen BJ, Janicke DM. The effects of weight management programs on self-esteem in pediatric overweight populations. *Journal of Pediatric Psychology* 2007; **32**: 1179–1195.

41. Ford AL, Hunt LP, Cooper A, Shield JPH. What reduction of BMI SDS is required in obese adolescents to improve body composition and cardiometabolic health? *Archives of Disease in Childhood* 2010; **95**: 256–261.

42. Wolfenden L, Wiggers J, Tursan d'Espaignet E, Bell AC. How useful are systematic reviews of child obesity interventions? *Obesity Reviews* 2009; **11**: 159–165.

Chapter 6.4

Residential programmes and weight loss camps in childhood obesity

Paul Gately
Leeds Beckett University, Leeds, UK

6.4.1 Introduction

Obesity has been described by the Foresight Report as a 'biological vulnerability to a toxic environment' [1]. Obesity coexists with deprivation [2] and clusters in families and social groups [3]. Current estimates are that there are 4.5 million overweight, 2.7 million obese and 140,000 severely obese children in the UK. Persistence of obesity is high – 85% of obese children become obese adults, as compared to approximately 12% of normal-weight children becoming obese adults [4–6].

The duration of obesity is also important, given data showing that, for every year a person is obese, their life expectancy is reduced by 6–7% [7], and the risk of type II diabetes is increased as well [8]. Obesity is strongly associated with depression, low self-esteem and quality of life, as well as poor mental health [9]. Studies have reported that obese children describe their quality of life as similar to that of children with terminal cancer [10]. The social consequences are less well recognised; however, the obese face greater social exclusion, bullying and stigma throughout their lives, and they also achieve lower levels of educational attainment and income [11]. There is now strong evidence that social networks assist in the maintenance of unhealthy behaviours [12].

Such issues provide a compelling case for action in families with serious obesity; however, it is worrying that mainstream services are not available in the UK. In fact, as outlined in the UK government strategy on obesity:

> … successful local strategies will need to strike a balance between 'treatment' interventions that help individuals to reach a healthier weight and sustained preventive effort to help to make healthy weight increasingly the norm. These are not alternatives – both are vital if we are to 'shift the curve'.

This is welcome, given that, from 2005 to 2010, 99.4% of the funding to tackle obesity focused on prevention of weight gain, with few (0.06%) resources spent to help promote weight loss and health improvement in the obese.

Recommendations [13] are that overweight and obese children should lose weight or achieve weight maintenance while they grow, but specific details are not available. While there is compelling evidence from the adult literature that a weight loss of 5–10% is important for improvement in health variables, without such guidance and concerns about the negative consequences of weight loss in children [14], encouragement for weight loss is likely to be limited. Of course, while caution is appropriate in addition to the physical consequences, it is important to recognise the psychological, social and emotional factors at this critical period in a young person's life. This is particularly true when the lifetime psychological, social and emotional factors are considered. For example, a study [15] has found that obese young women are 50% less likely to achieve higher education in

Advanced Nutrition and Dietetics in Obesity, First Edition. Edited by Catherine Hankey.
© 2018 John Wiley & Sons Ltd. Published 2018 by John Wiley & Sons Ltd.

Sweden. These additional factors suggest the need for more impactful and sustainable weight loss outcomes in children and young people.

The Cochrane [16] review on childhood obesity interventions shows that interventions are successful at achieving weight loss and weight loss maintenance. However, the degree of weight loss is small, with a BMI-SDS (a measure of relative weight change accounting for natural growth) change of 0.16 units across the 54 studies reviewed. This is not surprising, given that they were predominantly community-based interventions usually offering weekly contact with participants and their families over a 3–6 month period. Only three of the studies reported in this review were undertaken in a residential setting, highlighting both the lack of provision and research on residential treatment approaches. The high degree of cost involved in setting up residential weight loss programmes as well as the range of methodological challenges involved in ensuring a high degree of methodological rigour are the primary reasons for this lack of evidence.

6.4.2 Evidence base for residential programmes

In addition to the three residential weight loss programme studies in the Cochrane review [17–19], all undertaken in Northern Europe, there is a limited range of other published studies in residential settings. This demonstrates a lack of research evidence on these treatment options.

Residential programmes are primarily delivered in two settings: inpatient hospitals and weight loss camps. Inpatient programmes are delivered in hospital settings, with an average stay from 18 days to 12 months [20–23]. While all interventions report modification of dietary and physical activity behaviours, there are variations in the frequency, type and duration of physical activity promotions and dietary modifications (e.g. high-protein/low-energy, very-low-energy/calorie, liquid, high-fibre or low-energy diets). There are also large variabilities in the behaviour modification approaches used during the treatment period. This makes comparison between approaches difficult. The staff are typically a multidisciplinary team, involving paediatricians, dietitians, exercise specialists (or physiotherapists), psychologists and nurses. Weight loss camps are

residential camps run during the summer holiday period, and are discussed in later sections.

A primary strength of residential settings is that children can be removed from their obesogenic environments and can experience alternative environments that affect short- and long-term behaviours positively to support long-term weight management. The specific benefits and concerns of residential environments are summarised in Box 6.4.1.

Box 6.4.1 Potential benefits and concerns of residential environments for weight loss in children

Potential benefits

Weight loss: Given the ability to closely manage the environment, safe and sustainable weight loss can be achieved. In addition, weight loss in a controlled environment demonstrates to participants and families that their bodies respond in a predictable way to energy imbalance.

Health and well-being improvements: A range of health and well-being variables are improved by attending residential weight loss programmes.

Common goals: Relatedness is outlined as a key element of the self-determination theory [24]. Children often report that they are 'all in the same boat', suggesting a safe environment to try new activities. In addition, friendships are built that continue after the residential experience. This is particularly important, given the emerging evidence of the importance of social networks and their influence on behaviours and health.

Educational setting: The safe environment is maximised to educate children on a range of factors associated with their weight.

Behaviour change setting: In addition to educating children, residential environments provide an opportunity to shape behaviours directly (healthy eating, physical activity and reduced sedentary behaviours) as well as indirectly (teaching behaviour change skills such as goal setting, monitoring, etc.).

Potential concerns

Is weight loss sustained? There is concern that children return to their obesogenic environments, and that weight is hence typically regained.

Increased stigma of being sent to 'fat camp': There are concerns that attending weight loss camps may stigmatise children and young people [13].

Costs: In comparison to general health promotion, obesity prevention and community weight loss programmes, the costs of residential services are relatively high, which is a barrier.

6.4.3 Outcomes of residential programmes

Weight loss

Weight is significantly reduced during residential interventions. Rolland-Cachara et al. (2004) reported an average weight loss of 30 kg over a 9-month period, which corresponded to a change in BMI-SDS from 4.3 to 1.7 [19]. Braet et al. (2004) reported a 49% weight loss, with a wide variation in the weight loss of participants. Overall weight loss in residential inpatient programmes vary considerably, primarily due to their different durations and approaches [18].

Wider health benefits

Endo et al. (1992) reported significant improvements in a range of biochemical variables associated with atherosclerosis [20]. These include significant improvements in total cholesterol, triglyceride and apolipoprotein (A-I and B) levels, with no change in HDL cholesterol. Widhalm et al. (1983) have reported on the benefits of very-low-energy/calorie diets (VLCDs) on total cholesterol and LDL cholesterol [23].

Psychosocial benefits

Braet et al. (2004) reported significant improvements in global self-worth, school competence, athletic competence, social competence and physical appearance, with more positive outcomes found in boys and younger children [18]. In addition, improved eating pathology, with significant improvement in drive for thinness, occurance of bulimia, body dissatisfaction, external eating and eating, weight and shape concerns were observed. Braet et al. (2004) reported that the total number of binges per month reduced from 56% at baseline to 19% post-treatment [18]. These changes contrast with views that such interventions are likely to negatively impact on eating pathology [25,26].

Follow-up outcomes

Follow-up data is available on some but not all of the studies. Braet et al. (2004) reported significant increases in percentage overweight (another measure of relative weight) at 14 months post-intervention [18]. Rolland-Cachara et al. (2004) also reported a significant increase from post-treatment to follow-up at 2 years following intervention [19]. It should be noted that weight status was still significantly lower at the follow-up point. Deforche et al. (2005) [27] interviewed a number of participants involved in the study of Braet et al. (2004) at the end of the intervention, 1.5 years later [18]. The primary objective was to understand if there were differences in dietary and physical activity behaviours and their impacts. Deforche et al. (2005) categorised the children into four groups – undergoing healthy or unhealthy eating, and healthy or unhealthy physical activity [27]. At baseline, there was no difference in adjusted BMI between the groups. However, at follow-up, the adjusted BMI values were 138% (healthy physical activity and healthy eating), 150% (unhealthy physical activity and healthy eating), 183% (unhealthy physical activity, unhealthy eating) and 156% (healthy physical activity and unhealthy eating). This shows that, in some participants, behaviour changes can be sustained, and such sustained behaviour changes are associated with greater weight loss maintenance. It is unclear whether these changes are sufficient to be clinically important.

6.4.4 Weight loss camps

Residential weight loss camps are primarily active in the USA [28–30] and Europe [31,32]. Programmes run during the summer holiday period usually last 2–9 weeks. Most of the programmes involve dietary modification and physical activity promotion, while some include educational and behavioural change approaches. In addition, there are wide variations in the reporting of methods used by the weight loss camp programmes, which makes understanding and comparisons difficult.

Weight loss during weight loss camps

Significant weight loss during weight loss camps is reported by researchers, although the reported weight metric varies, with mean weight losses of

13.7 kg and 12.1 kg reported by Rohrbacher as far back as 1971 [29]. Gately et al. (2005) reported a mean weight loss of 6 kg and 2.4 BMI units [31]. There were no significant differences between age and gender, but a longer duration resulted in significantly greater weight loss.

Other health benefits during weight loss camps

King et al. (2008) reported significant improvements in metabolic variables, particularly LDL cholesterol, with the degree of LDL peak particle size significantly increased [33]. Hobkirk et al. (2012) also reported significant improvements in a range of cardiometabolic risk factors, which included fasting insulin, triglycerides, and systolic and diastolic blood pressures [34]. Gately et al. (2005) reported significant improvements in blood pressure (6% reduction in systolic and 7% reduction in diastolic) and in aerobic fitness (19% increase in relative VO_2) [31].

Psychosocial benefits

Numerous studies have all reported statistically significant improvements in psychological well-being variables following weight loss camps [31,35–37]. Walker reported positive changes in global self-worth and several other domains including athletic competence and physical appearance [37]. In addition, positive changes in body dissatisfaction, without any increase in worries about weight or appearance was observed. Barton reported significant cognitive changes, with reductions in negative automatic thoughts and increases in positive thoughts (primarily associated with exercise and appearance) [36]. Given the more holistic nature of weight loss camps, researchers have also reported improvements in a range of social factors. Holt reported a range of positive experiences; these included enjoyment and peer support, as well as staff support and a choice of activities [38]. In addition, close to half of the participants in the study reported that they were concerned about being bullied during the programme, although they reported that they did not experience any bullying once they had joined the programme.

Follow-up

Gately et al. showed weight loss maintenance during a 10-month follow-up period [39]. Mean BMI-SDS increased non-significantly during the follow-up period, and BMI-SDS was significantly lower as compared to baseline. This lead to 89% of participants having a lower BMI-SDS as compared to baseline. Hester also reported a range of positive outcomes following attendance at a weight loss camp programme [40]. These included continued weight loss or weight loss maintenance; employing new skills associated with behaviour change, in the form of planning, monitoring and goal setting; and the enjoyment of diet and physical activity. In addition, wearing new styles of clothes, making friends and improved achievements at school were reported. These qualitative outcomes are particularly important. Hester also reported on how camp participants faced challenges in their home environment after returning from camp, including conflicting messages from family, friends and medical practitioners, as compared to messages from the camp programme.

Non-evidence-based residential weight loss camps

Unfortunately, not all programmes are evidence based, and many involve poor practices, given that there are no quality standards, care or clinical governance required. The author had first-hand experience of such interventions in the USA. Despite the provision of a positive social climate, many programmes do not reflect best-practice in the provision of weight management. Many include little in the way of behaviour change therapy, and weight losses are often excessive, and dietary and physical activity practices extreme. There is clearly a need for such interventions to be better understood and systems established to ensure safe and effective practice.

6.4.5 Conclusion

Obesity and its duration are important public health issues. Early intervention is necessary, particularly for children with severe obesity. Residential interventions show promise with short- and long-term positive outcomes in weight- and health-related variables, with weight loss maintenance also being reported. However, there are a limited number of interventions that would be considered of high methodological quality.

The level of obesity/need and the quality of the intervention should be taken into consideration (given the availability of non-regulated commercial approaches). In addition, a balance must be struck between the more clinical hospital-based approaches as compared to the more holistic weight-loss-camp-based interventions. To date, we only have randomised controlled trial outcomes of hospital-based approaches, and, as yet, there is no study that has compared the outcomes of inpatient hospital programmes vs. residential camps.

Further research is necessary to understand the potential of residential approaches, although they show real promise as an alternative to surgical interventions or no treatment.

6.4.6 Summary box

Key points

- Reviews of childhood obesity interventions show that they achieve small weight losses, with a BMI-SDS change of 0.16 units across the 54 studies reviewed.
- Residential interventions show promise, with short- and long-term positive outcomes in weight- and health-related variables, only some interventions can be considered to possess high methodological quality.
- A balance is required between the more clinical hospital-based approaches and the more holistic weight-loss-camp-based interventions.
- To date, we only have randomised controlled trial outcomes of hospital-based approaches, and no study has yet compared the outcomes of inpatient hospital programmes vs. residential camps.

References

1. Government Office for Science. *Tackling Obesities: Future Choices – Project Report*, 2nd edn. London: HMSO, 2007.
2. Department of Health. National Child Measurement Programme: England, 2010/11 school year. The Health and Social Care Information Centre, 201.
3. Christakis NA, Fowler JH. The spread of obesity in a large social network over 32 years. *The New England Journal of Medicine* 2007; **357**: 370–379.
4. Wardle J, Brodersen NH, Cole TJ, Jarvis MJ, Boniface DR. Development of adiposity in adolescence: five year longitudinal study of an ethnically and socioeconomically diverse sample of young people in Britain. *BMJ* 2006; **332**: 1130–1135.
5. Singh AS, Mulder C, Twisk JWR, Van Mechelen W, Chinapaw MJM. Tracking of childhood overweight into adulthood: a systematic review of the literature. *Obesity Reviews* 2008; **9**: 474–548.
6. Johannsson E, Arngrimsson SA, Thorsdottir I, Sveinsson T. Tracking of overweight from early childhood to adolescence in cohorts born 1988 and 1994: overweight in a high birth weight population. *International Journal of Obesity* 2006; **30**(8): 1265–1271.
7. Abdullah A, Wolfe, R, Stoelwinder JU, De Courten M, Stevenson C, Walls HL, et al. The number of years lived with obesity and the risk of all-cause and cause-specific mortality. *International Journal of Epidemiology* 2011; **40**: 985–996.
8. Lee JM, Gebremariam A, Vijan S, Gurney JG. Excess body mass index-years, a measure of degree and duration of excess weight, and risk for incident diabetes. *Archives of Pediatrics and Adolescent Medicine* 2012; **166**(1): 42–48.
9. Andrew JH. Chapter 14: social and psychological factors in obesity. In: Williams G, Frühbeck G (eds) *Obesity Science to Practice*. Chichester UK: Wiley, 2009.
10. Schwimmer JB, Burwinkle TM, Varni JW. Health related quality of life of severely obese children and adolescents. *JAMA* 2003; **289**: 1813–1819.
11. Viner RM, Cole TJ. Adult socioeconomic, educational, social, and psychological outcomes of childhood obesity: a national birth cohort study. *BMJ* 2005; **330**: 1354–1359.
12. Centola D. An experimental study of homophily in the adoption of health behaviour. *Science* 2011; **334**: 1269–1272.
13. National Institute of Clinical Excellence. Obesity guidance on the prevention, identification, assessment and management of overweight and obesity in adults and children. NICE, 2006.
14. Neumark-Sztainer D, van den Berg P, Hannan PJ, Story M. Self-weighing in adolescents: helpful or harmful? Longitudinal associations with body weight changes and disordered eating. *Journal of Adolescent Health* 2006; **39**: 811–818.
15. Karnehed N, Rasmussen F, Hemmingsson T, Tynelius P. Obesity and attained education: cohort study of more than 700,000 Swedish men. *Obesity* 2006; **14**: 1421–1428.
16. Oude Luttikhuis H, Baur L, Jansen H, Shrewsbury VA, O'Malley C, Stolk RP, et al. Interventions for treating obesity in children (Review). *Cochrane Database of Systematic Reviews* 2009; **3**: 1–57.
17. Warschburger P, Fromme C, Petermann F, Wojtalla N, Oepen J. Conceptualisation and evaluation of a cognitive-behavioural training programme for children and adolescents with obesity. *International Journal of Obesity* 2001; **25**(1): S93–S95.
18. Braet C, Tanghe A, Decaluwe V, Moens E, Rosseel Y. Inpatient treatment for children with obesity: Weight loss, psychological well-being, and eating behavior. *Journal of Pediatric Psychology* 2004; **29**(7): 519–529.

19. Rolland-Cachera MF, Thibault H, Souberbielle JC, Souli D, Carbonel P, Deheeger M. Massive obesity in adolescents: dietary interventions and behaviours associated with weight regain at 2 y follow-up. *International Journal of Obesity and Related Metabolic Disorders* 2004; **28**(4): 514–519.

20. Endo H, Takagi Y, Nozue T, Kuwahata K, Uemasu F, Kobayashi A. Beneficial effects of dietary intervention on serum lipid and Apolipoprotein levels in obese children. *American Journal of Diseases of Children* 1992; **146**: 303–305.

21. Pena M, Bacallao J, Barta L, Amador M, Johnston FE. Fiber and exercise in the treatment of obese adolescents. *Journal of Adolescent Health Care* 1989; **10**: 30–34.

22. Wabitsch M, Braun U, Heinze E, Muche R, Mayer H, Teller W, et al. Body composition in 5–18-year-old obese children and adolescents before and after weight reduction as assessed by deuterium dilution and bioelectrical impedance analysis. *American Journal of Clinical Nutrition* 1996; **64**: 1–6.

23. Widhalm K, Zwiauer K, Weber H. Metabolic changes in a 3-week treatment with a low calorie protein-carbohydrate diet in massively obese adolescents. *Infusionsther Klin Ernahr* 1983; **10**(2): 82–89.

24. Deci EL, Ryan RM. *Intrinsic Motivation and Self-Determination in Human Behavior*. New York: Plenum Publishing Co, 1985.

25. Wing RR, Tate DF, Gorin AA, Raynor HA, Fava JL, Machan J. 'STOP regain': are there negative effects of daily weighing? *Journal of Consulting and Clinical Psychology* 2007; **75**(4): 652–656.

26. Shafran R, Fairburn CG, Robinson P, Lask B. Body checking and its avoidance in eating disorders. *International Journal of Eating Disorders* 2004; **35**: 93–101.

27. Deforche B, De Bourdeaudhuij I, Tanghe A, Debode P, Hills AP, Bouckaert J. Role of physical activity and eating behaviour in weight control after treatment in severely obese children and adolescents. *Acta Paediatrica* 2005; **94**(4): 464–470.

28. Cooper C, Sarvey S, Collier D. Willson C, Green I, Pories ML, et al. For comparison: experience with a children's obesity camp. *Surgery for Obesity and Related Diseases* 2006; **2**: 622–626.

29. Rohrbacher R. Influence of a special camp program for obese boys on weight loss, self-concept and body image. *Research Quarterly* 1973; **44**: 150–157.

30. Gately PJ, Cooke CB, Knight C, Carroll S. The acute effects of an 8-week diet, exercise, and educational camp program on obese children. *Pediatric Exercise Science* 2000; **12**: 413–423.

31. Gately PJ, Cooke CB, Barth JH, Bewick BM, Radley D, Hill AJ. Residential weight loss programs can work: A prospective cohort study of acute outcomes for overweight and obese children. *Pediatrics* 2005; **116**: 73–77.

32. Nowicka P, Lanke J, Pietrobelli A, Apitzsch E, Flodmark CE. Sports camp with six months of support from a local sports club as a treatment for childhood obesity. *Scandinavian Journal of Public Health* 2009; **37**(8): 793–800.

33. King RF, Hobkirk JP, Cooke CB, Radley D, Gately PJ. Low-density lipoprotein sub-fraction profiles in obese children before and after attending a residential weight loss intervention. *Journal of Atherosclerosis and Thrombosis* 2008; **15**(2): 100–107.

34. Hobkirk JP, King RF, Gately P, Pemberton P, Smith A, Barth JH, et al. Longitudinal factor analysis reveals a distinct clustering of cardiometabolic improvements during intensive, short-term dietary and exercise intervention in obese children and adolescents. *Metabolic Syndrome and Related Disorders* 2012; **10**: 20–25.

35. Braet C, VanWinckel M. Long-term follow-up of a cognitive behavioral treatment program for obese children. *Behavior Therapy* 2000; **31**: 55–74.

36. Barton SB, Walker LLM, Lambert G, Gately PJ, Hill AJ. Cognitive change in obese adolescents losing weight. *Obesity Research* 2004; **12**: 313–319.

37. Walker LM, Gately PJ, Bewick BM, Hill AJ. Children's weight loss camps: Psychological benefit or jeopardy? *International Journal of Obesity* 2003; **27**: 748–754.

38. Holt NL, Bewick BM, Gately PJ. Children's perceptions of attending a residential weight-loss camp in the UK. *Child: Care, Health and Development* 2005; **31**: 223–231.

39. Gately PJ, Cooke CB, Mackreth P, Carroll S. The effects of a children's summer camp program on weight loss, with a 10-month follow-up. *International Journal of Obesity* 2000; **11**: 1445–1452.

40. Hester JR, McKenna J, Gately PJ. Obese young people's accounts of intervention impact. *Patient Education and Counseling* 2010; **79**(3): 306–314.

Chapter 6.5

Pharmacological management of weight loss in childhood obesity

Jillian M Morrison and M Guftar Shaikh
Royal Hospital for Children, Glasgow, UK

The mainstay of the management of childhood obesity remains family-based behaviour change – that is, healthier eating, an increase in physical activity and a reduction in sedentary behaviour – as described in Chapter 6.1 (titled 'Diet in the management of weight loss in childhood obesity') and Chapter 6.2 (titled 'Physical activity in the management of weight loss in childhood obesity') in this book, and as recommended in guidelines published by a number of expert panels, including both the National Institute for Health and Care Excellence (NICE CG43) and the Scottish Intercollegiate Guidelines Network (SIGN Guideline 115) (Box 6.5.1) [1–3]. However, there are times when, despite intensive dietetic intervention and a motivated family, weight loss or even weight maintenance remains a challenge. As the prevalence of childhood obesity increases and risk of future medical complications that may lead to the beginning of a healthcare challenge for society and the health system, should drug therapy be considered? There are currently no anti-obesity medications licensed for use in children in the UK. However, both SIGN [1] and NICE [2] do offer guidelines for the restricted use of medications in adolescents (aged 12 years and above) with severe obesity and comorbidities (Box 6.5.1). Orlistat, biguanides and metformin are occasionally prescribed at paediatric obesity clinics, in combination with diet and lifestyle treatment plans [4].

Comorbidities such as hypertension, hyperinsulinaemia, dyslipidaemia, osteoarthritis and type 2 diabetes are risk factors in childhood obesity that may benefit from additional pharmacotherapy. However, childhood obesity can be aggravated by depression and other psychosocial problems, and the side effects of anti-obesity drugs mean that they need to be introduced with caution. Anti-obesity drugs work in one of three ways – either by increasing energy expenditure, by reducing gastrointestinal macronutrient absorption or by suppressing appetite and in turn reducing energy intake. Drugs are not a cure for obesity, and compliance with a healthy lifestyle remains a key component of therapy. However, drug treatment does remain an option, and NICE (2006) [2] and others suggest that pharmacotherapy be considered as a form of treatment for two groups of children – obese children who fail to respond to a formal programme of intensive lifestyle modification, or overweight children with comorbidities despite an intensive lifestyle modification programme.

As with other forms of treatment, drug therapy in childhood obesity involves behaviour change, and the family will need support from a multidisciplinary team to manage this form of treatment. A systematic review of pharmacological interventions for the treatment of obesity carried out by Gray et al. reports that modest weight reductions of up to 11 kg can be made using appropriate drug treatment [5]. However, most of the drugs described have been withdrawn due to adverse side effects. There may be a place for pharmacological interventions for the treatment of obesity if drugs can be developed that minimise the side effects; however, the evidence in children is limited [6]. A trial of pharmacotherapy can be considered for a period of 6–12 months in

---

Advanced Nutrition and Dietetics in Obesity, First Edition. Edited by Catherine Hankey.
© 2018 John Wiley & Sons Ltd. Published 2018 by John Wiley & Sons Ltd.

Box 6.5.1 NICE and SIGN guidelines relating to pharmacological management in childhood obesity

NICE Clinical Guideline 43

Consider drug treatment only after dietary, exercise and behavioural approaches have been started and evaluated.

Children <12 years

1. Drug treatment is not generally recommended.
2. Prescribe only in exceptional circumstances, if there are severe life-threatening comorbidities (e.g. sleep apnoea, raised intracranial pressure).
3. Prescribing should be started and monitored only in specialist paediatric settings.

Children ≥12 years

1. Drug treatment is recommended only if there are physical comorbidities – for example, orthopaedic problems, sleep apnoea or severe psychological comorbidities.
2. Prescribing should be started by specialist multidisciplinary teams with experience in prescribing for this age group. This comprises drug monitoring, psychological support, behavioural interventions, interventions to increase physical activity and interventions to improve diet.

Drug treatment started in specialist care, may be continued in primary care if local circumstances and/ or licensing allow.

Continued prescribing and withdrawal

1. Offer a 6–12-month trial of orlistat, with regular review of effectiveness, adverse effects and adherence.
2. Drug treatment may be used to help the child or young person to maintain weight loss, as well as to continue to lose weight.
3. If concerned about micronutrient intake, consider a supplement that provides the reference nutrient intake for all vitamins and trace elements.
4. If a child or young person's drug treatment is withdrawn because he or she has not reached the target weight, offer support to help maintain the weight loss, because his or her self-confidence and belief in the ability to make changes may be low.

SIGN Guideline 115

Orlistat should only be prescribed for severely obese adolescents (those with BMI ≥99.6th centile of the UK 1990 reference chart for age and sex) with comorbidities, or those with very severe to extreme obesity (BMI ≥3.5 SD above the mean of the UK 1990 reference chart for age and sex), attending a specialist clinic.
   There should be regular reviews throughout the period of use, including careful monitoring for side effects.

---

children over 12 years of age, but this must be in a specialist paediatric obesity clinic. Drug therapy may be considered in children under the age of 12 years if there are comorbidities, but local and national guidelines must be followed at all times.

6.5.1 Drugs used in childhood obesity

Orlistat

Orlistat (sold as Xenical, by Roche) acts by inhibiting gastrointestinal lipase activity, thus decreasing fat absorption. Orlistat has been shown to reduce BMI by 1.9 kg/m^2, with a weight loss of 4.4 kg over a 3-month treatment period [7]. A meta-analysis in adolescents shows a small response to orlistat [6]. It should only be continued beyond 3 months if there is >5% weight loss. There is a need for dietetic advice regarding how to identify foods high in fat to minimise gastrointestinal side effects such as flatulence and steatorrhoea, in addition to the dietary guidance provided alongside the medication. Young children may struggle to identify fatty foods, and steatorrhoea and abdominal pain may lead to food aversions and nutritionally compromised diets. As fat is poorly absorbed, there is a risk of low vitamin D and other fat-soluble vitamins. Despite multivitamin supplementation, vitamin D status was shown to be reduced after 1 month of orlistat treatment in obese adolescents [8]. There is also some evidence of low vitamin D status in obesity as increased blood concentrations are stored in adipose tissue, although the mechanism for this is poorly understood [9]. It is recommended that a multivitamin and mineral supplement containing adequate doses of fat-soluble vitamins be taken at least 2 hours after the orlistat dose to maximise absorption. Alternatively, the patients can be advised to take orlistat for 3 weeks out of 4 weeks, and, during the off week, to take a multivitamin preparation. A dose of 120 mg of orlistat before each main meal has been used. Side effects include hypertension, and the drug should be discontinued if blood pressure rises during treatment. Other side effects of this treatment include flatulence, abdominal distension and faecal incontinence, and it may adversely affect a child's quality of life, which is already compromised due to severe obesity – such as being forced to reduce participation in group activities and being subject to bullying. In older children, it is possible that compliance with medication may become an issue as they may stop taking the drug if they wish to consume high-fat foods.

Biguanides

Biguanides (metformin hydrochloride) reduce hepatic glucose production, decreases intestinal glucose absorption from the GI tract and enhances insulin sensitivity. Metformin is the drug of choice in children with type 2 diabetes, in whom adherence to dietary restrictions has failed to control diabetes. Most of the clinical literature on metformin deals with its use in the treatment and prevention of diabetes, but a frequently occurring side effect appears to be weight loss. A recent randomised controlled study using metformin for 6 months in obese children and adolescents demonstrated a beneficial effect on BMI-SDS as compared to placebo. The reduction in BMI-SDS was 0.1, which is relatively small, but this effect was sustained at 6 months, with improvements in fasting glucose and liver function, together with an increased adipocytokine ratio (adiponectin:leptin) [10]. Leptin and adiponectin are both secreted by adipose tissue, and leptin is involved in appetite regulation, while adiponectin improves insulin sensitivity [11,12]. Other studies have also shown metformin to aid weight loss of up to 4 kg, and metformin is increasingly being used in children [13]. Hsia et al. (2011) examined prescribing patterns in children and adolescents, and found that prescribing metformin had increased for children and adolescents, in particular for girls with polycystic ovarian syndrome. This is despite metformin not being licensed for weight loss in children [14]. Side effects of metformin include anorexia, abdominal pain, taste disturbances, nausea and vomiting.

To aid compliance and minimise side effects, the dose of metformin should be gradually increased, with dose increments of 250–500 mg/day every 2 weeks. A starting dose of 250 mg/day for young children and 500 mg/day for older children is recommended. The doses should be increased to 250 mg twice daily for young children and 500–1000 mg (maximum) twice daily for older children. Changing from standard metformin to modified-release metformin may help prevent children with significant gastrointestinal disturbances from discontinuing therapy.

A 6-month trial of metformin may halt the rise in BMI-SDS in this group of children, and will also improve the insulin glucose status, possibly acting as a catalyst and supporting more radical changes in lifestyle.

Octreotide

Hypothalamic obesity is a resistant form of obesity arising from damage to the satiety and appetite centres in the hypothalamus, resulting in hyperphagia and reduced energy expenditure. It occurs as a result of either brain tumours and/or cranial irradiation, such as craniopharyngioma, or genetic conditions such as Prader–Willi syndrome. Octreotide may play an important role in helping to manage rapid weight gain as a consequence of hyperphagia due to the cranial insult. Patients with hypothalamic obesity exhibit insulin hypersecretion, and octreotide acts by suppressing insulin production. In a study by Lustig et al. (2003), researchers were able to show a stabilisation of weight and BMI while on octreotide treatment [15]. Patients who demonstrated greater insulin hypersecretion seemed to benefit most after 6 months of treatment. However, this form of treatment requires regular subcutaneous injections, and side effects of diarrhoea, flatulence and vomiting can limit compliance. Long-acting preparations of octreotide have also been used with benefits in some, but not all, patients [16].

6.5.2 Future developments

A number of drugs are being developed, some with similar actions to those previously withdrawn (such as sibutramine), but which are more selective in their action and have fewer adverse effects. Some have gained approval for use in the USA [17–19]. Sibutramine, which is a serotonin reuptake inhibitor, was withdrawn due to concerns regarding its safety, despite displaying significant weight loss effects.

Qsymia

This drug is a combination of phentermine and topiramate, and was approved for use in the USA in 2012 for adults with BMI of >30 kg/m^2 and comorbidities, alongside diet and exercise [20]. Topiramate is an anticonvulsant that is approved for use in migraine and certain types of epilepsies, but a side effect is anorexia. Phentermine is thought to trigger the release of norepinephrine, which increases the blood concentrations of leptin, suppressing appetite. Used in combination, trials have shown positive results in weight reduction, with a mean weight loss of at least 10% [21,22]. This drug is not licensed for use in the UK yet.

Other combination therapies include bupropion and naltrexone, which in a Phase 2 trial demonstrated greater weight loss (4.3–5.5%) than with bupropion or naltrexone on its own (2.7% and 1.2%, respectively). Both these agents act on the satiety centres of the hypothalamus [23]. However, most trials thus far have been in adults, not children.

Belviq

Belviq (lorcaserin hydrochloride) has also been recently approved in the USA for use in adults. This is a centrally acting drug that works on serotonin receptors to reduce energy intake and body weight [24–26]. As with Qsymia, it is only licensed in adults at the moment, and may become available for use in children at some stage.

6.5.3 Bariatric surgery in children

If diet and pharmacotherapy fails, bariatric surgery should be considered. In adults, there have been increased success rates in those who have had bariatric surgery, but there is limited data in children. There have been very few adolescents who have undergone bariatric surgery in the UK, with most being morbidly obese, with body weights around 200 kg. The children need to be able to cope psychologically with the rigours of bariatric surgery and the consequences of such a radical procedure. Current guidelines suggest that there may be a role for surgery in adolescents who have completed puberty and who have a BMI of >40 kg/m^2, and in those with comorbidities who have failed both diet and pharmacotherapy [27].

6.5.4 Summary box

> **Key points**
> - Diet remains the cornerstone of the treatment of childhood obesity.
> - Limited drug treatments are available in paediatrics.
> - Behaviour change is a vital part of the treatment of childhood obesity, even in those who may benefit from additional drug treatment.

References

1. Scottish Intercollegiate Guidelines Network 115. Management of obesity – a national clinical guideline, NHS Quality Improvement Scotland, February 2010.
2. National Institute for Health and Care excellence CG43. Obesity: the preventions, identification, assessment and management of overweight and obesity in adults and children. NICE, 2006.
3. Speiser PW, Rudolf MC, Anhalt H, et al. Childhood obesity. *Journal of Clinical Endocrinology and Metabolism* 2005; **90**(3): 1871–1887.

4. Viner R, Nicholls D. Managing obesity in secondary care: a personal practice. *Archives of Disease in Childhood* 2005; **90**(4): 385–390.

5. Gray LJ, Cooper N, Dunkley A, et al. A systematic review and mixed treatment comparison of pharmacological interventions for the treatment of obesity. *Obesity Reviews* 2012; **13**(6): 483–498.

6. McGovern L, Johnson JN, Paulo R, et al. Clinical review: treatment of pediatric obesity: a systematic review and meta-analysis of randomized trials. *Journal of Clinical Endocrinology and Metabolism* 2008; **93**(12): 4600–4605.

7. McDuffie JR, Calis KA, Uwaifo GI, et al. Three-month tolerability of orlistat in adolescents with obesity-related comorbid conditions. *Obesity Research* 2002; **10**(7): 642–650.

8. McDuffie JR, Calis KA, Booth SL, Uwaifo GI, Yanovski JA. Effects of orlistat on fat-soluble vitamins in obese adolescents. *Pharmacotherapy* 2002; **22**(7): 814–822.

9. Han JC, Lawlor DA, Kimm SY. Childhood obesity. *Lancet* 2010; **375**(9727): 1737–1748.

10. Kendall D, Vail A, Amin R, et al. Metformin in obese children and adolescents: the MOCA trial. *Journal of Clinical Endocrinology and Metabolism* 2013; **98**(1): 322–329.

11. Arora S, Anubhuti. Role of neuropeptides in appetite regulation and obesity – a review. *Neuropeptides* 2006; **40**(6): 375–401.

12. Lihn AS, Pedersen SB, Richelsen B. Adiponectin: action, regulation and association to insulin sensitivity. *Obesity Reviews* 2005; **6**(1): 13–21.

13. Srinivasan S, Ambler GR, Baur LA, et al. Randomized, controlled trial of metformin for obesity and insulin resistance in children and adolescents: improvement in body composition and fasting insulin. *Journal of Clinical Endocrinology and Metabolism* 2006; **91**(6): 2074–2080.

14. Hsia Y, Dawoud D, Sutcliffe AG, Viner RM, Kinra S, Wong IC. Unlicensed use of metformin in children and adolescents in the UK. *British Journal of Clinical Pharmacology* 2012; **73**(1): 135–139.

15. Lustig RH, Hinds PS, Ringwald-Smith K, et al. Octreotide therapy of pediatric hypothalamic obesity: a double-blind, placebo-controlled trial. *Journal of Clinical Endocrinology and Metabolism* 2003; **88**(6): 2586–2592.

16. Lustig RH, Greenway F, Velasquez-Mieyer P, et al. A multi-center, randomized, double-blind, placebo-controlled, dose-finding trial of a long-acting formulation of octreotide in promoting weight loss in obese adults with insulin hypersecretion. *International Journal of Obesity* (London) 2006; **30**(2): 331–341.

17. Halford JC, Boyland EJ, Lawton CL, Blundell JE, Harrold JA. Serotonergic anti-obesity agents: past experience and future prospects. *Drugs* 2011; **71**(17): 2247–2255.

18. Johnson AM. Two new drugs approved for obesity. *South Dakota Medicine* 2012; **65**(9): 356–357.

19. Khan A, Raza S, Khan Y, et al. Current updates in the medical management of obesity. *Recent Patents on Endocrine, Metabolic & Immune Drug Discovery* 2012; **6**(2): 117–128.

20. Cameron F, Whiteside G, McKeage K. Phentermine and topiramate extended release (Qsymia): first global approval. *Drugs* 2012; **72**(15): 2033–2042.

21. Bays HE, Gadde KM. Phentermine/topiramate for weight reduction and treatment of adverse metabolic consequences in obesity. *Drugs Today* 2011; **47**(12): 903–914.

22. Cosentino G, Conrad AO, Uwaifo GI. Phentermine and topiramate for the management of obesity: a review. *Drug Design, Development and Therapy* 2013; **7**: 267–278.

23. Greenway FL, Dunayevich E, Tollefson G, et al. Comparison of combined bupropion and naltrexone therapy for obesity with monotherapy and placebo. *Journal of Clinical Endocrinology and Metabolism* 2009; **94**(12): 4898–4906.

24. Fidler MC, Sanchez M, Raether B, et al. A one-year randomized trial of lorcaserin for weight loss in obese and overweight adults: the BLOSSOM trial. *Journal of Clinical Endocrinology and Metabolism* 2011; **96**(10): 3067–3077.

25. Redman LM, Ravussin E. Lorcaserin for the treatment of obesity. *Drugs Today* 2010; **46**(12): 901–910.

26. O'Neil PM, Smith SR, Weissman NJ, et al. Randomized placebo-controlled clinical trial of lorcaserin for weight loss in type 2 diabetes mellitus: the BLOOM-DM study. *Obesity* (Silver Spring) 2012; **20**(7): 1426–1436.

27. August GP, Caprio S, Fennoy I, et al. Prevention and treatment of pediatric obesity: an endocrine society clinical practice guideline based on expert opinion. *Journal of Clinical Endocrinology and Metabolism* 2008; **93**(12): 4576–4599.

Surgical management of weight loss in childhood obesity

Kathleen B Hrovat, Linda M Kollar and Thomas H Inge
Cincinnati Children's Hospital Medical Center, Cincinnati, OH, USA

6.6.1 Introduction

Studies about surgical treatments for adult obesity were first published in the late 1960s. Bariatric procedures for adolescents with severe obesity were first reported in the 1970s and 1980s [1,2]. The procedures performed in this period included jejunoileal bypass, vertical-banded gastroplasty, Roux-en-Y gastric bypass (RYGB), biliopancreatic diversion and duodenal switch. These earlier experiences with a variety of procedures provided insight regarding the risks of surgical care, and have helped to shape current thinking about bariatric surgical procedures for adolescents [3].

The acceptance of bariatric surgery for paediatric populations varies across regions. A 2004 survey of European bariatric surgeons found that 39% offered laparoscopic surgery to patients less than 18 years of age [4]. The most common procedures included RYGB, adjustable gastric band (AGB) and vertical sleeve gastrectomy (VSG). These represent both restrictive (VSG and AGB) and malabsorptive/restrictive procedures (RYGB). The number of procedures performed yearly is rising; also, as evidence continues to show that bariatric procedures can be performed safely in the adolescent population, this trend is likely to continue [5]. With the expanding body of knowledge available about weight loss surgery in adolescents, several evidence-based guidelines are now available for clinicians treating obese children and adolescents [6].

Weight loss surgery for adolescents

There are unique factors specific to adolescents that must be addressed before surgery is offered to a morbidly obese teen. It would be advantageous to know precisely which preoperative and postoperative factors most influence successful outcome of surgery. Unfortunately, there are currently no established criteria for determining which adolescents will benefit most from weight loss surgery, and no evidence-based criteria to predict which patients are at highest risk for postoperative complications. In the absence of age-specific predictors of outcome, most specialists who conduct adolescent bariatric surgery empirically advise that candidates be referred to centres with multidisciplinary weight management teams experienced in meeting the distinct physical and psychological needs of adolescents. The many physical changes of the adolescent period are accompanied by a complicated psychosocial developmental process that is impacted by environmental and social factors, requiring thorough assessment in the context of bariatric surgery. The decisional capacity of the adolescent must be evaluated to assess the ability to understand the risks/benefits of an invasive, non-reversible, elective surgical procedure. Additionally, surgical care should be provided in conjunction with teams who are skilled in performing modern bariatric procedures.

The family is an important part of the preparation for surgery. The team should assess the 'family environment' and define who the adolescent considers as 'family' to determine if he or she has the

Advanced Nutrition and Dietetics in Obesity, First Edition. Edited by Catherine Hankey.
© 2018 John Wiley & Sons Ltd. Published 2018 by John Wiley & Sons Ltd.

support needed in order to be successful both preoperatively and postoperatively. The multidisciplinary team should encourage appropriate independence and plan for eventual transition to adulthood.

Eligibility criteria

Conventional wisdom holds that adolescents should achieve physical maturity prior to surgical weight loss treatment. This is generally assumed to be >13 years of age for girls and >15 for boys. Body mass index (BMI) is a useful inclusion criterion, with the minimum BMI threshold of 35 kg/m² in the setting of serious comorbidities of obesity (type 2 diabetes, obstructive sleep apnoea, benign intracranial hypertension, moderate non-alcoholic steatohepatitis). The American Society for Metabolic and Bariatric Surgery (ASMBS) supports further expansion of the eligibility criteria to those with a BMI of 30–35 kg/m² in the presence of type 2 diabetes. Those with a BMI of ≥40 kg/m² may be eligible with less serious comorbidities [3,7]. Additionally, the American Diabetes Association (ADA) recommends the following criteria for a surgical candidate:

- Should have experienced failure in at least 6 months of formal organised weight-loss treatment
- Should demonstrate commitment to comprehensive medical and psychological evaluations before and after weight loss surgery
- Should be capable and willing to adhere to nutritional guidelines postoperatively
- Should possess decisional capacity
- Should have a supportive family environment

Contraindications for surgical treatment of obesity in teens include pregnancy or breastfeeding, active substance abuse, inadequate social support and medically correctable causes of obesity.

6.6.2 Preoperative assessment

The preoperative evaluation includes a comprehensive medical history, physical examination and laboratory assessment for the causes and complications of obesity. Identification and medical management of comorbidities during the preoperative period

will assist in minimising surgical risk. A discussion on pregnancy prevention first begins in the preoperative period. It is commonly recommended to postpone pregnancy until 18 months after weight loss surgery. Therefore, an effective contraceptive method is essential [8].

All adolescents seeking weight loss surgery should receive a psychological assessment to assess developmental status, social support structure and presence of mental illness, and identify any behavioural conditions that could interfere with adherence to the diet and lifestyle changes required after surgery. The evaluation is generally conducted as a semi- structured interview, and may include screening inventories for depression, cognitive abilities and quality of life. Treatment of psychopathology and ongoing psychosocial support is essential prior to and after surgery [9] (Box 6.6.1).

Nutritional assessment

Nutritional management for adolescents considering weight loss surgery can be classified into three areas: nutritional assessment, education of the patient and family about nutritional requirements and postoperative monitoring of nutritional status. The multidisciplinary team should include a registered dietitian, preferably with experience in paediatric weight management and/or weight loss surgery.

The preoperative nutritional assessment may benefit from administration of a food/eating behaviours questionnaire and a review of the family/home environment. This can help identify any nutrient-poor food choices, lack of dairy foods, and the amount of fruits and vegetables and whole grains intake. The energy requirements of the patient, based on height, ideal body weight and age, should be determined. These energy requirements will be the basis for advising the patient on a preoperative eating pattern consisting of adequate high-quality protein (1–1.5 grams protein/kg of ideal body weight), fruits, vegetables and whole grains to achieve weight stability or weight loss [10]. At this time, behavioural strategies for healthy eating should be introduced, such as eating from smaller plates, measuring portions with measuring spoons and measuring cups, meal planning and grocery lists, and journaling or tracking

> **Box 6.6.1** Recommended tools to include in the assessment of adolescents undergoing weight loss surgery
>
> **Adolescent measures**
>
> *Beck Depression Inventory* (BDI-II): This is a 21-item multi-choice self-report inventory of physical and cognitive symptoms of depression, including assessment of suicidal ideation. Total score indicates moderate depressive symptoms in the clinically significant range.
>
> *Impact of Weight on Quality of Life* (IWQOL): This is a 73-item multi-choice self-report inventory that assesses the impact of weight on six domains: physical activity, body esteem, social life, distress, school and family relations. Domain-specific and total scores are obtained. Results indicate severe impairment in physical functioning, and moderate impairment in esteem, social, distress, and school and family functioning.
>
> *Pediatric Quality of Life Inventory* (Peds QL): This is a 23-item multi-choice self- and parent-report inventory of several domains of health-related quality of life, including physical, emotional, social and school functioning. Domain-specific and total-health-related quality-of-life scores are obtained. Results indicate severe impairment in physical functioning, moderate impairment in emotional functioning and mild impairment in social and school functioning.
>
> *Questionnaire on Eating and Weight Patterns – Revised* (QEWP-R): This is a 28-item self-report inventory that assesses a range of features associated with obesity and eating disorders, such as dieting and weight history, the presence or absence of binge episodes and features related to binge eating disorder. Results indicate symptoms of binge eating disorder.
>
> **Parent measures**
>
> *Peds QL* results indicate impairment in physical and emotional functioning, moderate impairment in social functioning and minimal impairment in school functioning.
>
> *Sizing Them Up*: This questionnaire is a 22-item, obesity-specific, parent-proxy measure of health-related quality of life. Six domains are assessed: emotional functioning, physical functioning, teasing/marginalisation, positive social attributes, mealtime challenges and school functioning. Results indicate moderate to severe impairment in physical, emotional functioning and minimal to mild impairment in all other domains.

daily intake of foods and fluids. The adolescent and family should receive information in written, visual and/or electronic form to accommodate different learning styles.

In order to better understand the adolescent's relationship to food and eating, an assessment of his or her 'mindful eating' habits should be evaluated. At its simplest, 'mindfulness' is the awareness of the present moment. Mindful eating is eating with intention and attention [11]. This information will allow the dietitian to set realistic goals that are measurable and attainable, and specific to the adolescent. A typical preoperative goal might be: 'I will drink water and sugar-free fluids daily with a goal of 2 litres each day, and quantify this amount with my water bottle'.

A preoperative liquid diet initiated 2 weeks prior to surgery introduces the adolescent to the postoperative dietary regimen, and may well improve the safety and efficiency of the surgical procedure by reduction of intra-abdominal fat stores and liver size [12]. Adolescents are capable of following individualised meal plans (approximately 1000–1200 kcal, or 4186–8373 kJ) provided by dietitians. Some centres, including our own (Surgical Weight Loss Program for Teens, Cincinnati, Ohio, USA), suggest choices for the liquid meal replacements for three daily meals, in conjunction with a portion-controlled typical solid evening meal of 400 kcal (1674 kJ). Liquid meal replacement is most readily accomplished as a defined and prepared product, such as a ready-to-drink protein shake, or a protein powder added to water or low-fat milk. Such a product, when substituted for a meal, should provide <200 kcal. Fluid goals and vitamin/mineral supplementation is also tracked during this preoperative liquid diet phase (1.8 litres of water and/or sugar-free liquids and a daily multivitamin supplement).

6.6.3 Surgical options

Important decisions about surgical procedure options are made in collaboration with the surgical team, the adolescent, key family members and/or caregivers. Individual factors to consider include BMI, comorbidities, surgeon experience and patient preference. Thorough preoperative education allows the adolescent and family to carefully weigh the risks and benefits of each of the surgical options. All bariatric procedures restrict dietary intake and result in a negative energy balance either through hypocaloric intake, altered energy expenditure or both. Malabsorption is not considered to be a major mechanism of weight regulation after RYGB, VSG or AGB. From clinical experience, the anticipated weight loss for adolescents in the year following RYGB or VSG is 25–35%, while results from AGB in adolescents is more variable, but may be 15–30%. A key principle to emphasise is that weight loss surgery is only a tool to help the adolescent lose weight; if the tool is used correctly (dietary and lifestyle recommendations are followed), then weight loss results can be remarkable. The concept of the surgery as a tool must be reiterated throughout the preoperative process and reinforced at every postoperative follow-up visit.

Restrictive procedures

Operations that reduce stomach size are known as 'restrictive procedures'. These procedures result in early satiety, limiting food intake, and can result in significant weight loss. These procedures are generally done laparoscopically.

The laparoscopic adjustable gastric band (LAGB) involves the placement of a silicone band with an inner inflatable balloon at the very top of the stomach, creating a small pouch. The second part of the operation involves the creation of a subcutaneous pocket for fixation of the port on the anterior rectus fascia. The key feature of this option is the adjustability. Fluid is injected or withdrawn through the

port to restrict or loosen the band. This requires frequent clinical follow-up for the band adjustments. Complications of LAGB include band slippage, reoperations for band or port replacement, erosion of the band, damage to the catheter tubing or port and dislodging of the port. One small randomised trial with adolescents in Australia found that 84% of them lost approximately 28% of their body weight (more than 50% of their excess weight) 2 years after LAGB [13], although the exact duration of follow-up varies according to hospital unit.

VSG is a subtotal gastric resection of the fundus and body of the stomach to create a long gastric tube based on the lesser curve of the stomach. Appetite is significantly reduced, and a feeling of fullness is reached after 1–1.5 cups of food. Complications of VSG include gastric leak along the long staple line, stricture, bleeding and nutritional deficiencies. Long-term data for this procedure are limited, but weight loss expectations are similar to RYGB. Adult studies have reported 25–30% BMI reduction (excess weight loss of 33–85%, with an overall mean of 55%) [14].

Malabsorptive procedures

In addition to the risks of restrictive surgeries, malabsorptive operations also carry greater risk for nutritional deficiencies. Biliopancreatic diversion with or without duodenal switch results in significant macronutrient and micronutrient malabsorption, and is not recommended for adolescents. RYGB is a commonly performed operation worldwide for adults and adolescents. A 15–30-ml gastric pouch is created just beyond the gastroesophageal junction. A Roux limb of jejunum is anastomosed to the gastric pouch, bypassing the remaining stomach, duodenum and a small portion of the jejunum. RYGB limits food intake and results in some micronutrient malabsorption, although most believe that no significant macronutrient malabsorption occurs. Complications of RYGB include gastric leak, stricture, internal hernia, bleeding, marginal ulcer and nutritional deficiencies. A longitudinal study of 61 adolescents who underwent RYGB found an average of 37% decrease in BMI, with those at lower initial BMI more likely to achieve non-obese BMI [15].

Table 6.6.1 Diet advancement protocols for weight loss surgery

Surgery type	Stage 1 (ice chips, water, sugar-free clear liquids)	Stage 2 (full liquids, high in protein)	Stage 3 (smooth-consistency foods and liquids)	Stage 4 (soft foods)	Stage 5 (all textures – healthy foods)
RYGB	30 ml/hour for the first 24–48 hours, then *ad lib* for 3–7 days	Weeks 2–4	Weeks 4–6	Weeks 7–9	Begins at week 9 for life
AGB	30 ml/hour for the first 24–48 hours	First 2 weeks after surgery	Weeks 3–4	Weeks 5–6	Week 7 and for life
VSG	30 ml/hour for the first 24–48 hours, then *ad lib* for 3–7 days	Weeks 1–5	Weeks 5–8	9–12 weeks postoperative	Week 13 and for life
Specific dietary advice	*Acceptable*: sugar-free clear liquids, including water, clear broth or bouillon, sugar-free gelatine, sugar-free fruit-flavoured drinks, fruit ice made with sugar-free fruit drinks, sugar-free popsicles. *Restrictions*: no carbonated beverages, no caffeine, no red dyes	*Energy*: 500–600 kcal/day (2093.4–2512 kJ). *Protein*: 50–60 g/day. *Fluids*: 2.4 litre/day, or based on estimated requirements. *Pattern*: 3–6 meals/day. *Volume*: ½ cup/meal for solid foods. *New foods introduced*: skimmed milk (1% fat), low-fat soya or Lactaid milk, high-protein drinks, light yogurt thinned with milk	*Energy*: 500–700 kcal/day (2093.4–2930.76 kJ). *Protein*: 60 g/day. *Fluids*: 2.4 litre/day, or based on estimated requirements. *Pattern*: 3–4 meals/day. *Volume*: ½ cup/meal for solid foods, or 180 ml/meal of protein drink. *Consistency*: Smooth foods. *New foods introduced*: Scrambled eggs, blended/minced turkey, chicken, flaked fish or mashed tofu, melted low-fat cheese, low-fat cottage cheese (small curd only), low-fat ricotta cheese. Try new foods one at a time every 2–3 days	*Energy*: 700–800 kcal/day (2930.76–3349.44 kJ). *Protein*: 60 g/day. *Fluids*: 2.4 litre/day, or based on estimated requirements. *Pattern*: 3–6 meals/day. *Volume*: ½–1 cup/meal for solid foods, or 360 ml/meal of protein drink. *New foods introduced*: *Protein foods*: shaved deli meats, low-fat cheese, lean pork, cooked beans. *Fruit*: soft or canned in own juice, no skin. *Vegetables*: soft cooked or canned. *Grains*: Toast, low-sugar cereal, crackers, oatmeal, rice, pasta, mashed potatoes (choose mainly whole grain products/foods)	*Energy*: 800–900 kcal/day (3349.44–3768.12 kJ). *Protein*: 60 g/day. *Fluids*: 2.4 litre/day, or based on estimated requirements. *Pattern*: 3–6 meals/day. *Volume*: ¾–1.5 cups/meal. *New foods introduced*: all healthy food choices
General long-term dietary advice	<ul><li>Avoid high-sugar foods and/or fat content to prevent dumping syndrome; symptoms may include cramping, clammy feeling, sweating, heart racing, vomiting and/or diarrhoea. Late dumping may occur up to 2 hours after eating foods high in sugar or fat.</li><li>Meals should be eaten in approximately 20 min.</li><li>Adolescents should be encouraged to stop drinking 30 min before a meal and not to drink until 30 min after a meal. Eating and drinking at the same time may decrease satiety and/or increase the incidence of vomiting.</li><li>Encourage eating slowly with small bites. Make sure food is cut into small pieces, and chew food well until it has a pureed consistency.</li><li>Do not eat or drink past the first feeling of fullness. When feeling full, stop eating and put food away, or discard what is left.</li><li>To prevent dehydration, encourage adolescents to continually sip fluids throughout the day, preferably water. Consider limiting caffeinated products</li><li>Do not lie down within 1 hour after meals.</li></ul>				

Source: Adapted from reference [17]. RYGB Roux-en-Y gastric bypass, AGB adjustable gastric band, VSG vertical sleeve gastrectomy.

6.6.4 Nutritional monitoring after surgery

The postoperative advancement of the diet for RYGB, ABG and VSG varies by the number of meals/day, as well as the consistency, texture and progression of the amount of food consumed at a meal. The diet is designed to restrict energy intake in order to produce the desired weight loss (Table 6.6.1). Every patient is different, and may not progress evenly at the stated time points. It is normal for a postoperative patient to experience food intolerances during the first 3–6 months after surgery. Over time, the patient will tolerate a variety of foods from each of the food groups.

Daily vitamin and mineral supplementation is essential throughout life after the common procedures. Education regarding the risks of vitamin/mineral deficits and the importance of continued monitoring of nutritional status will assist the adolescents in adherence. Table 6.6.2 outlines the suggested supplementation after weight loss surgery. Fibre intake has been identified as being very low postoperatively, far below the daily recommended intake. In the longer term, recommending fibre sources in the diet may be an important postoperative step to promote satiety and weight loss [16].

Table 6.6.2 Postoperative supplementation recommendations

Supplement	Restrictive procedures	RYGB	Comments
High-potency multivitamin	One daily	Two times daily	Begin with liquid or chewable formulas with at least 18 mg iron, 400 µg folic acid, and containing zinc and selenium Separate from calcium supplement by at least 2 hours Avoid enteric coating
Vitamin B$_{12}$	May be required	350–500 µg/day (tablet)	–
Optional B complex	One serving/day	One serving/day	Avoid time-released tablets May provide additional prophylaxis against thiamine deficiencies >1000 mg of supplemental folic acid could mask B$_{12}$ deficiency
Vitamin D	1000–2000 IU may be required	1000–2000 IU may be required	Screen for vitamin D deficiency Suggested dose for correction is 50,000 IU ergocalciferol weekly × 8 weeks (orally)
Elemental calcium	1500 mg/day	1500–2000 mg/day	Split into 500–600-mg doses Promote intake of dietary dairy sources in addition to supplements Calcium citrate is more effectively absorbed than calcium carbonate
Additional elemental iron	–	18–27 mg/day elemental	Recommended for menstruating females Consider exchanging multivitamins for prenatal vitamins in females Dosage may need to be adjusted based on biochemical markers Vitamin C may enhance absorption

Source: Adapted from reference [18].

6.6.5 Conclusion

Over the past three decades, scientific literature has reported positive outcomes of bariatric surgery in adolescents with severe obesity. There are factors unique to adolescents that must be addressed before surgery is offered as an option. The clinical team must consider an adolescent's cognitive, social and emotional development when considering his or her candidacy. Severe comorbid conditions associated with obesity in adolescents (type 2 diabetes, obstructive sleep apnoea, benign intracranial hypertension, non-alcoholic steatohepatitis and arterial hypertension) are resolved or significantly improved with surgery. In addition, adolescent patients can anticipate a 25–35% decrease in BMI. Behavioural strategies for healthy eating are introduced preoperatively, and reinforced at every postoperative visit. The concept of surgery as a tool is reiterated throughout the process. Institutions providing bariatric surgery to adolescents should only provide these services if a multidisciplinary team dedicated to providing both preoperative and postoperative care to this unique population is in place to ensure safety and excellent delivery of clinical care. As adolescent bariatric surgeries increase in number, continued research is necessary. Long-term outcome data are needed to base future treatment decisions for adolescents worldwide.

6.6.6 Websites

Weight-control Information Network: http://www.niddk.nih.gov/health/nutrit/win.htm

Cincinnati Children's Hospital: http://www.cchmc.org/weight

American Society for Metabolic and Bariatric Surgery: http://www.asmbs.org

6.6.7 Summary box

Key points

- Positive outcomes have been achieved through bariatric surgery in adolescents with severe obesity, including improvements in type 2 diabetes, obstructive sleep apnoea, benign intracranial hypertension, non-alcoholic steatohepatitis and arterial hypertension.

- Factors unique to adolescents must be addressed before surgery is offered as an option – especially those related to cognitive, social and emotional development.
- An adolescent patient can anticipate a 25–35% decrease in BMI – adequately supported using behavioural strategies for healthy eating.
- Institutions providing bariatric surgery to adolescents should only provide these services if they have available a multidisciplinary team dedicated to providing both preoperative and postoperative care to this unique population.
- Long-term outcome data are needed to base future treatment decisions for adolescents worldwide.

References

1. Randolph JG, Weintraub WH, Rigg A. Jejunoileal bypass for morbid obesity in adolescents. *Journal of Pediatric Surgery* 1974; **9**: 341–345.
2. Organ CH, Kessler E, Lane M. Long-term results of jejunoileal bypass in the young. *American Surgeon* 1984; **50**: 589–593.
3. Inge TH, Xanthakos SA, Zeller MH. Bariatric surgery for pediatric extreme obesity: now or later? *International Journal of Obesity* 2007; **31**: 1–14.
4. Rivas H, Martinez JL, Delgado S, Vidal J, Lacy AM. Current attitudes to the laparoscopic bariatric operations among European surgeons. *Obesity Surgery* 2004; **14**: 1247–1251.
5. Zwintshcer NP, Azarow KS, Horton JD, Newton CR, Martin MJ. The increasing incidence of adolescent bariatric surgery. *Journal of Pediatric Surgery* 2013; **48**: 2401–2407.
6. Aikenhead A, Lobstein T, Knai, C. Review of current guidelines on adolescent bariatric surgery. *Clinical Obesity* 2011; **1**: 3–11.
7. Mechanick JI, Youdim A, Jones DB, et al. Clinical practice guidelines for the perioperative nutritional, metabolic, and nonsurgical support of the bariatric surgery patient – 2013 update. *Obesity* 2013; **21**: S1–S27.
8. ACOG Committee Opinion Number 315. Obesity in pregnancy. *Obstetrics & Gynecology* 2005; **106**(September): 671–675.
9. Wadden TA, Sarwera DB. Behavioral assessment of candidates for bariatric surgery: a patient-oriented approach. *Surgery for Obesity and Related Diseases* 2006; **2**: 171–179.
10. US Department of Agriculture, National Agricultural Library. Dietary guidance. DRI tables.
11. Wansink B. *Mindless Eating*. New York: Bantam books, 2010.
12. Benotti PN, Still CD, Wood GC, et al. Preoperative weight loss before bariatric surgery. *Archives of Surgery* 2009; **144**(12): 1150–1155.
13. O'Brien PE, Sawyer SM, Laurie C, et al. Laparoscopic adjustable gastric banding in severely obese adolescents: a randomized trial. *JAMA* 2010; **303**: 519–526.
14. Clinical Issues Committee of the American Society for Metabolic and Bariatric Surgery. Updated position statement on sleeve gastrectomy as a bariatric procedure. *Surgery for Obesity and Related Diseases* 2010; **6**: 1–5.

15. Inge TH. Jenkins TM. Zeller M. Dolan L. Daniels SR. Garcia VF. Brandt ML. Bean J. Gamm K. Xanthakos SA. Baseline BMI is a strong predictor of nadir BMI after adolescent gastric bypass. *Journal of Pediatrics* 2010; **156**: 103–108.

16. Jeffreys RM, Hrovat K, Woo JG. Schmidt M, Inge TI, Xanthakos SA. Dietary assessment of adolescents undergoing laparoscopic Roux-en-Y gastric bypass surgery: macro and micronutrient, fiber and supplement intake. *Surgery for Obesity and Related Diseases* 2012; **8**(3, May): 331–336.

17. Fullmer M, Abrams S, Hrovat K, Mooney L, Scheimann A, Hillman J, Suskind D. Nutritional strategy for the adolescent patient undergoing bariatric surgery: report of a working group of the Nutrition Committee for the North American Society of Pediatric Gastroenterology, Hepatology and Nutrition and the National Association of Children's Hospital and Related Institutions. *Journal of Pediatric Gastroenterology and Nutrition* 2012; **54**: 125–135.

18. Aills L, Blankenship J, Buffington C, Furtado M, Parrott J. ASMBS allied health nutritional guidelines for the surgical weight loss patient. *Surgery for Obesity and Related Diseases* 2008; **4**: S73–S108.

Public health and the prevention of obesity

Chapter 7.1

National campaigns to modify eating behaviour in the prevention of obesity

Sandra Drummond

Queen Margaret University, Edinburgh, UK

Combating the rising level of obesity is probably the biggest health challenge of the twenty-first century in economically developed countries. However, the responsibility to make the appropriate healthy changes does not lie not solely with the individual, but across all levels of society. Hence, over the last 10–20 years, governments across the world have become increasingly aware of the importance of formulating effective policies that allow national campaigns to be put in place, in order to address the obesity problem.

The benefits of policy at the government level are wide ranging. A policy gives consensus on an issue, ensures consistency of information, provides a framework for action and promotes multi-agency and multi-disciplinary working. Further, it is a statement of intent; it outlines a programme of actions to achieve specific aims and objectives. In other words, it sets the guiding principles for the development of national campaigns that aim to address the issue of concern.

This chapter outlines and describes the key national campaigns in the UK and elsewhere that focus on reducing the prevalence of obesity.

7.1.1 National campaigns in the United Kingdom

National campaigns in England

In 2004, the UK government published the health improvement white paper titled 'Choosing Health' [1]. This paper aimed to support the general public by making it easier for them to become healthier. It addressed many target groups, including children, adults, the health service, the workplace and local communities. However, the focus was on health in general, with healthy weight as just one of the desired outcomes. In 2008, the Foresight Report on tackling obesity [2] highlighted the scale of the problem, and included projected obesity statistics for 2030 (Figure 7.1.1). These figures emphasised the urgent need for a response to the increasing levels of obesity from the society as a whole to enable individuals to make sustainable changes to their diet and activity levels. As a result, in 2008, the government published its response in a document titled 'Healthy Weight, Healthy Lives: A Cross-Government Strategy for England' [3]. This document focussed on five key areas. These were:

- To improve the healthiness of the diet by reducing high-energy-dense foods, to reduce foods high in salt and to increase fruit and vegetable intake
- To encourage habitual physical activity on a daily basis
- To prevent childhood obesity
- To make advice and support available for those with weight problems
- To give incentives for healthier lifestyles

The success of this campaign has been documented, and include better access to high-quality fruit and vegetables in low-income areas, schoolchildren being entitled to 5 hours of physical activity, improvements to school meals, improvements to the

Advanced Nutrition and Dietetics in Obesity, First Edition. Edited by Catherine Hankey.
© 2018 John Wiley & Sons Ltd. Published 2018 by John Wiley & Sons Ltd.

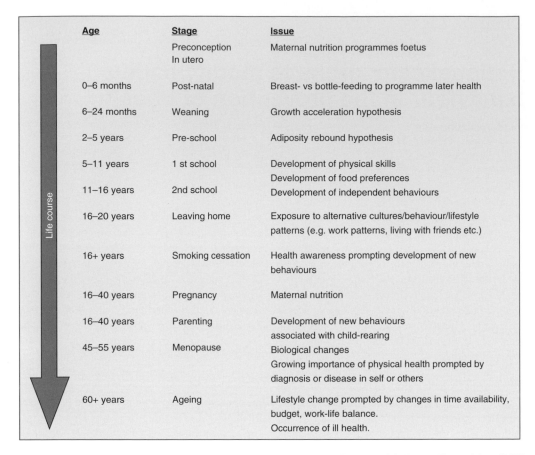

Age	Stage	Issue
	Preconception In utero	Maternal nutrition programmes foetus
0–6 months	Post-natal	Breast- vs bottle-feeding to programme later health
6–24 months	Weaning	Growth acceleration hypothesis
2–5 years	Pre-school	Adiposity rebound hypothesis
5–11 years	1 st school	Development of physical skills Development of food preferences
11–16 years	2nd school	Development of independent behaviours
16–20 years	Leaving home	Exposure to alternative cultures/behaviour/lifestyle patterns (e.g. work patterns, living with friends etc.)
16+ years	Smoking cessation	Health awareness prompting development of new behaviours
16–40 years	Pregnancy	Maternal nutrition
16–40 years	Parenting	Development of new behaviours associated with child-rearing
45–55 years	Menopause	Biological changes Growing importance of physical health prompted by diagnosis or disease in self or others
60+ years	Ageing	Lifestyle change prompted by changes in time availability, budget, work-life balance. Occurrence of ill health.

Figure 7.1.1   Life course stages where behavioural interventions are possible. Foresight Report Figure 4.1; p. 68 [2].

built environment with better facilities for activity and more opportunities for families to walk or cycle. It may be that these initiatives have been effective because they have specifically focussed on the target groups in most need for change (i.e. low-income groups and children), rather than assuming a blanket-style approach across the whole population. However, the key to the success of the Healthy Weight, Healthy Lives strategy is that it encourages not only individuals and families, but also communities as a whole to embrace the opportunities to make their lives healthier, and thus minimise the risk of weight gain.

Social marketing has been employed in the Change4Life campaign [4]. The aim of social

marketing is to integrate marketing concepts with other approaches – such as research and best practice – to influence behaviours that benefit individuals and communities for the greater social good. Social marketing is different from commercial marketing, where businesses and industries market their products for financial gain. The aim of social marketing is not necessarily financial, but rather to contribute to the achievement of 'social good'.

The 'Change4Life' national campaign was rolled out in 2009. It specifically addresses the rising obesity rates by encouraging families with children aged 5–11 years (and at risk of becoming overweight or obese) to get healthier by becoming more active and eating more healthily (Box 7.1.1). Its aim

> **Box 7.1.1** Change4Life: advice for families
>
> 1. Summer zone – ideas for summer activities
> 2. Up and about – how to get more active
> 3. 60 active min
> 4. Snack check
> 5. Five-a-day
> 6. Me-size meals
> 7. Cut back on fat
> 8. Sugar swap

> **Box 7.1.2** Change4Life: advice for adults ('Swap it – Don't stop it')
>
> 1. Activity swaps
>   a. Travel swap – cycle or walk instead of driving or taking the bus
>   b. Sitting down swap – get up and about rather than sitting
>   c. Hobby swap – choose an active rather than sedentary hobby (e.g. dancing, gardening)
>   d. TV swap: partake in some of the sports you watch on TV (e.g. pitch and putt, football in the park)
>   e. Swim/dance more
> 2. Portion swaps
> 3. Snack swap
> 4. Swap five-a-day
> 5. Fibre swap
> 6. Drink swap

is to get the whole of society involved in the prevention of weight gain, and therefore it also aims to engage with local authorities, community groups, the health service, places of work, schools, charities and local businesses. Recently, the campaign has expanded its target group to include families with younger children (aged 1–4 years) and also middle-aged adults (aged 45–65 years). The campaign has been advertised in TV commercials, posters, leaflets and pamphlets. There is also a dedicated website with online advertising, all with a distinctive logo, aimed at reaching a large target group and to get the information across to the target population. The campaign for families focuses on 'key challenges' ranging from consuming five-a-day fruit and vegetables, choosing healthier snacks, reducing sugar and fat intake, and becoming more active. The adult campaign is similar but includes challenges such as increasing the fibre in the diet and reducing the energy content of alcoholic drinks (Box 7.1.2). The emphasis is on making small changes, or making 'swaps', rather than promoting large, more substantial changes, which may not be perceived as achievable or sustainable in the long term.

At the outset, Change4Life was funded by the Department for Health, but funding was sought in 2011 from the food industry and charitable organisations. The aim of this new approach was for it to be less a government campaign, more a social movement and more backed by business, rather than by the government. This scheme involved companies providing up to £250 million in vouchers to families in return for swapping an unhealthy habit for a healthy one. Companies such as Unilever,

Uncle Ben's, Quorn, Cravendale, Asda and Mars Confectionery signed up to provide vouchers for their 'healthier' foods, with many of them displaying Change4Life's 'Be Food Smart' sub-brand, with advice on healthy meal options.

Targets were set for the first year, and an evaluation of the campaign was published after 1 year [5]. The results were promising, and expectations had been exceeded in some areas. It is of vital importance for evaluations to be carried out, as national campaigns are expensive – not only in economic terms, but also in terms of human resources, campaign materials and time. The Change4Life campaign was allocated a budget of £75 million over a period of 3 years. In the first year, the campaign reached 99% of the target group – 87% of the mothers with children aged 5–11 years were aware of the campaign and had seen the adverts, most of whom recognised the distinctive logo. The programme's targets were to generate 1.5 million responses from at-risk families, with 200,000 of those respondents converting into a customer relationship management (CRM) programme to support behaviour change. These targets were developed with help from their communications partners and the Central Office for Information, enabling them to forecast response and conversion rates based on media spend and mix. More than double the predicted number of families signed up for Change4Life (over 400,000), with more than the forecast numbers still engaged with the campaign. In the second year, it was reported that more families continued to join Change4Life, but the main marketing focus had shifted to supporting existing partners, rather than on recruitment [6]. Initial evidence suggests increased swapping to lower-fat dairy products and lower-sugar drinks, and reductions in sugary cereal consumption in the short term. However, there has been some suggestion that the interest may not be sustainable over the longer term. Ongoing evaluations are underway to determine the short- and long-term success of this campaign.

National campaigns in Scotland

In 2008, the Scottish government published 'Healthy Eating, Active Living: an action plan to improve diet, increase physical activity and tackle obesity (2008–2011)' [7]. The Scottish government allocated a total of £56 million to help achieve their objectives to reduce levels of obesity by enabling individuals to choose healthier diets and take part in more physical activities. This document focussed on several key areas, including:

• Targeting the disadvantaged, with the aim of reducing health inequalities
• Preschool children
• Pregnant women and women of child-bearing age

Part of the budget was allocated to supporting successful campaigns that were already up and running. For example, increased funding was provided for 'Paths for All' (www.pathsforall.org.uk) in order to induce greater participation in activities to increase energy expenditure. This is an example of partnership working, and many organisations have linked up to promote walking for health with the development of multi-use path networks in Scotland. Their overall aim is to reduce the number of physically inactive people by encouraging more people to walk more often. This campaign is already a success,

with over 20,000 individuals taking part in weekly organised walks. Other national campaigns that have benefited from increased support include 'Healthy Start'. This was a food voucher scheme for low-income pregnant women and mothers with infants. It also aims to increase the availability of advice on healthy eating, during and after pregnancy, with additional funds allocated to improving breast feeding rates, particularly in low socioeconomic groups. The 'Play@home' campaign focuses on the early years, from birth to 5 years of age, and promotes safe physical activity for toddlers and their families. Two school-based campaigns have also benefited – 'Active Schools' and Hungry for Success' – which together ensure that school children engage with appropriate levels of physical activity and are provided with healthy school meals. In addition to campaigns that help prevent increases in obesity, the Scottish government supports the 'Counterweight Programme' – an initiative to manage and treat overweight and obese patients in primary care. This extra funding has allowed Counterweight to increase its geographical spread across Scotland, with particular focus on areas of deprivation.

In addition to these campaigns, the Scottish government launched the 'Take Life On' campaign in 2008, which aimed to improve the health and wellbeing of all adults in Scotland [8]. Similar to the Change4Life campaign in England, Take Life On employs social marketing to engage with their target group. The aim is to make individuals feel able and empowered to make changes to their lifestyles that are sustainable in the long term, with subsequent long-term health benefits. A dedicated website and a series of advertisements on billboards, TV and radio have been employed to promote the campaign. The key messages include:

• Making healthy changes to the diet – encouraging five-a-day fruit and vegetables; consumption of more wholegrains and fish; less sugar, fat and salt
• To drink more water
• To drink less alcohol
• To increase levels of physical activity
• To encourage these changes across the family unit

National campaigns in Wales

In 2006, the Welsh government published a plan to deal with the rising obesity levels in a policy document titled 'Food and Fitness – Promoting Healthy Eating and Physical Activity for Children and Young People in Wales' [9]. This document focuses very much on the prevention of obesity in children and young adults, and includes action plans to improve school food provisions and to implement the MEND (Mind, Exercise, Nutrition … Do it!) programme, which specifically targets families with 7–13-year-old children [10]. MEND provides healthy lifestyle programmes in the community, focussing on weight management for families with children. The aim is to provide activity and nutrition programmes with information to empower both adults and children to become healthier and achieve healthy weights. This programme involves a participatory-based series of activity sessions and nutrition workshops, primarily for families with young children.

National campaigns in Northern Ireland

The government strategy to stop the increase in obesity in Northern Ireland is detailed in the 2005 policy document titled 'Fit Futures' [11]. The strategy here is to consider all ages in the plan to encourage healthy eating and increased physical activity, with the action plan developed in consultation with their target group. In 2011, *Safe*food, an organisation in Northern Ireland that aims to promote food safety, launched a campaign titled 'Stop the Spread' in an attempt to address the obesity epidemic in Northern Ireland. The focus of this national campaign is to encourage individuals to recognise overweight and obesity as being detrimental to health and not a normal state of affairs. *Safe*food's 2-year campaign involved social media networks, including TV and radio advertising, and a website where users can sign up to weight loss challenges and access information on how to lose weight – 'weigh2live' [12]. The website also has information on how to measure waist circumference, and hence enables individuals to assess the individual health risks related to their central obesity. Pharmacies and chemists have fully endorsed this initiative, and provide measuring tapes free of charge across the region.

7.1.2 National campaigns worldwide

To detail all campaigns that address the obesity problem worldwide is outside the scope of this chapter. However, some countries are more advanced than others in their public health campaigns, and these will be discussed briefly.

Epode International Network (EIN) claims to be the world's largest obesity prevention network – a claim that is justified as it has programmes in Europe (France, Belgium, Greece, the Netherlands, Portugal, Romania, Slovakia, Bulgaria, Italy, Spain, Hungary and the UK), North and South America, Israel, Australia, New Zealand, Taiwan and Singapore [13]. EIN supports community-based programmes to help prevent and reduce the prevalence of obesity and related diseases. By sharing best practice, putting science into practice, development of new strategies, generating more interest from the private sector and sharing information, the goal of EIN is to prevent childhood obesity and associated diseases through large-scale community programmes. The Netherlands, for example, has based their 'JOGG' initiative on the Epode methodology, focussing on achieving a healthy weight for all young people in the country [14]. JOGG involves a series of community-based initiatives that aim to encourage all people to make healthy food and exercise an easy and attractive choice. By taking a local approach and including shopkeepers, parents, health professionals, schools and local authorities, in addition to the target group – children and adolescents, the aim is to ensure that young people stay at a healthy weight. Measures such as including community involvement and commitment, and adapting projects and initiatives to suit the needs of each community, are key to their success.

Further afield, Australia's National Obesity Campaign has focused on making individuals aware of their body weight status by asking all Australian adults (aged 25–50 years) to measure their waist circumference. In order to assess their own health risks, Australians are encouraged to compare their own waist circumference with the recommended and upper limits for health. Titled 'Measure Up' [15], this campaign supports individuals at risk of obesity-related health complications by encouraging them to engage with a 12-week programme to 'kick start healthy habits'. Australia has also signed up to the 'MEND' programme in several of its states – New South Wales, Victoria, Queensland and Tasmania. The progress of Australia and New Zealand in obesity prevention over the last 20 years has come under the spotlight recently. Despite investments in policy development and anti-obesity programmes, Swinburn and Wood [16] blame the power of the food industry in limiting the implementation of many of the policy initiatives. However, some positives were highlighted, particularly in Australia, where they had implemented long-running 'whole of community' projects to reduce childhood obesity. These interventions took a community capacity building approach, and, over a 3-year period, saw improvements in unhealthy weight gain in children and adolescents. Swinburn and Wood firmly advocate this capacity building approach within each community, where local community centres, churches, schools and sports centres build capacity to enable them to engage better with families in promoting healthy lifestyles.

The USA, arguably the leader in the obesity statistics, launched an aggressive anti-obesity national campaign in 2011, optimistically entitled 'Campaign to End Obesity' [17]. At a national level, it aims to enable more Americans to become more active and to eat a healthier diet. This campaign is a joint effort, bringing together leaders from industry, academia and public health to drive forward initiatives to address the rising in levels of obesity. Some of the challenges of in this campaign included getting Americans to identify obesity as a disease; encouraging more widespread use of BMI as an indicator of obesity (with particular emphasis on children); and making healthy food affordable and available to disadvantaged groups. With these measures, the campaign aimed to make it easier for Americans to be active – by making the environment a safer place; by encouraging employers to promote health and

well-being in the work place; and by supporting ongoing obesity research.

7.1.3 Facilitating healthy change

By definition, national campaigns aim to engage with the nation's population. Many campaigns currently employ social marketing via websites, radio and TV to reach their target audience. However, the target audience should be made aware that they are, in fact, the target audience! Failing this, the health messages will fall on deaf ears. One evaluation of a mass media campaign run by the BBC, titled 'Fighting Fat, Fighting Fit', demonstrated that, although record numbers of individuals signed up to participate in the campaign, those who signed up were more likely to be educated women, and that there was less participation from men, individuals under the age of 25 years and those from lower socioeconomic groups [18]. The authors stated that this demographic was in line with BBC viewers, and not entirely unexpected. However, these findings illustrate the point that reaching the target group is a challenge for any campaign.

Even if there is wide awareness of a campaign, change in behaviour cannot be assumed. There are many factors involved in predicting behaviour change, such as whether individuals perceive there to be a risk or threat to their health if they do not make changes, and whether they believe that the recommended changes will reduce that threat. However, one of the most significant factors in predicting behaviour change is self-efficacy – that is, whether individuals believe themselves to be capable of making the change [19].

Predicting behaviour change is a challenging topic in itself, but there are two models that are most relevant to predicting dietary change. The Health Belief Model suggests that behaviour is based on the expected outcomes of the behaviour – whether an individual believes that he or she will benefit from the behaviour, and how much value the individual places on that benefit [20]. Focussing more specifically on behaviour *change* is the 'Stages of Change' framework [21]. This describes the discrete stages that an individual goes through in the process of making a change. These stages are:

(1) 'pre-contemplation', when the individual has not even started thinking about change – he or she may not even be aware of the need for change; (2) 'contemplation', when the individual is starting to think about making a change and has recognised that a change is needed, but has not done anything about it yet; (3) 'preparation', when the individual is taking small steps towards making a change in the near future; (4) 'action', when the individual is modifying his or her behaviour and has made the change to be more healthy; (5) 'maintenance', when these actions are being maintained, but effort is still required to prevent the final stage of change, which is (6) 'relapse', when the individual reverts back to his or her previous, less healthy behaviours. Understanding the motivation for behaviour change is a challenge. We cannot assume that the target population is a homogenous group, as not all individuals share the same motivations or beliefs, or at least not all at the same time. There is evidence to show that those most likely to respond to dietary change initiatives are older, well-educated women. Hence, it is recognised that there is a need for campaigns to address the gap between the healthy, motivated section of the population, and the less educated, more socially deprived section of the population. If the dietary changes recommended in public health campaigns were made less challenging, and require less effort, this could facilitate change for those in the 'contemplation' stage of change.

It may be that the simpler, smaller changes recommended in these campaigns will be the most achievable and successful, such as increasing the number of steps walked per day, or the simple 'swaps' detailed in the Change4Life campaign [4]. Campaigns that force individuals to recognise their health risks (by measuring their waist circumferences, for example) is also a way forward in gaining the attention of those who are currently overweight, but not yet obese, and perhaps not aware of their increased health risk.

However, campaigns that will be the most successful will be those which create environments that make it easy for individuals to make changes. In order to do this, there has to be collaboration among all sectors in the community, and the nation as a whole – for example, enabling easy access to local leisure facilities and play areas, to encourage physical activity; and ensuring that local shops and retail outlets make healthy foods available at reasonable costs. National campaigns that aim to do this are the way forward, as relying on the individual alone to be responsible for turning the obesity epidemic around is a risky strategy.

7.1.4 Summary box

Key points

- Several national and international initiatives have been designed to challenge obesity and weight gain.
- Change4Life was an early campaign using social marketing principles to engage families – with a long-term lifespan.
- Engaging the population and facilitating behaviour change are key to the success of any initiative.
- Formal evaluation has been challenging – but the EPODE and JOGG campaigns have shown early promise.
- Long-term public health approaches are required for achieving meaningful health changes – though evidence of effective programme content is accumulating.
- Long-term financial commitment is necessary to ensure change.

References

1. Choosing Health: Making Healthy Choices Easier, 2004. Available at http://webarchive.nationalarchives.gov.uk/+/www.dh.gov.uk/en/Publicationsandstatistics/Publications/PublicationsPolicyAndGuidance/DH_4094550, accessed November 2016.
2. Government Office for Science's Foresight Report: Tackling Obesities: Future Choices, 2008. Available at http://www.bis.gov.uk/foresight/our-work/projects/published-projects/tackling-obesities, accessed November 2016.
3. Healthy Weight, Healthy Lives: A Cross Government Strategy for England, 2008. Available at http://webarchive.nationalarchives.gov.uk/20100407220245/http:/www.dh.gov.uk/prod_consum_dh/groups/dh_digitalassets/documents/digitalasset/dh_084024.pdf, accessed November 2016.
4. Change4life. Department of Health, 2009. Available at http://www.nhs.uk/change4life/Pages/overview-policy-background.aspx?filter=OverviewAndPolicyBackground, accessed November 2016.

5. Change4Life: One Year On, 2010. Available at http://webarchive.nationalarchives.gov.uk/20130107105354/http://www.dh.gov.uk/prod_consum_dh/groups/dh_digitalassets/@dh/@en/documents/digitalasset/dh_115511.pdf, accessed November 2016.

6. Change4Life: Three Year Social Marketing Strategy, 2011. Available at https://www.gov.uk/government/uploads/system/uploads/attachment_data/file/213719/dh_130488.pdf, accessed November 2016.

7. Healthy eating, active living: an action plan to improve diet, increase physical activity and tackle obesity, 2008–2011. Available at www.scotland.gov.uk (http://www.scotland.gov.uk/Publications/2008/06/20155902/0, accessed November 2016.

8. Take Life On, 2008. Available at www.takelifeon.co.uk, accessed November 2016.

9. Food and Fitness – Promoting Healthy Eating and Physical Activity for Children and Young People in Wales. Available at http://www.physicalactivityandnutritionwales.org.uk/Documents/740/food-fitness-implement-e.pdf, accessed November 2016.

10. www.mendprogramme.org, accessed November 2016.

11. Fit Futures, 2005. Available at https://www.health-ni.gov.uk/publications/fit-futures, accessed November 2016.

12. Weigh2live. Available at http://weigh2live.safefood.eu/, accessed November 2016.

13. www.epode-international-network.com, accessed November 2016.

14. http://epode-international-network.com/programmes, accessed November 2016.

15. http://www.measureup.com.au, accessed November 2016.

16. Swinburn B, Wood A. Progress on obesity prevention over 20 years in Australia and New Zealand. *Obesity Reviews* 2013; **14**: 60–68.

17. www.obesitycampaign.org, accessed November 2016.

18. Miles A, Rapoport L, Wardle J, Afuape T, Duman M. Using the mass-media to target obesity: an analysis of the characteristics and reported behaviour change of participants in the BBC's 'Fighting Fat, Fighting Fit'. *Health Education Research* 2001; **16**: 357–372.

19. Cismaru M, Lavack AM. Social marketing campaigns aimed at preventing and controlling obesity. *International Review on Public and Non-Profit Marketing* 2007; **4**: 9–30.

20. Satia JA, Kristal AR, Curry S, Trudeau E. Motivations for healthful dietary change. *Public Health Nutrition* 2001; **4**: 953–959.

21. Prochaska JO, Velicer WF. The transtheoretical model of health behaviour change. *American Journal of Health Promotion* 1997; **12**: 38–48.

Chapter 7.2

Increasing physical activity to prevent childhood obesity

Gareth Stratton
Swansea University, Swansea, UK

The exponential increase in childhood obesity that started in the 1990s has now slowed but not receded. Much of the change in society – such as transport behaviour, the virtual world and technology, greater perceptions of danger and the penchant for a convenient lifestyle – has emerged among adults and children alike. These changes have reached the roots of families, and the resultant behaviours in diet and physical activity have resulted in a markedly different child phenotype than existed even 30 years ago. The obesogenic environment has promoted this change, and the childhood obesity phenotype has become commonplace across all sectors of society. Health professionals are concerned that this increase has left an indelible mark on society's perception of healthy weight, and that a return to the child phenotype of the 1980s is unlikely. This chapter considers evidence from systematic reviews where the relationships between physical activity, sedentary behaviour and overweight in children are discussed.

7.2.1 Definitions in exercise and health science

Before embarking on an analysis of these reviews, it is important to define the terms used in this area of study. 'Physical activity' is defined as any movement using the skeletal muscles that results in energy expenditure, such as walking to school, playing in the park, taking the stairs as opposed to the lift and so on. 'Exercise', on the other hand, is a subcategory of physical activity that is planned, structured, purposeful and repetitive – for example, playing sport, attending dance class, swimming or jogging. 'Sedentary behaviour' is defined as 'any waking activity characterized by an energy expenditure ≤ 1.5 metabolic equivalents *and* a sitting or reclining posture' [1].

Physical activity and sedentary behaviour are further categorised by intensity using metabolic equivalents (METs – the ratio of exercise to resting energy expenditure: EEE/REE), which are different in children as compared to adults [2]. For example, in children, moderate- and vigorous-intensity activities have been allocated MET values of 4.2 and 7.0, respectively, compared to 3 and 6 METs in adults, respectively. This confirms the long-held view that children are not simply mini-adults, and that growth and development add a layer of complexity to the science of childhood obesity [3]. Preventing, treating or managing unhealthy weight gain is also complicated by developmental pathways that are biopsychosocial and genetic. These factors require serious consideration when assessing the scientific literature on the prevention, management and treatment of unhealthy weight in children and youth. This chapter considers physical activity and sedentary time and their influence on the prevention of obesity, and also in its treatment, with a focus on children.

Advanced Nutrition and Dietetics in Obesity, First Edition. Edited by Catherine Hankey.
© 2018 John Wiley & Sons Ltd. Published 2018 by John Wiley & Sons Ltd.

7.2.2 International guidance on physical activity and sedentary behaviour in young people

As the volume and quality of literature related to health, physical activity and sedentary behaviour increases, dose–response recommendations have been updated. Most recently, the authors of these reports have gained greater confidence in making recommendations for preschoolers (under 5 years) and for children and adolescents (5–18 years). These recommendations include guidance on levels of sedentary behaviour, moderate to vigorous physical activity and musculoskeletal health (Table 7.2.1).

Details, however, vary between guidance documents. For example, the Australian guidance is split into three age groups (0–4, 5–12 and 13–17 years) and lists specific recommendations for sedentary time.

Physical activity recommendations for the overweight and obese

Physical activity guidelines are produced by teams consisting of academic, professional and public health experts who review the best-quality evidence on the relationships and effects of physical activity and sedentary time on the nation's health. Evidence statements supported by scientific research are drawn up and then used to create recommendations

Table 7.2.1 International examples of children and young people's physical activity and sedentary behaviour guidance

	Under 5 years	5–18 years
General	Physical activity should be encouraged from birth, particularly through floor-based play and water-based activities in safe environments.	–
Physical activity	Children of preschool age who are capable of walking unaided should be physically active for at least 180 min (3 hours) daily, spread throughout the day.	All children and young people should engage in moderate–vigorous-intensity physical activity for at least 60 min and up to several hours every day. Vigorously intense activities, including those that strengthen muscle and bone, should be undertaken on at least 3 days in a week.
Sedentary time	All children under age 5 years should minimise the amount of time spent being sedentary (being restrained or sitting) for extended periods (except time spent sleeping).	All children and young people should minimise the amount of time spent being sedentary (sitting) for extended periods.
Australian guidance	• *Children younger than 2 years of age* should not spend any time watching TV or using other electronic media (DVDs or video games). • *For children aged 2–5 years,* sitting and watching TV and the use of other electronic media (DVDs or video games) should be limited to less than 1 hour per day. • *Infants, toddlers and preschoolers (all children from birth to 5 years of age)* should not be sedentary, restrained or kept inactive for more than 1 hour at a time, with the exception of sleeping.	To reduce health risks, children aged 5–17 years should minimise the time spent being sedentary every day. To achieve this: • Limit the use of electronic media for entertainment (e.g. TV, seated video games and computer use) to no more than 2 hours a day – lower levels are associated with reduced health risks. • Break long periods of sitting as often as possible.

that are understandable to professionals and the public in general. The physical activity guidelines outlined in Table 7.2.1 are inclusive for all groups, regardless of ability/disability, weight status or age. The UK, US and Canadian guidance concur that the current literature does not yet allow for specific guidance to be made for overweight and obese young people. However, the World Health Organization suggests the following: inactive children and youth should progressively increase activity to eventually achieve 60 min [4]; inactive young people should start with smaller amounts of physical activity and gradually increase the duration, frequency and intensity over time; and, for children who are currently inactive, engaging in amounts below the recommended levels will bring more benefits than doing none at all.

Management of the childhood obesity epidemic would benefit from specific dose–response recommendations for physical activity and sedentary behaviour. For example, self-report of physical activity usually results in the majority of children who engage in 60 min of moderate to vigorous physical activity being classified as 'sufficiently active'; yet, childhood obesity remains perplexingly high. Reasons are attributed to (1) the overestimation of physical activity in self-reports as compared to objective measures [5]; (2) excess of energy intake over expenditure; (3) the activity levels remaining too low for a certain segment of children, given the contemporary lifestyles.

7.2.3 Epidemiology of overweight, physical activity, sedentary behaviour and cardiorespiratory fitness

Twenty-first-century lifestyles have resulted in children and young people having insufficient levels of physical activity and exercise [6], decreased endurance fitness [7–9] and increased sedentary time [10]. Figure 7.2.1 illustrates the changing nature of fitness and overweight in over 15,000 children in the 9–10 years age group from Liverpool (UK).

Recent data on physical activity among children in the UK was collected by self-reports during the Health Survey for England in 2012 [11]. Only 10% of boys and girls aged 2–4 years met the current

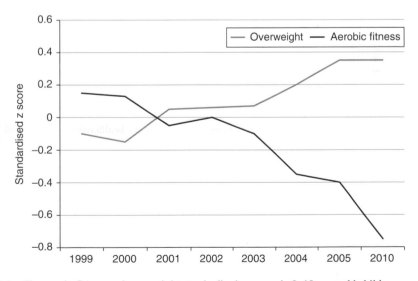

Figure 7.2.1 Changes in fitness and overweight standardised z-scores in 9–10-year-old children. Changes in BMI and fitness z-scores of 15,000 children in Liverpool (UK) between 1998 and 2004. The z-scores allow comparison of different measures using the same scale.

guidelines of at least 3 hours of physical activity per day for children under 5 years of age. Worryingly, just 21% of boys and 16% of girls aged 5–15 years were sufficiently active. Furthermore, the proportion of children who were sufficiently active decreased from 24% to 14% among 5–7-year-olds, and from 23% to 8% in 13–15-year-olds. The objectively measured physical activity levels in 7000 children aged 7 years recruited to the Millennium Cohort Study [12] found that the participants accumulated 27 min/day of moderate activity and 11 min/day of vigorous activity, and were sedentary for 5 hours/day; and that only 15% of all children were sufficiently active. Further, activity varied by ethnic group, with children of Indian and Bangladeshi origin being the least active and black children the most active. Interestingly a recent study in the UK found no significant variations in the proportions of children meeting current recommendations by BMI category – either among boys or girls, or among the 5–10, 11–15 and 5–15-year age groups [13].

The environment

For the purposes of this chapter, the physical and social environments will be considered in relation to childhood obesity. The social environment has an influence on children's physical activity and sedentary behaviours. In particular, peer influence, clustering of individuals into groups and family all combine to influence these behaviours. Salvy et al. [14] proposed four key factors that explain the effects of peers on physical activity among youth:

(1) Youth are more physically active in the presence of friends and peers than in the presence of family members or when alone.
(2) Peers and friends increase motivation to be active in overweight youth.
(3) Peer weight status does not have a moderating effect on physical activity.
(4) Experiencing negative peer interaction, such as bullying or social exclusion, decreases physical activity.

While Salvy and colleagues [14] offer a persuasive argument to support peer social context effects on physical inactivity, Lawman and Wilson concluded

that a systems approach – including parenting and physical environmental factors, particularly parental monitoring and neighbourhood context such as social cohesion – was important in the promotion of weight management in children and youth [15]. Further, another review reported that parental involvement and parenting strategies that used reward and positive reinforcement were effective in the treatment or the prevention of obesity [16]. For physical activity, behaviour-specific variables – such as activity of siblings, parental education, parent activity levels and logistical and emotional support – were associated [17]. On the other hand, 'permissive parenting' was related to increases in sedentary time and soft drink intake, and to reductions in breakfast consumption.

The home environment combines social and physical factors related to obesity. A review of 232 studies – in which 983,840 children participated – found that watching TV for more than 2 hours/day was associated with higher levels of adiposity, decreased fitness, lower scores for self-esteem and prosocial behaviour and decreased academic achievement [18]. Another review reported low-to-moderate-quality evidence relating increased television viewing to higher levels of adiposity in pre-schoolers [19].

In a review of the Home Physical Environment 'HomeSpace', media equipment in the home was positively associated with children's sedentary behaviour. However, in half the studies, physical activity equipment at home was not associated with physical activity, and was inversely associated with sedentary behaviours [20]. The role of parents in the social environment also influenced physical activity and sedentary time. TV-limiting devices decreased TV viewing, while the effect of active video games (that require physical activity for participation) on physical activity was inconclusive. In summary, the home environment is an influential setting for children's sedentary behaviour and physical activity. While changing or controlling the home physical environment shows promise for reducing screen-based sedentary behaviour, further interventions are needed to understand the broader impact of these changes. Future studies should prioritise investigating the influence of the home physical environment, and its interaction with the social environment, on objectively measured sedentary time and home context-specific behaviours, and ideally include technologies that allow objective measurement of physical activity and sedentary time.

Using data from the Sports for Liverpool's Next Generation (SportsLinx) project, the results from an analysis of the relationships between socioeconomic status, weight status and sex with children's participation in sedentary behaviours and sport were reported. More boys than girls watched TV, played video games and participated in sport, and more children of lower socioeconomic status spent time in sedentary behaviours than in sport participation. Overweight girls were more likely than normal-weight girls to use the Internet, although weight status was not consistently associated with sedentary behaviours. Proportionately more boys than girls watched TV, played video games and participated in sport, which suggests that boys find time for sedentary behaviours and physical activity [21]. From a preventive perspective, inequalities in the prevalence of sedentary behaviours and sport participation should be addressed for all children, regardless of socioeconomic status, weight status or sex.

In summary, the social environment – including the behaviours of parents, siblings and peers – influences physical activity and sedentary time. Importantly, these behaviours change with age and stage of development; thus, longitudinal studies are required to develop greater insight into this area. Furthermore, aspects of the home environment demonstrate relationships with overweight, physical activity and sedentary behaviour. The trends suggest that modifiable behaviours – such as passive parenting, use of electronic equipment and low sport engagement – are more prevalent in overweight children. In addition, the social environment may also be a precursor for gender differences in physical activity and sedentary behaviour.

Correlates of physical activity and sedentary behaviour have been used to inform prevention programmes for children. The problem to date is that few programmes have reported robust changes in weight status, and their effectiveness in promoting healthy weight is limited at best [22].

7.2.4 Interventions to increase physical activity and reduce sedentary time

Interventions to increase physical activity and reduce sedentary time can be implemented at the political, organisational, inter-individual or intra-individual level. No intervention claims to address all these levels at the same time. Most interventions are at the organisational, inter-individual or intra-individual level. For example, an organisation such as Play Wales may lobby for a policy on play. At the organisational level, Play Wales may use research evidence to promote active play as a school-level intervention by changing the playground environment [23]. Further, active play interventions can be delivered at an inter-individual level, where parents act as promoters of active play – for example, in pre-school children [24]. For older children, an intra-individual intervention may use active video games to increase physical activity at home [25].

There have been a wide variety of interventions that have aimed to increase physical activity, reduce sedentary time and decrease overweight. These include school, recess (play), childcare, family, community, educational, behavioural, active transport, parents, telemedicine and resistance exercise. Moreover, interventions using diet-only and diet plus exercise resulted in greater improvement in weight loss and metabolic profile [26]. Thus, interventions at all levels should focus on a combination of increased physical activity, reduced sedentary time and regulated diet.

Policies

Studies on the effects of school policy on obesity are in their infancy, and further research designs and approaches are required to verify results. However, in a review of the effects of policies related to school diet and physical activity on obesity, Williams found that, if the policies were implemented in isolation, then they would be insufficient to prevent or treat childhood overweight or obesity [27]. Policies that were effective were both developed and implemented as part of a multifaceted intervention programme.

Organisational

Mehtälä et al. systematically reviewed physical activity promotion in 2–6-year-old children in childcare settings [28]. Increases in physical activity levels or reductions in sedentary time were found in 14 studies, although the changes were modest. The data remain too limited to allow firm conclusions to be drawn on the effectiveness of the components that mediate physical activity interventions, although physical-activity-specific in-service teacher training seems a potential strategy. The findings of this review indicate that children's physical activity remained low and did not approach the 180 min/day criterion. A large, systematic review on school-based interventions included 32 studies involving over 55,000 participants [29]. Studies involving primary schools – unlike those involving high schools – reported significantly increased physical activity. Similar to Mehtälä et al.'s review on preschool studies, the interventions with the largest effects were comprehensive programmes that targeted nutrition and physical activity together [28]. Moreover, successful studies regularly monitored behaviour, modified the environment, included parents, used theoretical approaches to behaviour change and were at least 1 year in duration. Using the Cochrane methodology, Dobbins et al. [30] reported that children and adolescents exposed to an intervention spent (1) more time in moderate to vigorous physical activity (5–45 min more); (2) less time watching TV (5–60 min less per day); and (3) improved their aerobic fitness (from 1.6 to 3.7 ml/kg per min).

Stratton et al. have reported that physical activity during recess/playtime is low, and that overweight children were the least active during this time [31]. There have been a number of interventions that have investigated the effects of changing school recess/playtime on physical activity, particularly as children participate in school breaks for up to 600 times per year [31]. In a review of such interventions, Ickes et al. reported that 95% of studies demonstrated positive outcomes [32]. Further, most of these interventions were low cost, and included added equipment/materials, markings, zones, teacher involvement, active video games, activity of the week and activity cards (Figures 7.2.2 and 7.2.3).

The after-school period is a prime time for physical activity promotion. Many busy families utilise school programmes. Branscum and Sharma reviewed the effects of 20 interventions that included physical activity, diet or both [33]. These resulted in modest changes in behaviours and behavioural antecedents, but did not reduce indicators of obesity.

School-based interventions are generally reported to be the most effective in changing sedentary behaviour, physical activity and diet, although the long-term maintenance of these effects is questionable [34].

Individual

Sedentary time, inter-individual interventions: In a review of 10 systematic reviews of sedentary behaviour interventions, Biddle et al. reported a small but significant reduction in sedentary time effects, greater in children younger than 6 years [35]. Effective strategies included the involvement of family, behavioural interventions and electronic TV-monitoring devices. Meta-analyses of interventions aiming to reduce sedentary time reported a significant decrease in BMI of 0.81 kg/m^2 [18]. In an additional meta-analysis, van Grieken et al. calculated that a post-intervention reduction of 17.95 min/day in sedentary time resulted in a reduction in BMI of 0.25 kg/m^2[36]. No differences were found between single and multiple health behaviour interventions. Research into sedentary time is relatively new, and more analysis is required on interventions that target different types of sedentary behaviours or use specific behaviour change techniques in a variety of settings.

Parents, intra-individual interventions: General parenting skills and those specific to lifestyle behaviour seem to be effective in weight control interventions. In a review of 24 studies investigating the intensity of parental involvement in childhood obesity, medium- and high-intensity parental involvement were identified most frequently as being related to weight loss in intervention studies. However, in prevention studies, low-intensity parental involvement was identified most frequently. In summary the review concluded that the intensity of parental involvement and behaviour change techniques were key for effective long-term interventions for weight

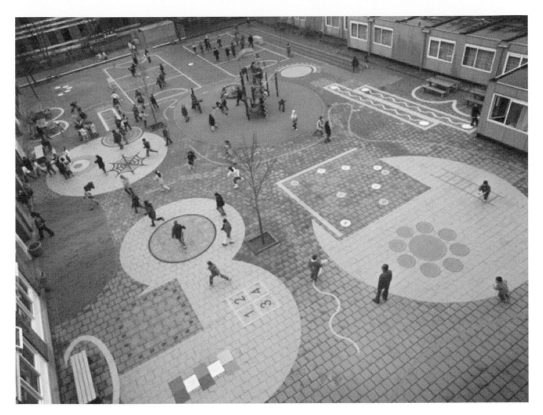

Figure 7.2.2 The Zonepark playground template.
The Zonepark template illustrating red (high activity/sports), blue (individual activity) and yellow (chill-out) zones.

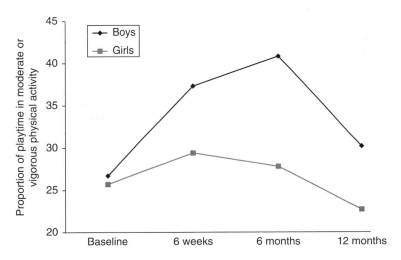

Figure 7.2.3 Changes in moderate and vigorous physical activity after a school playground intervention using multicolour markings.
Levels of moderate and vigorous physical activity in boys and girls at baseline, and then at 6 weeks, 6 months and 12 months after painting primary school playgrounds using the Zonepark template

control in childhood [37]. Niemeier and colleagues further reviewed 42 interventions that included parental involvement in nutrition education, physical activity education, physical activity sessions, behaviour education, behaviour therapy or a combination of these [38]. Significant differences existed among the levels of parent participation. In addition, intervention duration positively predicted intervention effectiveness, and the combination of parent participation and intervention duration significantly predicted intervention effectiveness. In summary, intra-individual interventions developed using behaviour change approaches that actively include parents are effective at reducing weight in children and youth. Furthermore, interventions of greater duration that involve parents are more successful.

Behaviour change interventions

In Martin et al.'s review, six behaviour change techniques were found to be effective components of weight management programmes and interventions [39]: (1) provision of information to individuals on the consequences of their behaviour, (2) environmental restructuring, (3) prompt practice, (4) prompt identification as role model/position advocate, (5) stress management/emotional control training and (6) general communication skills training. On the other hand, in weight management trials, providing information on the consequences of behaviour in general was a feature of non-effective interventions. In prevention trials, general information on the consequences of behaviour, such as rewarding successful behaviour and facilitating social comparison, was non-effective. A combination of effective behaviour change techniques identified in the prevention and management of childhood obesity should be a topic for further research [39]. Importantly, a staged approach to weight management for children with severe obesity has been recommended [40]. Rapid weight loss should not be pursued, because of sequential implications for healthy growth and pubertal development and the risk of inducing eating disorders.

There is also a developing literature about the health economics of inactivity and obesity in children. A report highlighted that physical inactivity in 11–25-year-olds will cost the UK economy £53 billion over their lifetimes, with the lowest-income households most likely to have the least active children. Indeed, figures suggest, that for every 11–15-year-old who becomes active, there is a potential cost-saving of £19,000 over his or her lifetime. On the other hand, the economic burden of childhood obesity is largely unknown [41]. Preventive and management interventions with acceptable health economics do exist, although locating the most cost-effective timing of preventive interventions during infancy and adolescence is a challenge. Data reporting their effects over longer periods are as yet unavailable. Physical activity programmes used to prevent obesity generate a range of cost-effectiveness ratios – in particular, the cost of the time required to exercise. However, there is a dearth of robust research in this area, and more competent simulation models are required to compare the cost-effectiveness of programmes used to prevent weight gain/obesity in youth [42].

7.2.5 Summary box

Key points

- Most children and adolescents are insufficiently active and spend too much time in sedentary behaviours.
- Insufficient levels of physical activity and changes in dietary behaviour have contributed to an upward trend in unhealthy weight in children.
- There are no specific physical activity recommendations for obese children, although experts suggest that children should build up to becoming sufficiently active.
- The social and physical environment, including the influence of technology using a virtual world, combine to impact on healthy weight development.
- Weight changes are affected by growth and development factors independent of food intake and exercise, particularly during adolescence.
- There is growing evidence that interventions are effective and cost-effective.
- The dose–response of physical activity and sedentary behaviour on healthy weight during the growing years is not fully understood.
- The long-term effects of behaviour change and obesity prevention and intervention programmes on healthy weight are largely unknown.

References

1. Sedentary Behaviour Research Network. Standardised use of the terms 'sedentary' and 'sedentary' behaviours. *Applied Physiology Nutrition and Metabolism* 2012; **37**: 540–542.

2. Harrell JS, McMurray RG, Baggett CD, Pennell ML, Pearce PF, Bangdiwala SI. Energy costs of physical activities in children and adolescents. *Medicine and Science in Sports and Exercise* 2005; **37**: 329–336.

3. Malina RM, Bouchard C, Bar-Or O. *Growth, Maturation, and Physical Activity*. Illinois: Champaign, 2004, pp. 1–17.

4. WHO. Global recommendations on physical activity for health. *Geneva: World Health Organization*, 2010, p. 60.

5. Health Survey for England. Physical activity and fitness, 2008. Available at http://digital.nhs.uk/catalogue/PUB00430/heal-surv-phys-acti-fitn-eng-2008-rep-v2.pdf, accessed September 2016.

6. Surveillance of physical activity in the UK is flawed: validation of the Health Survey for England Physical Activity Questionnaire. *Archives of Disease in Childhood* 2008; **93**: 1054–1058.

7. Tomkinson GR, Olds TS. Secular changes in pediatric aerobic fitness test performance: the global picture. *Medicine & Sports Science* 2007; **50**: 46–66.

8. Stratton G, Canoy D, Boddy LM, Taylor SR, Hackett AF, Buchan IE. Cardiorespiratory fitness and body mass index of 9–11-year-old English children: a serial cross-sectional study from 1998 to 2004. *International Journal of Obesity* 2007; **31**: 1172–1178.

9. Boddy LM, Fairclough SJ, Atkinson G, Stratton G. Changes in cardiorespiratory fitness in 9- to 10.9-year-old children: Sportslinx 1998–2010. *Medicine and Science in Sports and Exercise* 2012; **44**: 481–486.

10. Saunders LE, Green JM, Petticrew MP, Steinbach R, Roberts H. What are the health benefits of active travel? A systematic review of trials and cohort studies. *PLoS ONE* 2013; **8**: e69912.

11. Health Survey for England, 2012. Available at http://content.digital.nhs.uk/catalogue/PUB13218/HSE2012-Ch3-Phys-act-child.pdf, accessed October 2016.

12. Elwood P, Galante J, Pickering J, Palmer S, Bayer A, Ben-Shlomo Y, et al. Healthy lifestyles reduce the incidence of chronic diseases and dementia: evidence from the Caerphilly cohort study. *PLoS ONE* 2013; **8**: e81877.

13. Williams ED, Stamatakis E, Chandola T, Hamer M. Assessment of physical activity levels in South Asians in the UK: findings from the Health Survey for England. *Journal of Epidemiology and Community Health* 2011; **65**: 517–521.

14. Salvy SJ, Bowker JC, Germeroth L, Barkley J. Influence of peers and friends on overweight/obese youths' physical activity. *Exercise and Sport Sciences Reviews* 2012; **40**: 127–132.

15. Lawman HG, Wilson DK. A review of family and environmental correlates of health behaviors in high-risk youth. *Obesity* 2012; **20**: 1142–1157.

16. Cislak A, Safron M, Pratt M, Gaspar T, Luszczynska A. Family-related predictors of body weight and weight-related behaviours among children and adolescents: A systematic umbrella review. *Child: Care, Health and Development* 2012; **38**: 321–331.

17. Van Lippevelde W, Verloigne M, De Bourdeaudhuij I, Brug J, Bjelland M, Lien N, et al. Does parental involvement make a difference in school-based nutrition and physical activity interventions? A systematic review of randomized controlled trials. *International Journal of Public Health* 2012; **57**: 673–678.

18. Tremblay M, LeBlanc A, Kho M, Saunders T, Larouche R, et al. Systematic review of sedentary behaviour and health indicators in school-aged children and youth. *International Journal of Behavioral Nutrition and Physical Activity* 2011; **8**: 98–119.

19. Leblanc A, Spence J, Carson V, Gorber S, Dillman C, Janssen I, et al. Systematic review of sedentary behaviour and health indicators in the early years (aged 0–4 years). *Applied Physiology Nutrition and Metabolism* 2012; **37**: 753–772.

20. Maitland C, Stratton G, Foster S, Braham R, Rosenberg M. A place for play? The influence of the home physical environment on children's physical activity and sedentary behaviour. *International Journal of Behavioral Nutrition and Physical Activity* 2013; **10**: 99.

21. Rodgers N, Stratton G, Foweather L, Henaghan J, McWhannell N, Stone MR. The active City of Liverpool, Active Schools and SporstLinx (A-CLASS) Project. *Education and Health* 2006; **24**: 26–29.

22. Showell NN, Fawole O, Segal J, Wilson RF, Cheskin LJ, Bleich SN, et al. A systematic review of home-based childhood obesity prevention studies. *Pediatrics* 2013; **132**: e193–e200.

23. Ridgers ND, Timperio A, Crawford D, Salmon J. Five-year changes in school recess and lunchtime and the contribution to children's daily physical activity. *British Journal of Sports Medicine* 2012; **46**: 741–746.

24. O'Dwyer MV, Fairclough SJ, Ridgers ND, Knowles ZR, Foweather L, et al. Effect of a school-based active play intervention on sedentary time and physical activity in preschool children. *Health Education Research* 2013; **28**: 931–942.

25. Graves LEF, Ridgers ND, Atkinson G, Stratton G. The effect of active video gaming on children's physical activity, behavior preferences and body composition. *Pediatric Exercise Science* 2010; **22**: 535–546.

26. Ho M, Garnett SP, Baur LA, Burrows T, Stewart L, Neve M, et al. Impact of dietary and exercise interventions on weight change and metabolic outcomes in obese children and adolescents: a systematic review and meta-analysis of randomized trials. *JAMA Pediatrics* 2013; **167**: 759–768.

27. Williams AJ, Henley WE, Williams CA, Hurst AJ, Logan S, Wyatt KM. Systematic review and meta-analysis of the association between childhood overweight and obesity and primary school diet and physical activity policies. *International Journal of Behavioral Nutrition and Physical Activity* 2013; **10**: 101.

28. Mehtälä MAK, Sääkslahti AK, Inkinen ME, Poskiparta MEH. A socio-ecological approach to physical activity interventions in childcare: a systematic review. *International Journal of Behavioral Nutrition and Physical Activity* 2014; **11**: 1–112.

29. Sobol-Goldberg S, Rabinowitz J, Gross R. School-based obesity prevention programs: a meta-analysis of randomized controlled trials. *Obesity* 2013; **21**: 2422–2428.

30. Dobbins M, Husson H, DeCorby K, LaRocca RL. School-based physical activity programs for promoting physical

activity and fitness in children and adolescents aged 6 to 18. *Cochrane Database of Systematic Reviews (Online)* 2013. Available at http://onlinelibrary.wiley.com/doi/10.1002/14651858.CD007651.pub2/abstract;jsessionid=0585B3B586CFE0BA2520C68378682C67.f01t03, accessed October 2016.

31. Stratton G. Promoting children's physical activity in primary school: an intervention study using playground markings. *Ergon* 2000; **43**: 1538–1546.

32. Ickes MJ, Erwin J, Beighle A. Systematic review of recess interventions to increase physical activity. *Journal of Physical Activity and Health* 2013; **10**: 910–926.

33. Branscum P, Sharma M. After-school based obesity prevention interventions: a comprehensive review of the literature. *International Journal of Environmental Research and Public Health* 2012; **9**(4): 1438–1457.

34. Van Sluijs EMF, Kriemler S, McMinn AM. The effect of community and family interventions on young people's physical activity levels: a review of reviews and updated systematic review. *British Journal of Sports Medicine* 2011; **45**: 914–922.

35. Biddle SJH, Petrolini I, Pearson N. Interventions designed to reduce sedentary behaviours in young people: a review of reviews. *British Journal of Sports Medicine* 2014; **48**: 182–186.

36. Van Grieken A, Ezendam NP, Paulis WD, van der Wouden JC, Raat H. Primary prevention of overweight in children and adolescents: a meta-analysis of the effectiveness of interventions aiming to decrease sedentary behaviour. *International Journal of Behavioral Nutrition and Physical Activity* 2012; **9**: 61.

37. Van Der Kruk JJ, Kortekaas F, Lucas C, Jager-Wittenaar H. Obesity: a systematic review on parental involvement in long-term European childhood weight control interventions with a nutritional focus. *Obesity Reviews* 2013; **14**: 745–760.

38. Niemeier BS, Hektner JM, Enger KB. Parent participation in weight-related health interventions for children and adolescents: a systematic review and meta-analysis. *Preventive Medicine* 2012; **55**: 3–13.

39. Martin J, Chater A, Lorencatto F. Effective behaviour change techniques in the prevention and management of childhood obesity. *International Journal of Obesity* 2013; **37**: 1287–1294.

40. Valerio G, Licenziati MR, Tanas R, Morino G, Ambruzzi AM, Balsamo A, et al. Management of children and adolescents with severe obesity. *Minerva Pediatrica* 2012; **64**: 413–431.

41. John J, Wolfenstetter SB, Wenig CM. An economic perspective on childhood obesity: recent findings on cost of illness and cost effectiveness of interventions. *Nutrition* 2012; **28**: 829–839.

42. Gandjour A. Cost-effectiveness of preventing weight gain and obesity: what we know and what we need to know. *Expert Review of Pharmacoeconomics & Outcomes Research* 2012; **12**: 297–305.

Chapter 7.3

Designing public health initiatives for the prevention of obesity

Janet Cade
University of Leeds, Leeds, UK

Prevention and management of obesity is a priority, at both the strategic and policy levels, and in terms of practical delivery [1]. Due to the multifactorial nature of the causes of weight gain [2], designing and developing successful interventions present a challenge for public health practitioners. 'One size' does not fit all! Just as there are many elements in the development of the obesity system, there will be many potential routes towards one or more solutions. Only a long-term, broad and diversified approach will stem the rising prevalence of obesity. Intervention in just one area may lead to compensatory changes elsewhere, with unintended consequences, due to the complex interdependencies of the system. It is vital, therefore, to obtain accurate and comprehensive evidence of what works in which populations. This chapter will cover key elements that should be considered when designing obesity-related initiatives. These points should be considered by both researchers and obesity service commissioners. These design elements are the theory base, behavioural techniques, population characteristics, the scale/level of the intervention, outcome assessment, evaluation and the political/policy arena.

7.3.1 Theory and practice base for obesity-related public health initiatives

The design of a successful intervention requires a suitable and tested theory base, whether that is for interventions at the individual, local or national scale. This should be combined with the best available practical evidence of which intervention elements work. At the national level, the Foresight report [2] created a system map for obesity with seven key themes: physiology, individual activity, physical environment, food consumption, food production, individual psychology and social psychology. Each of these themes is interlinked, and may suggest areas that are ripe for intervention. Systematic reviews of interventions can identify key practical components for successful intervention design. A systematic review of controlled studies of childhood obesity prevention interventions found a broad range of promising intervention components [3]. These included targeting the school curriculum, increased physical activity sessions, improvements in school food and school environment, and support for teachers and parents. Interventions are not always explicitly described in publications, making it a challenge to base new initiatives on interventions that have been shown to work in other contexts [4].

There are many psychological theories that have been developed to support aspects of individual behaviour change through explaining concepts of behaviour initiation and maintenance. For example, the transtheoretical model of change (TTM) [5,6] highlights how different factors may be important in attempts to initially lose weight and then maintain the weight loss. Decisions regarding the initiation of a new behaviour depend on perceived future benefits, whereas maintaining a behaviour depends on

Advanced Nutrition and Dietetics in Obesity, First Edition. Edited by Catherine Hankey.
© 2018 John Wiley & Sons Ltd. Published 2018 by John Wiley & Sons Ltd.

Table 7.3.1 Taxonomy of different types of public health behaviour change interventions

	Intervention category	Examples of policy interventions
Regulation	Eliminate choice	Prohibiting goods or services (e.g. banning trans fats)
	Restrict choice	Restricting options available to individuals (e.g. only fruits during break at schools)
Fiscal measures	Disincentives	Fiscal policies to make behaviour costlier (e.g. taxation of high-fat foods)
	Incentives	Fiscal policies to make behaviour financially beneficial (e.g. tax breaks on fruit and vegetables)
Non-fiscal	Incentives and disincentives	Policies that reward or penalise behaviour (e.g. free bicycles for travel to work)
	Persuasion	Persuading individuals using arguments (e.g. counselling services or marketing campaigns)
Choice architecture including 'nudges'	Provision of information	Providing information (e.g. using leaflets, websites, front-of-pack nutrition labelling, energy information on food menus)
	Changes to physical environment	Altering environments (e.g. removing confectionery from checkout aisles, and restricting advertising of foods high in fat, salt and sugar)
	Changes to default situation	Changing default options (e.g. providing salad as a default side dish)
	Use of social norms and salience	Providing information about what others are doing (e.g. information about own energy intake as compared to similar others)

Based on Table 1 reference [10]

current satisfaction with the behaviour [7]. Other useful models in psychology include the health belief model (HBM), protection motivation theory (PMT), social cognitive theory (SCT) and the theory of planned behaviour (TPB) [8]. Interventions that are grounded in a theory base tend to be more successful than those not based on theory [9]. Development of interventions using multidisciplinary teams will facilitate appropriate translation of the background theory into practice.

Behavioural change techniques

Influences on behaviour can be classified according to genetics, individual thoughts, physical environment, social interaction, group interaction and the macrosocial environment [10]. Some actions are deliberate or consciously planned, whereas others are more automatic. The latter have been the focus of recent 'nudges', such as putting fruits at eye level in the refrigerator. The design of public health initiatives should consider the degree to which the intervention will have an impact on the individual, either consciously or unconsciously. A taxonomy of different types of interventions has been developed by the Science and Technology Committee, a select committee of the House of Lords in the UK Parliament [10]. This has been adapted for public health behaviour change interventions related to obesity (Table 7.3.1). Non-regulatory approaches to intervention relating to obesity are currently being emphasised politically, since there is less direct imposition on individuals and reduced burden on business. Social marketing principles are being used in the Change4Life programme in the UK. Commercial marketing techniques are used to promote behaviour change – for example, through product placement – and may be a useful tool in addition to regulation, education and the provision of real and appropriate choice. However, it is not clear whether this type of 'nudging' will work in practice, and a thorough evaluation of these techniques is required [11]. In addition, these approaches present some ethical considerations. The acceptability of an intervention may depend on how intrusive it is in an individual's life. Moreover, 'nudges' that enable and encourage choice by affecting non-deliberative processes also involve ethical issues, since people are not obviously aware that their behaviour is being changed.

7.3.2 Population

Consideration of the population who will be the focus of the initiative is important, owing to the different influences on the causation of obesity and the different needs relating to treatment. Specific population characteristics that may have an influence on the delivery and success of an intervention include age, gender, ethnicity, other associated morbidity, income/deprivation level and area of residence.

There are a number of points in the life course that may provide specific opportunities to influence behaviour. For example, preschool-age children may develop rebound adiposity [12], and interventions targeting parents of young children may help to reduce this effect. Women are more likely to take part in group-based weight management programmes than men [13]. The ability of common genetic variants to discriminate between obese and non-obese is too weak for clinical utility. Lifestyle factors were found to be more important [14]. The obesogenic environment may vary at a local level. Childhood obesity in an affluent ward was strongly associated with perceived neighbourhood safety and fruit and vegetable consumption. In a deprived ward, obesity was associated with expenditure on food, school meal purchase and multiple TV ownership. In all wards, perceived access to supermarkets and leisure facilities was associated with childhood obesity. This suggests that different interventions may be more appropriate in different areas [15].

A UK government policy paper titled *Healthy Lives, Healthy People: A Call to Action on Obesity in England* [16] has identified the empowerment of individuals to be a key component of the approach to reduce obesity levels. Elements of interventions to achieve this could include provision of guidance and information; encouragement (e.g. through Change4Life); and tailored support on weight management. At the individual level, interventions

should include self-monitoring and at least one other self-regulatory technique, such as goal-setting or feedback. Motivational interviewing is a technique that has been used with success [17]. A systematic review of potential mediators of energy-balance-related behaviour found limited high-quality research. However, self-efficacy and intention may be useful mediators of physical activity; there was also some indication that attitude, knowledge and habit strength were mediators of dietary behaviour intentions [18].

7.3.3 Intervention level

Initiatives to tackle obesity can be delivered at either the individual level or the population level. Public health initiatives are likely to incorporate both elements for a comprehensive strategy.

At the individual level, there is a range of existing commercial or primary-care-led weight reduction programmes. Results of a randomised controlled trial of six different weight management programmes found that commercially available approaches were more cost-effective and cheaper than primary-care-based services led by specialist staff [13]. Less is known about the successful design of population-based approaches. In a political climate where non-regulatory interventions are favoured, there is a role for national and local governments to encourage stakeholders to play a bigger part in developing healthier options. The call for voluntary initiatives on the part of the food and drink industry to reduce the national energy intake by 5 billion kcal/day has been criticised as being inadequate [19]. Others, however, point to the increase in reformulation of foods to be lower in energy, and that these businesses reach those groups of the population who may be particularly difficult to reach with conventional health messages [20]. Other nations, such as Denmark, have taken the bold stand of taxing foods that are high in fat. However, this tax was removed less than a year later (November 2012), owing to criticism that food prices had been inflated and jobs put at risk. Furthermore, the UK has agreed to introduce a sugar tax from 2018 that will comprise a taxable levy calculated according to the sugar content of soft drinks.

7.3.4 Evaluation

Before embarking upon a full-scale delivery or trial of an intervention, a feasibility study is vital. This explores, among other things, the acceptability, response, compliance and potential effect size of the intervention [21]. Public health initiatives related to obesity are, by their nature, complex interventions, and these require specific considerations in terms of evaluation. Following a systematic development of the intervention using the best available evidence and appropriate theory, this should be tested with pilot studies and, finally, with a full evaluation. There are many study designs that could be appropriate, but randomisation should always be considered, since it is the most robust method of preventing selection bias [21]. Unfortunately, evaluation of obesity interventions is often given second place to 'doing something', and many programmes have been commissioned without any adequate evidence of their likely success. Change4Life is an example. Evaluation after the first year focussed on project reach and brand awareness, rather than on providing evidence of behavioural change. However, recent evaluations suggest increased swapping to lower-fat dairy products and lower-sugar drinks and reductions in sugary cereal consumption in the short term. Longer-term evaluations on the impact on body weight and obesity are required.

7.3.5 Outcomes

The outcomes expected from an obesity-related intervention needs to be considered at the start of the programme. Different outcomes will be required for obesity prevention as compared to treatment. Studies evaluating complex interventions must state a primary outcome. There is usually a single primary outcome – it may be BMI, change in BMI or change in body weight. Only one of these should be chosen as the primary outcome, and the study should be powered to detect this change. The success or otherwise of the intervention will be measured against this primary outcome. Secondary outcomes can also be explored, such as change in diet or physical activity. However, these secondary outcomes should not be taken as measures of

success of the intervention if the primary outcome (e.g. weight change) was not effective. Process measures are also important to help explain findings related to the primary outcome [21] – for example, if a school-based intervention did not increase children's fruit and vegetable intake, this would be the result of poor implementation of the intervention by school staff [22]. This reflects the need for a thorough process evaluation to understand the impact of interventions, and to find what aspects are/are not effective.

Conclusions from systematic reviews of interventions to prevent weight gain have suggested that effectiveness might be more precisely demonstrated if study designs were improved – with more objective measures of physical activity and diet; more process-based outcomes; and longer follow-up periods [3,4,23]. Future intervention studies should report long-term post-intervention measures. Retention of knowledge, diet or physical activity patterns with long-term follow-up is unknown [23].

7.3.6 Political/policy arena

The design of public health initiatives must also consider the political context of the day. Otherwise, however brilliant the initiative, it will not be widely disseminated if it is out of line with the current political agenda. Initiatives should take account of the wider policy arena, such as policies relating to climate change or health inequalities, through engagement with key stakeholders [2].

7.3.7 Conclusion

Public health initiatives to tackle obesity must be many and varied to challenge the complex systems driving the upward trend. A number of key factors have been discussed that need to be considered when designing obesity-related initiatives. A good starting point is to learn from existing research that has been summarised in systematic reviews. These can point to the appropriate theory base and practical elements for success. Complex interventions will require input from a range of disciplines, including epidemiology, psychology, public health, environmental planning and others. Intervention design should include understanding how the intervention will result in behaviour change through conscious or unconscious actions. Tailoring of the initiative to the population is required, and may depend on a range of social, environmental and lifestyle factors. Fundamental to all initiatives will be an appropriate evidence base to demonstrate effectiveness. This can only be achieved through robust development, feasibility testing and trials. Evaluation including process measures will help understand what does or does not work. This should be built into any initiative to avoid wasting resources on ineffective programmes.

7.3.8 Summary box

Key points

- Public health policy is multi-factorial – and dependant on current government policy.
- Mandatory taxation has been introduced, although long term evaluation is required.
- Reformulation of current products is necessary to reach those resistant to health messages – and require food industry buy in.
- Interventions are often complex; process evaluation is key to determining how and why the intervention results were as they were.
- Delivery requires multidisciplinary input, and content adaption is often required. Depending on the location of the intervention, the intervention will result in behaviour change through conscious or unconscious actions.
- Tailoring of the initiative to the population is required, and may depend on a range of social, environmental and lifestyle factors.
- Fundamental to all initiatives will be an appropriate evidence base to demonstrate effectiveness, and robust evidence is still required.

References

1. National Institute for Health and Clinical Excellence. Obesity guidance on the prevention, identification, assessment and management of overweight and obesity in adults and children, 2006. London.

2. Foresight. *Tackling Obesities: Future Choices – Project Report*, 2nd edn. London: Government Office for Science, 2007.

3. Waters E, de Silva-Sanigorski A, Hall BJ, Brown T, Campbell KJ, Gao Y, et al. Interventions for preventing obesity in children. *Cochrane Database of Systematic Reviews* 2011; **12**: CD001871.

4. Hardeman W, Griffin S, Johnston M, Kinmonth AL, Wareham NJ. Interventions to prevent weight gain: a systematic review of psychological models and behaviour change methods. *International Journal of Obesity and Related Metabolic Disorders* 2000; **24**(2): 131–143.

5. Prochaska JO, DiClemente CC, Norcross JC. In search of how people change. Applications to addictive behaviors. *American Psychologist* 1992; **47**(9): 1102–1114.

6. Sutton S. Stage theories of health behaviour. In: Conner M, Norman P (eds) *Predicting Health Behaviour: Research and Practice with Social Cognition Models*, 2nd edn. Buckingham: Open University Press, 2005.

7. Rothman AJ. Toward a theory-based analysis of behavioral maintenance. *Health Psychology* 2000; **19**(1): 64–69.

8. Povey R, Conner M, Sparks P, James R, Shepherd R. The theory of planned behaviour and healthy eating: examining additive and moderating effects of social influence variables. *Psychology & Health* 2000; **14**(6): 991–1006.

9. Bluford DA, Sherry B, Scanlon KS. Interventions to prevent or treat obesity in preschool children: a review of evaluated programs. *Obesity* (Silver Spring) 2007; **15**(6): 1356–1372.

10. House of Lords Science and Technology Select Committee. *Behaviour Change*. London: The Stationery Office, 2011.

11. Change4Life brought to you by PepsiCo (and others). *Lancet* 2009; **373**(9658, Jan 10): 96.

12. Rolland-Cachera MF, Deheeger M, Maillot M, Bellisle F. Early adiposity rebound: causes and consequences for obesity in children and adults. *International Journal of Obesity (London)* 2006; **30**(4): S11–S17.

13. Jolly K, Lewis A, Beach J, Denley J, Adab P, Deeks JJ, et al. Comparison of range of commercial or primary care led weight reduction programmes with minimal intervention control for weight loss in obesity: lighten up randomised controlled trial. *BMJ* 2011; **343**: d6500.

14. Sandholt CH, Sparso T, Grarup N, Albrechtsen A, Almind K, Hansen L, et al. Combined analyses of 20 common obesity susceptibility variants. *Diabetes* 2010; **59**(7): 1667–1673.

15. Edwards KL, Clarke GP, Ransley JK, Cade J. The neighbourhood matters: studying exposures relevant to childhood obesity and the policy implications in Leeds, UK. *Journal of Epidemiology and Community Health* 2010; **64**(3): 194–201.

16. Department of Health. *Healthy Lives, Healthy People: A Call to Action on Obesity in England*. London: HM Government, 2011.

17. National Obesity Observatory. Brief interventions for weight management. NHS, 2011.

18. van Stralen MM, Yildirim M, te Velde SJ, Brug J, van MW, Chinapaw MJ. What works in school-based energy balance behaviour interventions and what does not? A systematic

review of mediating mechanisms. *International Journal of Obesity (London)* 2011; **35**(10): 1251–1265.

19. Mayor S. Specialists condemn government's obesity plan as too simplistic. *BMJ* 2011; **343**: d6688.

20. Hancock C. Change4life campaign. *Lancet* 2009; **373** (9665): 721.

21. Craig P, Dieppe P, Macintyre S, Michie S, Nazareth I, Petticrew M. Developing and evaluating complex interventions: the new Medical Research Council guidance. *BMJ* 2008; **337**: a1655.

22. Christian MS, Evans CE, Ransley JK, Greenwood DC, Thomas JD, Cade JE. Process evaluation of a cluster randomised controlled trial of a school-based fruit and vegetable intervention: Project Tomato. *Public Health Nutrition* 2011; **11**: 1–7.

23. Khambalia AZ, Dickinson S, Hardy LL, Gill T, Baur LA. A synthesis of existing systematic reviews and meta-analyses of school-based behavioural interventions for controlling and preventing obesity. *Obesity Reviews* 2011; **13**(3): 214–233.

Index